Maternal and Newborn **Success**

NCLEX®-Style Q&A Review

FOURTH EDITION

Nancy Beck Irland, DNP, MSN, RN
Certified Nurse Midwife (retired)
Policy Analyst for Nursing Education and Assessment (retired)
Oregon State Board of Nursing (OSBN)
Portland, OR

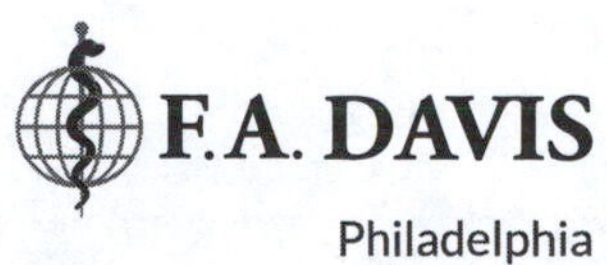

Philadelphia

F.A. Davis Company
1915 Arch Street
Philadelphia, PA 19103
www.fadavis.com

Printed in the United States of America

Last digit indicates print number: 10 9 8 7 6 5 4 3 2 1

Acquisitions Editor, Nursing: Jacalyn Sharp
Content Project Manager: Sean P. West
Electronic Project Manager: Sandra A. Glennie
Design and Illustrations Manager: Carolyn O'Brien

Library of Congress Cataloging-in-Publication Data

Names: Irland, Nancy Beck, 1951- author. | Maternal and newborn success.
Title: Maternal and newborn success: NCLEX-style Q & A review / Nancy Beck Irland.
Description: Fourth edition. | Philadelphia, PA: F.A. Davis Company, [2022] | Preceded by Maternal and newborn success / Margot R. De Sevo. Third edition. [2017] | Includes bibliographical references and index.
Identifiers: LCCN 2021022112 (print) | LCCN 2021022113 (ebook) | ISBN 9781719643061 (paperback) | ISBN 9781719646529 (ebook)
Subjects: MESH: Maternal-Child Nursing | Obstetric Nursing | Pregnancy Complications--nursing | Examination Questions
Classification: LCC RG951 (print) | LCC RG951 (ebook) | NLM WY 18.2 | DDC 618/.04231076--dc23
LC record available at https://lccn.loc.gov/2021022112
LC ebook record available at https://lccn.loc.gov/2021022113

This book is dedicated to the memory of my late parents, Ed and Jackie Beck, who warmly referred to me as "Nurse Nancy" throughout my life. It is also dedicated to my husband, Gary Irland, who has faithfully supported my writing and nursing careers, and to my children, Marcus Irland, David Irland (deceased), and Holly (Irland) Dovich, as well as our son-in-law, Adam Dovich. In addition, this dedication includes my delightful grandchildren Russell Dovich and Lucy Dovich, who I hope will one day find this book useful, should they choose nursing as a career.

More broadly, this dedication includes all nursing students and nurses new to obstetrics who share, with me, a profound amazement of reproduction and the incredible forces at work in pregnancy and birth. I am grateful to the experienced nurses who shared their knowledge and supported me when I was an obstetrical nurse-novice. No book can cover all the tips and tricks learned in a career that spans nearly 50 years, but this is a start. More importantly, it is my wish that beyond helping one to pass the NCLEX examination, the use of these tips and tricks and clinical judgments will assist learners beyond the examination.
I wish each of you a fulfilling and exciting nursing career as you deliver safe and satisfying client care.

Table of Contents

Author Biography

Dr. Irland has enjoyed a long obstetrical nursing career as both a staff nurse and a certified nurse-midwife. In addition, she has authored several professional articles in peer-reviewed nursing journals, and non-nursing books for children and adults. She recently retired from the Oregon State Board of Nursing, where she worked as program manager of nursing education in Oregon. In addition to national presentations, Dr. Irland has presented internationally at the Royal College of Surgeons in Dublin, Ireland. Dr. Irland was honored by the Oregon March of Dimes as Nurse Educator of the Year in 2013.

Acknowledgments

I would like to thank Terri Wood Allen for sharing a ride with me at the National Council of State Boards of Nursing (NCSBN) conference in September 2018, during which we discussed her work and my writing and nursing careers. That led to online introductions to Jacalyn Sharp and Sean West. Jacalyn and Sean, thank you for being so supportive and professional during the revisions and additions to this book. I have appreciated your insights, willingness to consider my suggestions, and your prompt responses to all of my questions. It has been a pleasure to work with all of you. Thank you.

1 Test-Taking

INTRODUCTION

This book is one of a series of books published by F.A. Davis that is designed to assist nurses in all phases of their careers. This text is an excellent supplement for a number of nursing school courses, including parent-child nursing, fetal growth and development, basic genetics, family processes, and women's health. It can serve as a guide for student nurses seeking success in nursing education and to assist in preparing for and taking the National Council of State Boards of Nursing (NCSBN) RN licensing exam. This exam is commonly referred to as the NCLEX-RN® examination (National Council Licensure Examination). Because this book includes nurse decision making, it can also be useful for registered nurses at the start of an obstetrical nursing career as a supplement for foundational information.

The learner who wishes to focus on specific content within obstetrical nursing can find a complete chapter on each of the perinatal phases, with questions focused on knowledge, communication, and clinical decision making in the antepartum, intrapartum, postpartum, and newborn periods. Each of these phases is further divided into *low risk* and *high risk* conditions in separate chapters. Other topics include fetal and neonatal development, genetics, women's health, sexually transmitted illnesses, domestic violence, rape, and contraceptive issues that affect women across the lifespan. In the Answers and Rationales sections of the chapters, an explanation for the correct answer as well as reasons why the distractors are incorrect are provided. Tips for decision making in the testing environment are also included.

GUIDELINES FOR USING THIS BOOK

The questions and answers in this book, including the rationales, are soundly referenced by peer-reviewed literature. They can serve as excellent learning tools. In addition, the case-study format within the Next Generation NCLEX (NGN) formatted questions may serve educators as springboards for classroom discussion to demonstrate the steps in clinical decision making. However, because these questions and responses have not been subjected to the rigor of the actual NCLEX-RN exam questions, they should not be used for testing and scoring, where a student's progression in the program or a nurse's evaluation for continued employment is at stake.

One or more questions in Next Generation NCLEX (NGN) format are included in most chapters, when applicable. This will help the test taker become familiar with the steps in the NCSBN's Clinical Judgment Measurement Model (NCJMM) and ultimately, to help the nurse to make appropriate clinical judgments in actual client care.

Concepts for the questions in this book are based on the guidelines of the 2019 NCLEX Test Plan prepared by the NCSBN (2019b, p. 4). These include four primary client needs as indicated below:

1. Safe and Effective Care Environment
   - Management of Care
   - Safety and Infection Control
2. Health Promotion and Maintenance
3. Psychosocial Integrity
4. Physiological Integrity

- Basic Care and Comfort
- Pharmacological and Parenteral Therapies
- Reduction of Risk Potential
- Physiological Adaptation

In addition, the test taker will note that the concepts of (1) nursing process, (2) caring, (3) communication and documentation, (4) teaching and learning, and (5) culture and spirituality are applied throughout the test. These are also from the NCSBN's 2019 Test Plan (NCSBN, 2019b, p. 5).

TEST-TAKING RESOURCE

For details on the RACE model, an important strategy for test taking, see another book in this series, *Fundamentals Success: NCLEX-Style Q&A Review*, 5th edition, by Patricia Nugent and Barbara Vitale.

USE THIS BOOK AS ONE EDUCATIONAL STRATEGY

Many strategies for learning and remembering are available on the internet and in the literature. Each learner must identify the best way they learn and take that approach. Most people learn best by teaching (or pretending to teach) someone else. State the information or explanation out loud, whether or not someone else is listening. Study in chunks of time every day, for 30 to 50 minutes. Handwriting the information is helpful for many learners. Include a review of the material that was covered 1 to 2 weeks ago to cement the information. Some learners prefer to use a textbook of questions like this one before the lecture, to identify the things they do not know, or need to know more about. The information then "sticks" because the brain is actively seeking the correct answer.

This book consists of 10 subsequent chapters by topic (Chapters 2–11), followed by a comprehensive exam in Chapter 12. Questions in each chapter include traditional knowledge questions and NGN clinical judgment questions where applicable. Each of these chapters consists solely of practice questions along with answers and rationales for each response. The rationales explain why a particular answer is correct when other answer options are incorrect. This information serves as a valuable learning tool for the nurse and helps to reinforce knowledge. Many answers include specific tips on how to approach answering the question when more than one answer may seem correct.

This first chapter focuses on the types of questions included in the NCLEX-RN examination, including Next Generation NCLEX (NGN) questions, although the NCSBN has indicated that NGN formats "will not be included in the test before 2023" (NCSBN, 2020). Chapters 2 through 11 consist of questions on topics related to maternity and women's health nursing. The Comprehensive Examination in Chapter 12 consists of an assortment of questions that cover topics from all the chapters in no particular order.

SUPPLEMENTARY APPENDIX

Rationales for clinical judgment require a firm understanding of physiology. The learner will note that the appendix in this book gives physiology in plain language and it re-tells the most challenging physiological conditions such as acid-base balance, gestational diabetes, and ABO incompatibility with the use of allegory. Research has shown that re-telling difficult concepts in story form can assist with understanding and retention (Day, 2009). This pedagogical approach puts a face on oxygen and insulin. Learners "see" them working (or not working) inside the village, and understand the negative effects of umbilical cord occlusion, anaerobic metabolism, hyperglycemia, and other dangerous conditions. The reader is also encouraged to refer to the material in the references for further information on topics of interest or concern.

NEXT GENERATION NCLEX-RN (NGN)

Although facts must be learned, nursing is not a fact-based profession. Nursing is an applied science that connects information in decision making. When a nurse enters a client's room, the client rarely asks the nurse to define a term or to recite a fact. Rather, the client presents the nurse with a set of data that the nurse must interpret, connect, and act on.

NCSBN Clinical Judgment Model (CJM)

Clinical judgment requires a nurse to "read between the lines" and apply fragmented pieces of information into a unified whole that may be unique to each client. The NCSBN has announced that in upcoming NCLEX-RN examinations, they will incorporate questions designed to assess and measure how well the graduate nurse can see those connections and can make appropriate clinical judgments. As indicated above, this format is referred to as "Next Generation NCLEX" (NGN), and will not be included in the test before 2023 (NCSBN, 2020). The NCSBN has indicated further that the NCLEX-RN exam will also include many of the current test question formats such as multiple choice, select all that apply, and so on. Because NGN questions are helpful in guiding the acquisition of effective clinical judgments whether or not they will be on a test, they are included in most of the chapters in this book. Students who take the test in 2023 or beyond will benefit from familiarity with the format, and nurses new to obstetrics will benefit by seeing the steps in obstetrical nurse decision making. Tips on clinical judgment in association with answering these questions are also included in this chapter.

The primary structure of the Next Generation NCLEX (NGN) questions is built on an unfolding case study that guides the test taker through the six steps of the NCSBN clinical judgment model (CJM) referred to as the NCSBN-CJM (Dickison et al., 2019). Each case study consists of six questions that guide the test taker through the six steps of clinical judgment and decision making identified by the NCSBN-CJM (NCSBN, 2020). These steps are as follows:

1. **Recognize cues.** What's abnormal? What puts the client at risk?
2. **Analyze cues.** What could be happening? Or, what might happen? Begin a list of hypotheses.
3. **Prioritize hypotheses.** What is most likely? Or, which hypothesis carries the highest risk to the client?
4. **Generate solutions.** What can I do?
5. **Take action.** Where shall I start?
6. **Evaluate outcomes.** Did it help?

Because the question for each of the six steps will be on its own page on the computerized test, the case study will be included with each step. In addition, on the NCLEX exam, test takers will be provided with the fictional client's electronic medical record with tabs to access as needed. Tabs may include the client's health history, nurses' notes, vital signs, and laboratory values. The test taker will be informed when nurses' notes have been updated and will be asked to refer to the latest information there.

One can see that the NCSBN-CJM is very similar to the traditional nursing process, which was used as a foundation to the NGN format but is not intended to replace the nursing process (Dickison et al., 2019). The nursing process is ongoing and ever-changing. Although the evaluation phase is identified as the last phase of the nursing process, it also can lead to another round of analyzing cues and so on. When nurses evaluate, they are reassessing clients to determine whether the actions taken met the needs of the client. If the goals were not met, the nurse asks "why?" and is obligated to start at the beginning by analyzing cues that indicate goals were not met and working down to develop new actions to meet the goals. If just some of the goals were met, priorities may need to be changed, and so on. For experienced nurses, this process is done quickly and intuitively. Novice nurses generally take the steps sequentially until the steps become innate and automatic.

NGN Question Formats

Formats for questions in each of the NGN steps may include a version of one of the following approved item types (NCSBN, 2019a):

1. **Extended Multiple Choice**. This is similar to current "Select all that apply" questions. The NCSBN has indicated that partial credit will be given for the right answers, but points are also deducted for the wrong answers, so the test taker must choose carefully (NCSBN, 2019a).
2. **Extended Drag and Drop.** The test taker drags items from one box to the other. This includes the standalone Bowtie item described below.
3. **Drop-down (Cloze).** This is very similar to fill-in-the-blanks in which the test taker chooses a word or phrase from a drop-down list to complete the sentence.
4. **Enhanced Hot Spot (Highlighting).** Test takers are asked to click on words or phrases in the nurses' notes to highlight such things as client risk, client conditions requiring follow-up, or client conditions that require advance preparation before receiving the client. When the test taker clicks on the selected section, it will show up yellow, as though highlighted manually with a felt-tipped pen.
5. **Matrix/Grid.** This is a table with 3 to 4 columns in which the test taker must consider such things as a list of potential orders and indicate if they are: (a) anticipated; (b) nonessential; or (c) contraindicated for the client in the case study. If used in an evaluation step, the test taker will be asked to indicate if the client's condition has (1) improved; (2) has not changed; or (3) has declined. A response is required in each column. Some questions will have two columns, some will have three, but all will require subjective assessments and decisions.
6. **Trend.** Addresses multiple steps of the NCJMM by having the candidate review information over time.
7. **Bowtie Diagram.** Another NGN format included in this book is the bowtie diagram question (NCSBN, 2021). In this shortened case study format, a case study is given, followed by just three questions. The test taker is first asked to select the *complication* of highest priority and drag it to the center box. In the next question, the test taker selects the best two *assessments* and drags each one into its own box on the left. Finally, the test taker selects the two most important *interventions* to take at that time and drags each of them into its own box on the right.

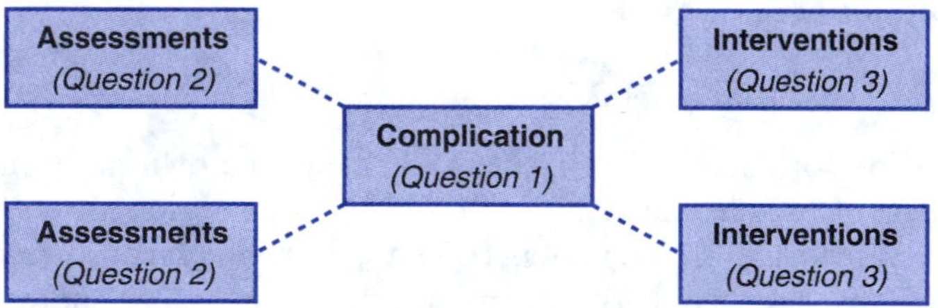

TRADITIONAL, NON-NGN QUESTIONS

While the new NCLEX-RN® exam will include a number of questions in the new NGN formats, the NCSBN has indicated that the exam will not be composed entirely of the NGN format (personal conversation, J. Schwartz; NCSBN, October, 2019). Most of the questions will still be traditional, "non-NGN," knowledge assessment questions discussed in this section, which are also important in assessing nursing knowledge. The types of questions and examples of each are discussed next.

1. Multiple-Choice Questions

In these questions, a stem is provided (a situation), and the test taker must choose among four possible responses. Sometimes the test taker will be asked to choose the best response, sometimes to choose the first action that should be taken, and so on. There are numerous ways that multiple-choice questions may be asked.

2. Fill-in-the-Blank Questions

These are calculation questions. The test taker may be asked to calculate a medication dosage, an intravenous (IV) drip rate, a minimum urinary output, or other factor. Included in the question will be the units that the test taker should have in the answer.

3. Drag-and-Drop Questions

In drag-and-drop questions, the test taker is asked to place four or five possible responses in chronological or rank order. The responses may be actions to be taken during a nursing procedure, steps in growth and development, etc. The items are called drag-and-drop questions because the test taker will move the items with their computer mouse. In this book, the test taker will simply be asked to write the responses in the correct sequence.

4. Multiple-Response Questions

The sentence "Select all that apply" following a question means that the examiner has included more than one correct response to the question. Questions will include up to five responses, and the test taker must determine which of the given responses are correct. There may be two, three, four, or even five correct responses.

5. Hot Spot Items

These items require the test taker to identify the correct response to a question about a picture, graph, or other image. For example, a test taker may be asked to place an "X" on the location where a complete placenta previa would be attached. It is important to be as precise as possible, such as placing the "X" on the RLQ of the drawing to indicate the likely location of a client's pain with appendicitis, rather than placing the "X" in the middle of the lower abdomen.

6. Items for Interpretation

Some questions may include an item to interpret. For example, the test taker may be asked to interpret the sound on an audio file as inspiratory stridor, recognize that a client is becoming progressively more anemic by interpreting laboratory results, or perform a calculation based on information given on an intake and output sheet.

HOW TO APPROACH EXAMINATION QUESTIONS

There are several techniques a test taker should use when approaching examination questions.

1. **Pretend the examination is a clinical experience**—First and foremost, test takers must approach critical-thinking questions as if they were in a clinical setting and the situation were developing on the spot. The student taking an examination and a nurse working on a clinical unit both need the same critical-thinking ability.

2. **Read the stem carefully before reading the responses**—As discussed above, there are several different types of questions on the NCLEX-RN® examination. Before answering any question, the test taker must be sure to identify what the question is asking—what is the "stem"?
3. **Read nothing into the stem**—The response reflects only the information given in the stem. For example, if the stem does not say the client is anxious, the test taker must not include an answer that includes anxiety.
4. **Consider possible responses before answering**—After clearly understanding the stem of the question, *but before reading the possible responses,* the test taker should consider possible correct answers to the question. Test question writers include only plausible answer options. A test writer's goal is to determine whether the test taker knows and understands the material. The test taker, therefore, must have an idea of what the correct answer might be before beginning to read the possible responses.
5. **Consider each possible response as a stand-alone true or false question.**
6. **When prioritizing answers, select either the client condition/s that threaten survival, and/or the answer/s that relate to CAB—circulation, airway, breathing.**
7. **Read the responses**—Only after clearly understanding what is being asked and after developing an idea of what the correct answer might be, the test taker reads the responses. The one response that is closest in content to the test taker's "guess" should be the answer that is chosen, and the test taker should not second-guess himself or herself. The first impression is almost always the correct response. Only if the test taker knows that he or she misread the question should the answer be changed.
8. **Read the rationales for each question**—In this book, rationales are given for each answer option. The learner should take full advantage of this feature. Read why the correct answer is correct. The rationale may be based on content, on interpretation of information, or on a number of other reasons. Understanding why the answer to one question is correct or is not correct is likely to transfer over to other questions with similar rationales. Next, read why the wrong answers are wrong. Again, the rationales may be based on a number of different factors, including the mistake of reading the question and/or answers too quickly.
9. **Finally, read all test-taking tips in this book and others**—Some of the tips relate directly to test-taking skills, whereas others include invaluable information in general.

SUMMARY

In the end, the person who knows the material and learns it consistently will do the best on the test. There is no substitute for studying and making sense of the information for oneself. The Appendix includes valuable re-telling of physiology that may assist in understanding and learning. If the test taker uses this text as recommended above, he or she should be well prepared to be successful when taking an examination in any or all of the content areas represented. As a result, the test taker should be fully prepared to function as a beginning registered professional nurse in the many areas of maternity and women's health.

Sexuality, Fertility, and Genetics

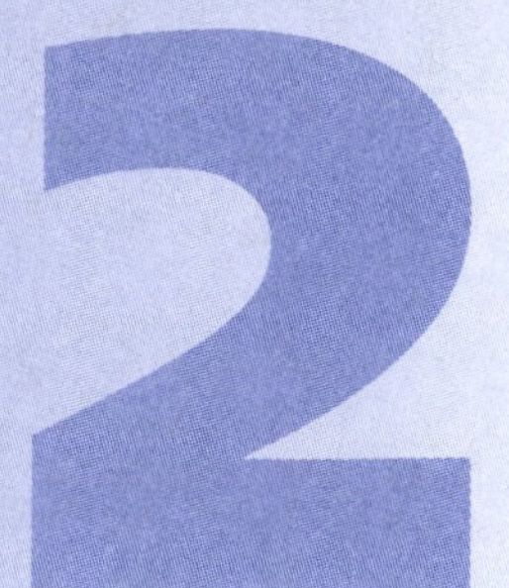

Reproduction is a superpower granted to humans, animals, and plants—the power to create in our likeness. In the quest for survival of the species, living things are driven by biological hormones to reproduce and make copies of themselves. For humans, pregnancy happens without any effort most of the time. This is considered both fortunate and unfortunate. It's fortunate if the "timing" is right, but it's unfortunate if it's not. Because we are so driven to complete this natural order of things, those who are infertile or sterile feel a profound sense of loss in their inability to accomplish this most primal instinct. Others, whose pregnancies result in the creation of a child with a genetic or physical handicap, also suffer a loss; the loss of their anticipated "perfect" child, and the loss of their dreams for this child.

But we're getting ahead of ourselves. Before pregnancy can begin, a sperm and an egg must unite and join forces in forming this new creature. The union of sperm and egg usually occurs as a result of sexual intercourse but can be accomplished via artificial insemination, most commonly intrauterine insemination (IUI), in-vitro fertilization, and a number of other procedures used in attempts to overcome infertility. Although the act of sexual intercourse is fairly well understood by teenagers and adults, the intricacies of the male and female reproductive systems, the hormones that drive us to mate, biological changes inside our bodies that support a pregnancy, and the magic of fertilization and genetics are complicated. The nurse with an understanding of all of these processes will have the necessary information to sort out and explain to clients what occurs in normal procreation and possible reasons why procreation does not take place. The informed nurse will have an understanding of what questions to ask the client, as the nurse serves to help clients understand reproduction and genetics.

This chapter includes questions on three related issues surrounding the process of reproduction: sexuality, infertility, and genetics. Since genetics involves much more than simply parents and their offspring, additional concepts are included in the genetics section.

KEYWORDS

The following words include English vocabulary, nursing/medical terminology, concepts, principles, or information relevant to content specifically addressed in the chapter or associated with topics presented in it. English dictionaries, your nursing textbooks, and medical dictionaries such as *Taber's Cyclopedic Medical Dictionary* are resources that can be used to expand your knowledge and understanding of these words and related information.

Allele
Amniocentesis
Aneuploidy
Artificial insemination
Autosomal dominant inheritance
Autosomal recessive inheritance
Autosome
Basal body temperature
Cell-free DNA
Chorionic villus sampling (CVS)
Chromosome
Clomiphene
Corpus cavernosum
Corpus luteum
Corpus spongiosum
Deoxyribonucleic acid (DNA)
Diploid
Down's syndrome
Duchenne muscular dystrophy
Ejaculatory duct
Endometrial biopsy
Epididymis

Estrogen
Expressivity
Fallopian tubes
Familial adenomatous polyposis (FAP)
Ferning capacity
Fertilization
Fimbriae
First trimester screen
Follicle-stimulating hormone (FSH)
Follicular phase
Fragile X syndrome
Gametes
Gametogenesis
Gene
Genetics
Genome
Genotype
GIFT (gamete intrafallopian transfer)
Glans
Gonadotropin-releasing hormone
Graafian follicle
Haploid
Hemophilia A
Human chorionic gonadotropin
Huntington disease
Hysterosalpingogram
Hysteroscopy
Infertility
In-vitro fertilization
Ischemic phase
Karyotype
Laparoscopy
Luteal phase
Luteinizing hormone (LH)
Meiosis
Menses
Menstrual cycle
Menstrual phase
Mitochondrial inheritance
Mitosis
Monosomy
Oogenesis
Ovary
Ovulation
Ovum
Pedigree
Penetrance
Phenotype
Phenylketonuria
Polycystic kidney disease (PKD)
Prepuce
Progesterone
Proliferative phase
Prostate
Ribonucleic acid (RNA)
Scrotum
Second trimester quad screen
Secretory phase
Seminal vesicle
Sex chromosome
Sexuality
Spermatogenesis
Spinnbarkeit
Sterility
Surrogate
Testes
Trisomy
Urethra
Uterus
Vagina
Vas deferens
X-linked recessive inheritance
Y-linked inheritance
ZIFT (zygote intrafallopian transfer)

QUESTIONS

Sexuality

1. A woman whose menstrual cycle is 35 days long states that she often has a slight pain on one side of her lower abdomen on day 21 of her cycle. She wonders whether she has ovarian cancer. Which of the following is the nurse's best response?
    1. "Women often feel a slight twinge on one side or the other when ovulation occurs."
    2. "You should seek medical attention as soon as possible since ovarian cancer is definitely a possibility."
    3. "Ovarian cancer is unlikely because the pain is not a constant pain."
    4. "It is more likely that such pain indicates an ovarian cyst because pain is more common with that problem."

2. A nurse is explaining to a client about monthly hormonal changes. Starting with day 1 of the menstrual cycle, please place the following four hormones in the chronological order in which they rise during the menstrual cycle.
   1. Follicle-stimulating hormone (FSH).
   2. Gonadotropin-releasing hormone (GnRH).
   3. Luteinizing hormone (LH).
   4. Progesterone.

3. A 54-year-old client calls her healthcare practitioner complaining of frequency and burning when she urinates. Which of the following factors that occurred within the preceding 3 days likely contributed to this client's problem?
   1. She had intercourse with her partner.
   2. She returned from a trip abroad.
   3. She stopped taking hormone replacement therapy.
   4. She started a weight-lifting exercise program.

4. A woman's temperature has just risen 0.4° F and will remain elevated during the remainder of her cycle. She expects to menstruate in about 2 weeks. Which of the following hormones is responsible for the change?
   1. Estrogen.
   2. Progesterone.
   3. Luteinizing hormone (LH).
   4. Follicle-stimulating hormone (FSH).

5. A woman is menstruating. If hormonal studies were to be done at this time, which of the following hormonal levels would the nurse expect to see?
   1. Both estrogen and progesterone are high.
   2. Estrogen is high and progesterone is low.
   3. Estrogen is low and progesterone is high.
   4. Both estrogen and progesterone are low.

6. A nurse teaches a woman who wishes to become pregnant that if she assesses for spinnbarkeit she will be able to closely predict her time of ovulation. Which technique should the client be taught to assess for spinnbarkeit?
   1. Take her temperature each morning before rising.
   2. Carefully feel her breasts for glandular development.
   3. Monitor her nipples for signs of tingling and sensitivity.
   4. Assess her vaginal discharge for elasticity and slipperiness.

7. In analyzing the need for teaching regarding sexual health in a client who is sexually active, which of the following questions is the most important for a nurse to ask?
   1. "How old are your children?"
   2. "Did you have intercourse last evening?"
   3. "With whom do you have intercourse?"
   4. "Do you use vaginal lubricant?"

8. When a nurse is teaching a woman about her menstrual cycle, which of the following information should be included as the most important change that happens during the follicular phase of the menstrual cycle?
   1. Maturation of the graafian follicle.
   2. Multiplication of the fimbriae.
   3. Secretion of human chorionic gonadotropin.
   4. Proliferation of the endometrium.

9. It is day 17 of a woman's menstrual cycle. She is complaining of breast tenderness and pain in her lower left quadrant. The woman states that her cycle is usually 31 days long. Which of the following is an appropriate reply by the nurse?
   1. "You are probably ovulating."
   2. "Your hormone levels should be checked."
   3. "You will probably menstruate early."
   4. "Your breast changes are a worrisome sign."

10. A man asks the nurse where his sperm are produced. On the diagram, please place an "X" on the site of spermatogenesis.

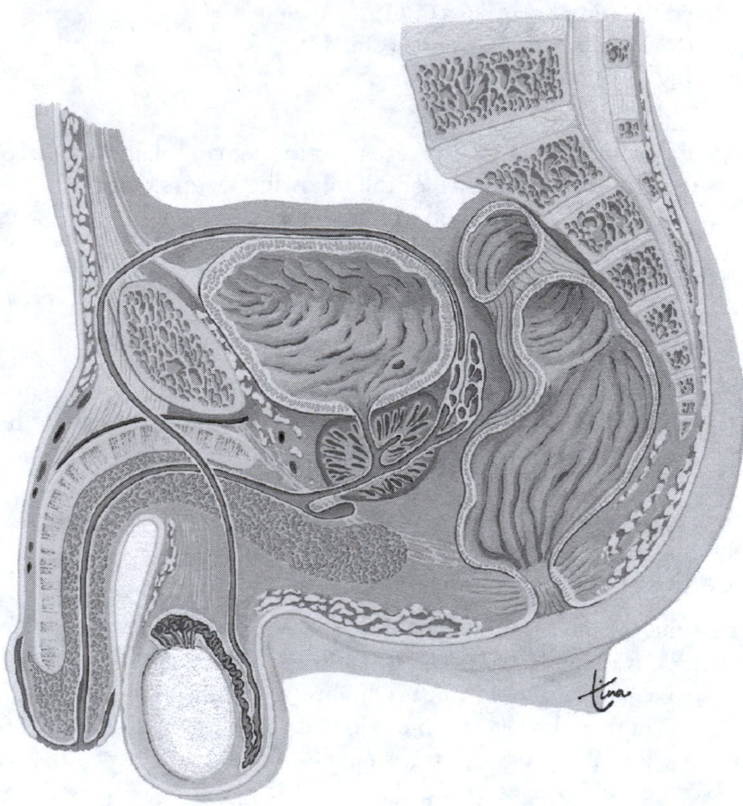

11. The nurse is teaching a class on reproduction. When asked about the development of the ova, the nurse would include which of the following?
1. Meiotic divisions begin during puberty in girls.
2. At the end of meiosis, four ova are created.
3. Each ovum contains the diploid number of chromosomes.
4. Like sperm, ova have the ability to propel themselves.

12. A client complaining of secondary amenorrhea is seeking care from her gynecologist. Which of the following may have contributed to her problem?
1. Athletic activities.
2. Vaccination history.
3. Pet ownership.
4. History of asthma.

13. What is the function of the highlighted region on the drawing below?
 1. It produces a fluid that nourishes the sperm.
 2. It secretes a fluid that neutralizes the acidic environment of the vagina.
 3. It is the reservoir where sperm mature.
 4. It contracts during ejaculation, forcing the sperm and fluid out of the urethra.

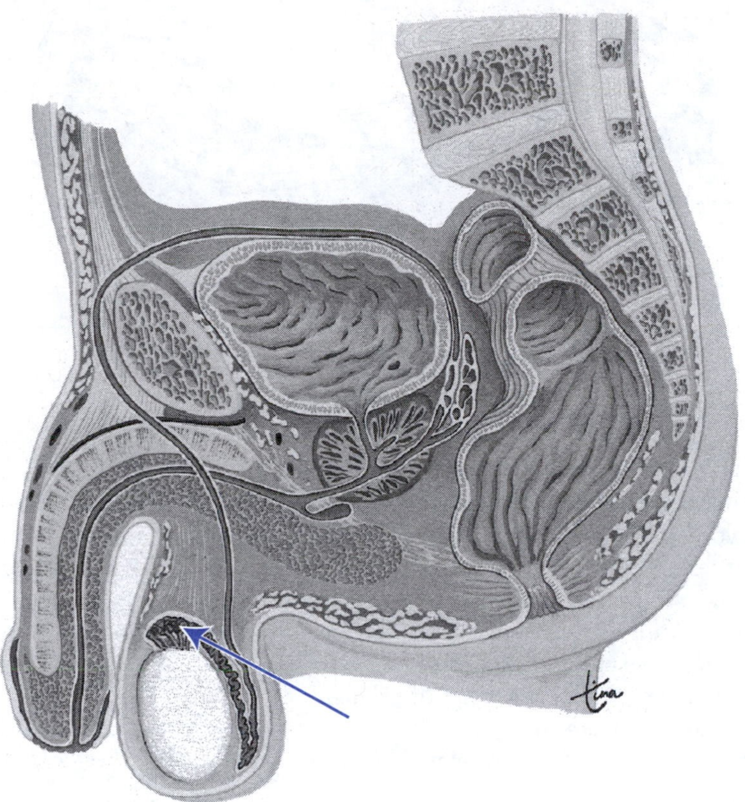

Infertility

14. A couple is seeking infertility counseling. During the history, it is noted that the man is a cancer survivor, drinks one beer every night with dinner, and takes a sauna every day after work. The response provided by the nurse should be based on which of the following?
 1. It is unlikely that any of these factors is affecting his fertility.
 2. Daily alcohol consumption could be altering his sperm count.
 3. Sperm may be malformed when exposed to the heat of the sauna.
 4. Cancer survivors have the same fertility rates as healthy males.

15. A nurse is teaching an infertile couple about how the sperm travel through the man's body during ejaculation. Please put the following five major structures in order, beginning with the place where spermatogenesis occurs and continuing through the path that the sperm and semen travel until ejaculation.
 1. Epididymis.
 2. Prostate.
 3. Testes.
 4. Urethra.
 5. Vas deferens.

16. A client has been notified that endometriosis is covering her fimbriae. She asks the nurse why that is such a problem. The nurse advises the woman that fertilization is often impossible when the fimbriated ends are blocked. Please place an "X" on the diagram to show the woman where fertilization takes place.

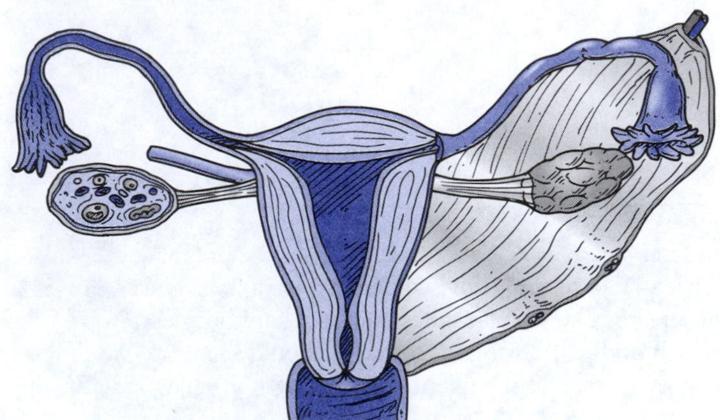

17. The nurse is providing counseling to a group of sexually active single women. Most of the women have expressed a desire to have children in the future but not within the next few years. Which of the following actions should the nurse suggest the women take to protect their fertility for the future? **Select all that apply.**
    1. Use condoms during intercourse.
    2. Refrain from smoking cigarettes.
    3. Maintain an appropriate weight for height.
    4. Exercise in moderation.
    5. Refrain from drinking carbonated beverages.

18. A couple is seeking advice regarding actions that they can take to increase their potential success in becoming pregnant. Which of the following recommendations should the nurse give to the couple?
    1. The couple should use vaginal lubricants during intercourse.
    2. The couple should delay having intercourse until the day of ovulation.
    3. The woman should refrain from douching.
    4. The man should be on top during intercourse.

19. A nurse working in an infertility clinic should include which of the following in her discussions with the couple?
    1. Adoption as an alternative to infertility treatments.
    2. The legal controversy surrounding intrauterine insemination.
    3. The need to seek marriage counseling before undergoing infertility treatments.
    4. Statistics regarding the number of couples who never learn why they are infertile.

20. A woman who is infertile has been diagnosed with endometriosis. She asks the nurse why that diagnosis has made her infertile. Which of the following explanations is appropriate for the nurse to make?
    1. "Scarring sometimes surrounds and blocks the ends of the fallopian tubes, preventing your eggs from being fertilized by your partner's sperm."
    2. "You are producing insufficient quantities of follicle-stimulating hormone that is needed to mature an egg every month."
    3. "Inside your uterus is a benign tumor that makes it impossible for the fertilized egg to implant."
    4. "You have a chronic infection of the vaginal tract that makes the secretions hostile to your partner's sperm."

21. Infertility increases a client's risk of which of the following diseases?
    1. Diabetes mellitus.
    2. Nystagmus.
    3. Cholecystitis.
    4. Ovarian cancer.

22. A client is to receive injections of menotropins for infertility prior to in-vitro fertilization. Which of the following is the expected action of this medication?
    1. Prolongation of the luteal phase.
    2. Stimulation of ovulation.
    3. Suppression of menstruation.
    4. Promotion of cervical mucus production.

23. A 35-year-old client is being seen for her yearly gynecological examination. She states that she and her partner have been trying to become pregnant for a little over 6 months and that a friend had recently advised her partner to take ginseng to improve the potency of his sperm. The woman states that they have decided to take their friend's advice. On which of the following information should the nurse base their reply?
    1. Based on their history, the client and her partner have made the appropriate decision regarding their fertility.
    2. Ginseng can cause permanent chromosomal mutations and should be stopped immediately.
    3. It is unnecessary to become concerned about this woman's fertility because she has tried to become pregnant for only a few months.
    4. Although ginseng may be helpful, it would be prudent to encourage the woman to seek fertility counseling.

24. A couple is seeking infertility counseling. The practitioner has identified the factors listed below in the woman's health history. Which of these findings may be contributing to the couple's infertility?
    1. The client is 36 years old.
    2. The client was 13 years old when she started to menstruate.
    3. The client works as a dental hygienist 3 days a week.
    4. The client jogs 2 miles every day.

25. A couple who has sought fertility counseling has been told that the man's sperm count is very low. The nurse advises the couple that spermatogenesis is impaired when which of the following occurs?
    1. The testes are overheated.
    2. The vas deferens is ligated.
    3. The prostate gland is enlarged.
    4. The flagella are segmented.

26. A man is being treated with sildenafil citrate for erectile dysfunction (ED). Which of the following is a contraindication for this medication?
    1. Preexisting diagnosis of herpes simplex 2.
    2. Nitroglycerin ingestion for angina pectoris.
    3. Retinal damage from type I diabetes mellitus.
    4. Complications after resection of the prostate.

27. A client has been notified that because of fallopian tube obstruction, her best option for becoming pregnant is through in-vitro fertilization. The client asks the nurse about the procedure. Which of the following responses is correct?
    1. "During the stimulation phase of the procedure, the physician will make sure that only one egg reaches maturation."
    2. "Preimplantation genetic diagnosis will be performed on your partner's sperm before they are mixed with your eggs."
    3. "After ovarian stimulation, intrauterine insemination (IUI) will be performed with your partner's sperm."
    4. "Any extra embryos will be preserved for you if you wish to conceive again in the future."

28. A client asks the nurse about the gamete intrafallopian transfer (GIFT) procedure. Which of the following responses would be appropriate for the nurse to make?
1. Fertilization takes place in the woman's body.
2. Zygotes are placed in the fallopian tubes.
3. Donor sperm are placed in a medium with donor eggs.
4. A surrogate carries the fetus.

29. A client who is undergoing ovarian stimulation for infertility calls the infertility nurse and states, "My abdomen feels very bloated, my clothes are very tight, and my urine is very dark." Which of the following is the appropriate statement for the nurse to make at this time?
1. "Please take a urine sample to the lab so they can check it for an infection."
2. "Those changes indicate that you are likely already pregnant."
3. "It is important for you to come into the office to be examined today."
4. "Abdominal bloating is an expected response to the medications."

30. Nurses employed in a midwifery office are attending a conference to learn about factors that increase a woman's risk of becoming infertile. To evaluate the nurses' learning, the conference coordinator tests the nurses' knowledge at the conclusion of the seminar. The nurses should know that which of the following problems increase/s a client's risk of developing infertility problems? **Select all that apply.**
1. Women who have menstrual cycles that are up to 30 days long.
2. Women who experience pain during intercourse.
3. Women who have had pelvic inflammatory disease.
4. Women who have excess facial hair.
5. Women who have menstrual periods that are over 5 days long.

31. An infertility specialist is evaluating whether a woman's cervical mucus contains enough estrogen to support sperm motility. Which of the following tests is the physician conducting?
1. Ferning capacity.
2. Basal body temperature.
3. Colposcopy.
4. Hysterotomy.

32. A couple who has been attempting to become pregnant for 5 years is seeking assistance from an infertility clinic. The nurse assesses the clients' emotional responses to their infertility. Which of the following responses would the nurse expect to find? **Select all that apply.**
1. Anger at others who have babies.
2. Feelings of failure because they can't make a baby.
3. Sexual excitement because they want so desperately to conceive a baby.
4. Sadness because of the perceived loss of being a parent.
5. Guilt on the part of one partner because they are not able to give the other a baby.

33. A client is to undergo a postcoital test for infertility. The nurse should include which of the following statements in the client's pre-procedure counseling?
1. "You will have the test the day after your menstruation ends."
2. "You will have a dye put into your vein that will show up on x-ray."
3. "You should refrain from having intercourse for the four days immediately before the test."
4. "You should experience the same sensations you feel when your doctor does your Pap test."

34. A client is to have a hysterosalpingogram. In this procedure, the physician will be able to determine which of the following?
1. Whether or not the ovaries are maturing properly.
2. If the endometrium is fully vascularized.
3. If the cervix is incompetent.
4. Whether or not the fallopian tubes are obstructed.

35. A client's basal body temperature (BBT) chart for one full month is shown below. Based on the temperatures shown, what can the nurse conclude?
1. It is likely that she has not ovulated.
2. The client's fertile period is between 12 and 18 days.
3. The client's period is abnormally long.
4. It is likely that her progesterone levels rose on day 15.

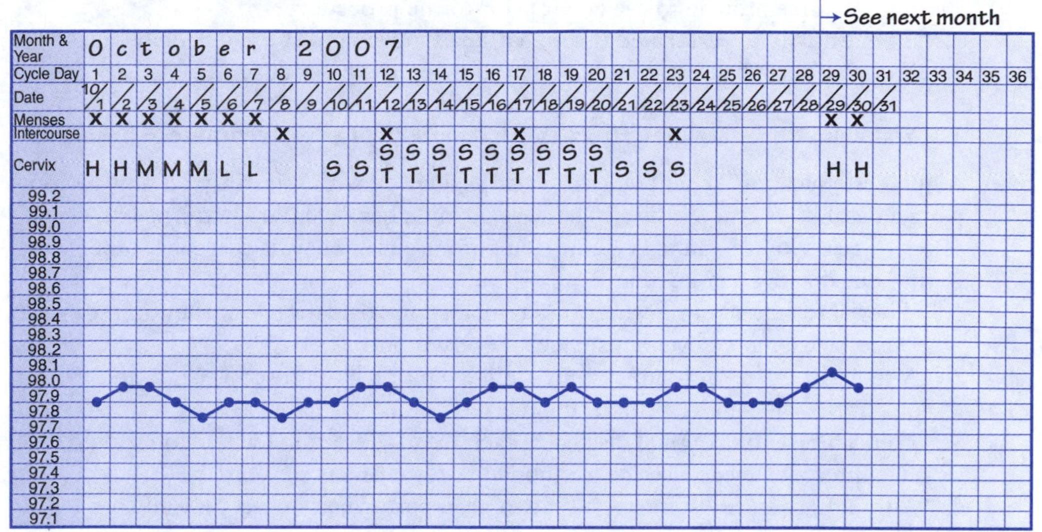

H–heavy period; **M**–moderate period; **L**–light period; **S**–sticky mucus; **SL**–slippery mucus; **T**–thick mucus; **Th**–thin mucus; **C**–clear mucus; **W**–white mucus

36. Which instruction by the nurse should be included in the teaching plan for an infertile woman who has been shown to have a 28-day biphasic menstrual cycle?
1. Douche with a cider vinegar solution immediately before having intercourse.
2. Schedule intercourse every day from day 8 to day 14 of the menstrual cycle.
3. Be placed on follicle-stimulating hormone therapy by the fertility specialist.
4. Assess the basal body temperature pattern for at least 6 more months.

37. A couple has been told that the male partner, who is healthy, is infertile "because he has cystic fibrosis." Which of the following explanations is accurate in relation to this statement?
1. Since the man is healthy, he could not possibly have cystic fibrosis.
2. Men with cystic fibrosis often have no epididymis.
3. Being infertile is not the same thing as being sterile.
4. Cystic fibrosis is a respiratory illness having nothing to do with reproduction.

38. A female client seeks care at an infertility clinic. Which of the following tests may the client undergo to determine what, if any, infertility problem she may have? **Select all that apply.**
1. Chorionic villus sampling.
2. Endometrial biopsy.
3. Hysterosalpingogram.
4. Serum progesterone assay.
5. Postcoital test.

39. A client is hospitalized in the acute phase of severe ovarian hyperstimulation syndrome. The nurse notes the client has fluid retention and 3+ pitting edema. Which of the following nursing goals is highest priority?
1. Client's weight will be within normal limits by date of discharge.
2. Client's skin will show no evidence of breakdown throughout hospitalization.
3. Client's electrolyte levels will be within normal limits within one day.
4. Client's lung fields will remain clear throughout hospitalization.

40. A client is receiving menotropins intramuscularly for ovarian stimulation. Which of the following is a common side effect of this therapy?
1. Piercing rectal pain.
2. Mood swings.
3. Visual disturbances.
4. Jerky tremors.

41. A client is to have a hysterosalpingogram. Which of the following information should the nurse provide to the client prior to the procedure?
1. "The test will be performed through a small incision next to your belly button."
2. "You will be on bedrest for a full day following the procedure."
3. "An antibiotic fluid will be instilled through a tube in your cervix."
4. "You will be asked to move from side to side so that x-ray pictures can be taken."

42. A nurse is educating a client who has been diagnosed with infertility on how to complete a basal body temperature chart to determine her ovulation pattern. The client states, "I really don't want to take my temperature every day. Is there any other way to find out if and when I ovulate?"
1. "There are a number of other ways to determine ovulation, but they all require you to be examined by an obstetrician every month."
2. "A test you can do at home requires you to spit on a microscopic slide and then look at the slide under a microscope."
3. "You can test your vaginal discharge each day to determine when you should have intercourse because the hormone progesterone is elevated."
4. "Although there are some tests that you can perform at home, they all cost well over a hundred dollars to purchase."

Genetics

43. The nurse is creating a pedigree from a client's family history. Which of the following symbols should the nurse use to represent a female?
1. Circle.
2. Square.
3. Triangle.
4. Diamond.

44. A woman has been advised that the reason she has had a number of spontaneous abortions is because she has an inheritable mutation. Which of the following situations is consistent with this statement?
1. A client developed skin cancer after being exposed to the sun.
2. A client developed colon cancer from an inherited dominant gene.
3. A client's genetic analysis report revealed a reciprocal translocation.
4. A client's left arm failed to develop when she was a fetus.

45. Which of the following client responses indicates that the nurse's teaching about care following chorionic villus sampling (CVS) has been successful?
1. If the baby stops moving, the woman should immediately go to the hospital.
2. The woman should take oral terbutaline every 2 hours for the next day.
3. If the woman starts to bleed or to contract, she should call her physician.
4. The woman should stay on complete bedrest for the next 48 hours.

46. A pregnant woman and her husband are both heterozygous for achondroplastic dwarfism, an autosomal dominant disease. The nurse advises the couple that their unborn child has which of the following probabilities of being of normal stature?
1. 25% probability.
2. 50% probability.
3. 75% probability.
4. 100% probability.

47. A couple inquire about the inheritance of Huntington disease (HD) because the prospective father's mother is dying of the illness. There is no history of the disease in his partner's family. The man has never been tested for HD. Which of the following responses by the nurse is appropriate?
   1. "Because HD is an autosomal dominant disease, each and every one of your children will have a 1 in 4 chance of having the disease."
   2. "Because only one of you has a family history of HD, the probability of any of your children having the disease is less than 10%."
   3. "Because HD is such a devastating disease, if there is any chance of passing the gene along, it would be advisable for you to adopt."
   4. "Because neither of you has been tested for HD, the most information I can give you is that each and every one of your children may have the disease."

48. A client with an obstetrical history of G4 P4004, states that her husband has just been diagnosed with polycystic kidney disease (PKD), an autosomal dominant disease. The husband is heterozygous for PKD, while the client has no PKD genes. The client states, "I have not had our children tested because they have such a slim chance of inheriting the disease. We intend to wait until they are teenagers to do the testing." The nurse should base the reply on which of the following?
   1. Because affected individuals rarely exhibit symptoms before age 60, the children should be allowed to wait until they are adults to be tested.
   2. The woman may be exhibiting signs of denial since each of the couple's children has a 50/50 chance of developing the disease.
   3. Because the majority of the renal cysts that develop in affected individuals are harmless, it is completely unnecessary to have the children tested.
   4. The woman's husband should be seen by a genetic specialist since he is the person who is carrying the affected gene.

49. A woman is a carrier for hemophilia A, an X-linked recessive illness. Her husband has a normal genotype. The nurse can advise the couple that the probability that their daughter will have the disease is:
   1. 0% probability.
   2. 25% probability.
   3. 50% probability.
   4. 75% probability.

50. At her first prenatal visit, a woman relates that her maternal aunt has cystic fibrosis (CF), an autosomal recessive illness. Which of the following comments is appropriate for the nurse to make at this time?
   1. "We can check to see whether or not you are a carrier for cystic fibrosis."
   2. "It is unnecessary for you to worry since your aunt is not a direct relation."
   3. "You should have an amniocentesis to see whether or not your child has the disease."
   4. "Please ask your mother whether she has ever had any symptoms of cystic fibrosis."

51. A woman asks the nurse, "My nuchal fold scan results were abnormal. What does that mean?" Which of the following comments is appropriate for the nurse to make at this time?
   1. "I am sorry to tell you that your baby will be born with a serious deformity."
   2. "The results show that your child will have cri du chat syndrome."
   3. "The test is done to see if you are at high risk for preterm labor."
   4. "An abnormal test indicates that your baby may have a chromosomal disorder."

52. A client who is 10 weeks pregnant states that her sister's son has been diagnosed with an X-linked recessive disease, Duchenne muscular dystrophy. She questions the nurse about the disease. Which of the following responses is appropriate for the nurse to make?
1. "Because Duchenne muscular dystrophy is inherited through the woman, it is advisable for you to see a genetic counselor."
2. "Duchenne muscular dystrophy usually occurs as a spontaneous mutation. It is very unlikely that your fetus is affected."
3. "Your child could acquire Duchenne muscular dystrophy only if both you and your husband carried the gene. You need to check your husband's family history."
4. "If you were to have an amniocentesis and it were to be positive for Duchenne muscular dystrophy, I could refer you to an excellent abortion counselor."

53. The genetic counselor informs a couple that they have a 25% probability of getting pregnant with a child with a severe genetic disease. The couple asks the nurse exactly what that means. Which of the following responses by the nurse is appropriate?
1. Their first child will have the genetic disease.
2. If they have four children, one of the children will have the disease.
3. Their fourth child will have the genetic disease.
4. Any baby they conceive may have the disease.

54. A client has just had an amniocentesis to determine whether her baby has an inheritable genetic disease. Which of the following interventions is highest priority at this time?
1. Assess the fetal heart rate.
2. Check the client's temperature.
3. Acknowledge the client's anxiety about the possible findings.
4. Answer questions regarding the genetic abnormality.

55. Once oogenesis is complete, the resultant gamete cell contains how many chromosomes?
1. 23.
2. 46.
3. 47.
4. 92.

56. Based on the karyotype shown below, which of the following conclusions can the nurse make about the female baby?
1. She has a genetically normal karyotype.
2. She has trisomy 21.
3. She has fragile X syndrome.
4. She has an autosomal monosomy.

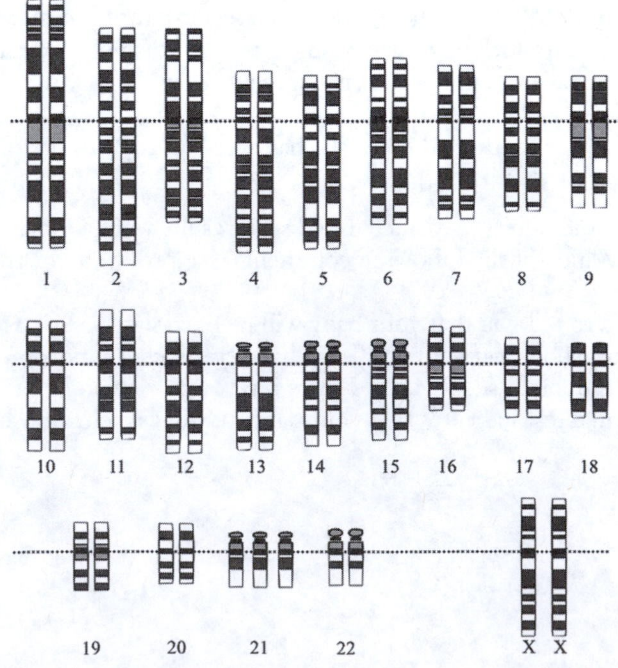

57. A genetic counselor's report states, "The genetic nomenclature for this fetus is 46, XX." How should the nurse who reads this report interpret the cytogenetic results?
1. The baby is female with a normal number of chromosomes.
2. The baby is an intersex male with female chromosomes.
3. The baby is male with an undisclosed genetic anomaly.
4. There is insufficient information to answer this question.

58. The nurse is analyzing the three generation pedigree below. In which generation is the proband?
1. I.
2. II.
3. III.
4. There is not enough information to answer this question.

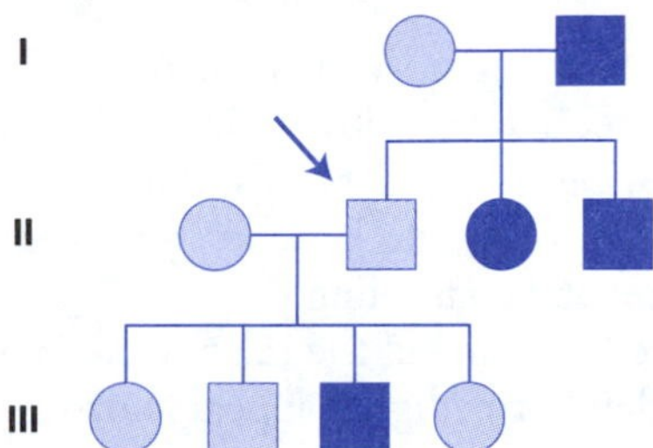

59. A woman is seeking genetic counseling during her pregnancy. She has a strong family history of diabetes mellitus. She wishes to have an amniocentesis to determine whether she is carrying a baby who will "develop diabetes." Which of the following replies would be most appropriate for the nurse to make?
1. "Doctors don't do amniocenteses to detect diabetes."
2. "Diabetes cannot be diagnosed by looking at the genes."
3. "Although diabetes does have a genetic component, diet and exercise can also influence whether or not someone develops diabetes."
4. "Even if the baby doesn't carry the genes for diabetes, the baby could still develop the disease."

60. A 25-year-old woman with no pregnancy history enters the infertility clinic stating that she has just learned she is positive for the *BRCA1* and the *BRCA2* genes. She asks the nurse what her options are for getting pregnant and breastfeeding her baby. The nurse should base her reply on which of the following?
1. Fertility of women who carry the *BRCA1* and *BRCA2* genes is similar to that of unaffected women.
2. Women with these genes should be advised not to have children because the children could inherit the defective genes.
3. Women with these genes should have their ovaries removed as soon as possible to prevent ovarian cancer.
4. Lactation is contraindicated for women who carry the *BRCA1* and *BRCA 2* genes.

61. A woman asks a nurse about pre-symptomatic genetic testing for Huntington disease. The nurse should base her response on which of the following?
1. There is no genetic marker for Huntington disease.
2. Pre-symptomatic testing cannot predict whether or not the gene will be expressed.
3. If the woman is positive for the gene for Huntington, she will develop the disease later in life.
4. If the woman is negative for the gene, her children should be tested to see whether or not they are carriers.

62. A woman who has undergone amniocentesis has been notified that her baby is XX with a 14/21 Robertsonian chromosomal translocation. The nurse helps the woman to understand which of the following?
1. The baby will have a number of serious genetic defects.
2. It is likely that the baby will be unable to have children when she grows up.
3. Chromosomal translocations are common and rarely problematic.
4. An abortion will probably be the best decision under the circumstances.

63. A woman who has had multiple miscarriages is advised to go through genetic testing. The client asks the nurse the rationale for this recommendation. The nurse should base their response on which of the following?
1. The woman's pedigree may exhibit a mitochondrial inheritance pattern.
2. The majority of miscarriages are caused by genetic defects.
3. A woman's chromosomal pattern determines her fertility.
4. There is a genetic marker that detects the presence of an incompetent cervix.

64. A nurse has just taken a family history on a client who is 10 weeks pregnant and has created the family pedigree shown below. Which of the following actions can the nurse anticipate the provider will take at this time?
1. Advise the woman that she should have an amniocentesis.
2. Send the client for genetic counseling.
3. Ask the woman if she knew any of the relatives who died.
4. Inform the woman that her pedigree appears normal.

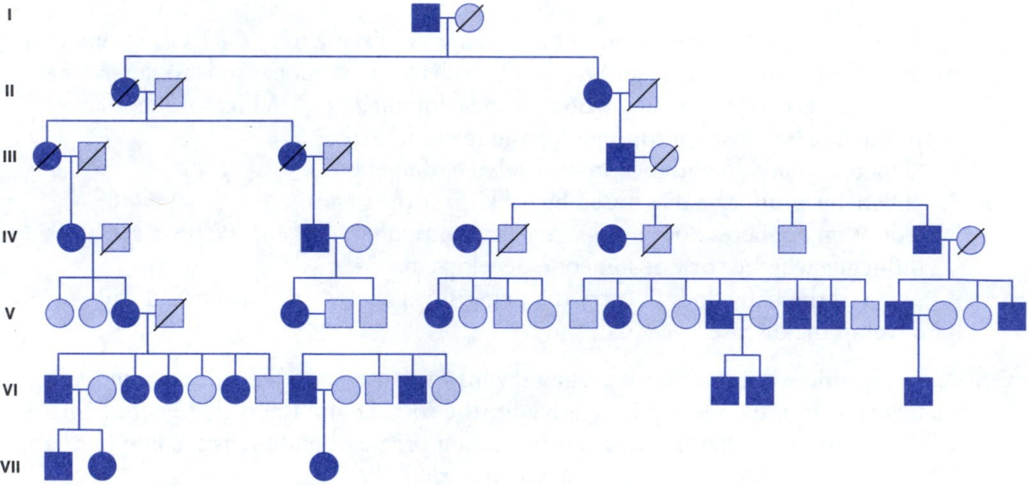

65. A woman is informed that she is a carrier for Tay-Sachs disease, an autosomal recessive illness. What is her phenotype?
1. She has one recessive gene and one normal gene.
2. She has two recessive genes.
3. She exhibits all symptoms of the disease.
4. She exhibits no symptoms of the disease.

66. During a genetic evaluation, it is discovered that a woman is carrying one autosomal dominant gene for a serious, late adult–onset disease, while her partner's history is unremarkable. Based on this information, which of the following family members should be considered high risk and in need of genetic counseling? **Select all that apply.**
1. The woman's fetus.
2. The woman's sisters.
3. The woman's brothers.
4. The woman's parents.
5. The woman's partner.

67. A man has inherited the gene for familial adenomatous polyposis (FAP), an autosomal dominant disease. He and his wife wish to have a baby. Which of the following would provide the couple with the highest probability of conceiving a healthy child?
1. Amniocentesis.
2. Chorionic villus sampling (CVS).
3. Preimplantation genetic diagnosis (PGD).
4. Gamete intrafallopian transfer (GIFT).

68. A woman asks the obstetrician's nurse about cord blood banking. Which of the following responses by the nurse would be best?
1. "I think it would be best to ask the doctor to tell you about that."
2. "The cord blood is frozen in case your baby develops a serious illness in the future."
3. "The doctors could transfuse anyone who gets into a bad accident with the blood."
4. "Cord blood banking is very expensive and the blood is rarely ever used."

69. A 3-month-old baby has been diagnosed with cystic fibrosis (CF). The mother says, "How could this happen? I had an amniocentesis during my pregnancy and everything was supposed to be normal!" What must the nurse understand about this situation?
1. Cystic fibrosis cannot be diagnosed by amniocentesis.
2. The baby may have an uncommon genetic variant of the disease.
3. It is possible that the laboratory technician made an error.
4. Instead of obtaining fetal cells, the doctor probably harvested maternal cells.

70. The nurse discusses the results of a three generation pedigree with the proband who has breast cancer. Which of the following information must the nurse consider?
1. The proband should have a complete genetic analysis done.
2. The proband is the first member of the family to be diagnosed.
3. The proband's first degree relatives should be included in the discussion.
4. The proband's sisters will likely develop breast cancer during their lives.

71. The nurse is analyzing the pedigree shown below. How should the nurse interpret the genotype of the individual in location II-4?
1. Affected male.
2. Unaffected female.
3. Stillborn child.
4. Child of unknown sex.

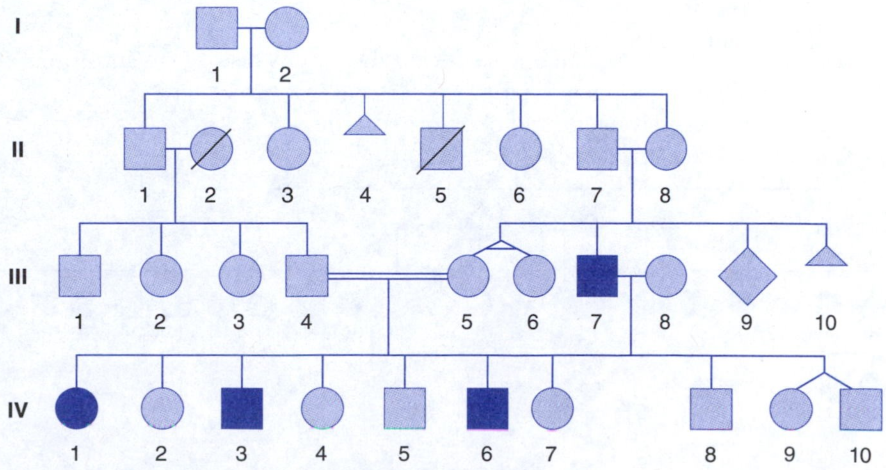

72. The nurse is analyzing the pedigree shown below. How should the nurse interpret the symbols of the individuals in locations IV-9 and IV-10?
1. Fraternal twins.
2. Unaffected couple.
3. Proband and sister.
4. Known heterozygotes.

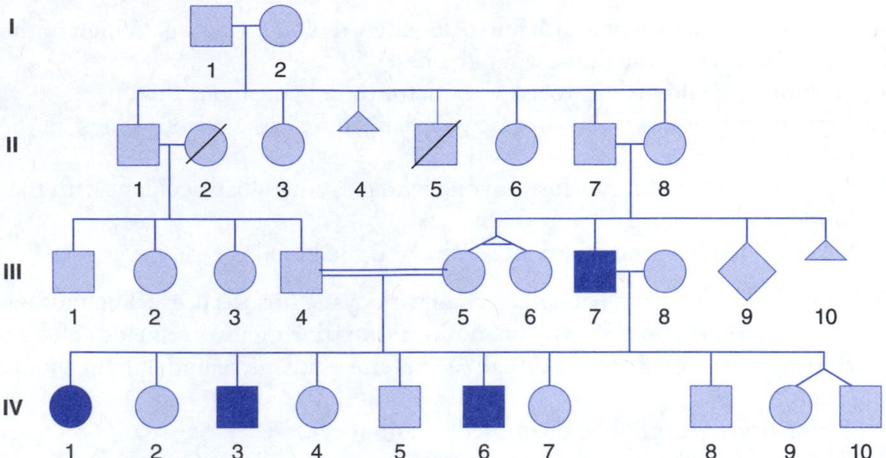

73. A woman who is a carrier for sickle cell anemia is advised that if her baby has two recessive genes, the penetrance of the disease is 100%, but the expressivity is variable. Which of the following explanations will clarify this communication for the mother? All babies with two recessive sickle cell genes will:
1. Develop painful vaso-occlusive crises during their first year of life.
2. Exhibit at least some signs of the disease while in the neonatal nursery.
3. Show some symptoms of the disease but the severity of the symptoms will be individual.
4. Be diagnosed with sickle cell trait but will be healthy and disease-free throughout their lives.

74. Analyze the pedigree below. Which of the following inheritance patterns does the pedigree depict?
1. Autosomal recessive.
2. Mitochondrial inheritance.
3. X-linked recessive.
4. Y-linked trait.

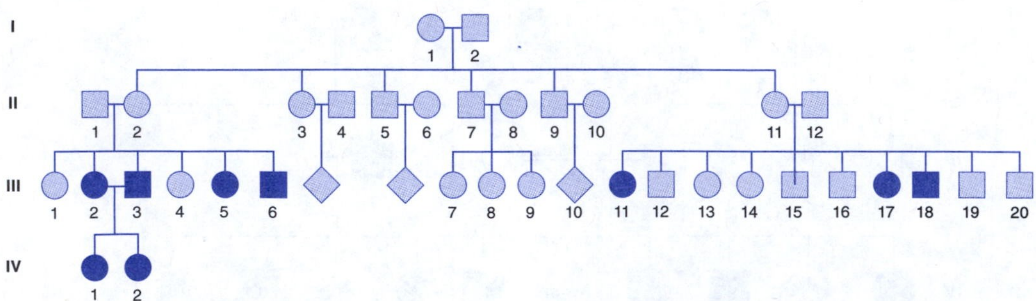

75. Analyze the pedigree below. Which of the following inheritance patterns does the pedigree depict?
1. Autosomal dominant.
2. Mitochondrial inheritance.
3. X-linked recessive.
4. Y-linked trait.

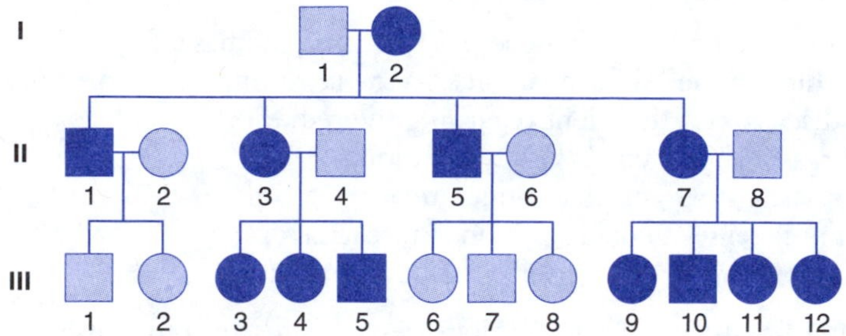

76. The nurse is counseling a pregnant couple who are both carriers for phenylketonuria (PKU), an autosomal recessive disease. Which of the following comments by the nurse is appropriate?
1. "I wish I could give you good news, but because this is your first pregnancy, your child will definitely have PKU."
2. "Congratulations, you must feel relieved that the odds of having a sick child are so small."
3. "There is a 2 out of 4 chance that your child will be a carrier like both of you."
4. "There is a 2 out of 4 chance that your child will have PKU."

77. A male client has green color blindness, an X-linked recessive genetic disorder. His wife has no affected genes. Which of the following statements by the nurse is true regarding the couple's potential for having a child who is color blind?
1. All male children will be color blind.
2. All female children will be color blind.
3. All male children will be carriers for color blindness.
4. All female children will be carriers for color blindness.

78. A woman whose blood type is O− (negative) states, "My husband is AB+ (positive)." The mother queries the nurse about what blood type the baby will have. Which of the following blood types should the nurse advise the mother that the baby may have? **Select all that apply.**
1. "Your baby could be type O+ (positive)."
2. "Your baby could be type O− (negative)."
3. "Your baby could be type AB− (negative)."
4. "Your baby could be type A+ (positive)."
5. "Your baby could be type B− (negative)."

79. A client's amniocentesis results were reported as 46, XY. Her obstetrician informed her at the time that everything "looks good." Shortly after birth the baby is diagnosed with cerebral palsy. Which of the following responses will explain this result?
1. It is likely that the client received the wrong amniocentesis results.
2. Cerebral palsy is not a genetic disease.
3. The genes that cause cerebral palsy have not yet been discovered.
4. The genes were never tested for cerebral palsy.

80. Most children born into families look similar but are not exactly the same. The children appear different because homologous chromosomes exchange genetic material at which of the following?
1. Centromere.
2. Chiasma.
3. Chromatid.
4. Codon.

81. A client is being interviewed prior to becoming pregnant. She states that she has a disease that is transmitted by mitochondrial inheritance. Which of the following statements is consistent with the client's disease?
    1. 100% of her children will be affected.
    2. Only her female children will be affected.
    3. Each fetus will have a 50% probability of being affected.
    4. A fetus will be affected only if it inherits a similar gene from its father.

82. A client wants to undergo amniocentesis because she has a family history of breast cancer. Which of the following choices is the most important information for the nurse to discuss with the client regarding the request?
    1. The breast cancer gene is highly penetrant.
    2. The breast cancer gene has moderate expressivity.
    3. The amniocentesis could result in a miscarriage.
    4. The majority of breast cancers are not inherited.

83. A woman is pregnant. During amniocentesis it is discovered that her child has Down's syndrome with a mosaic chromosomal configuration. She asks the nurse what that means. What is the nurse's best response?
    1. "Instead of two number 21 chromosomes, your child has three."
    2. "Your baby's number 21 chromosomes have black and white bands on them."
    3. "Some of your baby's number 21 chromosomes are longer than others."
    4. "Some of your baby's cells have two number 21 chromosomes and some have three."

84. Which of the following is an attainable short-term goal for a client who is 8 weeks pregnant and has a family history of cystic fibrosis?
    1. Have a sweat chloride test done.
    2. Seek out genetic counseling.
    3. Undergo chorionic villus sampling.
    4. Be seen by a pulmonologist.

85. What is the rationale for testing all neonates for maple syrup urine disease (MSUD) when only 1 in 100,000 to 300,000 children will be born with the disease?
    1. To encourage the parents to have genetic testing done.
    2. To prevent neurological disease in affected children.
    3. To reduce the amount of money insurance companies must pay for sick MSUD children.
    4. To persuade pharmaceutical companies to develop medications to treat children with MSUD.

86. A client who is planning to become pregnant tells the nurse, "I am so scared. My brother, who was born 2 years after I was, died a month after he was born. My mother says that he had a very serious genetic defect. I don't know what to do." Which of the following responses are appropriate for the nurse to make? **Select all that apply.**
    1. "It is almost impossible to figure out what happened way back then, but I'm sure everything will be fine with your baby."
    2. "Do you think your mother would allow your brother's body to be unearthed so that it could be tested for the genetic disease?"
    3. "There are a number of tests that can be performed during your pregnancy to screen the baby for genetic diseases."
    4. "I will discuss your concerns with your obstetrician. I am sure your doctor will refer you to a genetic counselor who hopefully will be able to help you."
    5. "I think your mother should make an appointment to meet with your obstetrician. I'm sure she knows a lot more about your brother's illness than she is telling you."

87. A client at 11 weeks' gestation, is being prepared for chorionic villus sampling (CVS). The woman is very anxious that the baby will be injured during the procedure. Which of the following statements would be appropriate for the nurse to make?
   1. "It is unlikely that the baby will be injured because before inserting the needle, the doctor will locate the baby and placenta using ultrasound."
   2. "I know how you feel. Every time I assist with the procedure I say a little prayer that the baby won't be hurt."
   3. "Has your doctor told you about all of the possible complications that can happen during the procedure?"
   4. "I understand how you feel, but you know how important it is to find out whether your baby has a genetic disease or not."

ANSWERS AND RATIONALES

The correct answer number and rationale for why it is the correct answer are given in **boldface blue type.** Rationales for why the other possible answer options are incorrect also are given, but they are not in boldface type.

Sexuality

1. **1. This statement is true, and the discomfort at the location of the ovary where ovulation occurs is called by the German word of "mittelschmerz" which means "middle pain." It is a one-sided pain related to ovulation. Ovulation usually occurs 14 days before the first day of the menses. It generally alternates between the left and right ovaries every month. The location of the pain indicates which ovary has ovulated that month.**

2. The history given by the woman is not indicative of ovarian cancer.
3. Ovarian cancer is not always painful, and symptoms would not occur on just one day of the month.
4. The timing of the pain is more significant than the type of pain, but it is not within the nurse's scope of practice to diagnose a condition.

TEST-TAKING HINT: Although the stem includes the fact that the woman is concerned about ovarian cancer, this question is actually testing what the test taker knows about ovulation.

2. **2, 1, 3, 4. Gonadotropin-releasing hormone stimulates the production of follicle-stimulating hormone (FSH) and luteinizing hormone (LH). FSH rises first and LH follows. After ovulation, progesterone rises.**

TEST-TAKING HINT: The menstrual cycle is governed by the rise and fall of estrogen within three phases: follicular phase (days 1–14); ovulatory phase (day 15); and luteal phase (days 16–28). The rise and fall of each hormone resembles the passing of a baton during a relay race. The menstrual cycle is counted by the number of days that pass from the first day of one bleeding episode to the next one. The average cycle lasts around 28 days.

During the follicular phase, which begins during the bleeding phase, both estrogen and progesterone are at low levels. The pituitary gland releases follicle-stimulating hormone (FSH) which begins maturing an egg. As the egg matures, it produces estrogen, which is highest just a day or two before ovulation. High levels of estrogen stimulate the hypothalamus, which releases gonadotropin-releasing hormone (GnRH) in pulsatile bursts. The GnRH, in turn, stimulates the pituitary to produce higher levels of FSH, and luteinizing hormone (LH). With that cocktail of FSH and LH, the mature egg is released and ovulation occurs. Within the now-empty follicle, a yellow corpus luteum develops to prepare the lining of the uterus for possible implantation of a fertilized egg. The estrogen level drops dramatically and progesterone soars as the uterus prepares for implantation. Progesterone gets its name from being in favor of gestation, or "pro" gestation and supports the pregnancy. If fertilization does not occur, the corpus luteum dies and menstruation begins approximately 14 days after ovulation, or mid-cycle.

3. **1. The fact that the client had intercourse in the last 3 days likely led to the symptoms she is reporting, which are symptoms of a urinary tract infection (UTI).**

2. Returning from a recent trip abroad is not likely related to the symptoms the client is reporting, which are symptoms of a UTI.
3. Stopping hormone replacement therapy is unlikely related to the symptoms reported by the client.
4. It is unlikely that starting a weight-lifting program is related to the symptoms of a UTI that the client is reporting.

TEST-TAKING HINT: Because of its location, the urinary meatus is at risk of bacterial contamination during intercourse. To prevent a UTI, women are encouraged to urinate immediately after having intercourse to flush any bacteria from the urethral opening.

4. 1. Estrogen begins to elevate before ovulation. It is not responsible for the temperature elevation.

2. Progesterone elevation occurs after ovulation and spikes at about 5 to 6 days after ovulation. Progesterone is thermogenic—that is, heat producing. Progesterone is the reason women's temperatures are elevated following ovulation.

3. LH spikes at the time of ovulation, but does not cause the spike in temperature.
4. FSH promotes the maturation of the ovum.

TEST-TAKING HINT: This question asks the test taker to explain a temperature rise that occurs 2 weeks prior to menstruation. It is essential

for the test taker to know that ovulation usually takes place approximately 14 days before the onset of menses. That eliminates estrogen and FSH, since the temperature would have been elevated much earlier in the cycle if those hormones were responsible. LH spikes and then drops at the time of ovulation, but because progesterone becomes elevated during the latter part of the menstrual cycle and is known to cause a rise in temperature (Steward & Raja, 2019), progesterone is the correct answer. If one remembers that progesterone induces inflammation, which brings warmth to the affected area, this can serve as a learning hack to remember the information.

5. 1. When the ovum is not fertilized, both estrogen and progesterone levels drop. The drop in hormones is followed by menstruation.
2. Estrogen rises before ovulation, not before menstruation.
3. Estrogen is low and progesterone is high after ovulation, when progesterone (being "pro gestation") prepares the uterine lining for possible implantation of a fertilized egg. Both progesterone and estrogen are low during menstruation.
4. When the ovum is not fertilized, both estrogen and progesterone levels drop. The hormonal drop is followed by menstruation.

TEST-TAKING HINT: Menstruation begins on day 1 of the menstrual cycle. Since pregnancy has not occurred, the test taker can deduce that the hormones of pregnancy did not remain elevated. Therefore, Option 4, that both estrogen and progesterone are low, is the correct response. The reproductive cycle is on clean-up as it prepares for another round.

6. 1. The temperature does elevate after ovulation, but the elevation is not defined as spinnbarkeit.
2. The breasts do become sensitive and some women do palpate tender nodules in the breasts at the time of ovulation, but those changes are not spinnbarkeit.
3. The nipples may tingle and become sensitive, but the sensations are not indicative of spinnbarkeit.
4. Spinnbarkeit is defined as the "thread" that is created when the vaginal discharge is slippery and elastic like raw egg white, at the time of ovulation. Sperm can penetrate it on their way to fertilize the egg. The changes are in response to high estrogen levels. The woman inserts her index and middle fingers into her vagina and touches her cervix. After removing her fingers, she separates her fingers and "spins a thread" between her fingers. When she is not in her fertile period, the mucus is thick and gluey.

TEST-TAKING HINT: It is important for the test taker to be familiar with self-help techniques to assist clients to understand their bodies. *Spinnbarkeit* is a German term that literally means "the ability to create a thread." When the woman is not fertile, the cervical mucus dries up, or becomes brittle.

7. 1. The ages of a client's children may be important, but it is not the most important information for the nurse to request.
2. Whether or not the client had intercourse the preceding night is important, but it is not the most important information for the nurse to solicit.
3. This question is the most important for the nurse to ask. The nurse is trying to learn whether or not the client is having intercourse with more than one partner and/or whether the client has intercourse with men or women or both.
4. Whether or not the client uses vaginal lubricant is important, but it is not the most important information for the nurse to ask about.

TEST-TAKING HINT: Clients who engage in sex with multiple sex partners are at high risk for infection and pregnancy. Women in lesbian relationships may be less likely to protect themselves from infection since there is no risk of pregnancy.

8. 1. FSH is elevated during the follicular phase and the graafian follicle (the site in the ovary where an ovum develops before ovulation) matures.
2. The fimbriae (finger-like tissues) are located at the ends of the fallopian tubes. They do not multiply in number.
3. The hormone hCG is not produced during the menstrual cycle. It is produced by the fertilized egg in early pregnancy.
4. Endometrial proliferation occurs during the secretory phase of the menstrual cycle.

TEST-TAKING HINT: The test taker should always try to find a clue in the stem for the answer to the question. In this question, the test taker is requested to choose "the most important change that happens during the follicular phase." In general, things are named logically, and this case is no different. The follicular phase is the period of the menstrual cycle when the follicle matures. Answers 2, 3, and 4 are false.

9. 1. **This statement is true. Breast tenderness and left-or-right-sided pelvic pain, referred to as *mittelschmerz*, often occur at the time of ovulation.**
2. Breast tenderness and mittelschmerz are symptoms of ovulation. They are not related to abnormal hormonal levels.
3. Menstruation occurs approximately 14 days after ovulation.
4. The breast changes are normal and often are felt by women at the time of ovulation.

TEST-TAKING HINT: There are two hints to the answer in this question. First, the woman has a 31-day cycle and it is day 17. It is, therefore, 14 days before the woman usually menstruates. Women usually ovulate 14 days before their menstrual periods begin. The one-sided lower quadrant pain is also a clue. Women often feel a twinge, called *mittelschmerz*, near the site of the ovary at the time of ovulation.

10. **The test taker should place an "X" on the testes.**

TEST-TAKING HINT: The test taker should be familiar with the anatomy and physiology of both the male and female reproductive systems. Spermatogenesis occurs in the testes, which is where the "X" should be placed. When the vas deferens is ligated during a vasectomy, the sperm are no longer able to migrate from the testes to the female reproductive tract, and the man becomes sterile.

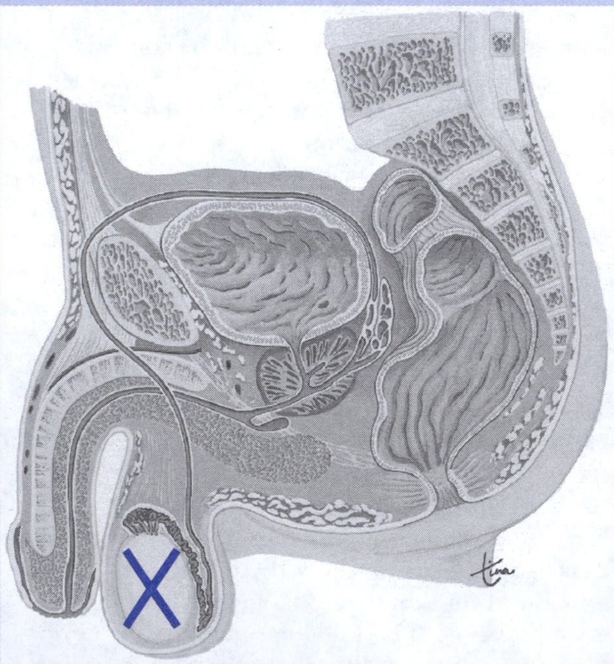

11. 1. **This answer is correct. Meiosis I occurs during puberty.**
2. This response is not true. At the completion of oogenesis only one ovum is created. At the completion of spermatogenesis, four sperm are created.
3. This response is not true. Each ovum contains the haploid number of chromosomes—a complete set of unpaired chromosomes, the mother's contribution to the baby's genetics.
4. This response is not true. Sperm have flagella that propel them through the woman's reproductive system. Ova, however, do not have the ability to propel themselves but rather are propelled externally by the cilia in the fallopian tubes.

TEST-TAKING HINT: Meiosis begins during puberty and the ova age during the following years. This is the likely reason why women who attempt to become pregnant after 35 years of age have an increased incidence of infertility as well as an increased probability of becoming pregnant with a trisomy chromosomal syndrome, for example, Down's syndrome.

12. 1. **If the young woman exercises excessively—for example, as a competitive gymnast or runner—her body fat index could become so low that she becomes amenorrheic.**
2. Vaccination history has not been shown to be related to secondary amenorrhea.
3. Pet ownership has not been shown to be related to secondary amenorrhea.
4. History of asthma has not been shown to be related to secondary amenorrhea.

TEST-TAKING HINT: If unsure of the definition, the test taker should be able to deduce what is meant by secondary amenorrhea. The prefix "a" means "not" and the remainder of the word refers to the menses. A problem that is labeled "primary" is one that occurs initially. A secondary problem occurs later. A client with primary amenorrhea, therefore, is a young woman who has never had a period. A client with secondary amenorrhea, as in this question, is a young woman who did have periods but whose periods have stopped. The most common cause of secondary amenorrhea is pregnancy. Many other causes, including a low body fat index such as can result from excessive or very strenuous exercises, can also lead to amenorrhea.

13. 1. The seminal vesicles, which are not highlighted in the diagram, produce a fluid that nourishes the sperm.
2. The prostate gland, which is not highlighted in the diagram, secretes a fluid that neutralizes the acidic environment of the vagina.
3. The highlighted organ is the epididymis, which is the reservoir where sperm mature.
4. The pubococcygeal muscles are not highlighted in the diagram. These muscles and others contract during ejaculation, forcing the sperm and fluid out of the urethra.

TEST-TAKING HINT: If the test taker is unfamiliar either with the location of the structures cited in the question or with the name and function of any of the components of the male reproductive system, he or she should review the anatomy and physiology of the male reproductive system.

Infertility

14. 1. This response is incorrect because exposing the testes to the heat of the sauna can alter the normal morphology of the sperm.
2. Alcohol consumed in excessive amounts can alter spermatogenesis, but one beer per day has not been shown to be a problem.
3. The high temperature of the sauna could alter the number and morphology of the sperm.
4. Chemotherapy has been shown to affect the ability of males to create sperm.

TEST-TAKING HINT: The test taker should try not to be intimidated by quantities and numbers when they are included in the stem or answer options. The stem states that the male client consumes one beer each evening. That is a distractor.

15. 3, 1, 5, 2, 4. The sperm are produced in the testes (3). They then proceed to the epididymis (1) where they mature. The vas deferens (5) is the conduit through which the sperm first travel during ejaculation. The prostate (2), encircling the neck of the urethra, produces a fluid that protects the sperm, and, finally, the sperm exit the male body via the urethra (4).

TEST-TAKING HINT: This is an alternate-form question. The test taker is required to place the items in the required sequence. In the NCLEX exam, this type of question is generally a "drag and drop" question in a numbered sequence. It is essential that the test taker knows and understands normal anatomy and physiology. If the normal functioning of the body is not understood, it will be very difficult for the test taker to learn and remember abnormalities. Although maternity is often viewed as a topic in women's health, it must be remembered that the male's contribution to the embryo is as important to a healthy pregnancy outcome as the woman's. Understanding the male reproductive system is, therefore, a necessary requirement.

16. The student should place an "X" on the outer third of the fallopian tube.

TEST-TAKING HINT: Although the question discusses the fimbriae or fimbriated ends, the question is actually asking where fertilization takes place—which is in the outer third of the tube. The test taker could place the "X" on either fallopian tube, as long as the location of the "X" is on the outer third of the fallopian tube. The test taker will note that the only difference in this drawing is that one tube and ovary are shown "open," and the other tube and ovary are shown "closed." Fertilization can take place in either tube, depending on which ovary released the egg.

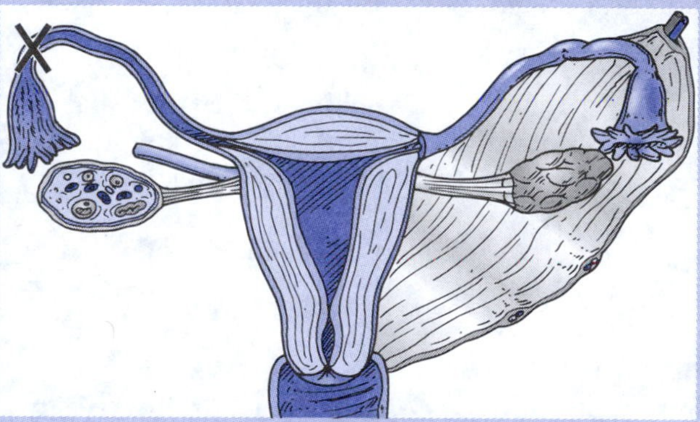

17. Answers 1, 2, 3, and 4 are correct.
1. Condoms should be worn during sexual contact to prevent infection with a sexually transmitted disease, which can affect the long-term health of the woman's reproductive system.
2. Women who smoke have a higher incidence of infertility than those who do not smoke.
3. Women who are either overweight or underweight have increased incidence of infertility.
4. Body mass index (BMI) is related to the amount of exercise a woman engages in.

Those who exercise excessively are more likely to have a very low BMI and those who rarely exercise, to be obese. Since fertility is related to body weight, it is recommended that women exercise in moderation.

5. There is some evidence that caffeine in large quantities may affect fertility, but decaffeinated carbonated beverages have never been cited as affecting one's fertility.

TEST-TAKING HINT: There are a number of factors that can affect fertility. Some of the factors are beyond a woman's control. For example, a woman may choose to delay childbearing until her 30s. Other factors, such as smoking cigarettes and exercising, are controllable.

18. 1. Use of vaginal lubricants is not recommended. Vaginal lubricants may alter the pH of the reproductive system, adversely affecting the couple's potential of becoming pregnant.

2. Delaying intercourse until the day of ovulation is a poor recommendation. The sperm live for about 3 days. If the couple has daily intercourse beginning 5 or 6 days before ovulation (the "fertile window") and continuing until the day of ovulation, they will maximize their potential of becoming pregnant.

3. **The woman should refrain from douching. Douching can change the normal flora and the pH in the vagina, making the environment hostile to the sperm.**

4. The position of the couple during intercourse will not affect the potential fertility of the woman.

TEST-TAKING HINT: There is a great deal of false information in the community regarding ways to maximize one's ability to become pregnant. For example, some couples believe that they should have intercourse less frequently when trying to become pregnant because sperm potency drops with frequent ejaculations. This notion has not been shown to be true. Clients need fact-based information regarding ways to maximize their ability to conceive.

19. 1. **It is important for the couple to be provided with all relevant information. Adoption is a viable alternative to infertility treatments.**

2. Although there are moral/ethical issues surrounding intrauterine insemination (IUI), there are no legal controversies. Artificial insemination is a legal procedure.

3. Although it is not without merit, marriage counseling is not mandatory before seeking infertility treatments.

4. This response is not true. Although up to 10% of couples appear to have no physical cause of their infertility, in the majority of cases a cause is found: one-third of cases are related to female problems, one-third of cases are related to male problems, and one-third of cases are a combination of male and female problems.

TEST-TAKING HINT: Whenever clients seek assistance from healthcare professionals, it is the obligation of the professional to provide the clients with all options of care. In the case of infertility, clients should be advised regarding infertility counseling, testing, and interventions as well as adoption strategies. The couple should determine for themselves which route(s) they wish to pursue.

20. 1. **Endometriosis is characterized by the presence of endometrial tissue outside the uterine cavity. The tissue may be on the tubes, ovaries, bladder, or colon. Adhesions develop from the monthly bleeding at the site of the misplaced endometrial tissue, causing pain and often resulting in infertility if scarring blocks the fallopian tube.**

2. Endometriosis is not characterized by hormonal imbalances. Hormonal imbalances can, however, lead to infertility.

3. A benign tumor of the muscle of the uterus is called a fibroid. It can interfere with pregnancy, but it is not related to endometriosis.

4. Endometriosis is not caused by an infection.

TEST-TAKING HINT: This question is essentially a knowledge-level question. All of the answer options relate to infertility problems, but only one is specifically related to endometriosis. It is important to have an understanding of gynecological issues since many do affect a woman's fertility.

21. 1. Diabetes has been shown to affect a woman's fertility, but infertility has not been shown to increase a woman's risk of developing diabetes.

2. Infertility has not been shown to increase a woman's risk of developing nystagmus, involuntary eye movements.

3. Infertility has not been shown to increase a woman's risk of developing cholecystitis.
4. **Infertility has been shown to increase a woman's risk of developing ovarian cancer.**

TEST-TAKING HINT: For a number of years, an association was noted between the long-term use of clomiphene to treat infertility and the incidence of ovarian cancer. It has also been shown that infertility itself is a contributing factor for ovarian cancer. The reason for the association is not yet known.

22. 1. The luteal phase occurs after ovulation. Menotropin injections are given to induce ovulation.
2. **Menotropin is administered to infertile women to increase follicular growth and maturation of the follicles and to stimulate ovulation.**
3. Menotropin does not suppress menstruation or promote cervical mucus production.
4. Menotropin does not suppress menstruation or promote cervical mucus production.

TEST-TAKING HINT: It is possible that the test taker would not know the action of menotropin. An educated guess can be made that a "tropin" is a substance that stimulates an organ to do something. The only answer that states that an organ is being stimulated is choice 2.

23. 1. On the Web, there are sites that promote the intake of ginseng as a therapy for both male and female infertility, although there is no strong evidence to show that either is true. In addition, there is nothing in the question to suggest that the infertility problem is caused by the poor quality of the man's sperm.
2. There is no evidence that ginseng causes mutations; rather, there is some evidence to show that it is antimutagenic.
3. There is cause for concern for this woman because she is 35 years old and has been unable to get pregnant for more than 6 months.
4. **Because fertility drops as a woman ages, it is advisable to encourage the couple to use conventional therapies in conjunction with the complementary therapy to maximize their potential of becoming pregnant.**

TEST-TAKING HINT: Complementary therapies are becoming more and more popular among clients. Although many have not been shown to have direct effects, it can be counterproductive to discourage clients from using complementary therapies. This may alienate the clients from the healthcare provider. Unless they are known to be dangerous, it is much better to encourage clients to discuss their use with an obstetrical provider and perhaps combine standard and complementary methods.

24. 1. **The client's age. For reproductive purposes, a woman aged 35+ years is considered to be "an older woman." Her fertility is reduced. If she does become pregnant, hers is considered to be a "geriatric pregnancy."**
2. Age 13 at the time of menarche is not a significant factor.
3. Working as a dental hygienist has not been shown to affect fertility.
4. Excessive exercise can interrupt hormonal function, but jogging 2 miles a day is a moderate exercise pattern and is not considered excessive.

TEST-TAKING HINT: The woman was 13 years old at menarche, an age that is well within normal limits. Working as a dental hygienist has not been shown to increase one's chances of developing infertility. An excessive exercise schedule is a problem, but jogging 2 miles a day is well within the definition of moderate exercise. When women are over 35 years of age, however, their fertility often drops.

25. 1. **Spermatogenesis occurs in the testes. High temperatures reduce the development of the sperm. Some experts recommend that the man wear boxers, not briefs, to avoid body heat.**
2. When the vas deferens is ligated, a man has had a vasectomy and is sterile. The sterility is not, however, due to impaired spermatogenesis, but rather to the inability of the sperm to migrate to the woman's reproductive tract.
3. The prostate does not affect spermatogenesis. An enlarged or hypertrophied prostate is usually a problem that affects older men.
4. The flagella are the "tails" of the sperm. They are normally divided into a middle and an end segment.

TEST-TAKING HINT: Knowledge of language will help the test taker to answer this question. The suffix "genesis" means "the beginning of, origin of, or the creation of." Therefore, the question is asking which of the factors listed will affect the creation of sperm.

26. 1. A diagnosis of herpes simplex 2 is not a contraindication for taking sildenafil citrate.
2. It is unsafe to take sildenafil citrate while also taking nitroglycerin for angina.
3. Sildenafil citrate is often prescribed for clients with erectile dysfunction (ED) from diabetes mellitus.
4. Sildenafil citrate is often prescribed for clients with ED from prostate resection.

TEST-TAKING HINT: Sildenafil citrate has been shown to increase the hypotensive effects of nitrate-containing medications because both Sildenafil and nitroglycerin work by relaxing the blood vessels. As such, Sildenafil should not be taken in conjunction with any medication that contains nitrates, including nitroglycerin.

27. 1. This response is not true. Physicians usually want a number of eggs to reach maturation.
2. Preimplantation genetic assessment, when done, is performed on the fertilized ova, not on the sperm or unfertilized ova.
3. Intrauterine insemination (IUI) will not be performed because the client's tubes are blocked. Although her ovaries will be stimulated, IUI will not be performed because the ova will be blocked from the uterus. Insemination will be performed in a petri dish.
4. This response is correct. Since multiple embryos are usually created during the in-vitro process, there are often more embryos created than are implanted. The couple may preserve the embryos.

TEST-TAKING HINT: The preserved embryos may be implanted in the future. For example, if the first transfer fails to result in a pregnancy, the remaining embryos may be transferred within a few months. If a pregnancy and a delivery do result, the couple may choose to implant the remaining embryos in the future when they decide to have another child.

28. **1. This statement is true. Although the gametes are placed in the fallopian tubes artificially, fertilization does occur within the woman's body.**
2. This statement is true of zygote intrafallopian transfer (ZIFT), not of gamete intrafallopian transfer (GIFT).
3. This statement is not true. Although donor eggs and sperm can be used, usually the couple's own gametes are used. When they are harvested, the gametes are placed directly into the fallopian tubes.
4. This statement describes surrogacy. A surrogate is usually impregnated via intrauterine insemination (IUI).

TEST-TAKING HINT: The processes for GIFT (gamete intrafallopian transfer) and ZIFT (zygote intrafallopian transfer) are similar to in vitro fertilization (IVF). GIFT may be considered when a couple has ethical concerns about fertilization occurring outside the body in a petri dish. With GIFT, the egg and sperm are mixed in a catheter, then implanted laparoscopically into the fallopian tube, where fertilization may or may not take place. The process of ZIFT, which is more like IVF, includes fertilizing the egg in a petri dish. However, unlike IVF, in which the fertilized eggs are monitored in the laboratory for 3 to 5 days before implantation, in ZIFT, the fertilized egg (now called a "zygote") is placed in the fallopian tube within 24 hours of fertilization.

The best way for the test taker to remember the various forms of infertility therapy is to remember the definitions of the components. For example, when GIFT is being discussed, the term "gamete" (G) refers to the male or female reproductive cell—that is, the sperm or ovum. When ZIFT is being considered, the term "zygote" (Z) refers to the fertilized ovum. The prefix "intra" means "within" and the term "fallopian" refers to the fallopian tube. When GIFT (or ZIFT) is discussed, the method of transfer into the fallopian tube is via laparoscope.

29. 1. It is unlikely that this woman has a urinary tract infection.
2. It is unlikely that the client is already pregnant.
3. This client should be seen by her infertility doctor.
4. Abdominal bloating is a sign of ovarian hyperstimulation.

TEST-TAKING HINT: This client is exhibiting signs of ovarian hyperstimulation. This is a serious complication. The client is likely third spacing her fluids (the fluids in her body are shifting into her interstitial spaces), resulting in abdominal distention, oliguria, and concentrated urine. The client should be evaluated by her physician.

30. **Answers 2, 3, and 4 are correct.**
1. A 30-day menstrual cycle is well within normal limits.
2. Dyspareunia, or pain during intercourse, may be a symptom of a sexually transmitted infection (STI)

or of endometriosis. Both STIs and endometriosis can adversely affect a woman's fertility.

3. **A woman who has had pelvic inflammatory disease (PID) is much more likely to have blocked fallopian tubes than a woman who has never had PID.**
4. **Women who have facial hair (hirsutism) often have polycystic ovarian syndrome (PCOS). PCOS clients frequently have irregular menses, elevated serum cholesterol, and insulin resistance. Women with PCOS are often infertile.**
5. A 5-day menstrual period is well within normal limits.

TEST-TAKING HINT: Women with PCOS have many symptoms: hirsutism, insulin resistance, high levels of circulating testosterone, and infertility, to name a few. To improve the chances of a woman with PCOS becoming pregnant, she is frequently prescribed clomiphene for the infertility and metformin for the insulin resistance. Sexually transmitted infections and endometriosis may also impair a woman's fertility.

31. 1. **When a woman's cervical mucus is estrogen rich, it is slippery and elastic (thread-like), and when assessed under a microscope, the practitioner will observe "ferning"—that is, an image that looks like a fern. The woman is then in her fertile period. When she is not in her fertile period, the mucus is thick and gluey.**
2. Basal body temperature assessments are performed to determine if and when ovulation occurs.
3. Colposcopy is a procedure performed to examine the cervix closely. It is not performed to evaluate the receptivity of a woman's cervical mucus to sperm.
4. A hysterotomy is a procedure in which an incision is made into the uterus.

TEST-TAKING HINT: When estrogen levels are high, a woman's cervical mucus is most receptive to a man's sperm. At that time, the pH of the vaginal and cervical environments is most conducive to the sperm's successful migration into the uterus and into the fallopian tubes, where it meets and fertilizes the egg.

32. Answers 1, 2, 4, and 5 are correct.
1. **Infertility clients often express anger at others who are able to conceive.**
2. **Infertility clients often express a feeling of personal failure.**
3. Infertility clients often express an aversion to sex because of the many restrictions/schedules/intrusions that are placed on their sexual relationship.
4. **Sadness is another common feeling expressed by infertility clients.**
5. **Guilt is commonly expressed by infertility clients.**

TEST-TAKING HINT: Couples who are experiencing infertility express many emotions. One common thread that connects all of the emotions is grief and loss. Infertile couples grieve their inability to conceive. They experience all of the stages of grief including denial, anger, bargaining, and depression. Acceptance, if it is ever reached, often takes many years.

33. 1. The postcoital test is done 1 or 2 days prior to ovulation.
2. No dye is administered and there are no x-ray pictures taken during a postcoital test.
3. The test is performed a few hours after a couple has intercourse.
4. **The client will undergo a speculum examination when cervical mucus will be harvested.**

TEST-TAKING HINT: The postcoital test is a simple assessment done to see whether the sperm are able to navigate the woman's cervical mucus to ascend into the uterus and fallopian tubes. A few hours postcoitus, in the days immediately prior to ovulation, the practitioner harvests cervical mucus to assess whether the sperm are still motile and to assess the ferning patterns of the mucus.

34. 1. Only the uterus and the fallopian tubes are evaluated during a hysterosalpingogram.
2. Tumors and other gross assessments of the uterus can be made out, but the vascularization of the endometrium is beyond the scope of the test.
3. The competency of the cervix cannot be evaluated during a hysterosalpingogram.
4. **The primary goal of a hysterosalpingogram is to learn whether or not the fallopian tubes are patent.**

TEST-TAKING HINT: During a hysterosalpingogram, a dye is inserted through the vagina into the uterine cavity. The dye, visualized on x-ray, then travels up into the fallopian tubes. If the tubes are blocked owing to scarring or endometriosis, the dye does not ascend.

35. 1. **When no temperature shifts are noted, it is likely that the client has not ovulated.**
2. If the client is not ovulating, she has no fertile period.
3. A 7-day menstrual period is not abnormally long.
4. There is no evidence of a progesterone elevation.

TEST-TAKING HINT: The test taker should be able to make basic interpretations of basal body temperature (BBT) charts. There is usually a slight dip in the temperature at the LH surge with a rise in temperature for the remainder of the cycle because of the inflammatory, thermogenic effect of progesterone. When no temperature changes are seen, it is likely that the client is not experiencing normal hormonal changes and is not ovulating.

36. 1. Unless medically indicated, douching should never be performed. A vinegar solution is especially inappropriate since sperm are unable to survive in an acidic environment.
2. **This action is recommended. Pregnancy is most likely to occur with daily intercourse from 6 days before ovulation up to the day of ovulation.**
3. If a client is experiencing a biphasic cycle, FSH therapy is probably not indicated.
4. The BBT chart does not need to be monitored for 6 more months, although it can be used to help time intercourse.

TEST-TAKING HINT: A biphasic cycle on a BBT chart is evidenced by a relatively stable temperature at the beginning of the cycle, a slight dip in temperature at the time of ovulation, and a sustained rise in temperature—of at least 0.4° F for the remainder of the cycle.

37. 1. The man may have both recessive genes for cystic fibrosis even though he is not ill.
2. This answer is incorrect. Some men with cystic fibrosis, however, have no vas deferens.
3. **This statement is correct. Not all men with cystic fibrosis are sterile, meaning they produce no sperm. Cystic fibrosis experts report that 90% of men with cystic fibrosis produce normal amounts of sperm (Henderson, 2017). Although the sperm may be unable to mix with the semen because of the absence of the vas deferens, fertilization is possible with assistive reproduction technology (ART) such as IVF.**
4. This statement is incorrect. Some men with cystic fibrosis have no vas deferens and, even if the vas is present, if the man is producing large amounts of thick mucus, the vas may become obstructed. Similarly, in women, the fallopian tubes may become obstructed with thick mucus.

TEST-TAKING HINT: Infertility and genetics are often related. A nurse employed in an infertility clinic must be aware of the differences between *infertility* and *sterility*. A client is considered infertile if she has not become pregnant after a year of trying to conceive. This window is shortened to 6 months if the woman is over 35 (ACOG, 2019b). The male factor is the cause of 40–50% of infertility cases (ACOG, 2019b). Sterility is the inability to create offspring. For a woman, this may be a chosen end result after a tubal ligation or hysterectomy. For a man, it may be related to low sperm count or poor motility. A woman who suffers miscarriages is not infertile. However, many miscarriages are caused by inborn genetic defects. In general, clients who are infertile should be referred for genetic counseling as part of the process.

38. **Answers 2, 3, 4, and 5 are correct.**
1. Chorionic villus sampling is done to assess for genetic disease in the fetus.
2. **Endometrial biopsy is performed about 1 week following ovulation to detect the endometrium's response to progesterone.**
3. **Hysterosalpingogram is performed after menstruation to detect whether or not the fallopian tubes are patent.**
4. **Serum progesterone assay is performed about 1 week following ovulation to determine whether or not the woman's corpus luteum produces enough progesterone to sustain a pregnancy.**
5. **Postcoital tests are performed about 1 to 2 days before ovulation to determine whether healthy sperm are able to survive in the cervical mucus.**

TEST-TAKING HINT: There are a number of tests that are performed to assess fertility in couples. It is important to remember that many of the assessments are invasive, painful, and embarrassing and, depending on the results, may label one of the partners as the cause of the infertility. The knowledge of who is responsible for the infertility can be very difficult for some clients to learn.

39. 1. This is an important goal, but it is not the priority nursing goal.
2. This is an important goal, but it is not the priority nursing goal.
3. This is an important goal, but it is not the priority nursing goal.
4. This is the priority nursing goal related to ovarian hyperstimulation syndrome.

TEST-TAKING HINT: A client who is suffering from ovarian hyperstimulation syndrome experiences intravascular hypovolemia and a related extravascular hypervolemia. Although the exact cause of the shift in fluids is unknown, the client may experience very serious complications, including pulmonary edema and ascites. Pulmonary edema can be life-threatening. The client is hospitalized and palliative therapy is provided until the client's fluid and electrolytes stabilize. It is essential throughout the client's acute phase to make sure that her pulmonary function remains intact.

40. 1. Piercing rectal pain has not been cited as a side effect of menotropins.
2. Mood swings and depression are common side effects of the hormonal therapy.
3. Visual disturbances have not been cited as a side effect of menotropins.
4. Jerky tremors have not been cited as a side effect of menotropins.

TEST-TAKING HINT: Not only is infertility itself a psychological stressor but the therapy used to treat it is also a stressor. The client is given daily injections of menotropins (a mixture of FSH and LH) for 10 days to 2 weeks. The impact of the hormonal injections can be very disruptive to the woman's psyche, leading to mood swings and, in some cases, severe depression.

41. 1. No incision is created when clients have hysterosalpingograms.
2. The client will be able to ambulate normally after the procedure.
3. A dye is instilled into the uterine cavity. Some doctors do prescribe oral antibiotics following the procedure to prevent infection.
4. This statement is correct. A number of pictures will be taken throughout the procedure. The client, who will be awake, is asked to move into positions for the x-rays.

TEST-TAKING HINT: A hysterosalpingogram is one of the many tests performed during a standard infertility work-up. The test taker should be familiar with the rationale for each of the tests as well as the procedures themselves and the information that should be conveyed to each client who is to undergo one of the procedures.

42. 1. This response is incorrect. There are a number of ovulation predictor tests that women can use at home to determine when they are ovulating.
2. This statement is correct. One of the at-home ovulation predictor kits requires women to place saliva on a microscopic slide and, after allowing the saliva to dry, to look at the slide under a microscope. If ovulation is occurring, the saliva appears ferned, that is, the image on the slide looks like the leaflets of a fern, indicating the presence of high levels of estrogen in the woman's body.
3. Although the vaginal discharge does change during women's menstrual cycles, there are no ovulation detection tests that require women to test their vaginal discharge.
4. Some of the ovulation detection kits are very expensive, while others require a minimal expense. The women may have to test their saliva and urine repeatedly over the course of many days or months, however, requiring them to purchase multiple test kits.

TEST-TAKING HINT: Women who wish to determine the timing of ovulation in order to maximize their potential of having intercourse at their most fertile period have many options available to them. They can monitor their BBT over a number of months to determine their pattern of ovulation. They can also employ a number of ovulation predictor tests that can be purchased without prescription. Some of the tests require women to test their urine, which will indicate when they are experiencing their LH surge, while others require women to test their saliva for high levels of estrogen.

Genetics

43. **1. The circle is the symbol used to represent the female.**
2. The square is the symbol used to represent the male.
3. The triangle is the symbol used to represent a stillborn.
4. The diamond is the symbol used to represent a child of unknown sex.

TEST-TAKING HINT: When the same symbols are used in all pedigrees, readers are able to analyze the results easily. Symbols that are light colored or completely uncolored depict healthy individuals. Those that are dark colored depict individuals with disease of some kind.

44. 1. The DNA in the client's skin cells did mutate, but the mutation will not affect the client's fertility because the woman's ovaries were not affected.
2. The inherited gene affects a client's risk of contracting colon cancer. It will not affect fertility.
3. A reciprocal translocation can result in infertility.
4. Failure of one arm to develop in utero is related to an environmental insult rather than a genetic insult.

TEST-TAKING HINT: Clients who have reciprocal translocations are usually phenotypically normal. When they produce gametes, however, the eggs (or sperm) have nuclei that are composed of an unbalanced amount of genetic material. Because their offspring are often nonviable, their pregnancies end in miscarriage.

45. 1. CVS is performed well before mothers feel quickening.
2. Tocolytics, such as terbutaline, are not routinely administered following CVS.
3. The mother should notify the doctor if she begins to bleed or contract.
4. It is unnecessary for the mother to stay on complete bedrest following a CVS.

TEST-TAKING HINT: The test taker, if familiar with normal pregnancy changes, can immediately eliminate choice 1 since CVS is performed between 10 and 12 weeks' gestation and quickening rarely occurs before 16 weeks' gestation, even in multiparous pregnancies. Spontaneous abortion is the most common complication of CVS; therefore, the woman should report any bleeding or contractions.

46. 1. The child has a 25% probability of being of normal stature.
2. The child has a 25% probability of being of normal stature.
3. The child has a 25% probability of being of normal stature.
4. The child has a 25% probability of being of normal stature.

After doing a Punnett square, it can be seen that the probability of the child being of normal stature is 1 in 4, or 25%.

	Father: A	a
Mother: A	AA	Aa
a	Aa	aa

TEST-TAKING HINT: Because both parents are heterozygous ("hetero" meaning "different"), they each have one dominant gene or allele (A) and one recessive gene or allele (a). Therefore, the genotype of each parent is Aa. Because achondroplasia is a dominant disease, the recessive allele in this scenario is the normal gene. Only one of the four boxes contains two recessive (normal) genes; therefore, their child has a 1 in 4, or 25%, chance of being of normal stature.

47. 1. If the prospective father possesses the gene, the probability of their children inheriting the gene is 1 in 2, or 50%. As the man has not been tested, it is impossible to determine the probabilities.
2. This statement is completely false.
3. It is improper for the nurse to recommend that the clients not have children. It is the couple's choice whether or not to get pregnant. It is the nurse's responsibility to give information that is as accurate as possible.
4. This statement is correct. No specific information can be given until or unless the potential father decides to be tested.

TEST-TAKING HINT: It is important for the test taker to know the clinical course of Huntington disease (HD), a deteriorating disease of the brain. Affected clients slowly succumb to abnormal movements, behavioral changes, and dementia. There is no cure for this devastating disease. Many clients are reluctant to be tested for the gene since they then end up waiting for the dreaded symptoms to appear. It is not uncommon, therefore, for clients to have no definitive knowledge of their genetic makeup in relation to HD.

48. 1. Symptoms usually appear in affected individuals in their 30s or 40s, but the symptoms can appear as early as childhood.
2. This response is correct. As can be seen by the Punnett square results, the children have a 50/50 chance of developing PKD. Since the capital A connotes the dominant gene, the child needs only one affected gene to exhibit the disease.

	Father: A	a
Mother: a	Aa	aa
a	Aa	aa

3. This statement is untrue. PKD can be a very serious illness. Some clients with the disease will require dialysis and/or kidney transplants.
4. This statement is inappropriate. The husband's genotype is already known.

TEST-TAKING HINT: Remember to clarify which inheritance pattern is being discussed in the stem and ALWAYS complete a Punnett square before answering a question. It is very easy to become confused when being asked about Mendelian inheritance patterns.

49. 1. **The probability of the couple having a daughter with hemophilia A is 0%.**
2. The probability of the couple having a daughter with hemophilia A is 0%.
3. The probability of the couple having a daughter with hemophilia A is 0%.
4. The probability of the couple having a daughter with hemophilia A is 0%.

After doing a Punnett square, it can be seen that the probability of the couple having a daughter with hemophilia A is 0%; in recessive X-linked inheritance, females would have to have two affected "x" genes to exhibit the disease.

	Father: X	Y
Mother: X	XX	XY
"x"	X"x"	"x"Y

(Affected X is depicted as "x")

TEST-TAKING HINT: It is essential when discussing X-linked recessive inheritance that the probability of males and females be assessed separately. Because males carry only one X, they only need one affected "x" to exhibit the X-linked recessive disease. The four offspring depicted in the Punnett square include one unaffected female (XX), one female who carries the gene but does not have the disease since the gene is recessive (X"x"), one healthy male (XY), and one male who has the affected gene and therefore the disease ("x"Y). Females must carry the affected gene on two "x" chromosomes to exhibit the disease. Thus, the probability of a female in the scenario having the disease is 0. It is important to note, however, that the probability of the daughters being carriers is 1 in 2, or 50%.

50. 1. **It is possible that this woman is a carrier for cystic fibrosis (CF). A genetic evaluation can be done to determine that possibility.**
2. The affected gene could have been transmitted both to the woman's mother and to the aunt.
3. Only if both this woman and her partner are carriers is there a possibility of their child having CF. And even if that were the case, the probability of the fetus having the disease would be 1 in 4, or 25%, because CF is an autosomal recessive disease.
4. This response is inappropriate. The mother could be a carrier of the CF gene (carriers are symptom-free) so the client should be tested.

TEST-TAKING HINT: The nurse must remember that just because there is a history of a genetic disease in the family, it does not mean that every member of the family will be affected. It is much less invasive as well as much less expensive to do a test on the client's blood to see whether she is carrying the CF gene than to do an amniocentesis to see whether the baby is affected. If both the father and the mother were found to be carriers, then it would be advisable to offer fetal genetic counseling to the couple.

51. 1. This response is inappropriate. The nuchal fold scan is done either late in the first trimester or with the second trimester quad screen. A fetal genetic evaluation must be done before a definitive diagnosis can be made. A genetic analysis is the only absolute diagnostic tool.
2. Cri du chat syndrome is caused by a deletion on chromosome 5. Among other complications, children with cri du chat suffer from severe intellectual disability.
3. The first trimester assessment screens for Down's syndrome and other trisomy chromosomal syndromes. It does not screen for preterm labor risk.
4. **This statement is true, but the definitive diagnosis can be made only via genetic testing.**

TEST-TAKING HINT: The first trimester screen is performed to assess for Down's syndrome and other trisomy chromosomal syndromes. It is important for the nurse to remember that screening tests are NOT diagnostic. They are relatively inexpensive tests that are performed on the majority of clients to identify those who are likely to exhibit a disease process. If screening test results are positive, more sophisticated diagnostic tests are performed to make definitive diagnoses.

52. 1. **Because Duchenne muscular dystrophy is X-linked, if her sister is a carrier, she too may be a carrier. She should see a genetic counselor.**
2. It is unlikely that Duchenne muscular dystrophy developed as a spontaneous mutation.
3. Duchenne muscular dystrophy is X-linked, so the father's genetics will not affect the outcome.
4. This response is inappropriate. The decision to abort a child with a disease is up to the parents. Each set of parents must be allowed to make the decision for themselves. Their decision is likely to be based on many things, including their ability to care for a child with a developmental disability and the knowledge that their child is affected by a genetic disease. The nurse cannot make the assumption that the parents will decide to abort, or deliver, an affected child.

TEST-TAKING HINT: It is important for the nurse to remember that clients who find out that their child has a genetic disease through amniocentesis do not learn of the results until well into the second trimester. These clients, therefore, may need to decide whether or not to abort the pregnancy once they have felt fetal movement. Even for clients who are pro-choice, the decision to have an abortion so late in the pregnancy can be a very difficult one.

53. 1. Each pregnancy has its own probability so it is impossible to predict which, if any, child will or will not have the disease.
2. Each pregnancy has its own probability so it is possible for all or none of the children to have the disease.
3. Each pregnancy has its own probability so it is impossible to predict which, if any, child will or will not have the disease.
4. **This is true. Every time the woman gets pregnant, there is a possibility (25% chance) that she is carrying a child with the disease.**

TEST-TAKING HINT: The term "probability" refers to the likelihood of something occurring rather than to whether something definitely will occur. This concept is often misunderstood by a layperson. It is very important that nurses communicate to parents who carry gene mutations that every time the woman is pregnant, she has the possibility, or risk, of carrying a baby with the defect.

54. 1. **Assessing the fetal heart rate is the highest priority since, although rare, the fetus may have been injured during the procedure.**
2. Taking the client's temperature is not the most important action to take at this time.
3. Psychosocial issues are always significant, but they must take a backseat to physiological assessments.
4. It is important to answer all questions posed by clients but, again, these should be answered only after physiological interventions are completed.

TEST-TAKING HINT: This is a prioritizing question. All answers, therefore, are correct. It is the test taker's responsibility to determine which response is of highest priority. When answering prioritizing questions, the test taker should remember the importance of Maslow's hierarchy of needs and established procedures for providing first aid and CPR. The answer that relates to one or both of these priorities—that is, survival (Maslow's first step on the hierarchy), circulation, airway, or breathing—is generally the correct answer.

55. 1. **The haploid number of chromosomes—a complete string of unpaired chromosomes—is 23, the normal number of chromosomes in the gamete—in this case, in the ovum.**
2. The diploid number of chromosomes is 46, the normal number of chromosomes in the somatic cells of human beings. The ovum and sperm each contribute 23 chromosomes that pair up.
3. Aneuploidy is characterized by a chromosomal number that is not equal to a multiple of the haploid number—that is, the number of chromosomes in the cell is NOT equal to 23, 46, 69, 92, and so on. Trisomy 21 (47 chromosomes) is an example of an aneuploid number, as is a chromosome number of 48 or 49.
4. Polyploidy is characterized by a chromosomal number that is equal to twice, three times, four times, and so on, of the diploid number—that is, the number of chromosomes in the cell is equal to 92 (2×46), 138 (3×46), and so on.

TEST-TAKING HINT: The test taker should use their understanding of language to answer the question. Oogenesis is the development of the female egg, or ovum. (Spermatogenesis is

the development of the male sperm.) In order for the fertilized egg (which is created once the ovum and sperm combine) to have the diploid or normal number of chromosomes, the ovum and sperm must each have the haploid number of chromosomes, or 23 in each.

56. 1. This response is incorrect. The baby has Down's syndrome.
2. This response is correct. The baby has three number 21 chromosomes.
3. This response is incorrect. The fetus has an aneuploid number of chromosomes. There is no evidence of a fragile segment on the long arm of the X chromosome.
4. This response is incorrect. All of the autosomes are paired.

TEST-TAKING HINT: Karyotypes that show translocations, deletions, and other abnormalities can be very difficult to interpret, but it is relatively easy to discern monosomy and trisomy defects. The test taker must simply count the number of chromosomal pairs. If any chromosome is missing its mate or if there are three of any of the chromosomes, the fetus will usually exhibit a distinct syndrome. One exception to the rule is the fetus that carries multiple Y chromosomes with 1 X—for example, XYY or XYYY. In that situation, the baby will appear healthy and, in the vast majority of cases, act normally.

57. 1. This response is correct. The normal number of chromosomes is present—46—and the child is a female—XX.
2. This response is incorrect. Intersex individuals exhibit both male and female organs and characteristics. Intersexuality may be caused by a number of things, including an environmental insult or a genetic mutation.
3. This response is incorrect. An example of a male with a genetic defect is 46, XY, 16p13.3. The child is a male—XY—and the defect, as indicated in the nomenclature, is on the p arm of the 16th chromosome at location 13.3.
4. There is sufficient information to answer this question.

TEST-TAKING HINT: When reading genetic nomenclature, the test taker should first look for the number of chromosomes in the cells and then the sex makeup of the cells. If there is a mosaic genotype, the information will be separated by a slash mark. If there is a genetic defect, the information will follow the baseline data.

58. 1. The proband is not in generation I.
2. The proband is in generation II. The proband, or first member of a family to be diagnosed with a specific medical/genetic problem, is identified in a pedigree by an arrow.
3. The proband is not in generation III.
4. There is sufficient information to answer the question. The proband is the member of the family who is identified by an arrow.

TEST-TAKING HINT: There are symbols that have been accepted in the scientific community for labeling pedigrees. The arrow pointing to one member in a pedigree labels the proband, or the first member of the family to be diagnosed with the specific medical/genetic problem.

59. 1. Although this response is accurate, it is an inappropriate response for the nurse to make.
2. Although this response is accurate, it is an inappropriate response for the nurse to make.
3. This response is accurate. Diabetes is one of the many diseases that has both a genetic and an environmental component.
4. Although this response is accurate, it is an inappropriate response for the nurse to make.

TEST-TAKING HINT: Although virtually 100% of some diseases are genetically determined, most diseases have both genetic and environmental components. In other words, they have multifactorial etiologies. Diseases such as diabetes mellitus, cancer, and asthma are examples of diseases with multifactorial etiologies.

60. 1. This statement is true. Female clients who are *BRCA1* or *BRCA2* positive have similar fertility rates to those who are *BRCA1* or *BRCA2* negative.
2. This statement is incorrect. Nurses provide information and the client decides whether or not to have children. It is inappropriate for nurses to counsel clients whether or not to have children based on the client's genotype.
3. The decision to have an oophorectomy is the client's. The nurse's role is to provide the client with information regarding the genetic profile.
4. Lactation is not contraindicated for these women.

TEST-TAKING HINT: Many women who have been found to carry a *BRCA* gene decide to have mastectomies and/or oophorectomies. Other women choose to have children and then have the procedures and still others choose to have frequent diagnostic tests to monitor for the development of cancer. The client must make her decision based on accurate information provided by healthcare professionals.

61. 1. There is a genetic marker for Huntington's disease.
2. In the case of Huntington's disease, if a person has the gene and lives long enough, there is virtually a 100% probability he or she will develop the disease. The gene has a high degree of expressivity or, in other words, people who carry the gene will develop the disease.
3. This answer is correct, if a person has the gene and lives long enough, virtually 100% of the time the disease will develop and progress.
4. There is no carrier state when a disease is transmitted via a dominant inheritance pattern as Huntington's disease is.

TEST-TAKING HINT: The test taker must understand the difference between recessive and dominant illnesses. There is a carrier state in recessive illnesses because two affected genes must be present in the genome for the disease to be expressed. Only one affected gene must be present for a dominant disease to be expressed.

62. 1. This response is incorrect. The child will likely be a normal-appearing female.
2. Because there is a translocation in the child's chromosomal pattern, the child's gametes will likely contain an abnormal amount of genetic material and the child will likely be infertile.
3. Translocations are usually not problematic for the first generation, but they can lead to significant defects and/or infertility in the next generation.
4. The client must decide for herself whether or not to abort the fetus.

TEST-TAKING HINT: When a reciprocal translocation has occurred, part of the chromosomal material from one chromosome improperly attaches to another chromosome and vice versa. In the case of a Robertsonian translocation, the affected individual is aneuploid, with an abnormal number of chromosomes in the sperm or ovum, since the centromeres of two chromosomes fuse while the genetic material from the short arms of the chromosomes is lost. Affected individuals usually appear normal and will develop normally even, as in the case of the Robertsonian translocation, some genetic material is lost. When the child's gametes develop via meiosis, however, each of the eggs will contain an abnormal quantity of genetic material.

63. 1. The pedigree should be analyzed for any and all abnormal inheritance patterns.
2. This is true. The incidence of miscarriage is very high—about one out of every five pregnancies—and the majority of miscarriages are related to a genetic defect.
3. A woman's fertility is determined by many factors.
4. This statement is not true. There is no genetic marker for incompetent cervix.

TEST-TAKING HINT: If a client has had more than two miscarriages, she and her partner should be referred to a genetic counselor. Either one of them may have a genetic anomaly that is affecting the viability of the fetus. In addition, a DNA sample of the products of each miscarriage should be sent for genetic analysis. Frequently a diagnosis can be made from the analyses.

64. 1. It is too soon to advise a client to have an amniocentesis. Although the pedigree shows an autosomal dominant inheritance pattern, a genetic counselor should analyze the pedigree.
2. This is appropriate. Although nurses and primary care providers should have a basic understanding of genetic information, genetic counselors are the experts in this area.
3. This information may be relevant but should be asked carefully within a counseling session. It is best for a genetic counselor to ask the questions.
4. This response is inappropriate. The pedigree shows an autosomal dominant inheritance pattern.

TEST-TAKING HINT: The nurse should anticipate that clients' primary healthcare providers will refer clients to specialists when indicated. The area of genetics is one that is highly specialized and new information is being developed each day. A genetic counselor possesses the specialized knowledge.

65. 1. This is the woman's genotype. It is not the woman's phenotype.
2. This is the genotype of a person with Tay-Sachs disease.

3. This is the phenotype of a person with Tay-Sachs disease.
4. **This is the woman's phenotype.**

TEST-TAKING HINT: A person's genotype refers to a person's genetic code. A person who is a carrier for an autosomal recessive disease will have a heterozygous genotype—Aa. A person's phenotype refers to the person's observable characteristics. A person who is a *carrier* for an autosomal recessive disease will have a normal phenotype, with no observable symptoms of the disease. Only persons who have a genotype of aa would express the disease.

66. Answers 1, 2, 3, and 4 are correct.
1. **The woman's fetus has a 1 in 2, or 50%, probability of having the gene.**
2. **The woman's sisters have a 1 in 2, or 50%, probability of having the gene.**
3. **The woman's brothers have a 1 in 2, or 50%, probability of having the gene.**
4. **One of the woman's parents definitely has the gene. Since the age of onset can be as late as age 50, the parents' symptoms may not yet have appeared.**
5. It is unlikely that the woman's partner has the gene.

TEST-TAKING HINT: This question requires the test taker to do a reverse genetic analysis. If a woman is carrying one autosomal dominant gene, then her genotype is Aa. She received the affected gene from one of her parents and a normal gene from her other parent. One of her parents, therefore, definitely carries the gene. Because one of her parents carries the gene, each of her siblings has a 50/50 probability of carrying the gene. Because she carries the gene, her fetus has a 50/50 probability of carrying the gene. Since the woman's partner's history is unremarkable, it is unlikely that he carries the gene.

67. 1. Amniocentesis is performed in the second trimester to provide the couple with information regarding the genetics of a fetus in utero.
2. CVS is performed in the first trimester to provide the couple with information regarding the genetics of a fetus in utero.
3. **Preimplantation genetic diagnosis will provide the couple with the highest probability of conceiving a healthy child.**
4. GIFT is a type of infertility procedure, not a genetic test.

TEST-TAKING HINT: Preimplantation genetic diagnosis (PGD) is a form of genetic assessment that is done with in-vitro fertilization (IVF). The assessment is performed prior to the transfer of the embryo into the woman's fallopian tubes. Since only healthy embryos are implanted, a couple will not have to decide whether or not to terminate affected pregnancies.

68. 1. This response is inappropriate. The client has asked the nurse for information regarding cord blood banking.
2. **This statement is correct. The baby's umbilical cord blood is kept by a cord blood bank to be used if and when the baby should develop a serious illness such as leukemia.**
3. The blood is not used in the same way that general blood donations are used. It is used to treat catastrophic illnesses.
4. This response is true, but it does not provide the client with the information she needs to make an informed decision.

TEST-TAKING HINT: Umbilical cord blood contains stem cells that are used to treat cancers and other catastrophic illnesses such as sickle cell anemia. It is administered in the same way that a bone marrow transplant is administered.

69. 1. This statement is not accurate. Cystic fibrosis can be detected via amniocentesis.
2. **This response is likely. The genetic tests that are performed check only for the most common genetic variants of many diseases, including CF. If the baby were positive for an uncommon variant, it would be missed.**
3. It is unlikely that the laboratory technician made a mistake.
4. Although it is possible, it is unlikely that maternal cells were harvested rather than fetal cells.

TEST-TAKING HINT: There are more than 1,000 genetic variants of CF, so it is impossible to test for all the variants. Unfortunately, clients do not realize that amniocentesis is not 100% reliable in identifying genetic problems. In addition, not all variants are tested on the newborn screen.

70. 1. Until the pedigree is fully analyzed, the need for a complete genetic analysis is uncertain.
2. **This statement is true. The proband is the first individual in any family to be identified with a disorder.**
3. This is not correct. Genetic information is confidential. Only if the proband agrees can others be included in the discussion. Plus, the proband's relatives may or may not be interested in discussing their potential of acquiring a genetic disease.

4. It is virtually impossible to determine if and when someone will develop breast cancer, even if a genetic screen has been performed.

TEST-TAKING HINT: Per HIPAA (Health Insurance and Portability Accountability Act of 1996), a nurse who works for a healthcare organization must not discuss any information about a client's health information unless given express permission to do so by the client. A client's right to privacy includes the right to keep information confidential from relatives as well as strangers. In addition, anyone who has a genetic disease is further covered by GINA (Genetic Information Nondiscrimination Act of 2008), which requires that insurance companies and employers not discriminate against those with genetic illnesses (U.S. Department of Health and Human Services, n.d.). It is important to remember that the genetic information of one family member may affect others in the family since they, too, may carry defective genes. This knowledge can be very difficult for some family members as well as for the proband. In essence, the nurse must remember that client information must be kept confidential.

71. 1. An affected male would be depicted as a darkened square without a slash mark.
2. An unaffected female would be depicted as a light-colored or uncolored circle without a slash mark.
3. A stillborn child is depicted as a triangle. If the child is known to have had the defect, the triangle would be a darkened triangle.
4. A child of unknown sex is depicted as a diamond. If the child is known to have had the defect, the symbol would be a darkened diamond.

TEST-TAKING HINT: For nurses to interpret pedigrees, they must be familiar with the symbols and terminology used. The Roman numerals at the left of pedigrees depict the generations pictured. Each individual in each generation is then numbered from left to right. The fourth individual from the left in the second generation, therefore, is at location II-4. A slash mark (/) through a symbol indicates that the individual is deceased.

72. 1. The individuals are fraternal twins.
2. An unaffected couple would be depicted as a square and circle connected by a single line. The square and circle would both be light colored or uncolored.
3. The proband is always identified by an arrow.
4. Known heterozygotes are half dark colored and half light colored. For example, a male who is a known heterozygote would be depicted as a square, half of which is dark colored and half of which is light colored.

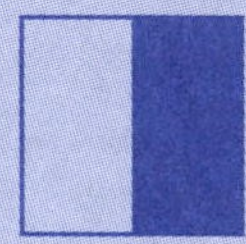

TEST-TAKING HINT: As seen in the pedigree, a y-connector is used to attach the twins to their parents' offspring line. If the twins were monozygotic, they would be of the same sex and there would be an additional line between the legs of the "y," as seen in the individuals in locations III-5 and III-6.

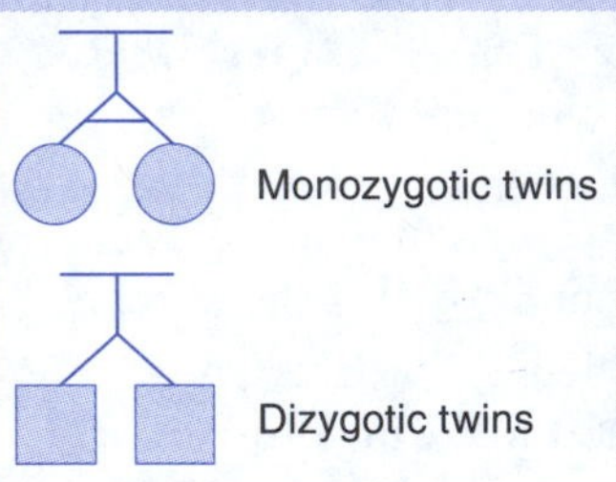

73. 1. This response is incorrect. No one can make such a prediction.
2. Neonates virtually never exhibit signs of sickle cell because fetal hemoglobin does not sickle.
3. This response is correct. Babies with two recessive sickle cell genes will show some symptoms of the disease but the severity of the symptoms will be individual.
4. This response is incorrect. Virtually all children with sickle cell anemia will exhibit some symptoms during their lives.

TEST-TAKING HINT: The test taker must be familiar with common terms used to describe genetic diseases, such as "penetrance" and "expressivity." ***Penetrance:*** **When a disease is 100% penetrant, 100% of the individuals who have the gene(s) for the disease will exhibit the disease. Similarly, if a disease is 80% penetrant, only 80% of the individuals who have the gene(s) for the disease will exhibit the disease.** ***Expressivity:*** **This term refers to the range of severity—or phenotypes—of a particular genetic disease.**

74. 1. **The pedigree is an example of autosomal recessive inheritance.**
2. The pedigree is not an example of mitochondrial inheritance.
3. The pedigree is not an example of X-linked recessive inheritance.
4. The pedigree is not an example of Y-linked trait inheritance.

TEST-TAKING HINT: An autosomal recessive inheritance pattern is characterized by four things: (1) parents of affected children are usually disease-free; (2) about one out of every four children in large families exhibits the disease; (3) boys and girls are affected equally; and (4) all the children are affected when both parents have the disease.

75. 1. The pedigree is not an example of autosomal dominant inheritance.
2. **The pedigree is an example of mitochondrial inheritance.**
3. The pedigree is not an example of X-linked recessive.
4. The pedigree is not an example of Y-linked trait.

TEST-TAKING HINT: Mitochondrial DNA is transmitted only from mothers. None of an affected man's children are ever affected. A mitochondrial inheritance pattern is characterized by the fact that all of an affected woman's children, whether male or female, exhibit the disease.

76. 1. This response is inappropriate. Each pregnancy carries the same probability of being affected.
2. This response is inappropriate. It is impossible for a nurse to know how a couple will respond to the probability that their fetus will be affected.
3. **This response is accurate.**
4. This response is inaccurate. There is a 1 out of 4 chance that the baby will inherit both recessive genes and have the disease.

	Father: A	a
Mother: A	AA	Aa
a	Aa	aa

TEST-TAKING HINT: As can be seen by the Punnett square, there is a 3 out of 4 probability that their child will be healthy (AA and Aa)—a 1 out of 4 probability that their child will carry no abnormal genes for PKU (AA)—a 2 out of 4 probability that their child will be a carrier (Aa)—and a 1 out of 4 probability that their child will have the disease (aa).

77. 1. This response is incorrect. None of their male children will be green color blind.
2. This response is incorrect. None of their female children will be green color blind.
3. This response is incorrect. Males do not carry X-linked recessive traits.
4. **This response is correct. All of the females will be carriers.**

TEST-TAKING HINT: The male client has a genotype of "x"Y, the "x" being the recessive gene responsible for green color blindness. The female has a genotype of XX; both of her genes are normal.

As can be seen by the Punnett square, all of the daughters will carry one affected "x" gene from their father, but none of the sons will carry an affected "x" gene.

	Father: "x"	Y
Mother: X	X"x"	XY
X	X"x"	XY

(Affected X is depicted as "x")

78. **Answers 4 and 5 are correct.**
1. This response is incorrect. The baby will be either type A or type B. Type O is the recessive.
2. This response is incorrect. The baby will be either type A or type B. Type O is the recessive.
3. This response is incorrect. The offspring cannot be type AB since the mother is type O.
4. **The baby could be blood type AO (type A) and, if the father is heterozygous for the Rh factor, the baby could be either Rh+ (positive) or Rh− (negative).**
5. **The baby could be type BO (type B) and, if the father is heterozygous for the Rh factor, the baby could be either Rh+ (positive) or Rh− (negative).**

TEST-TAKING HINT: Each biological parent contributes to the baby's blood type. Blood types A and B are dominant and type O is recessive. To answer this question, the test taker must be familiar with the concept of codominance. In addition, the test taker must create separate Punnett squares. Codominance refers to the fact that both blood type A and type B dominate. If a person possesses the gene for both types, he or

she will, therefore, be type AB. In this question, because the mother is type O, the baby will receive either type A or B from the father. As such, the baby cannot be type AB. Three Punnett squares are needed to determine the answer to this question because the father's Rh genotype could be either homozygous or heterozygous and because a person's blood type is independent of a person's Rh factor. Punnett square to determine blood type:

	Father: A	B
Mother: O	AO (type A)	BO (type B)
O	AO (type A)	BO (type B)

If father is homozygous for Rh+ (positive):

	Father: +	+
Mother: −	+ −(Rh+)	+ −(Rh+)
−	+ −(Rh+)	+ −(Rh+)

If father is heterozygous for Rh:

	Father: +	−
Mother: −	+ −(Rh+)	− −(Rh−)
−	+ −(Rh+)	− −(Rh−)

79. 1. This information is unsupported by the scenario. Cerebral palsy is not a genetic defect and is not detected through amniocentesis.
2. Cerebral palsy is not a genetic disease. It is caused by a hypoxic injury that can occur at any time during pregnancy, labor and delivery, or the postdelivery period.
3. Cerebral palsy is not a genetic disease. It is caused by a hypoxic injury that can occur at any time during pregnancy, labor and delivery, or the postdelivery period.
4. Cerebral palsy is not a genetic disease. It is caused by a hypoxic injury that can occur at any time during pregnancy, labor and delivery, or the postdelivery period.

TEST-TAKING HINT: Some couples believe that if an amniocentesis result shows that the chromosomes and genes are normal, then the baby will be normal. This is not true. Some problems are caused by teratogens, some are caused by birth injuries, and some genetic diseases are not tested for. Although whole genome analysis may be performed in the future, at this time only a discreet number of defects are assessed during amniocentesis.

80. 1. The centromere is the site where sister chromatids attach during cell division.
2. A chiasma is the site where crossing over between non-sister chromatids takes place. At this site, genetic material is swapped between the chromatids.
3. A chromatid is one strand of a duplicated chromosome. Sister chromatids are attached at the chromosome's centromere.
4. A codon is a triad of messenger RNA that encodes for a specific amino acid in a protein.

TEST-TAKING HINT: Crossing over at the chiasmata is an essential process during meiosis. DNA is exchanged between non-sister chromatids—one from the mother and one from the father. This results in the genetic variance of the species.

81. **1. This statement is accurate. All of the woman's children will be affected.**
2. This statement is incorrect. All of the woman's children will be affected.
3. This statement is incorrect. All of the woman's children will be affected.
4. This statement is incorrect. All of the woman's children will be affected.

TEST-TAKING HINT: Mitochondrial DNA is inherited through the mother only. Since all of the woman's gametes contain her mitochondrial DNA, all of her offspring will be affected.

82. 1. The breast cancer genes are highly penetrant, but this is not the most important information.
2. The breast cancer genes are moderately expressive, but this is not the most important information.
3. Amniocentesis does, although rarely, end in miscarriage, but this is not the most important information.
4. The most important information for the nurse to provide the client is that the vast majority of cases of breast cancer are not inherited.

TEST-TAKING HINT: Every year, about 200,000 cases of breast cancer are diagnosed, but only 5% to 10% of the cases are inherited. It would be inappropriate to perform an amniocentesis for breast cancer unless the mother has been found to carry one of the genes. In addition, it must be remembered that even inherited breast cancer has a strong environmental component.

83. 1. This is the definition of Down's syndrome but not of Down's syndrome with mosaic chromosomal configuration.
2. All chromosomes are banded.
3. The number 21 chromosomes are of normal length in Down's syndrome.
4. Mosaicism is characterized by the fact that some of the cells of the body have the abnormal number of chromosomes but some of the cells have the normal number. This may happen with rapid disjunction. In Down's syndrome, it means that some of the cells have three number 21 chromosomes and some have the normal number of two number 21 chromosomes. Mosaicism is not specific to Down's syndrome but can occur with other chromosomal abnormalities.

TEST-TAKING HINT: The concept of mosaicism can be remembered by thinking about a mosaic piece of art. Mosaic tiles are bits of glass or ceramic that are different colors and shapes but, when put into a design, create a piece of art. In genetics, mosaicism refers to the fact that various cells of the body have different numbers of chromosomes.

84. 1. This goal is inappropriate. The client has a family history of cystic fibrosis. She does not have the disease.
2. This goal is appropriate. Since the client has a family history of the disease, she should seek genetic counseling.
3. This goal is inappropriate. It is unnecessary to have CVS unless both the mother and the father are found to be carriers of cystic fibrosis.
4. This goal is inappropriate. The client has a family history of cystic fibrosis. She does not have the disease.

TEST-TAKING HINT: Cystic fibrosis is an autosomal recessive disease. If the woman has a family history of CF, she may be a carrier for the disease. If her partner also is a carrier, there would be a 1 in 4, or 25%, probability of the fetus having the disease and a 1 in 2, or 50%, chance of the child being a carrier. It is important for the woman to seek genetic counseling.

85. 1. Although the parents should seek genetic counseling before getting pregnant in the future, this is not the rationale for newborn testing.
2. This is the rationale for newborn testing for maple syrup urine disease. It is done to prevent neurological disease in affected children.
3. This is a benefit of many of the newborn tests, but it is not the primary rationale. The cost-benefit ratio (in terms of money) does not always support newborn testing. In very rare diseases like MSUD, the cost of testing is often higher than the cost of care for any affected children.
4. This is not a rationale for newborn testing.

TEST-TAKING HINT: When children with inborn metabolic diseases follow strict diets, they have the potential to grow into normal adulthood. It is essential that the tests be performed during the neonatal period because the children's diets must be altered as quickly as possible to prevent the adverse effects. When children with MSUD eat restricted foods, their brains are severely affected, leading to mental retardation, coma, and death.

86. Answers 3 and 4 are correct.
1. This response is inappropriate. The woman's baby may not "be fine."
2. Even though performing a genetic analysis on the woman's brother's tissue is the only accurate way to determine exactly what genetic disease the baby had, it is inappropriate for the nurse to suggest disinterring the woman's brother's body.
3. There are a number of tests that can be performed during a pregnancy to screen the baby for genetic diseases: cell-free DNA analysis, first trimester screen, second trimester quad screens, CVS, and amniocentesis.
4. This is an appropriate response. This client should be referred for genetic counseling.
5. Although the woman may suggest having her mother meet with the obstetrician or the genetic counselor, it is inappropriate for the nurse to suggest that the mother meet with the obstetrician.

TEST-TAKING HINT: Cell-free DNA analysis, which tests fetal DNA, is a test performed on the mother's blood during gestation week 10 or later. The first-trimester screen, performed between weeks 11 and 14, is a two-step assessment. The mother's blood is tested for the presence of two proteins—human chorionic gonadotropin (hCG) and pregnancy-associated plasma protein-A (PAPP-A), both of which are produced by the products of conception—and an ultrasound is performed to analyze the clarity of the space at the back of the baby's neck, called the nuchal translucency. The mother's blood is tested for the second-trimester quad

screen, performed between 15 and 20 weeks' gestation. Four substances are evaluated: alpha-fetoprotein (AFP), a protein made by the developing baby; human chorionic gonadotropin (hCG), a hormone made by the placenta; estriol, a hormone made by the placenta and the baby's liver; and inhibin A, another hormone made by the placenta. Depending on the results of any of the three assessments, a prediction is made regarding the probability of presence of a fetal chromosomal defect, specifically trisomy 13, 18, or 21. If a positive result is obtained, chorionic villus sampling, a first-trimester genetic assessment, or amniocentesis, performed during the second trimester, can be performed to make a diagnosis. The diagnostic tests can also be performed to determine whether a specific hereditary defect is present in the fetus but, at the present time, only a small number of those diseases are assessed via CVS or amniocentesis.

87. 1. **This statement is correct. It is unlikely that the baby will be injured because, before inserting the needle, the doctor will locate the products of conception using ultrasound.**
2. Not only is it inappropriate for the nurse to acknowledge that he or she has fears regarding the procedure, it is inappropriate for the nurse to refer to a religious action as the client may have religious beliefs that differ from those of the nurse.
3. This statement does nothing to help to dispel the fears of the client.
4. This statement is not appropriate. The nurse's assumptions regarding the client's motivation for having a CVS may be completely incorrect.

TEST-TAKING HINT: CVS is performed in the first trimester, earlier than amniocentesis. The results are, therefore, obtained earlier in the pregnancy. Placental tissue is extracted using a needle inserted through the abdomen or transvaginally. Ultrasound is used to locate the position of the fetus and the placenta. Chromosomal, as well as inheritable genetic diseases, can be diagnosed with CVS.

3 Women's Health Issues

Women who present for pregnancy care are often affected by other issues at the same time. These issues may include domestic violence, eating disorders, and sexually transmitted infections. After the birth, questions about contraception and breastfeeding are of importance and the nurse will want to be familiar with the most up-to-date information to share with these clients. This chapter focuses on some of the more common non-pregnancy-related issues requiring clinical judgment by nurses caring for women across the lifespan. It also includes a review of statistics in interpreting public health studies in the literature.

KEYWORDS

The following words include English vocabulary, nursing/medical terminology, concepts, principles, or information relevant to content specifically addressed in the chapter or associated with these topics. For enhanced understanding, you might enjoy comparing definitions and the histories of some of these terms, principles, and concepts in English dictionaries, your nursing textbooks, and medical dictionaries such as *Taber's Cyclopedic Medical Dictionary.*

Anorexia nervosa
Bacterial vaginosis
Bilateral tubal ligation
Birth control pills
Bone density
Breast cancer
Breast self-examination
Bulimia
Calendar method
Cervical cancer
Cervical cap
Child abuse
Chlamydia
Confidence interval
Contraceptive patch
Contraceptive sponge
Dental dam
Domestic violence
Endometriosis
Endometritis
Ethinyl estradiol and levonorgestrel
Etonogestrel/ethinyl estradiol vaginal ring
Female condom
Fibrocystic breasts
Flunitrazepam
GHB (*gamma*-hydroxybutyric acid)
Gonorrhea
Hepatitis B
Herpes simplex 2
Hormone replacement therapy
Human immunodeficiency virus (HIV)
Human papillomavirus (HPV)
Intrauterine device (IUD)
Lactation amenorrhea method (LAM)
Lesbian
Levonorgestrel
Male condom
Mammogram
Maternal mortality rate
Medroxyprogesterone acetate
Mifepristone/misoprostol (formerly RU-486)
Osteoporosis
Ovarian cancer
Pelvic inflammatory disease (PID)
Perimenopause
Pubic lice
Rape (including date rape)
Risk ratio
Sexual assault
Sexually transmitted infections
Significant difference
Syphilis
Toxic shock syndrome
Trichomoniasis
Vasectomy
Withdrawal (coitus interruptus)

QUESTIONS

1. A 19-year-old client with multiple sex partners is being counseled about the hepatitis B vaccination. During the counseling sessions, which of the following should the nurse advise the client to receive?
   1. Hepatitis B immune globulin before receiving the vaccine.
   2. Vaccine booster every 10 years.
   3. Complete series of three intramuscular injections.
   4. Vaccine as soon as she becomes 21.

2. A postpartum client has decided to use medroxyprogesterone acetate as her contraceptive method. What should the nurse advise the client regarding this medication?
   1. Take the pill at the same time each day.
   2. Refrain from breastfeeding while using the method.
   3. Expect to have no periods as long as she takes the medicine.
   4. Consider switching to another birth control method in a year or so.

3. The nurse is administering medroxyprogesterone acetate to a postpartum client. Which of the following data must the nurse consider before administering the medication?
   1. The patch must be replaced at the same time each week.
   2. The client must be taught to use sunscreen whenever in the sunlight.
   3. The medicine is contraindicated if the woman has lung or esophageal cancer.
   4. The client must use an alternate form of birth control for the first two months.

4. Which statement by the client indicates that she understands the teaching provided about the intrauterine device (IUD)?
   1. "The IUD can remain in place for a year or more."
   2. "I will not menstruate while the IUD is in."
   3. "Pain during intercourse is a common side effect."
   4. "The device will reduce my chances of getting infected."

5. A client has been diagnosed with pubic lice. Which of the following signs/symptoms would the nurse expect to see?
   1. Macular rash on the labia.
   2. Pruritus.
   3. Hyperthermia.
   4. Foul-smelling discharge.

6. The nurse is teaching a client regarding the treatment for pubic lice. Which of the following should be included in the teaching session?
   1. The antibiotics should be taken for a full 10 days.
   2. All clothing should be pretreated with bleach before wearing.
   3. Shampoo should be applied for at least 2 hours before rinsing.
   4. The pubic hair should be combed after shampoo is removed.

7. The parent of a newborn angrily asks the nurse, "Why would the doctor want to give my baby the vaccination for hepatitis B? It's a sexually transmitted disease, you know!" Which of the following is the best response by the nurse?
   1. "The hepatitis B vaccine is given to all babies. It is given because many babies get infected from their mothers during pregnancy."
   2. "It is important for your baby to get the vaccine in the hospital because the shot may not be available when your child gets older."
   3. "Hepatitis B can be a life-threatening liver infection that is contracted not only by sexual contact but also by contact with contaminated blood. An infected family member or caregiver can unknowingly pass the virus to your baby."
   4. "Most parents want to protect their children from as many serious diseases as possible. Hepatitis B is one of those diseases."

8. A nurse is reading the research article "Efficacy of Informational Letters on Hepatitis B Immunization Rates in University Students" (Marron et al., 1998). In the article, the researchers analyzed the means by which the students learned about the hepatitis B vaccine and compared that information with whether or not the students actually received the vaccine. Table 3-1 describes the data. Which of the following interpretations of the data from Table 3-1 is correct?
   1. When one considers those who "read/heard" about the vaccine, there is no significant difference between the percentage of students who received the immunization and those who did not receive the immunization.
   2. The likelihood of students who received the vaccine when they learned about it from the "health history form" was about 1.6 times that of the "health history form" students who did not receive the vaccine.
   3. Of those who were not vaccinated, 44.4% received their information from "Letters."
   4. The largest percentage of students who received the vaccine learned about it from the "University Health Service (UHS) providers."

Table 3-1. Comparison of Self-Reported Sources of Hepatitis B Virus Information by Group

Source	Group Intervention—% Who Received the Vaccine (n = 137)	Control—% Who Did Not Receive the Vaccine (n = 126)	Risk Ratio	95% Confidence Interval (CI)	*p*-value
Read/Heard	87.7	70.2	1.25	1.12–1.40	Less than 0.001
School paper	11.7	11.9	0.98	0.51–1.90	0.95
Mass media	24.8	36.5	0.68	0.47–0.99	0.4
Bulletin board	38.7	42.9	0.90	0.67–1.21	0.49
Fliers	50.4	44.4	1.13	0.88–1.46	0.34
Letters	48.9	11.1	4.40	2.61–7.42	Less than 0.001
Parents	33.6	21.4	1.57	1.04–2.36	0.03
University Health	2.2	5.6	0.39	0.10–1.49	0.15 Service Providers
Family doctor	25.5	29.4	0.87	0.59–1.29	0.49
Friends	20.4	34.1	0.60	0.40–0.90	0.01
Health History Form	38.7	23.8	1.62	1.11–2.37	0.01

From: Marron, R. L., Lanphear, B. P., Kouides, R., Dudman, L., Manchester, R. A., & Christy, C. (1998). Efficacy of informational letters on hepatitis B immunizations rates in university students. *Journal of American College Health, 47*(3), 123–127. https://doi.org/10.1080/07448489809595632

9. A nurse is reading a research article on the incidence of sexually transmitted diseases in one population as compared with a second population. The relative risk (RR) is reported as 0.80 and the 95% confidence interval (CI) is reported as 0.62 to 1.4. How should the nurse interpret the results?
   1. Because the CI of the RR includes the value of 1, the difference between the groups is meaningless.
   2. A 95% confidence interval is a statistically significant finding.
   3. A relative risk of 0.80 is moderately powerful.
   4. Because there is no *p*-value reported for the CI, the nurse is unable to make any conclusions about the data.

10. A client at 24 weeks' gestation is found to have bacterial vaginosis. Her primary healthcare provider has ordered metronidazole to treat the problem. Which of the following educational information is important for the nurse to provide to the client at this time?
1. The client must be careful to observe for signs of preterm labor.
2. The client must advise her partner to seek therapy as soon as possible.
3. A common side effect of the medicine is a copious vaginal discharge.
4. A repeat culture should be taken 2 weeks after completing the therapy.

11. A nonpregnant young woman has been diagnosed with bacterial vaginosis (BV). The nurse questions the woman regarding her sexual history, including her frequency of intercourse, how many sexual partners she has, and her use of contraceptives. What is the rationale for the nurse's questions?
1. Clients with BV can infect their sexual partners.
2. The nurse is required by law to ask the questions.
3. Clients with BV can become infected with HIV and other sexually transmitted infections more easily than uninfected women.
4. The laboratory needs a full client history to know for which organisms and antibiotic sensitivities it should test.

12. A client is noted to have multiple soft warts on her perineum and rectal areas. The nurse suspects that this client is infected with which of the following sexually transmitted infections?
1. Human papillomavirus (HPV).
2. Human immunodeficiency virus (HIV).
3. Syphilis.
4. Trichomoniasis.

13. A client is to receive 2.4 million units of penicillin G benzathine IM to treat syphilis. The medication is available as 1,200,000 units/mL. How many mL should the nurse administer?

_______ mL

14. Four women who use superabsorbent tampons during their menses are being seen in the medical clinic. The client with which of the following findings would lead the nurse to suspect that the client's complaints are related to her use of tampons rather than to an unrelated medical problem?
1. Diffuse rash with fever.
2. Angina.
3. Hypertension.
4. Thrombocytopenia with pallor.

15. A client seen in the emergency department is diagnosed with pelvic inflammatory disease (PID). Before discharge, the nurse should provide the client with health teaching regarding which of the following?
1. Endometriosis.
2. Menopause.
3. Ovarian hyperstimulation.
4. Sexually transmitted infections.

16. A client has contracted herpes simplex 2 for the first time. Which of the following signs/symptoms is the client likely to complain of?
1. Flu-like symptoms.
2. Metrorrhagia.
3. Amenorrhea.
4. Abdominal cramping.

17. Which of the following sexually transmitted infections is characterized by a foul-smelling, yellow-green discharge that is often accompanied by vaginal pain and dyspareunia?
1. Syphilis.
2. Herpes simplex.
3. Trichomoniasis.
4. Condylomata acuminata.

18. The nurse is educating a group of adolescent clients regarding bacterial sexually transmitted infections (STIs). The nurse knows that learning was achieved when a group member states that they can expect the following, if they contract a sexually transmitted infection.
1. Menstrual cramping.
2. Heavy menstrual periods.
3. Flu-like symptoms.
4. Lack of signs or symptoms.

19. A client has been diagnosed with pelvic inflammatory disease (PID). Which of the following organisms are the most likely causative agents? **Select all that apply.**
1. *Gardnerella vaginalis.*
2. *Candida albicans.*
3. *Chlamydia trachomatis.*
4. *Neisseria gonorrhoeae.*
5. *Treponema pallidum.*

20. The public health nurse calls a client and states, "I am afraid that I have some disturbing news. A man who has been treated for gonorrhea by the health department has told them that he had intercourse with you. It is very important that you seek medical attention." The client replies, "There is no reason for me to go to the doctor! I feel fine!" Which of the following replies by the nurse is appropriate at this time?
1. "I am sure that you are upset by the disturbing news, but there is no reason to be angry with me."
2. "I am sorry. We must have received the wrong information."
3. "That certainly could be the case. People often report no symptoms."
4. "All right, but please tell me your contacts because it is possible for you to pass the disease on even if you have no symptoms."

21. A client has been diagnosed with primary syphilis. Which of the following physical findings would the nurse expect to see?
1. Cluster of vesicles.
2. Pain-free lesion.
3. Macular rash.
4. Foul-smelling discharge.

22. A client has been diagnosed with syphilis. Which of the following nursing interventions is appropriate?
1. Counsel the client about how to live with a chronic infection.
2. Inquire about symptoms of other sexually transmitted infections.
3. Assist the primary healthcare practitioner with cryotherapy procedures.
4. Educate the client regarding the safe disposal of menstrual pads.

23. After a sex education class, the school nurse overhears an adolescent discussing safe sex practices. Which of the following comments by the young person indicates that teaching about infection control was effective?
1. "I don't have to worry about getting infected if I have oral sex."
2. "Teen women are at highest risk for sexually transmitted infections (STIs)."
3. "The best thing to do if I have sex a lot is to use spermicide each and every time."
4. "Boys get human immunodeficiency virus (HIV) easier than girls do."

24. An asymptomatic woman is being treated for HIV infection at the women's health clinic. Which of the following comments by the client shows that she understands her care?
1. "If I get pregnant, my baby will be HIV positive."
2. "I should have my viral load and antibody levels checked every day."
3. "Since my partner and I are both HIV positive, we use a condom."
4. "To be safe, my partner and I engage only in oral sex."

25. A female client asks the nurse about treatment for human papilloma viral warts. The nurse's response should include which of the following?
1. An antiviral injection cures approximately 50% of cases.
2. Aggressive treatment is required to cure warts.
3. Warts often spread when an attempt is made to remove them surgically.
4. Warts often recur a few months after a client is treated.

26. A triage nurse answers a telephone call from the male partner of a client who was recently diagnosed with cervical cancer. The man is requesting to be tested for human papillomavirus (HPV). The nurse's response should include which of the following?
1. There is currently no approved test to detect HPV in men.
2. A viral culture of the penis and rectum is used to detect HPV in men.
3. A Pap smear of the meatus of the penis is used to detect HPV in men.
4. There is no need for a test because men do not become infected with HPV.

27. A client who is sexually active is asking the nurse about vaccines administered to prevent human papillomavirus (HPV). Which of the following should be included in the counseling session?
1. The vaccines are not recommended for women who are already sexually active.
2. The vaccines protect recipients from all strains of the virus.
3. The most common side effect from the vaccines is pain at the injection site.
4. Anyone who is allergic to eggs is advised against receiving the vaccines.

28. A couple seeking contraception and infection-prevention counseling state, "We know that the best way for us to prevent both pregnancy and infection is to use condoms plus spermicide every time we have sex." Which of the following is the best response by the nurse?
1. "That is correct. It is best to use a condom with spermicide during every sexual contact."
2. "That is true, except if you have intercourse twice in one evening. Then you do not have to apply more spermicide."
3. "That is not true. It has been shown that condoms alone are very effective and that spermicide can increase the transmission of some viruses."
4. "That is not necessarily true. Spermicide has been shown to cause cancer in men and women who use it too frequently."

29. The nurse is teaching an uncircumcised male to use a condom. Which of the following information should be included in the teaching plan?
1. Apply mineral oil to the tip and shaft of the condom-covered penis.
2. Pull back the foreskin before applying the condom.
3. Create a reservoir at the tip of the condom after putting it on.
4. Wait five minutes after ejaculating before removing the condom.

30. The nurse is teaching a young woman how to use the female condom. Which of the following should be included in the teaching plan?
1. Reuse female condoms no more than five times.
2. Refrain from using lubricant because the condom may slip out of the vagina.
3. Wear both female and male condoms together to maximize effectiveness.
4. Remove the condom by twisting the outer ring and pulling gently.

31. A client has a history of toxic shock syndrome. Which of the following forms of birth control should she be taught to avoid?
    1. Diaphragm.
    2. Intrauterine device.
    3. Birth control pills (estrogen-progestin combination).
    4. Medroxyprogesterone acetate.

32. During a counseling session on natural family planning techniques, how should the nurse explain the consistency of cervical mucus at the time of ovulation?
    1. It becomes thin and elastic.
    2. It becomes opaque and acidic.
    3. It contains numerous leukocytes to prevent vaginal infections.
    4. It decreases in quantity in response to body temperature changes.

33. A client is learning about the care and use of the diaphragm. Which of the following comments by the woman shows that she understands the teaching that was provided?
    1. "I should regularly put the diaphragm up to the light and look at it carefully."
    2. "This is one method that can be used during menstruation."
    3. "I can leave the diaphragm in place for a day or two."
    4. "The diaphragm should be well powdered before I put it back in the case."

34. The nurse teaches a couple that the diaphragm is an excellent method of contraception providing that the woman does which of the following?
    1. Does not use any cream or jelly with it.
    2. Douches promptly after its removal.
    3. Leaves it in place for 6 hours following intercourse.
    4. Inserts it at least 5 hours prior to having intercourse.

35. The nurse is working with a client who states that she has multiple sex partners. Which of the following contraceptive methods would be best for the nurse to recommend to this client?
    1. Intrauterine device.
    2. Female condom.
    3. Bilateral tubal ligation.
    4. Birth control pills.

36. A client is pregnant with a Copper T intrauterine device (IUD) in place. The physician has ordered an ultrasound to be done to evaluate the pregnancy. The client asks the nurse why this is so important. The nurse should tell the client that the ultrasound is done primarily for which of the following reasons?
    1. To assess for the presence of an ectopic pregnancy.
    2. To check the baby for serious malformations.
    3. To assess for pelvic inflammatory disease.
    4. To check for the possibility of a twin pregnancy.

37. An adolescent client confides to the school nurse that she is sexually active. The client asks the nurse to recommend a "very reliable" birth control method, but she refuses to be seen by a physician or nurse practitioner. Which of the following methods would be best for the nurse to recommend?
    1. Contraceptive patch.
    2. Withdrawal method.
    3. Female condom.
    4. Contraceptive sponge.

38. As a preceptor, you are observing a newly employed nurse answering questions from a pregnant client who is considering a bilateral tubal ligation in the hospital after the birth of her baby. Which of the following instructions by the nurse requires follow-up? **Select all that apply.**
1. The surgical procedure is easily reversible.
2. Menstruation usually ceases after the procedure.
3. Libido should remain the same after the procedure.
4. The incision will be made endocervically.
5. The procedure cannot be done at the time of a cesarean section.

39. The nurse is selecting educational materials for clients seeking contraception information. Which of the following issues about each client must the nurse consider before suggesting contraceptive choices? **Select all that apply.**
1. Age.
2. Ethical and moral beliefs.
3. Sexual patterns.
4. Socioeconomic status.
5. Childbearing plans.

40. A client is being issued a new prescription for a low-dose combination birth control pill. What advice should the nurse give the client about next steps if she ever forgets to take a pill?
1. Take it as soon as she remembers, even if that means taking two pills in one day.
2. Skip that pill and refrain from intercourse for the remainder of the month.
3. Wear a pad for the next week because she will experience vaginal bleeding.
4. Take an at-home pregnancy test at the end of the month to check for a pregnancy.

41. A couple is seeking family planning advice. They are newly married and wish to delay childbearing for at least 3 years. The woman, age 26, has never been pregnant, has no medical problems, and does not smoke. She states, however, that she is very embarrassed when she touches her vagina. Which of the following methods would be most appropriate for the nurse to suggest to this couple?
1. Diaphragm.
2. Cervical cap.
3. Intrauterine device (IUD).
4. Birth control pills (BCPs).

42. What is essential for the nurse to teach a woman who has just had an intrauterine device (IUD) inserted?
1. "Palpate your lower abdomen each month to check the patency of the device."
2. "Remain on bedrest for 24 hours after insertion of the device."
3. "Report any complaints of painful intercourse to the physician."
4. "Insert spermicidal jelly within 4 hours of every sexual encounter."

43. A 16-year-old client who had unprotected intercourse 24 hours ago has entered the emergency department seeking assistance. Which of the following responses by the nurse is appropriate?
1. "You can walk into your local pharmacy and buy a morning after pill."
2. "I am sorry but because of your age I am unable to assist you."
3. "The emergency department doctor can prescribe high-dose birth control pills (BCPs) for you."
4. The nurse's response is dependent upon which state they are practicing in.

44. A young client is seen in the emergency department. She states, "I took a pregnancy test today. I'm pregnant. My parents will be furious with me!! I have to do something!" Which of the following initial responses by the nurse is most appropriate?
1. "You can take medicine to abort the pregnancy so your parents won't know."
2. "Let's talk about your options."
3. "The best thing for you to do is to have the baby and to give it up for adoption."
4. "I can help you tell your parents."

45. A breastfeeding client is requesting that she be prescribed an ethinyl-estradiol-and-levonorgestrel-combined pill as a birth control method. Which of the following information should be included in the client teaching session?
1. The client will menstruate every 8 to 9 weeks.
2. The pills are taken for 3 out of every 4 weeks.
3. Breakthrough bleeding is a common side effect.
4. Breastfeeding is compatible with the medication.

46. Five women, aged 35 to 39, wish to use a contraceptive skin patch containing a combination of female hormones (ethinyl estradiol and norelgestromin) for family planning. Which of the women should be carefully counseled regarding the safety considerations of the method? **Select all that apply.**
1. The client who smokes 1 pack of cigarettes each day.
2. The client with a history of lung cancer.
3. The client with a history of deep vein thrombosis.
4. The client who runs at least 50 miles each week.
5. The client with a history of cholecystitis.

47. A postpartum client plans to use the lactational amenorrhea method of birth control. The nurse should advise the client that the method is effective only if which of the following conditions are present? **Select all that apply.**
1. Being less than 6 months postpartum.
2. Being amenorrheic since delivery of the baby.
3. Supplementing with formula no more than once per day.
4. Losing less than 10% of weight since delivery.
5. Sleeping at least 8 hours every night.

48. A client is being taught how to use the diaphragm as a contraceptive device. Which of the following statements by the client indicates that the teaching was effective? **Select all that apply.**
1. Petroleum-based lubricants may be used with the device.
2. The device must be refitted if the client gains or loses 10 pounds or more.
3. The anterior lip must be pushed under the symphysis pubis.
4. Additional spermicide must be added if the device has been in place over 6 hours.
5. The diaphragm should be cleaned with a 10% bleach solution after every use.

49. Four women with significant health histories wish to use the diaphragm as a contraceptive method. Which of the following clients should be counseled that the diaphragm may lead to a recurrence of her problem?
1. Urinary tract infections.
2. Herpes simplex infections.
3. Deep vein thromboses.
4. Human papilloma warts.

50. A woman is using the contraceptive sponge as a birth control method. Which of the following actions is it important for her to perform to maximize the sponge's effectiveness?
1. Insert the sponge at least 1 hour before intercourse.
2. Thoroughly moisten the sponge with water before inserting.
3. Insert spermicidal jelly at the same time the sponge is inserted.
4. Replace the sponge with a new one if intercourse is repeated.

51. The nurse is providing education to a couple regarding the proper procedure for male condom use. The nurse knows that the teaching was effective when the couple states that which of the following procedures should be taken before the man's penis becomes flaccid after ejaculation?
1. The woman should douche with white vinegar and water.
2. The woman should consider taking a postcoital contraceptive.
3. The man should hold the edges of the condom during its removal.
4. The man should apply spermicide to the upper edges of the condom.

52. The nurse is developing a standard care plan for the administration of mifepristone/misoprostol for pregnancy termination. Which of the following information should the nurse include in the plan?
    1. Women should be evaluated by their healthcare practitioners 2 weeks after taking the medicine.
    2. This is the preferred method for terminating an ectopic pregnancy when an intrauterine device is in place.
    3. The only symptom clients should experience is bleeding 2 to 3 days after taking the medicine.
    4. Women who experience no bleeding within 3 days should immediately take a home pregnancy test.

53. The nurse is providing an unmarried, perimenopausal woman with a pregnancy history of G3 P2012, with contraceptive counseling. The client has four sex partners and smokes 1 pack of cigarettes per day. Which of the following methods is best suited for this client?
    1. Male condom.
    2. Intrauterine device.
    3. Etonogestrel/ethinyl estradiol vaginal ring.
    4. Oral contraceptives.

54. A client who has been taking birth control pills for 2 months calls the clinic with the following complaint: "I have had a bad headache for the past couple of days and now I have pain in my right leg." Which of the following responses should the nurse make?
    1. "Continue the pill, but take one aspirin tablet with it each day for the remainder of the month."
    2. "Stop taking the pill, and start using a condom for contraception."
    3. "Come to the clinic this afternoon so that we can see what is going on."
    4. "Those are common side effects that should disappear in a month or so."

55. The nurse has taught a couple about the temperature rhythm method for birth control. Which of the following behaviors would indicate that the teaching was effective?
    1. The client takes her basal body temperature before retiring each evening.
    2. The couple charts information from at least six menstrual cycles before using the method.
    3. The couple resumes having intercourse as soon as they see a rise in the basal body temperature.
    4. The client assesses her vaginal discharge daily for changes in color and odor.

56. A nurse is providing contraceptive counseling to a perimenopausal client with an obstetrical history of G3 P2012, who is in a monogamous relationship. Which of the following comments by the client requires follow-up?
    1. "The calendar method is the most reliable method for me to use."
    2. "If I use the IUD, I am at minimal risk for pelvic inflammatory disease."
    3. "I should still use birth control even though I had only 2 periods last year."
    4. "The contraceptive patch contains both estrogen and progesterone."

57. The nurse is interviewing a client regarding contraceptive choices. Which of the following client statements would most influence the nurse's teaching?
    1. "I have 2 children."
    2. "My partner and I have sex twice a week."
    3. "I am 25 years old."
    4. "I feel funny touching my private parts."

58. Which of the following clients, who are all seeking a family planning method, is the best candidate for birth control pills?
1. 19-year-old with multiple sex partners.
2. 27-year-old who bottle feeds her newborn.
3. 29-year-old with chronic hypertension.
4. 37-year-old who smokes one pack per day.

59. The nurse is meeting four sexually active clients in the family planning clinic today. It would be most appropriate for the nurse to recommend the intrauterine device (IUD) to which of the clients? **Select all that apply.**
1. 16-year old, high school student.
2. 20-year-old, recent college graduate.
3. 24-year-old, G0 P0000.
4. 28-year-old, recent history of chlamydia.
5. 30-year-old, G3 P2102.

60. A nurse is educating a group of women in her parish about osteoporosis. The nurse should include in her discussion that which of the following is a risk factor for the disease process?
1. Multiparity.
2. Increased body weight.
3. Late onset of menopause.
4. Heavy alcohol intake.

61. A client is taking alendronate for osteoporosis. The nurse should advise the client about which of the following when taking the medication?
1. Remain upright for 30 minutes after taking the medication.
2. Take only after eating a full meal.
3. Take medication in divided doses 3 times each day.
4. Do not break or crush the capsule.

62. A client is put on calcium supplements to maintain bone health. To maximize absorption, the client is also advised to take which of the following supplements?
1. Vitamin D.
2. Vitamin E.
3. Folic acid.
4. Iron.

63. A client asks a nurse to express an opinion on the value of taking hormone replacement therapy (HRT). The nurse should be aware that it is recognized that HRT is effective in which of the following situations?
1. No client should ever take hormone replacement therapy.
2. Women experiencing severe menopausal symptoms.
3. Women with severe coronary artery disease.
4. Women with a history of breast cancer.

64. A client states that she feels "dirty" during her menses so she often douches to "clean myself." The nurse advises the client that it is especially important to refrain from douching while menstruating because douching will increase the likelihood of her developing which of the following gynecological complications?
1. Fibroids.
2. Endometritis.
3. Cervical cancer.
4. Polyps.

65. The nurse is counseling a client who has been diagnosed with mild osteoporosis. Which of the following lifestyle changes should the nurse recommend? **Select all that apply.**
1. Eat yellow and orange vegetables.
2. Go on daily walks.
3. Stop smoking.
4. Consume dairy products.
5. Sleep at least 8 hours a night.

66. The nurse should suspect that a client is bulimic when the client exhibits which of the following signs/symptoms?
1. Significant weight loss and hyperkalemia.
2. Respiratory acidosis and hypoxemia.
3. Dental caries and scars on her knuckles.
4. Hyperglycemia and large urine output.

67. A client has been admitted to the hospital with a diagnosis of bulimia from forced vomiting. Which of the following serum laboratory reports would the nurse expect to see? **Select all that apply.**
1. Potassium 3 mEq/L.
2. Bicarbonate 30 mmol/L.
3. Platelet count 450,000 cells/mcl.
4. Hemoglobin A1C 9%.
5. Sodium 150 mEq/L.

68. A client has been admitted to the hospital with a diagnosis of bulimia. Which of the following physical findings would the nurse expect to see?
1. Mastoiditis.
2. Hirsutism.
3. Gynecomastia.
4. Esophagitis.

69. A school nurse notices that a young woman with scars on the knuckles of her right hand runs to the bathroom each day immediately after eating a high-calorie lunch. Which of the following actions by the nurse is appropriate at this time?
1. Nothing, because her behavior is normal.
2. Question the young woman to see if she is being abused.
3. Recommend that the young woman be seen by her doctor.
4. Follow the young woman to the bathroom.

70. The clinic nurse is interviewing a client preceding her annual checkup. Which of the following findings would make the nurse suspicious that the client has anorexia nervosa?
1. Food allergies and an aversion to exercise.
2. Significant weight loss and amenorrhea.
3. Respiratory distress and thick oral mucus.
4. Cardiac arrhythmias.

71. An 18-year-old client is being evaluated for school soccer by the school nurse. The expected weight for the young woman's height is 120 lb. Her actual weight is 96 lb. The client states that she runs 6 miles every morning and swims 5 miles every afternoon. Which of the following actions should the nurse take at this time?
1. Ask the client the date of her last menstrual period.
2. Encourage the client to continue her excellent exercise schedule.
3. Congratulate the client on her ability to maintain such a good weight.
4. Advise the client that she will have to stop swimming once soccer starts.

72. A client is being seen in the gynecology clinic. The nurse notes that the client has a swollen eye and a bruise on her cheek. Which of the following is an appropriate statement for the nurse to make?
1. "I am required by law to notify the police department of your injuries."
2. "Women who are abused often have injuries like yours."
3. "You must leave your partner before you are injured again."
4. "It is important that you refrain from doing things that anger your partner."

73. Which of the following questions should be asked of women during all routine medical examinations? **Select all that apply.**
1. "Has anyone ever forced you to have sex?"
2. "Are you sexually active?"
3. "Are you ever afraid to go home?"
4. "Does anyone you know ever hit you?"
5. "Have you ever breastfed a child?"

74. The nurse suspects that a client has been physically abused. The client refuses to report the abuse to the police. Which statement by the client suggests to the nurse that the relationship may be in the "honeymoon phase"?
1. "My partner said that he will never hurt me again."
2. "My partner drinks alcohol only on the weekends."
3. "My partner yells less than he used to."
4. "My partner has frequent bouts of insomnia."

75. A client who has been abused for a number of years is finally seeking assistance in leaving her relationship. Identify the actions that the nurse should take at this time. **Select all that apply.**
1. Comment that the victim could have left long ago.
2. Assist the victim to develop a safety plan.
3. Remind the victim that the abuse was not her fault.
4. Help the victim to contact a domestic violence center.

76. A client with multiple bruises on her arms and face is seen in the emergency department accompanied by her partner. When asked about the injuries, the partner states, "She ran into a door." Which of the following actions by the nurse is of highest priority?
1. Take the client's vital signs.
2. Interview the client in private.
3. Assess for additional bruising.
4. Document the location of the bruises.

77. Which of the following behaviors would indicate to a nurse that a pregnant client might be in an abusive relationship? **Select all that apply.**
1. Denies that any injuries occurred, even when bruising is visible.
2. Gives an implausible explanation for any injuries.
3. Gives the nurse eye contact while answering questions.
4. Allows her partner to answer the nurse's questions.
5. Frequently calls to change appointment times.

78. A client is being seen following a sexual assault. A rape examination is being conducted. Which of the following specimens may be collected from the victim during the examination? **Select all that apply.**
1. Buccal swab for genetic analysis.
2. Samples of pubic hair.
3. Toenail scrapings.
4. Samples of head hair.
5. Sputum for microbiological analysis.

79. The nurse is conducting a seminar with young adolescent women regarding actions they can take to protect themselves from date rape. Which of the following guidelines are essential to include in the discussion? **Select all that apply.**
1. The girls should consume drinks from enclosed containers.
2. The girls should keep extra money in their shoes or bras.
3. The girls should keep condoms in their pocketbooks.
4. The girls should meet a new date in a public place.
5. The girls should go on group dates whenever possible.

80. A young client in a disheveled state is admitted to the emergency department. She states that she awoke this morning without her underwear on but with no memory of what happened the evening before. She thinks she may have been raped. Which of the following assessments by the nurse is most likely accurate?
1. The client is spoiled and is exhibiting attention-seeking behavior.
2. The client is experiencing a psychotic break.
3. The client regrets having had consensual sex.
4. The client unknowingly ingested a date rape drug.

81. A client has just entered an emergency department after a stranger rape. Which of the following interventions is of highest priority at this time?
1. Create a safe environment.
2. Offer postcoital contraceptive therapy.
3. Provide sexually transmitted disease prophylaxis.
4. Take a thorough health history.

82. The nurse at Victims Assistance Services is speaking with a young client who states that she was sexually assaulted at a party the evening before. The victim states, "I ran home and took a shower as soon as it happened. I felt so dirty." Which of the following responses should the nurse make first?
1. "The evidence kit may still reveal important information."
2. "It was important for you to do that for yourself."
3. "Have you washed your clothes? If not, we might be able to obtain evidence from them."
4. "Do you remember what happened? If not, someone may have put a drug in your drink."

83. A young client was a victim of a sexual assault. After the rape examination has been completed, the client requests to be given emergency contraception (EC). Which of the following information should the nurse teach the client regarding the therapy?
1. EC is illegal in all 50 states.
2. The most common side effect of EC is excessive vaginal bleeding.
3. The same medicine that is used for EC is used to induce abortions.
4. EC is best when used within 72 hours of contact.

84. A nurse is caring for a client who states that she is a lesbian. Which of the following should the nurse consider when caring for this client?
1. Lesbian women are usually less sexually active than straight women.
2. Lesbian women need not be asked about domestic violence issues.
3. Lesbian women should be tested for cervical cancer every 3 to 7 years.
4. Lesbian women should be monitored for sexually transmitted infections.

85. The nurse advises the women to whom she is providing healthcare teaching at a local church that they should see their healthcare provider to be assessed for ovarian cancer if they experience which of the following signs/symptoms?
1. Vaginal bleeding and weight loss.
2. Frequent urination, breast tenderness, and extreme fatigue.
3. Abdominal pain, bloating, and a constant feeling of fullness.
4. Hardness on one side of the abdomen.

86. A client states that she has been diagnosed with fibrocystic breast disease. She asks the nurse, "Does that mean that I have breast cancer?" Which of the following statements by the nurse is appropriate at this time?

1. "I am so sorry. I am sure that the doctor will do everything possible to cure you of the cancer."
2. "I am not the best person to ask about your diagnosis. I suggest that you ask the doctor."
3. "If your lumps are round and mobile they are not cancerous, but if they are hard to the touch you probably do have cancer."
4. "You do not have cancer, but it is especially important for you to have regular mammograms to monitor for any changes."

87. The nurse is educating a group of women on how to perform a breast self-examination (BSE). Which of the following actions should the nurse advise the women to take? **Select all that apply.**

1. Use the flat part of their index, middle, and ring fingers.
2. Use pressure in three intensities: light, moderate, and deep.
3. Look for dimpling while bending forward from the waist.
4. Feel for lumps throughout the entire breast, including the tail of Spence.
5. Check for nipple discharge.

88. A school nurse is conducting a class on the transmission of human papillomavirus (HPV) for middle school students. Which of the following information should be included in the discussion?

1. The enzymes in the mouth effectively metabolize and destroy HPV.
2. To prevent oral infection, sexually active individuals should wear dental dams when engaging in oral intercourse.
3. HPV vaccines effectively prevent oral as well as genital and rectal HPV infections.
4. When cultured routinely, oropharyngeal excretions accurately predict the likelihood of the development of HPV-induced cancer.

ANSWERS AND RATIONALES

The correct answer number and rationale for why it is the correct answer are given in **boldface blue type.** Rationales for why the other possible answer options are incorrect also are given, but they are not in boldface type.

1. 1. The immune globulin is not administered before giving the vaccine.
   2. The vaccine is administered in a series of three injections. Booster shots are not recommended for otherwise healthy people with noncompromised immune systems.
   3. **To be immunized against hepatitis B, a three-injection vaccine series is administered.**
   4. The vaccine can be administered at any age.

TEST-TAKING HINT: The current recommendation by the Centers for Disease Control and Prevention (CDC) is that the hepatitis B vaccine series be started during the neonatal period before discharge from the hospital (Schillie et al., 2018). The second and third shots are administered 1 month and 6 months after the first shot, respectively. For adults who have not received the vaccine in infancy the series can be administered at any age.

2. 1. Medroxyprogesterone acetate is either administered via intramuscular or subcutaneous injection every 3 months.
   2. Medroxyprogesterone acetate is a progesterone-based contraceptive. It is safe for use and should not adversely affect the ability to breastfeed.
   3. Both amenorrhea and menorrhagia are side effects of the medication. The client should be advised to notify her healthcare practitioner regarding any significant menstrual pattern changes.
   4. **Many women who use medroxyprogesterone acetate for over 2 years have been found to suffer from loss of bone density. Some of the changes in bone density may be irreversible.**

TEST-TAKING HINT: There is a black box recommendation on the medroxyprogesterone acetate label. A black box warning is placed on some prescription medications that have been found to have significant side effects. In the case of medroxyprogesterone acetate, the black box warning is related to an increased risk of osteoporosis if use of this medication is prolonged. The Food and Drug Administration (FDA) has the power to require pharmaceutical companies to include a black box on a medication that, although approved for use, carries risks when taken.

3. 1. Medroxyprogesterone acetate is administered via intramuscular injection or subcutaneously every 3 months.
   2. **The client should use sunscreen while receiving medroxyprogesterone acetate for birth control.**
   3. The medication is contraindicated for use by women who have breast cancer or who are pregnant. It is not contraindicated for use by those suffering from lung or esophageal cancer.
   4. After the first injection, it is often recommended that the client use an alternate form of birth control for at least a week, but not for 2 months. The client should know that medroxyprogesterone acetate will not protect her from sexually transmitted infections.

TEST-TAKING HINT: Women can develop dark patches on their skin when using medroxyprogesterone acetate. The patches often become darker in women who are in the sun without protection. It is strongly recommended that women who use medroxyprogesterone acetate use sunscreen whenever they are exposed to the sun.

4. 1. **IUDs can remain in place for extended periods of time.**
   2. The client should expect to menstruate regularly while the IUD is in place.
   3. If dyspareunia occurs, the client should contact her healthcare practitioner.
   4. Women who have IUDs in place are at slightly higher risk of developing pelvic infections.

TEST-TAKING HINT: Women who have multiple sex partners or who have had a recent history of a sexually transmitted infection should be considered at highest risk for infection. The risk for all women is most pronounced during the 20 days immediately following IUD insertion.

5. 1. A macular rash is not indicative of pubic lice.
   2. **Pruritus is, by far, the most common symptom of pubic lice.**

3. Hyperthermia is not commonly seen with an infestation of pubic lice.
4. Foul-smelling discharge is not commonly seen with an infestation of pubic lice.

TEST-TAKING HINT: Pubic lice, not to be confused with head lice, are commonly called crabs. They are insects, usually sexually transmitted, that invade the pubic hair. Although they are not the same as head lice, the pubic infestation is treated with the same pediculicidal shampoos. (For information regarding the recommended medical treatment of clients with pubic lice, see https://www.cdc.gov/parasites/lice/pubic/treatment.html)

6. 1. Lice are not treated with antibiotics.
2. After lice treatment, clothing should be washed thoroughly in hot water (at or hotter than 130° F (54.4° C)) and dried in a hot dryer for at least 20 minutes.
3. The over-the-counter shampoo should be applied for 10 minutes or as stated in the package insert, and then rinsed off.
4. To remove the nits, or eggs, the pubic hair may be combed with a fine-tooth nit comb after the shampoo is removed.

TEST-TAKING HINT: Nits are very small, white, lice eggs that are about the size of a period at the end of a sentence. They adhere firmly to the shaft of the pubic hair and take about 1 week to hatch. It is very helpful, therefore, to remove the nits with a fingernail or a fine-tooth nit comb to prevent reinfestation.

7. 1. This statement is inappropriate. The hepatitis B vaccine is not administered to prevent all babies from contracting hepatitis B vertically. The majority of babies receive the vaccine to prevent them from contracting the virus in the future. If a pregnant client is hepatitis B positive, her baby would also receive the hepatitis B immune globulin (HBIG), in addition to the vaccine, within 12 hours of delivery. This protocol minimizes the incidence of vertical transmission.
2. This statement is inappropriate. Vaccines are not administered simply because they are available.
3. This is the best answer. Hepatitis B is a very serious disease that can be transmitted sexually or via contact with blood and blood products.
4. This response implies that the mother in the scenario is not interested in protecting her child. That is very unlikely.

TEST-TAKING HINT: A number of individuals who contract the hepatitis B virus become long-term carriers of the disease and are able to transmit it to others. They are also at high risk for the development of chronic liver disease and liver cancer. Hepatitis B is spread through contact with blood of an infected person (even if they show no symptoms). Hepatitis B can spread through open cuts or sores, sharing toothbrushes or other personal items, and through food chewed for a baby, to name a few. The virus can live on objects for 7 days or more (Schillie et al., 2018).

8. 1. There was a significant difference between the vaccinated and unvaccinated students in the "read/heard" group—$P < 0.001$.
2. This is true. The risk ratio for the "Health History form" category is 1.62.
3. Of those who learned about the vaccine from "Letters," 11.1% were not vaccinated.
4. The smallest percentage of students in both the vaccinated and unvaccinated groups learned about the vaccine from the UHS providers.

TEST-TAKING HINT: To provide evidence-based nursing, it is very important to be able to read tables and interpret data from scholarly articles. Risk ratios, confidence intervals, and significance data are especially critical and must be understood. It is of interest to note that in the study in question, the healthcare providers were the poorest source of information about the hepatitis B vaccine. Remember that *p*-values determine the strength or weakness of research results. If you imagine a statistical curve with vertical lines, the *p*-value is the area on either side of the curve, where the line comes down and merges into the straight line (see diagram on next page). The smaller that area is, the more confident we can be in the research results. It indicates visually that there's only a minute chance the differences we found were random. In order to accept a test result, we want the *p*-value to be at least 0.05 or lower. When research results show a *p*-value of 0.05 or lower (0.04 to 0.01), we can say that we are 95% (or 96% or 99%) confident that there is an actual difference between the two approaches in the research project as opposed to random variations. The null hypothesis says there is no difference between the approaches and our research amounts to nothing. The *p*-value says the null hypothesis is wrong and our research *did make a statistically significant difference*. As a result, we have reasonable grounds to reject the null hypothesis

that our change hasn't made any difference and to have confidence in our results.

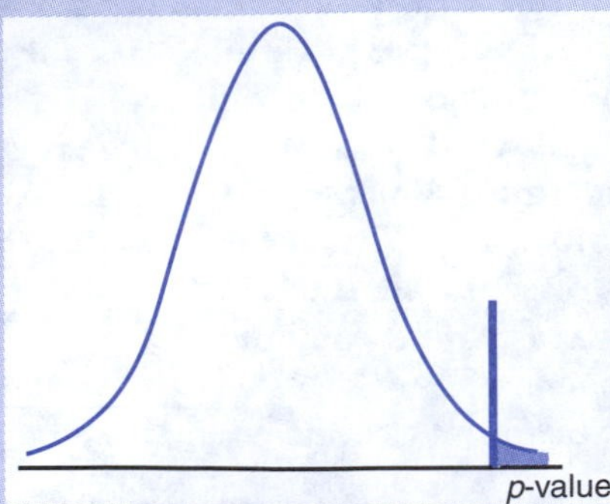

9. 1. This is true. Relative risk connotes the probability of an experimental event occurring in relation to the control. An RR = 1 means that the rate of an experimental event occurring is the same as the rate of the control event occurring. An RR less than 1 means that the rate of an experimental event occurring is less than the rate of the control event occurring. An RR greater than 1 means that the rate of an experimental event occurring is greater than the rate of the control event occurring.
2. The values in a 95% confidence interval provide the reader with a range of possible results for the information being given. For example, as in the scenario, although the researchers report the result as one number—0.80—they are 95% confident that the result is between 0.62 and 1.4.
3. An RR of 0.80 means that the rate of an experimental event occurring is only 80% as likely as the likelihood of the control event occurring.
4. This is false. When the RR and CI values are provided for the reader, an interpretation of the data can be made.

TEST-TAKING HINT: Confidence intervals are often reported in relation to relative risk (also called risk ratios) or odds ratios. They also are often reported to interpret raw data. For example, a mean may be reported as 15 with a 95% CI of 10 to 17. The researchers are then stating that the calculated mean is 15 and they are 95% confident that the actual mean is between 10 and 17. Consulting a statistics text when reading research studies is an excellent practice.

10. 1. Clients with bacterial vaginosis are at high risk for preterm labor.
2. Male partners rarely need treatment. Females may, however, need to be treated.
3. Bacterial vaginosis is characterized by a discharge that is often foul-smelling. The discharge is not related to the therapy.
4. An initial, diagnostic microscopic and culture assessment is done. It is not required that a repeat test be done 2 weeks later.

TEST-TAKING HINT: Bacterial vaginosis (BV) is quite common. The problem is characterized by a shift in the bacterial flora of the vagina, resulting in a copious, foul-smelling, "fishy" vaginal discharge. BV can be diagnosed by clinical criteria that include the fishy odor of vaginal discharge, "clue cells" on microscopic exam, and a pH of greater than 4.5. A gram stain is the gold standard for laboratory diagnosis. The usual findings show a decrease in lactobacilli with an increase in *Gardnerella vaginalis* or other anaerobic bacteria.

11. 1. Unless the partner is female, the transmission to partners is low.
2. There is no law that requires the nurse to ask these questions.
3. This statement is true. The change in normal flora increases the client's susceptibility to other organisms.
4. There is no need to provide the laboratory with this information.

TEST-TAKING HINT: Once the information regarding the client's history and lifestyle is gathered, the nurse must provide needed care and teaching. Questions regarding intercourse with multiple partners as well as previous sexually transmitted illnesses (STIs), including HIV, should be asked and, when indicated, additional testing should be considered. If the client is sexually active, the nurse should discuss the client's use of contraceptive methods that will protect her from infection as well as pregnancy.

12. 1. Human papillomavirus (HPV) is characterized by flat warts on the vaginal and rectal surfaces.
2. HIV/AIDS is characterized by nonspecific symptoms like weight loss, dry cough, and fatigue.
3. Primary syphilis is characterized by a nonpainful lesion, called a chancre.
4. Trichomoniasis is characterized by a yellowish green vaginal discharge. Like bacterial vaginosis, it usually has a very strong, fishy smell.

TEST-TAKING HINT: The nurse should be familiar with the primary symptoms of sexually transmitted infections. A client may confide in the nurse about symptoms that she

is experiencing. The nurse must be able to determine when symptoms require medical attention.

13. 2 mL

There are two different methods that may be used to solve the problem: ratio and proportion method and dimensional analysis method.

Ratio and proportion method:

The formula for determining the quantity of the medication that must be given using ratio and proportion is:

$$\frac{\text{Known dosage}}{\text{Known volume}} = \frac{\text{Ordered dosage}}{\text{Needed volume}}$$

$$\frac{1{,}200{,}000 \text{ units}}{1 \text{ mL}} = \frac{2{,}400{,}000 \text{ units}}{x \text{ mL}}$$

$$12 : 1 = 24 : x$$

$$x = 2$$

Dimensional analysis method:

The formula for determining the quantity of the medication that must be given using dimensional analysis is:

$$\frac{\text{Known volume}}{\text{Known dosage}} = \frac{\text{Ordered dosage}}{\text{Ordered volume}}$$

$$\frac{1 \text{ mL}}{1{,}200{,}000 \text{ units}} = \frac{2{,}400{,}000 \text{ units}}{2 \text{ mL}}$$

TEST-TAKING HINT: The important lesson for the test taker to learn from this example is that math principles do not change simply because numbers are large. Penicillin is ordered in millions of units. Simply proceed slowly with each step of the process to find the correct result.

14. 1. **A diffuse rash with fever should be taken very seriously. These are symptoms of toxic shock syndrome (TSS).**
    2. Angina is not related to tampon use.
    3. Hypertension is not related to tampon use. Hypotension, however, may be related.
    4. Thrombocytopenia is not related to tampon use.

TEST-TAKING HINT: This client is likely developing TSS. It is associated with the use of superabsorbent tampons. *Staphylococcus aureus*, a bacterium that colonizes the skin, proliferates in the presence of the tampons in the warm and moist environment of the vagina. Women with the disorder develop a rash, fever, severe vomiting and diarrhea, muscle aches, and chills. The problem must be treated quickly. It is important to note that the mortality rate from TSS approaches 50% (see https://medlineplus.gov/ency/article/000653.html).

15. 1. PID is not related to endometriosis.
    2. PID is not related to menopause.
    3. PID is not related to ovarian hyperstimulation.
    4. **PID usually occurs as a result of an ascending sexually transmitted infection.**

TEST-TAKING HINT: The most common organisms to cause PID are the organisms that cause gonorrhea and chlamydia. In the early stages of these infections, women often experience only minor symptoms. It is not uncommon, therefore, for the organisms to proliferate and ascend into the uterus and fallopian tubes. The client must be taught healthcare practices to decrease her likelihood of a recurrence of the problem (see http://cdc.gov/std/PID/STDFact-PID.htm).

16. 1. **The initial infection of herpes simplex 2 is often symptom-free but, if symptoms do occur, the client may complain of flu-like symptoms as well as vesicles at the site of the viral invasion.**
    2. Metrorrhagia is not associated with herpes simplex 2.
    3. Amenorrhea is not associated with herpes simplex 2.
    4. Abdominal cramping is not associated with herpes simplex 2.

TEST-TAKING HINT: Both herpes simplex 1 and herpes simplex 2 can infect the mucous membranes of the gynecological tract and the oral cavity. The viruses can be transmitted when a vesicle comes in contact with broken skin or mucous membranes. Although outbreaks do resolve, the virus stays dormant in the body and recurrences are often seen during periods of physical and/or emotional stress.

17. 1. Syphilis is caused by the spirochete *Treponema pallidum*. If untreated, syphilis is a three-stage illness. The primary symptom is a pain-free lesion called a chancre.
    2. The primary symptom of herpes simplex is the presence of a cluster of painful vesicles.
    3. **Trichomoniasis is characterized by a yellowish green, foul-smelling discharge.**
    4. Condylomata are vaginal warts.

TEST-TAKING HINT: Trichomoniasis is a sexually transmitted infection caused by a protozoan. Women who develop the infection during pregnancy may develop preterm labor. Women who are infected with trichomoniasis have an increased risk of contracting HIV if exposed (see

https://www.cdc.gov/std/trichomonas/stdfact-trichomoniasis.htm).

18. 1. Menstrual cramping is not usually related to sexually transmitted infections.
2. Heavy menstrual periods are not usually related to sexually transmitted infections.
3. Flu-like symptoms are not usually related to sexually transmitted infections.
4. Most commonly, women experience no signs or symptoms when they have contracted a sexually transmitted infection.

TEST-TAKING HINT: Women are usually symptom-free when they initially contract gonorrhea or chlamydia. In women infected with syphilis, the chancre of a primary infection is pain-free, so women may not realize they have been infected with the spirochete. As a result, it is very important that women—especially those with multiple sex partners—be seen yearly by a gynecologist or nurse practitioner to be tested for STIs.

19. Answers 3 and 4 are correct.
1. *Gardnerella vaginalis* does not cause PID.
2. *Candida albicans* does not cause PID.
3. *Chlamydia trachomatis* is a common cause of PID.
4. *Neisseria gonorrhoeae* is a common cause of PID.
5. *Treponema pallidum* does not cause PID.

TEST-TAKING HINT: It is important for the nurse to have a working knowledge of pathogens that cause infectious diseases. PID is caused by a bacterium. *Candida* is a yeast, and *Treponema*, the agent that causes syphilis, is a spirochete. The two bacterial organisms listed—*Chlamydia trachomatis* and *Neisseria gonorrhoeae*—are the most common causes of PID. Although *Gardnerella vaginalis* is a bacterium, it is not a common cause of PID.

20. 1. This is not appropriate. The nurse should not assume knowledge of how the client feels.
2. This is not appropriate. The nurse must pursue the discussion since women often have no symptoms when infected with gonorrhea.
3. This is true. Women often have no symptoms when infected with gonorrhea.
4. This is not appropriate. The client has not been diagnosed with gonorrhea.

TEST-TAKING HINT: This client is exhibiting signs of denial or knowledge deficit related to STIs. The nurse must respectfully educate and persuade the client to seek care. Giving her the information that many women have no signs or symptoms of disease is essential.

21. 1. A cluster of vesicles is consistent with a diagnosis of herpes, not primary syphilis.
2. A pain-free lesion, called a chancre, is consistent with a diagnosis of primary syphilis.
3. A macular rash is not seen with primary syphilis. A reddish brown rash is seen with stage 2 syphilis.
4. A foul-smelling discharge is not seen with primary syphilis.

TEST-TAKING HINT: Syphilis is caused by a spirochete and, like other spirochetal illnesses, has a three-stage course. The first stage of the disease is the chancre stage. A chancre is a small, round, painless lesion that will disappear, even without treatment, after a month or so. If the client is not treated, the disease will progress to stage 2, during which a reddish brown rash develops, usually on the palms and soles, sores on the mucous membranes, or flu-like symptoms develop. If the client is still left untreated, the disease will progress to stage 3, the symptoms of which often appear years later and include: dementia, paralysis, numbness, and blindness. The damage resulting from the tertiary stage of syphilis is not reversible.

22. 1. Syphilis is treatable. The treatment of choice is penicillin.
2. Any time someone is infected with one sexually transmitted infection (STI), it is recommended that he or she be assessed for other STIs.
3. Cryotherapy is not performed on clients with syphilis.
4. This is unrelated.

TEST-TAKING HINT: Clients who have become infected with an STI may be innocent victims of an unfaithful partner, or may be engaging in risk-taking behavior. If either they or their partner/s are sexually intimate with at least one other person, they run the risk of exponentially greater exposure. It is important, therefore, that clients who have one disease be further evaluated for the presence of other infections.

23. 1. This is a fallacy. Both men and women can become infected from oral sex.
2. This is true. The mucous membranes of females and of the teenagers are more permeable to STIs than the mucous membranes of adults and males.
3. The best thing a sexually active man or woman can do is to use a condom—male or

female—during intercourse. The only way to stay absolutely disease-free is to practice celibacy.
4. This is a fallacy. Females are more susceptible to disease than are males.

TEST-TAKING HINT: A number of fallacies related to sexual activity are often shared in society. One of the most common fallacies is that oral sex is safe. It is not. Rather than infecting the reproductive system, the STI will infect the mucous membranes of the mouth. For example, genital warts have been seen in the mouth and throat, and herpes simplex 2 can infect the oral cavity. It is recommended that dental dams be used to minimize the transmission of STIs to the oral cavity if oral sex is practiced.

24. 1. This is not true. When clients with HIV receive therapy during pregnancy and throughout labor and delivery and their babies receive oral therapy after delivery, the transmission rate of HIV is almost zero.
2. The viral load and CD4 counts should be monitored regularly, but they do not need to be assessed daily.
3. This is true. She and her partner should use condoms during sexual intercourse.
4. Even though the transmission of HIV via oral sex is likely much lower than it is from genital or rectal intercourse, it is still a dangerous practice.

TEST-TAKING HINT: The human immunodeficiency virus is prone to mutation. It is important that clients use condoms whenever they have intercourse because if the virus mutates and the client becomes infected with two strains of the virus, the progression to AIDS is hastened.

25. 1. There are no injections for treating warts. There are gels and creams that can be applied to the warts.
2. This statement is incorrect. Warts usually spontaneously disappear after a period of time.
3. This statement is incorrect. It is a common practice to remove warts surgically.
4. This statement is true. It is not uncommon for warts to return a few months after an initial treatment.

TEST-TAKING HINT: Genital warts are caused by the human papillomavirus. There are more than 100 viral types of HPV. Most of them are harmless, but some high-risk types result in genital warts while others can cause cancer. Some of the topical treatments for genital warts can be applied at home by the individual or can be administered by a practitioner. Surgery and cryotherapy, also used to treat warts, must be performed by a skilled practitioner.

26. 1. This is true. The CDC has not approved any tests to detect HPV in men.
2. The CDC has not approved any tests to detect HPV in men.
3. The CDC has not approved any tests to detect HPV in men.
4. The CDC has not approved any tests to detect HPV in men.

TEST-TAKING HINT: Some gay men do have anal Pap smears done to attempt to detect cancer cells in the rectum. For more information, see https://www.cdc.gov/std/hpv/stdfact-hpv-and-men.htm).

27. 1. This statement is not true. The vaccine can be administered to women as young as 9 and up to age 26, whether sexually active or not.
2. This statement is not true. The vaccine does not protect against many strains of HPV.
3. This statement is true. There are very few side effects experienced by those who receive the vaccine.
4. This statement is not true.

TEST-TAKING HINT: The CDC Advisory Committee on Immunization Practices recommends that all young men and women between the ages of 11 and 12, or as young as age 9 and up to age 26, be immunized against HPV. There are two vaccines available in the United States.

28. 1. This statement is false. Spermicidal creams have been shown actually to increase the transmission of some sexually transmitted infections.
2. This statement is false. Spermicidal creams have been shown actually to increase the transmission of some sexually transmitted infections.
3. This statement is true. Spermicidal creams have been shown to actually increase the transmission of some sexually transmitted infections.
4. This statement is false. Spermicidal creams have not been shown to be cancer-causing agents.

TEST-TAKING HINT: This question is a lesson in changing practice. For many years, it was recommended that men and women always use condoms with spermicide to prevent the spread of STIs, including HIV. It has been shown, however, that latex and polyurethane condoms without added spermicide are effective. In

addition, there is evidence that some spermicides can actually increase the permeability of the mucous membranes to HIV.

29. 1. Oil- and petroleum-based products can destroy the latex in condoms.
2. The foreskin should be pulled back before applying the condom.
3. Before beginning to put the condom on, a reservoir should be created by pinching the end of the condom.
4. The condom should be removed immediately after ejaculation.

TEST-TAKING HINT: Latex condom use is an excellent means of infection control as well as the prevention of an unwanted pregnancy. However, this is true only when the condom is applied correctly. In addition to the items noted previously, the condom should be applied before any contact between partners has been made, the rim of the condom should be held when removed to keep the semen from spilling, and the male and female condoms should not be used simultaneously because the friction that is caused by the two devices can cause one of them to come off or break.

30. 1. Female condoms, like male condoms, should be used only once.
2. Water-based lubricants can be used with female condoms. The same is true of male condoms.
3. Using both the male and female condom together is not recommended.
4. The female condom should be removed by twisting the outer ring and pulling gently.

TEST-TAKING HINT: The goal of condom use is to prevent sperm from ascending into the uterine cavity and for sperm and/or infectious secretions from coming in contact with mucous membranes. The best way to prevent these situations from happening is by preventing leakage of the fluid in the condom as quickly as possible. The woman should twist and hold the rim of her condom while removing it from the vagina.

31. **1. Toxic shock syndrome (TSS) is associated with diaphragm use.**
2. TSS is not associated with IUD use.
3. TSS is not associated with the use of birth control pills.
4. TSS is not associated with the use of medroxyprogesterone acetate.

TEST-TAKING HINT: TSS is associated with women who use tampons, especially superabsorbent tampons, and those who use barrier types of contraceptives. It is important, therefore, that anyone who has already experienced an episode of TSS be warned against using those items (Allen, 2004).

32. **1. The cervical mucus becomes thin and elastic at the time of ovulation in order for sperm to enter the uterus.**
2. The cervical mucus becomes almost transparent and alkaline at the time of ovulation.
3. The mucus is leukocyte poor.
4. The quantity of cervical mucus increases at the time of ovulation.

TEST-TAKING HINT: At the time of ovulation, the cervical mucus is most receptive to the migration of sperm into the uterine cavity. It is thin, slippery, and alkaline, making it most hospitable to the sperm. Women can monitor the consistency of their cervical mucus daily to predict their most fertile periods.

33. **1. The woman should regularly check the diaphragm by looking at it with a good light source.**
2. The diaphragm should not be used during menstruation.
3. If the diaphragm is left in place for extended periods of time, the woman is at much higher risk for serious complications, especially toxic shock syndrome.
4. The diaphragm should never be powdered because of the possibility of irritation, infection, or cancer.

TEST-TAKING HINT: The diaphragm is only as good as the barrier it creates. If there are any holes or breaks in the material, sperm will be able to ascend into the uterine cavity. The woman, therefore, must carefully check for pin-sized holes by regularly examining the diaphragm with a good light source.

34. 1. The diaphragm provides insufficient protection when used without spermicide.
2. It is recommended that women not douche unless medically advised to do so.
3. The diaphragm should be left in place for at least 6 hours after intercourse has ended.
4. The diaphragm should be inserted no earlier than 4 hours before intercourse. If put in place before that time, additional spermicide must be inserted before intercourse begins.

TEST-TAKING HINT: Although spermicide is not recommended to be used with condoms, diaphragms that are being used for contraception

are not effective without the addition of spermicidal gels or creams.

35. 1. The intrauterine device is an effective contraceptive device, but it will not protect against sexually transmitted infections.
2. The female condom is recommended both for contraception and for infection control.
3. Bilateral tubal ligation is an effective contraceptive method, but it will not protect against sexually transmitted infections.
4. Birth control pills are effective contraceptive methods, but they will not protect against sexually transmitted infections.

TEST-TAKING HINT: The key to answering this question is the fact that the client has multiple sex partners. The client is at high risk for becoming pregnant but she is also at high risk for acquiring a sexually transmitted infection. It is important for the nurse to consider that fact when providing family planning information.

36. **1. When pregnancy occurs with an IUD in place, an ectopic pregnancy should be ruled out.**
2. Malformations of the fetus are uncommon.
3. Symptoms of PID are not similar to those of early pregnancy. The most common symptoms of PID are abdominal pain, dyspareunia, foul-smelling vaginal discharge or bleeding, and fever.
4. Twin pregnancies are no more common with a failed IUD than in general.

TEST-TAKING HINT: Pregnancies do not often occur with an IUD in place. When they do, they are often ectopic pregnancies implanted in the fallopian tubes. This is thought to be related to the IUD's effects on the uterine endometrium, making it less receptive to the embryo. The IUD is also thought to reduce the motility of the cilia at the opening of the fallopian tube. Copper-containing IUDs assist in birth control by continuously releasing a small amount of copper, resulting in prostaglandin release within the uterus. The formation of what is referred to by some experts as a "biologic foam" within the uterine cavity, has a toxic effect on sperm and ova and impairs implantation. If fertilization occurs, the combination of the biologic foam and reduced motility of the fallopian tube cilia can result in the fertilized egg implanting in the fallopian tube, outside of the uterus.

37. 1. To obtain the contraceptive patch, the client must obtain a prescription for the device from a healthcare practitioner.
2. The withdrawal method (coitus interruptus) is an unreliable method, especially for teenage males.
3. The female condom is about 95% effective as a contraceptive device and is also effective as an infection-control device.
4. Although no prescription is needed to use the contraceptive sponge, it is only about 80% effective. In addition, since the contraceptive sponge uses a spermicide as its means of contraception and infection control, its use may actually be dangerous.

TEST-TAKING HINT: Because this client refuses to see a physician or nurse practitioner, her contraceptive options are limited. Adolescents' sex practices are often different from those of adults. Teens rarely plan to have intercourse. Sexual intercourse often happens on the spur of the moment. It is important, therefore, that adolescents use a method that is immediately effective. In addition, it is not uncommon for adolescents to have more than one sexual partner. Infection control must be an additional consideration. Female condoms meet both needs. The most important elements of using the female condom are (1) always having it with you and (2) knowing how to use it effectively. Clients should also be informed about options available if the condom slips out of place or breaks.

38. **Answers 1, 2, 4, and 5 require follow-up with both the client and the nurse.**
1. This is not true. The surgical procedure is not easily reversible. It should be considered permanent sterilization.
2. This is not true. Menstruation will not cease.
3. The client's libido should remain unchanged.
4. This is not true. The procedure is performed at the umbilicus through an incision approximately 1 inch wide. It is not done through the cervix.
5. This is not true. The procedure can easily be done at the same time as a cesarean section after the baby's birth.

TEST-TAKING HINT: The NCLEX exam may ask the test taker to identify information that "requires follow-up." This indicates the test-taker must identify the statements or actions that are not appropriate or that are not true.

In this question, all of these statements are untrue except for statement #3. As such, all statements except statement #3 require "follow-up." The test taker must remember that

in a bilateral tubal ligation, surgery merely blocks the sperm from traveling to the egg to complete fertilization. There is more than one method to ligate the tube. A common method is to pull the fallopian tube into a loop, tie the loop off, then cut it off and cauterize the exposed ends. The ovary and uterus are untouched. As such, the client's hormones are unaffected, libido remains the same, and menstruation does not stop.

39. All choices—1, 2, 3, 4, and 5—are correct.
   1. The client's age should be considered.
   2. The client's ethical and moral beliefs should be considered.
   3. The client's sexual patterns should be considered.
   4. The client's socioeconomic status should be considered.
   5. The client's childbearing plans should be considered.

TEST-TAKING HINT: Each of these factors must be considered when providing family planning counseling. The age of the client will affect, for example, natural family planning, which is not the most appropriate means for women desiring reliable contraception or for women who are perimenopausal and have irregular menstrual cycles. The client's beliefs can markedly affect her choices. If the client has multiple sex partners, an infection-control device should be considered. Some choices are quite expensive and, depending on the client's access to insurance, may not be feasible. If a client has completed her family, she may wish a permanent form of birth control versus a client who is young and still interested in having children. Although the nurse selects the most appropriate options for the client from a medical perspective, however, the final decision is up to the client. As such, the client must be informed about the pros and cons of each method in order to make an informed choice.

40. 1. This is correct. To maintain the hormonal levels in the bloodstream, the client should take the pill as soon as she remembers.
   2. This is incorrect. If one pill is missed, it should be taken as soon as possible. If two or more pills are missed, an alternate form of contraception should be used for the remainder of the month.
   3. Breakthrough bleeding can happen at any time, but it rarely happens when one pill is taken a little late.
   4. A pregnancy test is not necessary unless the client is concerned that she may have become pregnant.

TEST-TAKING HINT: Women who take low-dose birth control pills experience fewer side effects than women who take high-dose pills. It is important, however, that the pills be taken regularly, ideally at the same time each day. If one pill is missed, it should be taken as soon as possible. If two or more are missed, an alternate form of contraception should be used for the rest of the month until her next period, and the client should contact her healthcare provider to determine whether or not the rest of the pills should be taken.

41. 1. Diaphragm is not appropriate. The client must touch her vagina to insert the device.
   2. Cervical cap is not appropriate. She must touch her vagina to insert the device.
   3. Although the intrauterine device is effective and the client is in a monogamous relationship, it is recommended that the client palpate for the string after each menses. This requires vaginal manipulation.
   4. The birth control pill would be the best choice for this client. She has no medical contraindications to the pill, she wishes to bear children in the future, and it requires no vaginal manipulation.

TEST-TAKING HINT: Multiple factors must be considered before suggesting a particular contraception choice for a client. Because of the number of choices available, the client benefits if the nurse narrows the recommended choices to those that are best in each situation, with the reasons the nurse feels they might not be desirable to the client. In the end, however, it is the client's choice.

42. 1. The client should palpate for the presence of the string at the external cervical os after each menses.
   2. It is not necessary to go on bedrest after an IUD insertion.
   3. Reports of dyspareunia (painful intercourse) should be communicated to the physician.
   4. There is no need to insert spermicidal jelly when an IUD is in place. The IUD is effective immediately.

TEST-TAKING HINT: The sudden onset of dyspareunia may indicate the development of Pelvic Inflammatory Disease (PID). The client should be examined to determine whether or not she has developed an infection.

43. 1. A woman may buy a morning-after pill at any pharmacy without a prescription in some states but not in all.

2. There are some states, like New York, that enable adolescents to obtain contraception, including emergency contraception, without a parent's consent. However, that is not true in all states.
3. An emergency room physician may be able to prescribe a high-dose BCP in some states but not in all. The high-dose BCP works similarly to the morning-after pill.
4. **This statement is true. Access to health care by adolescents, including access to birth control methods, is determined by individual states.**

TEST-TAKING HINT: It is essential that the nurse knows and understands the rights of clients in their state. It is important to note, however, that because the NCLEX-RN® is an international examination, state-specific information will not be asked. (For state-specific information, see www.guttmacher.org/statecenter/spibs/spib_OMCL.pdf.)

44. 1. This response is inappropriate. The nurse must provide the client with all of her options.
2. **This is correct. The nurse should discuss with the young client all of her possible choices.**
3. This response is inappropriate. The nurse must provide the client with all of her options.
4. This is an appropriate follow-up comment. Once the options are provided for the young woman, she may decide to maintain the pregnancy and be in need of assistance to tell her parents. However, it is not appropriate as an initial response.

TEST-TAKING HINT: Unless working in an environment that precludes the nurse from discussing the possibility of an abortion, the nurse is obligated to provide the young client with all of her choices—maintaining the pregnancy and keeping the baby, maintaining the pregnancy and planning an adoption, and terminating the pregnancy. The nurse with a personal bias against abortion should refer the client to another nurse who will discuss the option.

45. 1. Women who take the ethinyl-estradiol-and-levonorgestrel-combined pill menstruate every 3 months.
2. An ethinyl-estradiol-and-levonorgestrel-combined pill is a daily birth control pill.
3. **Women who take an ethinyl-estradiol-and-levonorgestrel-combined pill do experience breakthrough bleeding fairly often.**
4. Breastfeeding is not compatible with this pill.

TEST-TAKING HINT: Women who wish to breastfeed can take some types of birth control pills (BCPs) but not pills that contain an estrogen medication, such as this one. Estrogen inhibits milk production. If they wish to take BCPs, breastfeeding women should take progestin-only pills.

46. Answers 1 and 3 are correct.
1. **Women who smoke should be counseled against using the patch.**
2. A history of lung cancer is not a contraindication to the patch.
3. **Women who have a history of deep vein thrombosis (DVT) should be counseled against using the patch.**
4. Being a runner is not a contraindication to the patch.
5. A history of cholecystitis is not a contraindication to the patch.

TEST-TAKING HINT: Estradiol is a form of estrogen. Estrogen contributes to blood clot (thrombin) formation. Women 35 years and older who use the patch are at particularly high risk for the development of thrombi. Women with certain medical conditions such as diabetes or DVT or with lifestyle issues such as smoking that place them at high risk for thrombi should be counseled against use of the patch.

47. Answers 1 and 2 are correct.
1. **The lactational amenorrhea method (LAM) can be effective until 6 months postpartum.**
2. **As long as the client has had no period since delivery, the LAM can be effective.**
3. If the mother gives any supplementation, the LAM is not reliable.
4. There are no weight loss restrictions when using the LAM.
5. There are no sleep requirements when using the LAM.

TEST-TAKING HINT: The LAM is a natural family planning method that is highly effective for postpartum women. However, there are three criteria that must be in place for the method to be effective: (1) The client must be exclusively breastfeeding her baby; (2) the client's baby must be less than 6 months old; (3) the client must not yet have regained her menses after the delivery (see https://www.waba.org.my/resources/lam/index.htm#LAM).

48. Answers 2, 3, and 4 are correct.
1. This response indicates that further teaching is needed. Only water-based lubricants should be used with the diaphragm.
2. **This is true. If a client's weight either increases or decreases by 10 lb or more, the device must be refitted.**

3. **This is true. For the diaphragm to fit appropriately, the upper part of the rim must be pushed snugly under the symphysis.**
4. **This is true. Although the device is a type of barrier, it is ineffective without spermicide and the action of spermicide is only effective for 6 hours.**
5. This response indicates that further teaching is needed. The diaphragm should be cleaned with mild soap and water after each use.

TEST-TAKING HINT: The diaphragm is an excellent device if it is used properly. In addition to the factors cited in the question, the following guidelines apply: (1) the device must be refitted after a client has given birth; (2) it must remain in place for at least 6 hours after intercourse; (3) if the couple should decide to engage in intercourse again within the 6-hour period, additional spermicide must be inserted into the vagina without removing the diaphragm, before penile penetration.

49. 1. **Women who use the diaphragm have increased incidence of urinary tract infections.**
2. A diaphragm may be used by a woman with a history of herpes simplex infections, but the device will not protect the woman's partner from contracting the virus.
3. A woman with a history of DVT can safely use the diaphragm.
4. A diaphragm may be used by a woman with a history of HPV, but the device will not protect the woman's partner from contracting the virus.

TEST-TAKING HINT: Because the rim of the diaphragm must be inserted under the symphysis, the woman's urethra is sometimes occluded by the pressure of the ring within the vagina. This makes it difficult to completely empty the bladder when urinating. As a result, the woman is at high risk for developing urinary tract infections (Davis, 2011).

50. 1. The sponge may be inserted any time between 24 hours and a few minutes before intercourse.
2. **The sponge must be moistened with water until it is foamy.**
3. Additional spermicide need not be used.
4. This is not true. The sponge offers contraceptive protection for up to 24 hours no matter how many times a couple has intercourse.

TEST-TAKING HINT: Because of its ability to protect a woman from becoming pregnant for up to a full day no matter how many times a couple has intercourse, the sponge is a very popular method. It must be remembered, however, that the sponge does not protect against sexually transmitted infections and its effectiveness is not as high as the effectiveness of other methods such as condoms.

51. 1. Douching is not only ineffective as a contraceptive method, it can also adversely change the pH in the vagina, contributing to the risk of infection.
2. A post-coital contraceptive is not necessary if the man carefully removes the condom.
3. **This is true. The man should carefully remove the condom while holding its edges.**
4. Applying spermicide to the upper edges of the condom is not appropriate. While attempting to apply the spermicide, sperm could easily spill from the condom.

TEST-TAKING HINT: The penis becomes flaccid very rapidly after ejaculation. The man should carefully remove the penis from the vagina before the penis becomes flaccid while holding the edges of the condom. If it does become flaccid, he should be especially careful during its removal.

52. 1. **This is true. It is very important that women be evaluated to make sure that the pregnancy is terminated. Even when bleeding occurs, the pregnancy may still be intact.**
2. This is not true. Mifepristone/misoprostol should not be used when an IUD is in place. The IUD should be removed before the medication is administered.
3. This is not true. Bleeding is not the only symptom women experience. Women usually complain of cramping, nausea, vomiting, and fatigue. A number of other complaints have also been made.
4. This can cause unnecessary delay. If there is no bleeding, the woman should be seen by the physician for additional treatment.

TEST-TAKING HINT: Mifepristone/misoprostol is available for use in terminating unwanted pregnancies, for completing incomplete spontaneous abortions, and for terminating ectopic pregnancies. If the medicine proves to be ineffective and the pregnancy survives, there is a strong possibility that the fetus will be damaged. It is very important, therefore, that the client be assessed to make sure that she truly aborted the conceptus.

53. 1. **The male condom is the best device for this client.**
2. Because she has multiple sex partners, the IUD is not the best choice for this client.

3. The etonogestrel/ethinyl estradiol vaginal ring is a hormonal device. Because this client is over 35 years old and is a smoker, the etonogestrel/ethinyl estradiol vaginal ring is not the best choice for her.
4. Oral contraceptives are hormonally based. Because this client is over 35 years old and is a smoker, birth control pills are not the best choice for her.

TEST-TAKING HINT: Even when perimenopausal clients are being counseled, the nurse must ask about drug use, smoking, sexual patterns, and so forth. It cannot be assumed that simply because a client is in her 50s or more that she is asexual or that she is engaging in safe lifestyle choices.

54. 1. This is inappropriate. This client should be seen by her healthcare practitioner.
2. This is inappropriate. This client should be seen by her healthcare practitioner.
3. This is an appropriate statement. This client should be seen by her healthcare practitioner.
4. This is inappropriate. This client should be seen by her healthcare practitioner.

TEST-TAKING HINT: Clients who use hormonally based contraceptive methods are at high risk for clot formation. This client is communicating symptoms that may indicate the presence of a clot. She should be seen by her practitioner to rule out deep vein thrombosis that could lead to stroke.

55. 1. This is not appropriate. The basal body temperature (BBT) should be taken upon awakening in the morning.
2. This is correct. The couple should chart temperatures for at least 6 months.
3. This is not appropriate. The couple should wait to engage in intercourse until the client's temperature has been elevated above preovulation baseline for at least 3 days.
4. An additional action that can be taken as a complement to the temperature rhythm method is cervical mucus assessment, but it is not required. The elasticity of the mucus should be assessed, not the color or odor of the mucus.

TEST-TAKING HINT: It is essential that a full 6 months of information be obtained before using the rhythm method as a birth control device. All activities should be recorded on the BBT sheet. For example, the couple should document when the client has a period, when they have intercourse, when they sleep late, and when the client feels ill. Each of these situations, and many more, can affect the client's temperature.

56. 1. This is not true. The menstrual cycle of perimenopausal women is very irregular. It is very difficult to identify safe and unsafe periods for these women.
2. This is true. This client is a multigravida in a monogamous relationship. She is low risk for infections as well as spontaneous expulsion of the device.
3. This is true. Even with very irregular menses the client may still be ovulating.
4. This is true. The patch contains both an estrogen and a progesterone medication.

TEST-TAKING HINT: After providing any kind of teaching, including teaching about contraceptive measures, it is very important to evaluate the client's understanding. A client's misunderstanding could easily result in unexpected pregnancy, injury to her or, if she were to become pregnant, to the unborn baby.

57. 1. The fact that the client has two children will not necessarily affect her contraceptive choice. Some couples with two children have completed their childbearing, while others wish to have many more children.
2. The frequency of intercourse is usually not a consideration unless the client has intercourse with a number of partners.
3. This particular client's age does not preclude her from using any device. However, clients over age 35, especially if they smoke, should not use any of the hormonally based contraceptive methods.
4. This statement is very important. If the client refuses to touch her genital area, she is an unlikely candidate for a number of contraceptive devices: female condom, diaphragm, sponge, cervical cap, and IUD.

TEST-TAKING HINT: It is very important for the nurse to listen very carefully to clients' comments. Many of their statements will influence the nurse's teaching in only minor ways, while other client comments will dramatically affect the nurse's birth control suggestions. However, all appropriate methods must be offered, as the final decision belongs to the client. The nurse must share the pros and cons of each method and explain why some options are medically contraindicated. In this client scenario, the nurse might not know that the client is willing to learn how to overcome her current discomfort with touching her "private parts."

58. 1. Although this client has no medical contraindications to using birth control pills, she is having intercourse with a number of partners and, therefore, needs a method that will protect her from infection.

2. **Of the four clients listed, this client is the best candidate for the use of the birth control pill.**
3. This client has chronic hypertension. She is already at high risk for thrombus formation and stroke and birth control pills would increase her risk.
4. This client is over 35 years old and smokes. She is already at high risk for thrombus formation and stroke and the birth control pill would increase her risk.

TEST-TAKING HINT: Birth control pills that contain both estrogen and progesterone are inappropriate for clients who breastfeed because the estrogen inhibits milk production. There is no such contraindication for mothers who bottle feed. It is important to remember, however, that women who breastfeed can use progestin-only pills and still maintain their milk supply.

59. Answers 1, 2, 3, and 5 are correct.

1. **It would be appropriate to recommend the IUD to a high school student.**
2. **It would be appropriate to recommend the IUD to a recent college graduate.**
3. **It would be appropriate to recommend the IUD to a 24-year-old nullip.**
4. This client has a recent history of a sexually transmitted infection. She is not the best candidate for the IUD.
5. **It would be appropriate to recommend the IUD to a client who has two children.**

TEST-TAKING HINT: The American Academy of Pediatrics has published a policy statement recommending that pediatricians counsel sexually active adolescents to choose contraceptive options that are the most effective and require the least amount of adherence, that is, progestin implants and IUDs (American Academy of Pediatrics, 2014). Teens should be counseled also to use a condom for infection control and to consider celibacy. Although in the past, nulliparous clients who had IUDs inserted often complained of pain and many expelled the devices, nulliparous women prescribed IUDs currently on the market usually experience few, if any, side effects.

60.
1. Multiparity is not a risk factor for osteoporosis.
2. Not only does obesity not cause osteoporosis, but some believe that obesity is a protective factor against loss of bone density.
3. Early-onset menopause is a risk factor for osteoporosis.
4. **Alcohol consumption is a contributing factor to osteoporosis.**

TEST-TAKING HINT: Daily consumption of alcohol is a contributing factor to the development of osteoporosis because alcohol interferes with the absorption of vitamin D and calcium in the body. An adequate consumption of vitamin D and calcium is essential for strong bones, and alcohol should be consumed in moderation. Because estrogen promotes bone density, early onset of menopause and the accompanying reduction in estrogen is a risk factor for osteoporosis.

61.
1. **This is a true statement. Clients are to take the medication on an empty stomach immediately after awakening and remain upright for at least 30 minutes.**
2. This statement is incorrect. Clients should take the medication on an empty stomach.
3. Depending on the dosage, the medication is given either once weekly or once daily.
4. This statement is not true. The medication comes in tablet form with no precautions against breaking or crushing.

TEST-TAKING HINT: Alendronate must be consumed with a full glass of water on an empty stomach. It is especially important that the client sit upright for at least 30 minutes after taking the medication because severe upper gastrointestinal irritation can result when reclining. Esophageal irritation, ulceration, and erosions can develop when the medication is taken improperly.

62.
1. **Calcium absorption is enhanced dramatically when vitamin D is also consumed.**
2. Calcium absorption is not directly related to vitamin E consumption.
3. Calcium absorption is not directly related to folic acid consumption.
4. Calcium consumption can inhibit iron absorption.

TEST-TAKING HINT: To maintain proper bone health, it is important for clients, especially women, to consume sufficient quantities of both calcium and vitamin D. The recommended intake of vitamin D from age 1 to 70 is 600 international units per day; after the age of 70, 800 international units per day. The recommended calcium intake for individuals in the young adult to age 50 group is 1,000 mg per day and after the age of 50, 1,200 mg per day.

63.
1. This is not true. There are situations when hormone replacement therapy (HRT) is recommended.

2. **Women who are experiencing severe menopausal symptoms can benefit from HRT. However, it is recommended that they not be on the medication for an extended period of time.**
3. HRT should not be given to women to prevent or treat coronary artery disease.
4. Women with a history of breast cancer should not take HRT.

TEST-TAKING HINT: Although it was once thought that HRT protected women from coronary artery disease, new evidence shows that it is not the case. HRT does help to protect women from osteoporosis, but the incidence of breast cancer in women who take the medication does increase. The recommendation by the FDA is that women who need to take HRT for menopausal symptom relief should do so at the lowest dose possible for the shortest period of time possible. Those who are prone to osteoporosis should use other means—for example, exercise, plus calcium and vitamin D intake—to prevent bone loss.

64. 1. Fibroids are benign tumors of the myometrium. Douching does not increase the incidence of fibroids.
2. **Douching can increase a client's potential for endometritis (pelvic inflammatory disease).**
3. Cervical cancer is almost exclusively caused by the human papillomavirus that is contracted through sexual contact.
4. Polyps are abnormal tissue growths. They do not develop as a result of douching.

TEST-TAKING HINT: Endometritis, an inflammation of the lining of the uterus (the endometrium), is also called pelvic inflammatory disease (PID) when the condition is not associated with pregnancy, as in this question. Endometritis is not the same thing as *endometriosis.* The act of douching can cause serious gynecological infections up to and including PID. When a client douches, she disrupts the normal flora in her vagina. Pathogens can then invade the area and the douching solution can push the pathogens into the upper gynecological system. Douching should never be performed unless ordered by a healthcare practitioner.

65. Answers 2, 3, and 4 are correct.
1. Yellow and orange vegetables are rich in vitamin A. There is no recommendation to increase one's intake of vitamin A to prevent osteoporosis.
2. **Daily exercise does help to prevent the development of osteoporosis, since it strengthens the bones.**
3. **Smoking is associated with the development of osteoporosis.**
4. **Dairy products contain calcium and many have vitamin D added. Both of these nutrients are essential for preventing osteoporosis.**
5. There is no evidence that the lack of sleep is a contributing factor to the development of osteoporosis.

TEST-TAKING HINT: There are a number of factors that clients are unable to control in relation to the development of osteoporosis—for example, gender (women are more at risk than men), age (older women are more at risk than younger women), and genetics (family history plays a role). Any client who is at risk because of the preceding factors should be especially counseled to eat well, stop smoking, drink alcohol in moderation, and get daily exercise.

66. 1. Clients with bulimia often show little fluctuation in weight and are usually hypokalemic.
2. Bulimia is not related to respiratory acidosis or hypoxemia.
3. **Dental caries and scars on the knuckles are classic signs of bulimia.**
4. Hyperglycemia with polyuria is associated with diabetes mellitus.

TEST-TAKING HINT: Clients with bulimia force themselves to vomit in an effort to expel ingested calories after eating. Teeth are adversely affected because of the contact of stomach acids with the teeth due to frequent and repeated vomiting. The knuckle scarring, called Russell's sign, develops from tissue injury during the act of jamming the fingers down the throat to force vomiting. Clients with this condition may also take large quantities of cathartics.

67. Answers 1 and 2 are correct.
1. **The nurse would expect to see a low potassium level. The Merck Manual lists the normal potassium levels as 3.5 to 5 mEq/L.**
2. **The nurse would expect to see a high bicarbonate level. The Merck Manual lists the normal bicarbonate level as 23 to 28 mmol/L.**
3. The nurse would not expect to see a high platelet count.
4. Unless the client was a diabetic, the nurse would not expect to see a high glycosylated hemoglobin level.
5. The nurse would not expect to see a high sodium level.

TEST-TAKING HINT: By forcing themselves to vomit, clients with bulimia lose electrolytes and hydrochloric acid from their stomachs. The primary electrolytes that become skewed are potassium, sodium, chloride, and bicarbonate. The large volume loss of gastric secretions leads to secretion of bicarbonate into the blood (Brinkman & Sharma, 2020), driving it well above the normal levels of 20 mmol/L. To review the physiology, if the client is vomiting repeatedly, the loss of stomach acids upsets the acid–base balance. All acids produced must equal all acid that's lost. Parietal cells in the stomach create and replace the hydrochloric acid (HCL). The "payment" for the acid ingredients is bicarbonate ions. The location of the parietal cells, between the stomach and the veins gives them a convenient "front door" to the stomach and a "back door" to the veins (or pantry) that service the stomach. For each hydrogen (H) and chlorine (CL) ion the cells pull from the blood (the pantry) to replace the HCL that was vomited, they create and "exchange" one bicarbonate (base) ion, putting it into the blood as payment (Heitzmann & Warth, 2007). This is sometimes referred to as the "alkaline tide." The blood now has a higher level of bicarbonate (HCO_3) than normal, leading to a higher pH and higher bicarbonate levels. Resulting low potassium levels put clients at high risk for cardiac arrhythmias. Their cardiac status should be carefully monitored. (For normal lab values see https://www.merckmanuals.com/en-pr/professional/resources/normal-laboratory-values/blood-tests-normal-values).

68. 1. Mastoiditis is inflammation of the mastoid bones. This usually results from the progression of a middle ear infection.
2. Hirsutism is characterized by excessive hair growth. Alopecia, or loss of hair, is commonly seen in bulimic clients.
3. Gynecomastia is the hypertrophy of the breast tissue in males. This is not related to bulimia.
4. Esophagitis is a common finding in people with bulimia.

TEST-TAKING HINT: Because clients with bulimia repeatedly induce vomiting, the client's esophagus is repeatedly exposed to stomach acids. As a result, they may develop a variety of upper gastrointestinal complications, including esophagitis. Clients who also abuse laxatives may have guaiac-positive stools.

69. 1. The nurse should follow up on her observations.
2. The evidence does not suggest that the young woman is being abused.
3. The nurse should not simply refer the young woman to a doctor.
4. The nurse should follow the young woman into the bathroom to see if she is vomiting.

TEST-TAKING HINT: This young woman is exhibiting presumptive signs of bulimia such as Russell's sign (knuckle scarring), gorging (eating a large, calorie-filled meal), and proceeding to the bathroom immediately after eating. It is very likely that the young woman will purge herself of the large meal by self-induced vomiting. The nurse should then discuss her observations with the young woman and, if appropriate, with her parents.

70. 1. People with anorexia commonly engage in excessive exercise regimes.
2. Significant weight loss and amenorrhea are characteristic signs of anorexia.
3. These symptoms are related to severe upper respiratory illnesses, such as cystic fibrosis.
4. Cardiac arrhythmias are more characteristic of bulimia than anorexia.

TEST-TAKING HINT: The diagnostic criteria for anorexia nervosa are a body weight that is less than 85% of that expected, a pathological fear of gaining weight, a disturbed body image, and the failure to have a menstrual period for three or more cycles. Clients who are anorexic are usually women, and are often high achievers who also exercise to excess.

71. 1. Asking the client for the date of her last menstrual period is the best response. The school nurse should also note that the client's weight is very low and that her exercise schedule is extreme.
2. Encouraging the client to continue her exercise schedule is inappropriate. This young woman is exhibiting clear signs of anorexia nervosa.
3. Congratulating the client on her weight maintenance is inappropriate. This young woman is exhibiting clear signs of anorexia nervosa.
4. Advising the client to choose between swimming or soccer is inappropriate. This young woman is exhibiting clear signs of anorexia nervosa and it should not be normalized.

TEST-TAKING HINT: This question requires the test taker to calculate the percentage of the young woman's weight in relation to her expected weight. Once it is noted that she is more than 15% below her expected weight ($120 - \frac{96}{120} \times 100 = 20\%$) and that she exercises excessively, the nurse needs to assess whether or not she is exhibiting another sign of anorexia nervosa—namely, amenorrhea.

72. 1. The nurse is not required by law to report the injuries.
2. **This is an appropriate statement.**
3. The nurse must develop a rapport with the client before accusing the partner of abuse.
4. This statement implies that the partner was justified in abusing the client. This is inappropriate.

TEST-TAKING HINT: **Women (or men) who are being abused will often deny the abuse. It is not uncommon for abused women to enter the healthcare system a number of times before making the decision to terminate the relationship with the abuser. The nurse must discuss observations of concern with the young woman—always in private—and provide the client with possible options at each visit. It is essential that the nurse not ignore the signs, no matter how many times the client denies that she is being abused.**

73. Answers 1, 2, 3, and 4 are correct.
1. **"Have you ever been forced to have sex?" is a question that should be asked at each healthcare contact.**
2. **"Are you sexually active?" is a question that should be asked at each healthcare contact.**
3. **"Are you afraid to go home?" is a question that should be asked at each healthcare contact.**
4. **"Does anyone you know ever hit you?" is a question that should be asked at each healthcare contact.**
5. It is not necessary to ask a client if she has ever breastfed every time she is seen for a healthcare visit.

TEST-TAKING HINT: **Women (or men) who are being abused rarely discuss their relationships unless asked directly. To identify clients who are being threatened, physically abused, and/or sexually abused, it is essential that nurses query them at each visit. The questioning can be done during a face-to-face interview or via a paper-and-pencil questionnaire. If the client states that she is being abused, the nurse should be ready to provide information on safe environments, police contacts, etc. To be able to provide comprehensive care, the nurse should also inquire about whether or not the client is sexually active in order to inform the client of possible risk factors as indicated.**

74. 1. **A promise to never hit someone again is an example of a comment made during the "honeymoon phase."**
2. Some abusers have set patterns to their behavior, like drinking and abusing only on weekends.
3. During the "tension-building" phase, abusers often abuse verbally and may even engage in some physical abuse.
4. Insomnia is not typically part of the "cycle of violence."

TEST-TAKING HINT: **The nurse must understand that an abusive relationship cycles through stages of love and commitment (the honeymoon phase), followed by abuse, and then once again enters a honeymoon phase of apology and commitment and promises to never abuse again. The initial love and commitment phase lasts well into the time when the relationship becomes violent. The feelings generated by both parties during the "honeymoon phase" revisit that early period of the relationship, but do not guarantee that the violence will not occur again. It is essential, therefore, for the nurse to develop a rapport with the victim and to remind her that no one deserves to be abused. Options must then be provided to her. Even if she refuses to acknowledge her situation at first, the nurse must revisit the discussion every time the client revisits the healthcare system, making sure not to stigmatize or alienate the client.**

75. Answers 2, 3, and 4 are correct.
1. Telling the client she should have left earlier is inappropriate. The victim should be praised for making the decision to leave even if it took many years.
2. **It is very important to assist the victim to develop a safety plan. The victim will likely be in danger once the abuser learns that she has decided to leave.**
3. **It is very important to remind the victim that the abuse was not her fault. Many victims believe that they deserve the violence.**
4. **It is very important to help the victim to contact a domestic violence center. This is a very difficult step for victims to take.**

TEST-TAKING HINT: **After many years of abuse, victims often have very low self-esteem and are very frightened of their abusers. They need a great deal of emotional support as well as clear, structured guidance in how to leave the relationship. Nurses must be prepared to supply the support (see http://mysistersplacedc.org).**

76. 1. Taking the client's vital signs is not the highest priority.
2. **This is essential. The client must be interviewed in private.**
3. Assessing for additional bruising is not the highest priority.

4. Documenting the location of the bruises is not the highest priority.

TEST-TAKING HINT: This client is exhibiting classic signs of physical abuse. The partner is domineering and the client has injuries that are not supported by the history. To obtain a more accurate history, the nurse must interview the client alone. This can often take place in the women's restroom since, unless the partner is a woman, the partner is unable to follow.

77. Answers 1, 2, 4, and 5 are correct.
   1. **Healthcare providers should be suspicious that a client is a victim of abuse when the client denies the severity of injuries, or denies that injuries occurred.**
   2. **The history should be assessed very carefully. Often the injuries are not supported by the story.**
   3. Victims of abuse frequently refuse to make eye contact with healthcare practitioners.
   4. **Abusers frequently dominate conversations with their victims. When asked questions by the nurse, abusers frequently respond rather than allowing their partners to respond.**
   5. **Women who frequently skip prenatal or other follow-up appointments must be queried regarding the reason for the absences. There are many possible explanations—for example, they may have no transportation to the site or they may be forced to remain at home because of visible injuries. If prudent, a visiting nurse might be sent to the home to determine the reason for the absences.**

TEST-TAKING HINT: Nurses must use all their senses when interviewing clients. A physical assessment should be conducted and questions about presumptive evidence of abuse must be discussed. In addition, the client's communications must be critically assessed. Women who always defer to their partners may be exhibiting a sign of abuse. In addition, the history provided by the client and/or her partner must be evaluated for its credibility. If any injuries do not coincide with the story provided, the nurse must investigate the situation further while always keeping in mind the risk to the client if the partner suspects she has been "saying too much."

78. Answers 1, 2, and 4 are correct.
   1. **A buccal swab may be taken. The client's DNA must be ruled out when compared to any specimens obtained.**
   2. **Pubic hair samples may be obtained. These are compared with any specimens taken from the crime scene.**
   3. Toenail scrapings are not usually obtained, but fingernail scrapings may be.
   4. **Head hair samples are obtained. These are compared with any specimens taken from the crime scene.**
   5. Sputum is usually not analyzed.

TEST-TAKING HINT: In many ways, a rape examination is another form of invasion for a client who has been raped. Prior to the exam, the examiner must request permission by the victim to obtain samples. It is important to explain the process of obtaining the sample and what the client will be asked to do to assist in obtaining the sample. Other samples that may be obtained include vaginal smears. The examiner may request to keep any or all clothing worn by the victim, and may request to take pictures of the injuries, if present. If the perpetrator were to go to trial, it would be far in the future. By that time the victim will no longer have any outward signs of assault. It is important to provide the prosecution with as much evidence as possible if a conviction is to be obtained. It is essential to remember, however, that the victim must be allowed to refuse any part of the examination (see www.rainn.org).

79. Answers 1, 4, and 5 are correct.
   1. **It is essential that young women remember to drink liquids only from containers that they have opened themselves and that have never been out of their possession.**
   2. Although keeping extra money in one's shoes or bra is a good idea, it will not protect a young client from a sexual assault.
   3. It is an excellent idea for young women to keep condoms in their pocketbook in case they decide, unexpectedly, to engage in consensual sexual intercourse. However, this is not a suggestion that should be given as a protection against sexual assault.
   4. **Young women should be encouraged to meet new dates in a public place. It is unlikely that an assault will occur in a place where others are present.**
   5. **When a mixed group goes out together, it is unlikely that an assault will take place.**

TEST-TAKING HINT: It is very important that young women protect themselves from date rape. Being in a crowd is one excellent way to prevent the potential for being a victim of sexual assault. And because odorless and tasteless date rape drugs can be added to beverages, it is important for

young women to consume drinks that have not been out of their sight.

80. 1. It is likely that this client has been a victim of a sexual assault rather than showing signs of being spoiled.
 2. It is likely that this client has been a victim of a sexual assault rather than someone having a psychotic break.
 3. It is likely that this client has been a victim of a sexual assault, not consensual sex.
 4. It is likely that this client has been a victim of a sexual assault after ingesting a date rape drug.

TEST-TAKING HINT: Women who have ingested date rape drugs often experience some amnesia afterward. Date rape drugs can decrease a woman's ability to resist sexual aggression. The medications can be detected in urine samples up to 72 hours after ingestion.

81. **1. This client has just been violated. It is essential that she be treated kindly, in a location where she feels safe.**
 2. The young client should be offered postcoital contraception, but this is not the priorityaction at this time.
 3. The young client should be offered sexually transmitted infection prophylaxis, but this is not the priority action at this time.
 4. A health history should be taken, but this is not the priority action at this time.

TEST-TAKING HINT: The initial action the nurse must perform when caring for a client who has just been sexually assaulted is to provide the client with an environment that enables them to regain a feeling of control. The nurse should ask permission for all care, including history taking. And the care should take place in a secure location. Only after the client has given permission for care should the nurse and other caregivers discuss other issues like history, postcoital contraception, and prophylaxis for infections.

82. 1. Benefits of the evidence kit should be made only after the nurse has told the client that her actions were appropriate.
 2. This statement acknowledges the fact that the client needed to regain some control over her situation.
 3. Only after telling the client that her actions were appropriate should the nurse ask if the client washed her clothes.
 4. Only after the nurse has asked the client if it is all right to ask questions about the assault should the client be asked if she remembers anything about the incident.

TEST-TAKING HINT: A very common response by women to a sexual assault is the need to cleanse their bodies. They frequently state that they feel "dirty." This action does destroy much of the evidence needed if the case were to go to trial, but the nurse must communicate to the client an understanding and acceptance of the young woman's decisions without making her feel guilty or fearful that she has done something wrong.

83. 1. This statement is not true. EC is available and legal in all of the United States.
 2. This statement is not true. The most common side effects from EC are nausea, vomiting, and headache.
 3. This statement is not true. EC medications are essentially high-dose birth control pills.
 4. This statement is true. Although EC works up to 5 days after unprotected intercourse, it is most effective when taken within 72 hours of the exposure.

TEST-TAKING HINT: It is essential that the nurse understand the differences between EC and an abortifacient. EC is used to prevent pregnancy after unprotected intercourse. If the woman is unknowingly pregnant at the time she takes EC, she will not abort the fetus. EC is used up to 5 days following exposure, while an abortifacient such as mifepristone/misoprostol is used to abort a fetus and is used up to 70 days from the first day of the last menstrual period.

84. 1. This statement is incorrect. Lesbian women are neither more nor less sexually active than straight women.
 2. This statement is incorrect. Domestic violence can occur in any relationship, straight or gay.
 3. This statement is incorrect. Gay women should have Pap tests at the same frequency as straight women.
 4. This statement is true. All women who are sexually active should be monitored for sexually transmitted infections.

TEST-TAKING HINT: The special needs of gay clients are often ignored by healthcare workers. When caring for clients, one question that should be asked is the client's sexual orientation and preferred pronouns. Unless the nurse asks the question, important issues may be missed.

85. 1. This statement is incorrect but, although unexpected vaginal bleeding and weight loss are not related to ovarian cancer, the symptoms should be assessed by a healthcare provider.

2. This statement is incorrect. Frequent urination, breast tenderness, and extreme fatigue are seen in early pregnancy.
3. **This statement is correct. Abdominal pain, bloating, and feeling of fullness are early symptoms of ovarian cancer.**
4. This statement is incorrect but, although a firm area on the abdomen is not related to ovarian cancer, the symptom should be assessed by a healthcare provider.

TEST-TAKING HINT: Ovarian cancer is often called the silent killer because it is rarely diagnosed in its early stages. The following signs/symptoms, in addition to those listed above, have been identified as early signs of the disease: pelvic pain, abdominal growth, and difficulty eating. Women should be advised to seek care from their healthcare providers if they experience the symptoms.

86.
1. Stating the doctor will cure the client's cancer is inappropriate. The client does not have cancer at this time.
2. Deferring all information to the doctor is inappropriate. The nurse should provide information about fibrocystic breast disease as requested by the client.
3. Describing criteria for diagnosis is inappropriate. Although breast cysts are usually round and mobile, any nodule felt by a client should be assessed by a healthcare practitioner.
4. **Recommending regular mammograms is the best response. This client does not have cancer but should be carefully monitored.**

TEST-TAKING HINT: Because women who have fibrocystic breast disease have very dense and nodular breasts, it is very difficult to detect cancerous lesions by simple palpation. It is very important, therefore, that these women have regular mammograms and ultrasounds and magnetic resonance images (MRIs), if recommended, to monitor for malignant changes.

87. Answers 1, 2, 4, and 5 are correct.
1. **The flat part of the fingers should be used to palpate the breast.**
2. **The breast should be palpated using three pressure depths—light, middle, and deep.**
3. Evidence of dimpling should be assessed while looking in a mirror.
4. **The women should feel for lumps throughout the entire breast, including the tail of Spence, while standing and while lying down.**
5. **Women should assess for nipple discharge.**

TEST-TAKING HINT: The nurse should be familiar with BSE and be able to teach women how to perform the skill. Clients are then able to take an active role in their own health. In addition, however, it is important for the nurse to advise women that neither BSE nor a palpation examination performed by a healthcare practitioner has been shown to increase survival rates in clients with breast cancer. Only mammography has been shown to increase survival rates.

88.
1. This statement is false. Oral enzymes do not eradicate HPV from the mouth.
2. **This statement is correct. To prevent oral infection, sexually active individuals should wear dental dams when engaging in oral intercourse.**
3. There is insufficient research to determine whether HPV vaccines effectively prevent oral as well as genital and rectal HPV infections.
4. There is no diagnostic test to detect HPV in the oropharyngeal cavity that has been approved by the FDA.

TEST-TAKING HINT: Sequelae related to oral HPV such as warts and cancer, are on the rise. It has been estimated that up to 80% of adolescents engage in oral intercourse, falsely assuming that unprotected oral intercourse is safe. This is thought to be related to the rise in oral HPV. To prevent transmission of HPV to the oropharyngeal cavity, it is recommended that individuals wear a dental dam—a piece of latex inserted into the mouth—whenever engaging in oral intercourse.

4 Low Risk Antepartum

Pregnancy is divided broadly into three phases: (1) antepartum, the period of time from conception to the onset of labor; (2) intrapartum, the phase that includes the onset of labor through delivery of the placenta; and (3) postpartum, also known as the puerperium, the 6-week period of time after delivery in which maternal physiological changes of pregnancy return to their pre-pregnant state. This chapter covers normal prenatal care during the antepartum phase of pregnancy.

Each of these phases is further divided into more discrete time frames. The antepartum phase is divided by thirds into trimesters with each trimester counting approximately 12 weeks of the 40-week pregnancy. The first trimester, counted from conception to 12 weeks' gestation, is often a period of physical discomfort that includes nausea, vomiting, fatigue, and urinary frequency. This trimester is the most important one for fetal development as all the frameworks and structures for body systems are formed. Before taking medication or natural supplements of any kind, the woman should confirm with her provider that the medication or herbs will not interfere with fetal and placental development.

The second trimester, from week 13 through week 26, is generally one of excitement and anticipation. The mother feels well, is no longer nauseated, and begins to feel a connection with the fetus as she feels it moving inside. Fetal body systems are growing and maturing steadily after being formed in the first trimester.

By the time women complete their third trimester, weeks 29 through delivery at around 40 weeks' gestation, they are often very uncomfortable, dealing with backaches, trouble breathing because of the size of the uterus against the diaphragm, and frequent urination as a result of less bladder capacity. By the time the baby is ready to be born, mothers are usually more than ready for labor to begin.

The nurse must be prepared to counsel, support, and provide anticipatory guidance to the client throughout the antepartum period to inform the clients about what to expect, what is normal, and danger signs to report. The nurse must never assume, however, that all clients wish to receive the information in the same way, or with the same detail. Care must be individualized and guided by each client's needs and understanding of pregnancy.

KEYWORDS

The following words include English vocabulary, nursing/medical terminology, concepts, principles, or information relevant to content specifically addressed in the chapter or associated with topics presented in it. English dictionaries, your nursing textbooks, and medical dictionaries such as *Taber's Cyclopedic Medical Dictionary* are resources that can be used to expand your knowledge and understanding of these words and related information.

Ambivalence
Amnion
Amniotic fluid
Antepartum
Birth plan
Blastocyst
Chadwick's sign
Chloasma
Chorion
Chorionic villi
Corpus luteum
Couvade

Decidua
DHA (docosahexaenoic acid)
Dizygotic twins
Embryo
Estrogen
Fetal development
Fetus
Fundal height
Fundus
Gravida
Hegar's sign
Human chorionic gonadotropin
Human placental lactogen
Kyphosis
Lanugo
Lightening
Linea nigra
Listeria
Medication pregnancy category
Melasma
Monozygotic twins
Montgomery glands
Morula
Mucous plug
Multigravida
Certified nurse midwife (CNM)
Oral glucose tolerance test (OGTT) fasting and non-fasting
Organogenesis
Physiological anemia of pregnancy
Pica
Placenta
Positive signs of pregnancy
Pregnancy
Presumptive signs of pregnancy
Primigravida
Probable signs of pregnancy
Progesterone
Prostaglandin
Quickening
Spider nevi
Striae gravidarum
Surfactant
Symphysis
Teratogen
Trimester
Umbilicus
Vegan
Vernix caseosa
Xiphoid process

QUESTIONS

CASE STUDY: *The first three questions are part of a case study. This is based on a bowtie question format that nursing graduates may see in the Next Generation NCLEX© (NGN) exam (National Council of State Boards of Nursing, 2021). On the computerized test, the test taker will drag the appropriate answer into the appropriate box. Note that the first answer applies to the center box, with answers to question 2 in the boxes on the left, and answers to question 3 in the boxes on the right. For the purposes of this book, the test taker can select the correct answers as in any multiple-choice question. The bowtie diagram is given to provide familiarity with the format.*

(National Council of State Boards of Nursing [NCSBN], 2020). For more information on the Next Generation NCLEX (NGN) question formats, see NGN quarterly newsletters at https://www.ncsbn.org.
NCLEX questions assume the nurse has a provider's order for listed interventions, unless noted otherwise.

A client with newly diagnosed type 2 diabetes mellitus is seeking preconception counseling.

1. Before actively trying to become pregnant, the client is strongly encouraged to stabilize her blood glucose to reduce the possibility of her baby developing which of the following?
1. Port wine stain.
2. Cardiac defect.
3. Hip dysplasia.
4. Intussusception.

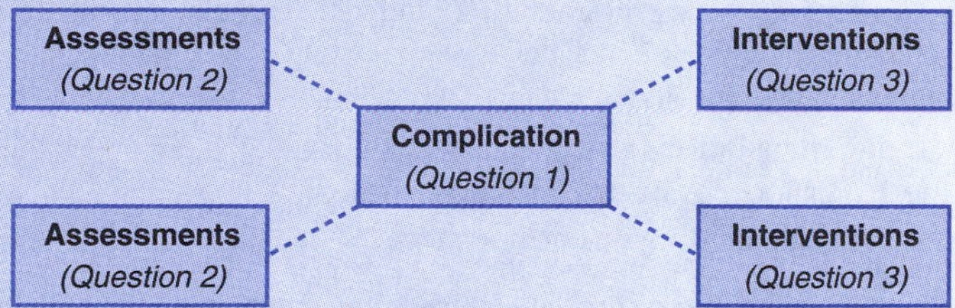

2. Which of the following assessments can the nurse anticipate that the provider will monitor to reduce the risk of the identified complication? **Select two.**
1. Glycosylated hemoglobin (HgbA1c) level.
2. Blood pressures.
3. Weight.
4. Pre-prandial blood sugar assessments.

3. Specify two interventions the nurse should recommend to the client as a way to reduce the risks of the identified complication. **Select two.**
1. Regular blood pressure monitoring.
2. Carbohydrate counting.
3. Regular exercise.
4. Support stockings.

4. An antenatal client is informing the nurse of her prenatal signs and symptoms. Which of the following findings would the nurse determine are presumptive signs of pregnancy? **Select all that apply.**
1. Amenorrhea.
2. Breast tenderness.
3. Quickening.
4. Frequent urination.
5. Uterine growth.

5. The nurse is assessing the laboratory report of a client at 40 weeks' gestation. Which of the following values would the nurse expect to find elevated above pre-pregnancy levels? **Select all that apply.**
1. Glucose.
2. Fibrinogen.
3. Hematocrit.
4. Bilirubin.
5. White blood cells.

6. When analyzing the need for health teaching of a prenatal client who is a multigravida, the nurse should ask which of the following questions?
1. "What are the ages of your children?"
2. "What is your marital status?"
3. "Do you ever drink alcohol?"
4. "Do you have any allergies?"

7. A woman whose prenatal weight was 105 pounds weighs 109 pounds at her 12-week visit. Which of the following comments by the nurse is appropriate at this time?
   1. "We expect you to gain about 1 lb per week, so your weight is a little low at this time."
   2. "Most women gain no weight during the first trimester, so I would suggest you eat fewer desserts for the next few weeks."
   3. "You entered the pregnancy well underweight, so we should check your diet to make sure you are getting the nutrients you need."
   4. "Your weight gain is exactly what we would expect it to be at this time."

8. Because nausea and vomiting are such common complaints of pregnant women, the nurse provides anticipatory guidance to a client at 6 weeks' gestation by telling her to do which of the following?
   1. Avoid eating greasy foods.
   2. Drink orange juice before rising.
   3. Consume 1 teaspoon of nutmeg each morning.
   4. Eat three large meals plus a bedtime snack.

9. A client enters the prenatal clinic. She states that she missed her period yesterday and used a home pregnancy test this morning. She states that the results were negative, but "I still think I am pregnant." Which of the following statements would be appropriate for the nurse to make at this time?
   1. "Your period is probably just irregular."
   2. "We could do a blood test to check."
   3. "Home pregnancy test results are very accurate."
   4. "You should repeat the test in one week."

10. A client with an obstetrical history of G1 P0000, is having her first prenatal physical examination. Which of the following assessments should the nurse inform the client that she will have that day? **Select all that apply.**
    1. Pap smear.
    2. Mammogram.
    3. Glucose tolerance test.
    4. Biophysical profile.
    5. Complete blood count.

11. The nurse plans to provide anticipatory guidance to a client at 10 weeks' gestation who is being seen in the prenatal clinic. Which of the following information would be appropriate for the nurse to provide?
    1. Pain management during labor.
    2. Methods to relieve backaches.
    3. Breastfeeding positions.
    4. Characteristics of the newborn.

12. A client asks the nurse what was meant when the provider told her she had a positive Chadwick's sign. Which of the following information about the finding would be appropriate for the nurse to convey at this time?
    1. "It is a purplish stretch mark on your abdomen."
    2. "It means that you are having heart palpitations."
    3. "It is a bluish coloration of your cervix and vagina."
    4. "It means the doctor heard abnormal sounds when you breathed in."

13. A client enters the prenatal clinic. She states that she believes she is pregnant. Which of the following hormone elevations will indicate a high probability that the client is pregnant?
    1. Chorionic gonadotropin.
    2. Oxytocin.
    3. Prolactin.
    4. Luteinizing hormone.

14. A 16-year-old, G1 P0000, is 10 weeks pregnant. She is being seen for a prenatal visit. She tells the nurse that she felt the baby move that morning. Which of the following responses by the nurse is appropriate?
1. "That is very exciting. The baby must be very healthy."
2. "Can you describe what you felt?"
3. "That is impossible. The baby is not big enough yet."
4. "Would you please let me see if I can feel the baby?"

15. A 20-year-old client states that the at-home pregnancy test that she took this morning was positive. Which of the following comments by the nurse is appropriate at this time?
1. "Congratulations, you and your family must be so happy."
2. "Have you told the baby's father yet?"
3. "How do you feel about that?"
4. "Please tell me when your last menstrual period was."

16. A client is in the 10th week of her pregnancy. Which of the following symptoms would the nurse expect the client to exhibit? **Select all that apply.**
1. Backache.
2. Urinary frequency.
3. Dyspnea on exertion.
4. Fatigue.
5. Diarrhea.

17. The certified nurse midwife has just palpated the fundal height at the location noted on the picture below. It is likely that the client is how many weeks pregnant?
1. 12.
2. 20.
3. 28.
4. 36.

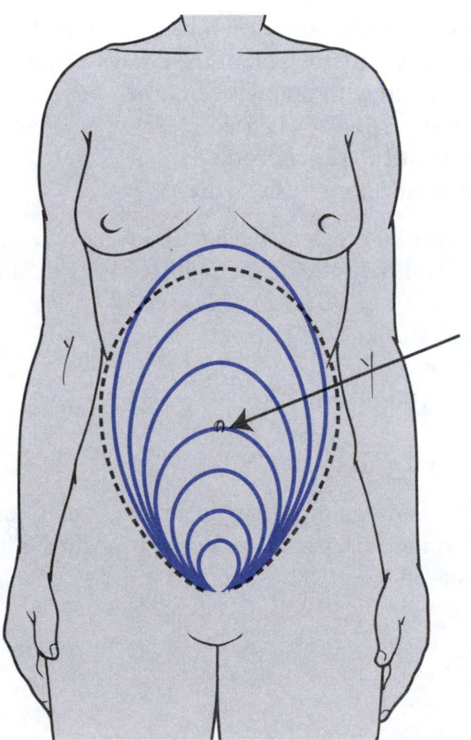

18. When assessing the psychological adjustment of a client at 8 weeks' gestation, which of the following would the nurse expect to see signs of?
1. Ambivalence.
2. Depression.
3. Anxiety.
4. Ecstasy.

19. A client makes the following statement after finding out that her pregnancy test is positive, "This is not a good time. I am in college and the baby will be due during final exams!" Which of the following responses by the nurse would be most appropriate at this time?
1. "I'm absolutely positive that everything will turn out all right."
2. "I suggest that you e-mail your professors to set up an alternate plan."
3. "It sounds like you're feeling a little overwhelmed right now."
4. "You and the baby's father will find a way to get through the pregnancy."

20. The nurse reviews each of the following findings in a client at 10 weeks' gestation. Which of the findings would enable the nurse to tell the client that she is positively pregnant?
1. Fetal heart rate via Doppler.
2. Positive pregnancy test.
3. Positive Chadwick's sign.
4. Montgomery gland enlargements.

21. The nurse takes the history of a new client at her first prenatal visit. Her obstetrical history is G2 P1001. Which of the following statements would indicate that the client should be referred to a genetic counselor?
1. "My first child has cerebral palsy."
2. "My first child has hypertension."
3. "My first child has asthma."
4. "My first child has cystic fibrosis."

22. The nurse has taken a health history on four primigravid clients at their first prenatal visits. It is high priority that which of the clients receives nutrition counseling?
1. The woman diagnosed with phenylketonuria.
2. The woman who has Graves' disease.
3. The woman with Cushing's syndrome.
4. The woman diagnosed with myasthenia gravis.

23. Which of the following findings in a client at 8 weeks' gestation with an obstetrical history of G2 P1001, should the nurse highlight for the nurse midwife? **Select all that apply.**
1. Body mass index of 17 kg/m^2.
2. Rubella titer of 1:8.
3. Blood pressure of 100/60 mm Hg.
4. Hematocrit of 30%.
5. Hemoglobin of 13.2 g/dL.

24. A client who is 6 weeks pregnant is having a pelvic examination. Which of the following would the primary healthcare provider expect to find?
1. Thin cervical muscle.
2. An enlarged ovary.
3. Thick cervical mucus.
4. Pale pink vaginal wall.

25. A pregnant client's primary healthcare provider has ordered a 100-gram glucose solution for a 3-hour oral glucose tolerance test (OGTT) to test the client for gestational diabetes. The nurse is providing pre-procedure counseling to the client. Which of the following must the client do? **Select all that apply.**
1. Fast for 8 to 16 hours prior to the test.
2. Bring a first void urine specimen to the laboratory for testing.
3. Consume a solid sugar cube immediately upon awakening.
4. Drink 16 ounces of water 1 hour prior to the test.
5. Smoke no cigarettes the day of the test.

26. The nurse working in an outpatient obstetric office assesses four clients who are pregnant for the first time. Which of the client findings should the nurse highlight for the physician? **Select all that apply.**
1. 17 weeks' gestation; denies feeling fetal movement.
2. 24 weeks' gestation; fundal height at the umbilicus.
3. 27 weeks' gestation; salivates excessively.
4. 34 weeks' gestation; experiences uterine cramping.
5. 37 weeks' gestation; complains of hemorrhoidal pain.

27. The following four changes occur during pregnancy. Which of them usually increases the father's interest and involvement in the pregnancy?
1. Learning the results of the pregnancy test.
2. Attending childbirth education classes.
3. Hearing the fetal heartbeat.
4. Meeting the obstetrician or midwife.

28. The nurse midwife tells a client that the baby is growing and that ballottement was evident during the vaginal examination. How should the nurse explain what the nurse midwife means by ballottement?
1. The nurse midwife saw that the mucous plug was intact.
2. The nurse midwife felt the baby rebound after being pushed.
3. The nurse midwife palpated the fetal parts through the uterine wall.
4. The nurse midwife assessed that the baby is head down.

29. A multigravid client is 22 weeks pregnant. Which of the following symptoms would the nurse expect the client to exhibit?
1. Nausea.
2. Dyspnea.
3. Urinary frequency.
4. Leg cramping.

30. A 75-gram oral glucose tolerance test (OGTT) is ordered at or after 24 weeks' gestation for a pregnant client to assess her physiological response to which of the following pregnancy hormones?
1. Estrogen.
2. Progesterone.
3. Human placental lactogen.
4. Human chorionic gonadotropin.

31. A client is 15 weeks pregnant. She calls her obstetrical provider's office to request medication for a headache. The nurse answers the telephone. Which of the following is the nurse's best response?
1. "Because the organ systems in the baby are developing right now, you may take no medication."
2. "You can take any of the over-the-counter medications because they are all safe in pregnancy."
3. "The physician will prescribe a medication for you that has been shown not to cause any fetal injuries."
4. "The physician will prescribe a rectal suppository because the medicine will not enter your blood stream."

32. A client who was seen in the prenatal clinic at 20 weeks' gestation weighed 128 lbs at that time. Approximately how many pounds would the nurse expect the client to weigh at her next visit at 24 weeks' gestation?
1. 129 to 130 lb.
2. 131 to 132 lb.
3. 133 to 134 lb.
4. 135 to 136 lb.

33. A client at 18 weeks' gestation telephones the obstetrician's office stating, "I'm really scared. I think I have breast cancer. My breasts are filled with tumors." The nurse should base the response on which of the following?
1. Breast cancer is often triggered by pregnancy.
2. Nodular breast tissue is normal during pregnancy.
3. The woman is exhibiting signs of a psychotic break.
4. Anxiety attacks are especially common in the second trimester.

34. A woman states that she frequently awakens with "painful leg cramps" during the night. Which of the following assessments should the nurse make?
1. The woman's exercise schedule.
2. Her Goodell's sign.
3. Her Hegar's sign.
4. The woman's dietary intake.

35. Which of the following exercises should be taught to a pregnant woman who complains of backaches?
1. Kegel exercises.
2. Pelvic tilting.
3. Leg lifting.
4. Crunching.

36. A woman in her third trimester indicates that she wishes to breastfeed her baby, "but I don't think my nipples are right." Upon examination, the nurse notes that the client has inverted nipples. Which of the following actions should the nurse take at this time?
1. Advise the client that it is unlikely that she will be able to breastfeed.
2. Refer the client to a lactation consultant for advice.
3. Call the labor room and notify them that a client with inverted nipples will be admitted.
4. Teach the woman exercises to evert her nipples.

37. Which of the following vital sign changes should the nurse highlight for a pregnant woman's obstetrician?
1. Pre-pregnancy blood pressure (BP) 100/60 and third trimester BP 140/90.
2. Pre-pregnancy respiratory rate (RR) 16 rpm and third trimester RR 22 rpm.
3. Pre-pregnancy heart rate (HR) 76 bpm and third trimester HR 88 bpm.
4. Pre-pregnancy temperature (T) 98.6° F (37° C) and third trimester T 99.2° F (37.3° C).

38. A nurse midwife has advised a client at 40 weeks' gestation to take evening primrose oil 2,500 mg daily as a complementary therapy. This suggestion was made because evening primrose has been shown to perform which of the following actions?
1. Relieve back strain.
2. Improve development of colostrum.
3. Ripen the cervix.
4. Reduce the incidence of hemorrhoids.

39. A client at 40 weeks' gestation with a Bishop score of 1, is advised by her nurse midwife to take evening primrose daily. The office nurse advises the client to report which of the following side effects that has been attributed to the oil?
1. Skin rash.
2. Pedal edema.
3. Blurred vision.
4. Tinnitus.

40. A client at 37 weeks' gestation states that she noticed a "white liquid" leaking from her breasts during a recent shower. Which of the following nursing responses is appropriate at this time?
1. Advise the woman that she may have a galactocele.
2. Encourage the woman to pump her breasts to stimulate an adequate milk supply.
3. Assess the liquid because a breast discharge is diagnostic of a mammary infection.
4. Reassure the mother that this is normal in the third trimester.

41. A client at 36 weeks' gestation is complaining of dyspnea when lying flat. Which of the following is the likely clinical reason for this complaint?
1. Maternal hypertension.
2. Fundal height.
3. Hydramnios.
4. Congestive heart failure.

42. The nurse is providing anticipatory guidance to a woman in her second trimester regarding signs/symptoms that are within normal limits during the latter half of the pregnancy. Which of the following comments by the client indicates that teaching was successful? **Select all that apply.**
1. "During the third trimester I may experience frequent urination."
2. "During the third trimester I may experience heartburn."
3. "During the third trimester I may experience nagging backaches."
4. "During the third trimester I may experience persistent headache."
5. "During the third trimester I may experience blurred vision."

43. A client in her third trimester is concerned that she will not know the difference between labor contractions and normal aches and pains of pregnancy. How should the nurse respond?
1. "Don't worry. You'll know the difference when the contractions start."
2. "The contractions may feel just like a backache, but they will come and go."
3. "Contractions are a lot worse than your pregnancy aches and pains."
4. "I understand. You don't want to come to the hospital before you are in labor."

44. Which finding would the nurse view as normal when evaluating the laboratory reports of a client at 34 weeks' gestation?
1. Mild anemia.
2. Thrombocytopenia.
3. Polycythemia.
4. Hyperbilirubinemia.

45. The nurse asks a client at 31 weeks' gestation to lie on the examining table during a prenatal examination. In which of the following positions should the client be placed?
1. Orthopneic.
2. Lateral-recumbent.
3. Sims.
4. Semi-Fowler.

46. A third-trimester client is being seen for routine prenatal care. Which of the following assessments will the nurse perform during the visit? **Select all that apply.**
1. Blood glucose.
2. Blood pressure.
3. Fetal heart rate.
4. Urine protein.
5. Pelvic ultrasound.

47. A nurse is working in the prenatal clinic. Which of the following findings seen in third-trimester clients would the nurse consider to be within normal limits? **Select all that apply.**
1. Leg cramps.
2. Varicose veins.
3. Hemorrhoids.
4. Fainting spells.
5. Lordosis.

48. A client at 36 weeks' gestation is lying flat on her back. Which of the following maternal signs/symptoms would the nurse expect to observe?
1. Hypertension.
2. Dizziness.
3. Rales.
4. Chloasma.

49. The nurse is interviewing a Muslim client at 38 weeks' gestation. Which of the following questions could be inappropriate for the nurse to ask?
1. "Do you plan to breastfeed your baby?"
2. "What do you plan to name the baby?"
3. "Which pediatrician do you plan to use?"
4. "How do you feel about having an episiotomy?"

50. A woman is at 36 weeks' gestation. Which of the following tests will be done during her prenatal visit?
1. Oral glucose tolerance test.
2. Amniotic fluid volume assessment.
3. Vaginal and rectal cultures.
4. Karyotype analysis.

51. A client at 34 weeks' gestation calls the obstetric office stating, "Since last night I have had three nosebleeds." Which of the following responses by the nurse is appropriate?
1. "You should see the doctor to make sure you are not becoming severely anemic."
2. "Do you have a temperature?"
3. "One of the hormones of pregnancy makes the nasal passages prone to bleeding."
4. "Do you use any inhaled drugs?"

52. The nurse asks a woman about how the woman's husband is dealing with the pregnancy. The nurse concludes that counseling is needed when the woman makes which of the following statements?
1. "My husband is ready for the pregnancy to end so that we can have sex again."
2. "My husband has gained quite a bit of weight during this pregnancy."
3. "My husband seems more worried about our finances now than before the pregnancy."
4. "My husband plays his favorite music for my belly so the baby will learn to like it."

53. The blood of a pregnant client was initially assessed at 10 weeks' gestation and reassessed at 38 weeks' gestation. Which of the following results would the nurse expect to see?
1. Rise in hematocrit from 34% to 38%.
2. Rise in white blood cells from 5,000 cells/mm^3 to 15,000 cells/mm^3.
3. Rise in potassium from 3.9 mEq/L to 5.2 mEq/L.
4. Rise in sodium from 137 mEq/L to 150 mEq/L.

54. A client is at 35 weeks' gestation. Which of the following findings would the nurse expect to see?
1. Nausea and vomiting.
2. Maternal ambivalence.
3. Fundal height 35 cm above the symphysis pubis.
4. Pitting edema.

55. A client at 26 weeks' gestation calls the triage nurse stating, "I'm really scared. I tried not to but I had an orgasm when we were making love. I just know that I will go into preterm labor now." Which of the following responses by the nurse is appropriate?
   1. "Lie down and drink a quart of water. If you feel any back pressure at all call me back right away."
   2. "Although oxytocin was responsible for your orgasm, it is very unlikely that it will stimulate preterm labor."
   3. "I will inform the doctor for you. What I want you to do is to come to the hospital right now to be checked."
   4. "The best thing for you to do right now is to take a warm shower and then do a fetal kick count assessment."

56. A couple is preparing to interview obstetric primary care providers to determine who they will go to for care during their pregnancy and delivery. To make the best choice, which of the following actions should the couple perform first?
   1. Take a tour of hospital delivery areas.
   2. Develop a preliminary birth plan.
   3. Make appointments with three or four obstetric care providers.
   4. Search the Internet for the malpractice histories of the providers.

57. During a prenatal visit, a pregnant client is complaining of ptyalism. Which of the following nursing interventions is appropriate?
   1. Encourage the woman to brush her teeth carefully.
   2. Advise the woman to have her blood pressure checked regularly.
   3. Encourage the woman to wear supportive hosiery.
   4. Advise the woman to avoid eating rare meat.

58. A pregnant woman reports she has never been vaccinated for any illness. An injection to prevent which of the following communicable diseases should be administered to the woman during her pregnancy?
   1. Influenza.
   2. Mumps.
   3. Rubella.
   4. Varicella.

59. A pregnant woman and her husband inform the nurse that they have just moved into a three-story home that was built in the 1930s. Which of the following is critical for the nurse to advise the woman to protect the unborn child?
   1. Stay out of any rooms that are being renovated.
   2. Drink water only from the hot water tap.
   3. Refrain from entering the basement.
   4. Climb the stairs only once per day.

60. After nutrition counseling, a woman with an obstetrical history of G3 P1101, states emphatically that she certainly won't eat any strawberries during her pregnancy. Which of the following is the likely reason for this statement?
   1. The woman is allergic to strawberries.
   2. Strawberries have been shown to cause birth defects.
   3. The woman believes in old wives' tales.
   4. The premature baby died because the woman ate strawberries.

61. The nurse discusses sexual intimacy with an expectant couple. Which of the following should be included in the teaching plan?
   1. Vaginal intercourse should cease by the beginning of the third trimester.
   2. Breast fondling should be discouraged because of the potential for preterm labor.
   3. The couple may find it necessary to experiment with alternate positions.
   4. Vaginal lubricant should be used sparingly throughout the pregnancy.

62. Which of the following skin changes should the nurse highlight for a pregnant woman's healthcare practitioner?
    1. Linea nigra.
    2. Melasma.
    3. Petechiae.
    4. Spider nevi.

63. A pregnant woman informs the nurse that her last normal menstrual period was on September 20, 2021. Using Nagele's rule, the nurse calculates the client's estimated date of delivery as:
    1. May 30, 2022.
    2. June 20, 2022.
    3. June 27, 2022.
    4. July 3, 2022.

64. A father experiencing couvade syndrome is likely to exhibit which of the following symptoms/behaviors? **Select all that apply.**
    1. Heartburn.
    2. Promiscuity.
    3. Hypertension.
    4. Bloating.
    5. Abdominal pain.

65. A nurse is advising a pregnant woman about the danger signs of pregnancy. The nurse should teach the mother that she should notify the physician immediately if she experiences which of the following signs/symptoms? **Select all that apply.**
    1. Convulsions.
    2. Double vision.
    3. Epigastric pain.
    4. Persistent vomiting.
    5. Polyuria.

66. A woman provides the nurse with the following obstetrical history: Delivered a son, now 7 years old, at 28 weeks' gestation; delivered a daughter, now 5 years old, at 39 weeks' gestation; had a miscarriage 3 years ago; and had a first-trimester abortion 2 years ago. She is currently pregnant. Which of the following portrays an accurate picture of this woman's gravidity and parity?
    1. G4 P2121.
    2. G4 P1212.
    3. G5 P1122.
    4. G5 P2211.

67. The nurse is caring for a pregnant client who is a vegan. Which of the following foods should the nurse suggest the client consume as substitutes for restricted foods?
    1. Tofu, legumes, broccoli.
    2. Corn, yams, green beans.
    3. Potatoes, parsnips, turnips.
    4. Cheese, yogurt, fish.

68. When assessing the fruit intake of a pregnant client, the nurse notes that the client usually eats one piece of fruit per day and drinks a 12 oz glass of fruit juice per day. Which of the following is the most important communication for the nurse to make?
    1. "You are effectively meeting your daily fruit requirements."
    2. "Fruit juices are excellent sources of folic acid."
    3. "It would be even better if you were to consume more whole fruits and less fruit juice."
    4. "Your fruit intake far exceeds the recommended daily fruit intake."

69. A client states that she is a strong believer in vitamin supplements to maintain her health. The nurse advises the woman that it is recommended to refrain from consuming excess quantities of which of the following vitamins during pregnancy?
1. Vitamin C.
2. Vitamin D.
3. Vitamin B2 (niacin).
4. Vitamin B12 (cobalamin).

70. A vegan client is being counseled regarding vitamin intake. It is essential that this woman supplement her intake of which of the following B vitamins?
1. B1 (thiamine).
2. B2 (niacin).
3. B6 (pyridoxine).
4. B12 (cobalamin).

71. A client informs the nurse that she is "very constipated." Which of the following foods would be best for the nurse to recommend to the client?
1. Pasta.
2. Rice.
3. Yogurt.
4. Celery.

72. A pregnant client is lactose intolerant. Which of the following foods could this woman consume to meet her calcium needs?
1. Turnip greens.
2. Green beans.
3. Cantaloupe.
4. Nectarines.

73. A nurse who is providing nutrition counseling to a new, pregnant client advises the woman that a serving of meat is approximately equal in size to which of the following items?
1. Deck of cards.
2. Paperback book.
3. Clenched fist.
4. Large tomato.

74. Which of the following choices can the nurse use to teach a prenatal client about a 1 oz nonmeat serving of protein?
1. 2 tbsp peanut butter.
2. 1 egg.
3. 1 cup cooked lima beans.
4. 3 ounces mixed nuts.

75. A nurse is discussing the serving sizes in the grains food group with a new prenatal client. Which of the following foods equals a 1 oz serving from the grain group? **Select all that apply.**
1. 1 bagel.
2. 1 slice of bread.
3. 1 cup cooked pasta.
4. 1 tortilla.
5. 1 ounce dry cereal.

76. A woman asks the nurse about consuming herbal supplements during pregnancy. Which of the following responses is appropriate?
1. Herbals are natural substances, so they are safely ingested during pregnancy.
2. It is safe to take licorice and cat's claw, but no other herbs are safe.
3. A federal commission has established the safety of herbals during pregnancy.
4. The woman should discuss everything she eats with a healthcare practitioner.

77. A nurse is discussing diet with a pregnant woman. Which of the following foods should the nurse advise the client to avoid consuming during her pregnancy?
1. Bologna.
2. Cantaloupe.
3. Asparagus.
4. Popcorn.

78. A client at 12 weeks' gestation tells the nurse that she and her husband eat sushi at least once per week. She states, "I know that fish is good for me, so I make sure we eat it regularly." Which of the following responses by the nurse is appropriate?
1. "You are correct. Fish is very healthy for you."
2. "You can eat fish, but sushi is too salty to eat during pregnancy."
3. "Sushi is raw. Raw fish is especially high in mercury."
4. "It is recommended that fish be cooked to destroy harmful bacteria."

79. The nurse is caring for a prenatal client who states she is prone to developing anemia. Which of the following foods should the nurse advise the client is the best source of iron?
1. Raisins.
2. Hamburger.
3. Broccoli.
4. Molasses.

80. It is discovered that a pregnant woman practices pica. Which of the following complications is most often associated with this behavior?
1. Hypothyroidism.
2. Iron-deficiency anemia.
3. Hypercalcemia.
4. Overexposure to zinc.

81. A woman confides in the nurse that she practices pica. Which of the following alternatives could the nurse suggest to the woman?
1. Replace laundry starch with salt.
2. Replace ice with frozen fruit juice.
3. Replace soap with cream cheese.
4. Replace soil with uncooked pie crust.

82. A pregnant client is experiencing nausea and vomiting every afternoon. The ingestion of which of the following spices has been shown to be a safe complementary therapy for this complaint?
1. Ginger.
2. Sage.
3. Cloves.
4. Nutmeg.

83. A woman tells the nurse that she would like suggestions for alternate vitamin C sources because she isn't very fond of citrus fruits. Which of the following suggestions is appropriate?
1. Barley and brown rice.
2. Strawberries and potatoes.
3. Buckwheat and lentils.
4. Wheat flour and figs.

84. A nurse is providing diet counseling to a new prenatal client. Which of the following dairy products should the client be advised to avoid eating during the pregnancy?
1. Frozen yogurt.
2. Parmesan cheese.
3. Gorgonzola cheese.
4. Chocolate milk.

85. A nurse has explained the function of amniotic fluid to a client. Which of the following statements by the woman indicates that the teaching was successful? **Select all that apply.**
   1. The fluid provides fetal nutrition.
   2. The fluid cushions the fetus from injury.
   3. The fluid enables the fetus to grow.
   4. The fluid provides the fetus with a stable thermal environment.
   5. The fluid enables the fetus to practice swallowing.

86. Why is it essential that women of childbearing age be counseled to plan their pregnancies?
   1. Much of the organogenesis occurs before the missed menstrual period.
   2. Insurance companies must preapprove many prenatal care expenditures.
   3. It is recommended that women be pregnant no more than three times during their lifetime.
   4. The cardiovascular system is stressed when pregnancies are less than 2 years apart.

87. A woman has just completed her first trimester of pregnancy. Which of the following fetal structures can the nurse tell the woman are well formed at this time? **Select all that apply.**
   1. Genitals.
   2. Heart.
   3. Fingers.
   4. Alveoli.
   5. Kidneys.

88. An ultrasound of a fetal heart shows that normal fetal circulation is occurring. Which of the following statements should the nurse interpret as correct in relation to the fetal circulation?
   1. The foramen ovale is a hole between the ventricles.
   2. The umbilical vein contains oxygen-poor blood.
   3. The right atrium contains both oxygen-rich and oxygen-poor blood.
   4. The ductus venosus lies between the aorta and pulmonary artery.

89. The nurse is teaching a couple about fetal development. Which statement by the nurse is correct about the morula stage of development?
   1. "The fertilized egg has yet to implant into the uterus."
   2. "The lung fields are finally completely formed."
   3. "The sex of the fetus can be clearly identified."
   4. "The eyelids are unfused and begin to open and close."

90. A client is carrying dizygotic twins. She asks the nurse about the babies. Which of the following explanations is accurate?
   1. During a period of rapid growth, the fertilized egg divided completely.
   2. When the client ovulated, she expelled two mature ova.
   3. The babies share one placenta and a common chorion.
   4. The babies will definitely be the same sex and have the same blood type.

91. A mother has just experienced quickening. Which of the following developmental changes would the nurse expect to occur at the same time in the woman's pregnancy?
   1. Fetal heart begins to beat.
   2. Lanugo covers the fetal body.
   3. Kidneys secrete urine.
   4. Fingernails begin to form.

92. A woman who is seen in the prenatal clinic is found to be 8 weeks pregnant. She confides to the nurse that she is afraid her baby may be "permanently damaged because I had at least five beers the night I had sex." Which of the following responses by the nurse would be appropriate?
1. "I would let the doctor know that if I were you."
2. "It is unlikely that the baby was affected."
3. "Abortions during the first trimester are very safe."
4. "An ultrasound will tell you if the baby was affected."

93. A pregnant client's fundal height is noted to be at the xiphoid process. The nurse is aware that which of the following fetal changes is likely to be occurring at the same time in the pregnancy?
1. Surfactant is formed in the fetal lungs.
2. Eyes begin to open and close.
3. Respiratory movements begin.
4. Spinal column is completely formed.

94. Below are four important landmarks of fetal development. Please place them in chronological order:
1. Four-chambered heart is formed.
2. Vernix caseosa is present.
3. Blastocyst development is complete.
4. Testes have descended into the scrotal sac.

95. Which of the following developmental features would the nurse expect to be absent in a 41-week gestation fetus?
1. Fingernails.
2. Eyelashes.
3. Lanugo.
4. Milia.

96. A woman delivers a stillborn baby that has lanugo covering the entire body, nails that are present on the fingers and toes, but eyes that are still fused. Prior to the death, the mother stated that she had felt quickening. Based on this information, the nurse knows that the baby is about how many weeks' gestation?
1. 15 weeks.
2. 22 weeks.
3. 29 weeks.
4. 36 weeks.

97. A client asks the nurse, "Could you explain how the baby's blood and my blood separate at delivery?" Which of the following responses is appropriate for the nurse to make?
1. "When the placenta is born, the circulatory systems separate."
2. "When the doctor clamps the cord, the blood stops mixing."
3. "The separation happens after the baby takes the first breath. The baby's oxygen no longer has to come from you."
4. "The blood actually never mixes. Your blood supply and the baby's blood supply are completely separate."

98. The nurse is reading an article that states that the maternal mortality rate in the United States in the year 2020 was 14. Which of the following statements would be an accurate interpretation of the statement?
1. In the year 2020, there were 14 maternal deaths in the United States per 100,000 live births.
2. In the year 2020, there were 14 maternal deaths in the United States per 100,000 women of childbearing age.
3. In the year 2020, there were 14 maternal deaths in the United States per 100,000 pregnancies.
4. In the year 2020, there were 14 maternal deaths in the United States per 100,000 women in the country.

99. A pregnant client is counseled by her primary healthcare provider to have a vaccination during her third trimester of pregnancy. The client questions the healthcare provider's recommendation. Which of the following statements would be appropriate for the nurse to give the client?
   1. "When received during pregnancy, the rotavirus vaccine helps to prevent dehydration in newborns."
   2. "If you receive the tetanus, diphtheria, and acellular pertussis vaccine, your baby will be protected against whooping cough."
   3. "When received during pregnancy, the human papillomavirus vaccine helps to prevent newborns from acquiring the sexually transmitted infection."
   4. "If you receive the varicella vaccine, your baby will be protected from the chickenpox virus."

100. A nurse is providing health education to a group of women who are planning to become pregnant. Which of the following actions should the nurse advise the women to take throughout their pregnancies? **Select all that apply.**
   1. The women should avoid consuming well done meat.
   2. The women should avoid traveling to locations where the Zika virus is endemic.
   3. The women should engage in a daily exercise program.
   4. The women should drink beer and wine instead of spirits like whiskey and vodka.

ANSWERS AND RATIONALES

The correct answer number and rationale for why it is the correct answer are given in **boldface blue type.** Rationales for why the other possible answer options are incorrect also are given, but they are not in boldface type.

1.
    1. Port wine stains are not a complication of maternal hyperglycemia.
    2. **Maternal hyperglycemia can contribute to fetal cardiac defects.**
    3. Hip dysplasia is not a complication of maternal hyperglycemia.
    4. Intussusception is not a complication of maternal hyperglycemia.

2. **Answers 1 and 4 are correct.**
    1. **The maternal HgbA1c level reflects the average maternal blood sugars over a 3-month period of time to indicate glycemic control. If the level is high, the client may be advised to delay pregnancy until the levels are within a more normal range in order to avoid fetal cardiac defects.**
    2. Maternal blood pressures do not affect fetal cardiac defects.
    3. Maternal weight does not directly affect fetal cardiac defects.
    4. **The mother's pre-prandial blood sugar readings may be assessed to determine appropriate interventions.**

3. **Answers 2 and 3 are correct.**
    1. Regular blood pressure monitoring will not affect fetal cardiac defects.
    2. **Carbohydrate counting can help to reduce hyperglycemia and maintain normoglycemia to prevent fetal cardiac defects.**
    3. **Regular exercise can contribute to normoglycemia.**
    4. Support stockings will not affect fetal cardiac defects.

Assessments (Question 2) Maternal Hemoglobin A1c		Interventions (Question 3) Carbohydrate Counting
	Complication (Question 1) Fetal Cardiac Defects	
Assessments (Question 2) Preprandial Blood Sugar Assessments		Interventions (Question 3) Regular Exercise

TEST-TAKING HINT: The stem of this question indicates this client has a problem with maintaining normoglycemia. The most serious complication in the list in the first question is a cardiac defect associated with hyperglycemia. All of the answers that follow will relate to hyperglycemia assessments in particular, as in question 2. The answers in question 3 are also related to the stem, which is achievement or maintenance of normoglycemia.

4. **Answers 1, 2, 3, and 4 are correct.**
    1. **Amenorrhea is a presumptive sign of pregnancy.**
    2. **Breast tenderness is a presumptive sign of pregnancy.**
    3. **Quickening is a presumptive sign of pregnancy.**
    4. **Frequent urination is a presumptive sign of pregnancy.**
    5. Uterine growth is a probable sign of pregnancy.

TEST-TAKING HINT: There are three classifications for signs of pregnancy: presumptive, probable, and positive. Signs that are totally subjective, or *presumptive*, are those that are usually noted by the client and compel her to make an appointment with a provider. These include amenorrhea, breast tenderness, quickening, and frequent urination. Signs that one can see are objective, but not totally absolute. These are termed *probable* and include uterine growth, and changes in the cervix such as Chadwick's sign, a bluish discoloration. Signs that are absolute, or *positive*, include hearing the fetal heartbeat and seeing ultrasound images of the embryo or fetus.

5. **Answers 2 and 5 are correct.**
    1. Glucose levels should be within normal limits.
    2. **Fibrinogen levels will be elevated slightly in a 40-week pregnant woman because coagulation factors like fibrinogen increase to help prevent excessive blood loss during delivery.**
    3. Hematocrit levels are usually slightly lower because of increased plasma volume.
    4. Bilirubin levels should be within normal limits.
    5. **A woman's white blood cell count will be elevated above normal at 40 weeks' gestation as a means of protecting her body (and ultimately the fetus) from infection.**

TEST-TAKING HINT: During the latter part of the third trimester, coagulation factors increase in preparation for delivery. It is the body's means of protecting itself against a large loss of blood following delivery of the placenta. In addition, the white blood cell count rises as a means of protecting the body from infection.

6. 1. The ages of her children is important information, but it is not associated with health teaching.
   2. Her marital status is important to know, but it is not associated with health teaching.
   3. **Alcohol use is important information to determine a prenatal client's health teaching needs.**
   4. A client's allergies are important to know, but the information is not associated with health teaching.

TEST-TAKING HINT: When answering test questions, the test taker should focus on the specific information that is being requested. In this question, although several of the possible responses are questions that should be asked of a pregnant multigravid client at some point, only one is related to the client's needs for health teaching.

7. **Answers 1 and 4 are correct.**
   1. **Weight gain of 0.8 to 1 lb per week is expected during the second and third trimesters only.**
   2. A weight gain of 3 to 5 lb is expected during the entire first trimester.
   3. Since the client's height is not stated, there is no way to know whether or not the client is underweight.
   4. **The weight gain is normal for the first trimester.**

TEST-TAKING HINT: One of the assessments that aids healthcare practitioners in assessing the health and well-being of antenatal clients and their babies is weight gain. For women who enter the pregnancy with a normal weight for height, the expected weight gain is 3 to 5 lb for the entire first trimester and approximately 0.8 to 1 lb per week from weeks 13 to 40. Women with a normal BMI, therefore, should gain between 25 and 35 lb during the entire pregnancy (American College of Obstetricians and Gynecologists [ACOG], 2013a).

8. 1. **Greasy foods should be avoided.**
   2. Saltine crackers may be eaten before rising. Drinking orange juice has not been recommended.
   3. Although consuming ginger may help to alleviate the nausea and vomiting of pregnancy, neither cinnamon nor nutmeg has been shown to alleviate the symptoms.
   4. It is recommended that mothers eat small frequent meals throughout the day.

TEST-TAKING HINT: Although many women experience nausea and vomiting or morning sickness upon rising, many women complain of nausea and/or vomiting at other times of the day. One theory that has been offered to explain this problem is that the body is ridding itself of ingested foods that could potentially harm the fetus, or the body is protecting the woman from having an appetite and eating foods that could harm the fetus during its crucial development phase.

9. 1. This response is inappropriate. It does not acknowledge the client's concerns.
   2. **This response is correct. Serum pregnancy tests are more sensitive than urine tests.**
   3. This statement is correct, but because the woman's period is only 1 day late, the test may not be sensitive enough to detect the pregnancy.
   4. The client could repeat the test, but since the more accurate serum test is available, it would be better for the nurse to recommend that action. At-home tests are reliable only if used correctly.

TEST-TAKING HINT: Because quantitative pregnancy tests measure the exact quantity of human chorionic gonadotropin (HCG) in the bloodstream, they are more accurate than urine tests that simply measure whether or not the hormone is present in the urine. Similar to the urine tests on the market, qualitative serum tests only detect whether or not the hormone is present, but they are still considered to be more accurate than urine tests.

10. **Answers 1 and 5 are correct.**
    1. **The client will have a Pap smear done.**
    2. A mammogram will not be performed.
    3. A glucose assessment will likely be performed at the end of the second trimester.
    4. A biophysical profile may be done but not until the third trimester.
    5. **A complete blood count will be performed.**

TEST-TAKING HINT: At the first prenatal visit, pregnant clients will undergo complete obstetrical and medical physical assessments. The assessments are performed to provide the healthcare practitioner with baseline data regarding the health and well-being of the woman as well as to inform the healthcare practitioner of any medical problems that the mother has that might affect the pregnancy. A breast examination will be performed by the

practitioner to assess for abnormalities, but since mammograms are potentially harm-producing x-rays, they are ordered only in emergent cases during pregnancy.

11. 1. It is too early in the pregnancy to provide anticipatory guidance about pain management during labor.
2. It is appropriate for the nurse to provide anticipatory guidance regarding methods to relieve back pain.
3. It is too early in the pregnancy to provide anticipatory guidance about breastfeeding positions.
4. It is too early in the pregnancy to provide anticipatory guidance about characteristics of the newborn.

TEST-TAKING HINT: Anticipatory guidance looks ahead to what can be anticipated. This client will be entering the second trimester in a couple of weeks. It will likely be a month before she is seen again, when she is around 14 weeks' gestation. As the uterus grows, the client often begins to change her posture, leaning back a bit to adjust to the added weight of the pregnancy in front. She is likely to begin experiencing backaches. It is appropriate for the nurse to provide information about this possibility and appropriate ways to relieve the backaches.

12. 1. Purplish stretch marks are called abdominal striae.
2. Chadwick's sign is not related to the heart muscle.
3. A positive Chadwick's sign means that the client's cervix and vagina are a bluish color. It is a probable sign of pregnancy.
4. Chadwick's sign is not related to the respiratory system.

TEST-TAKING HINT: Chadwick's sign is a probable sign of pregnancy. The bluish coloration is a result of the increase in vascularization of the area in response to the high levels of circulating estrogen in the pregnant woman's system.

13. 1. High levels of the hormone chorionic gonadotropin in the bloodstream and urine of the woman is a probable sign of pregnancy.
2. Oxytocin is the hormone of labor. It is not measured as a sign of pregnancy.
3. Prolactin is the hormone that stimulates lactogenesis immediately after delivery. It is not measured as a sign of pregnancy.
4. Luteinizing hormone is the hormone that stimulates ovulation. It is not measured as a sign of pregnancy.

TEST-TAKING HINT: Human chorionic gonadotropin is produced by cells surrounding the growing embryo. Its presence in the bloodstream signals the body to keep the corpus luteum alive. Until the placenta takes over the function of producing progesterone and estrogen, the corpus luteum produces the hormones that are essential to the maintenance of the pregnancy.

14. 1. This is an inappropriate statement to make.
2. The nurse should query the young woman about what she felt.
3. Even though this statement is correct, it is inappropriate to dismiss the young woman so abruptly.
4. This is an inappropriate statement to make.

TEST-TAKING HINT: Quickening, or subjective fetal movement, occurs between 16 and 20 weeks' gestation. At 10 weeks' gestation it would be impossible for the young woman to feel fetal movement. The nurse, therefore, should elicit more information from the teen to determine what she had felt. Sometimes intestinal gas bubbles can mimic fetal movement. However, the client should not be made to feel insulted or embarrassed for reporting this symptom.

15. 1. It is inappropriate to assume that the client and her family are happy about the pregnancy.
2. It is inappropriate to assume that the baby's father is still in the young woman's life.
3. It is important for the nurse to ask the young woman how she feels about being pregnant. She may decide not to continue with the pregnancy.
4. This information is important, but it is not the best statement to make initially.

TEST-TAKING HINT: Some pregnant women are happy about their pregnancy, some are worried, and still others are frightened. At the initial interview, it is essential that the nurse not assume that the woman will respond in any particular way. The nurse must ask open-ended questions to elicit the woman's feelings about the pregnancy.

16. Answers 2 and 4 are correct.
1. Backaches usually do not develop until the second trimester of pregnancy.
2. The woman will likely complain of urinary frequency.
3. Dyspnea is associated with the third trimester of pregnancy.
4. Most women complain of fatigue during the first trimester.
5. Diarrhea is not a complaint normally heard from prenatal clients.

TEST-TAKING HINT: During the first trimester, the mother's body undergoes a number of important changes. The embryo is developing, many maternal hormones are increasing, and the maternal blood supply is increasing. To accomplish each of the tasks, her body uses additional energy. The mother is fatigued not only because her body is undergoing great change but also because her thyroid gland has not yet caught up with the increasing energy demands. In addition, because her organs are confined within the bony pelvis, her enlarging uterus prevents her bladder from expanding adequately as it fills with urine. As a result, the woman needs to urinate much more frequently than she did prior to becoming pregnant.

17. 1. It is not likely the nurse midwife can feel the fundus at 12 weeks' gestation.
2. **The fundus is at the level of the umbilicus at 20 weeks' gestation.**
3. The fundus is between the umbilicus and the xiphoid process at 28 weeks' gestation.
4. The fundus is at the level of the xiphoid process at 36 weeks' gestation.

TEST-TAKING HINT: The fundal height is assessed at every prenatal visit. It is an easy, noninvasive means of assessing fetal growth after 20 weeks' gestation. The nurse should know that the top of the fundus is at the level of the umbilicus, or approximately 20 cm from the top edge of the pubic bone, at 20 weeks' gestation. From then on, the fundal height should match the weeks of gestation quite closely.

18. **1. It is common for women to be ambivalent about their pregnancy during the first trimester.**
2. The nurse should be concerned if a client at 8 weeks' gestation exhibited signs of depression.
3. The nurse should be concerned if a client at 8 weeks' gestation exhibited signs of anxiety.
4. It is unusual for women at 8 weeks' gestation to exhibit signs of ecstasy. This is not to say they won't exhibit signs of happiness or elation, especially if they have anticipated a pregnancy for some time.

TEST-TAKING HINT: Even women who stop taking birth control pills to become pregnant are often startled and ambivalent when they actually get pregnant. This is not pathological. Usually, the women slowly accept the pregnancy and by 20 weeks' gestation, when they feel the baby moving inside, they are happy and enthusiastic about the prospect of becoming a mother.

19. 1. This comment is inappropriate. First of all, everything may not turn out all right. In addition, the comment ignores the client's concerns.
2. Talking with professors for exam scheduling is a possible plan for the future, but first the nurse should acknowledge the client's feelings.
3. **Acknowledging the presence of overwhelming feelings is the best comment. It acknowledges the concerns that the client is having.**
4. This comment is inappropriate. First of all, it assumes that the father of the baby is in the picture and, second, it ignores the client's concerns.

TEST-TAKING HINT: Nurses have two roles when clients express concerns to them. First, the nurse must acknowledge the client's concerns so that the client feels accepted and understood. Second, the nurse must help the client to think through possible solutions to cope with the situation. It is very important, however, that acceptance of the client's feelings precedes the period of problem solving.

20. **1. Hearing a fetal heart rate is a positive sign of pregnancy.**
2. A positive pregnancy test is a probable sign of pregnancy.
3. A positive Chadwick's sign is a probable sign of pregnancy.
4. Montgomery gland enlargement is a presumptive sign of pregnancy.

TEST-TAKING HINT: Positive signs of pregnancy are signs that irrefutably show that a fetus is in utero. An ultrasound of a fetus is one positive sign and the fetal heartbeat is another positive sign.

21. 1. Cerebral palsy is not a genetic disease.
2. Hypertensive conditions can be genetically based, but a family history of hypertension does not warrant referral to a genetic counselor.
3. Asthma can be genetically based, but a family history of asthma does not warrant referral to a genetic counselor.
4. **Cystic fibrosis is an autosomal recessive genetic disease, so the client with a family history of cystic fibrosis should be referred to a genetic counselor.**

TEST-TAKING HINT: Virtually all diseases—chronic and acute—have some genetic component, but the ability for the genetic counselor to predict the recurrence of certain conditions in subsequent fetuses is very poor. Those illnesses with clear hereditary patterns, however, do warrant referral to genetic counselors in order to prepare for the birth of another child with the same condition.

Cystic fibrosis is inherited via an autosomal recessive inheritance pattern.

22. 1. **The client with phenylketonuria (PKU) must receive counseling from a registered dietitian.**
 2. The client with Graves' disease does not require strict nutrition counseling.
 3. The client with Cushing's syndrome does not require strict diet counseling.
 4. The client with myasthenia gravis does not require strict diet counseling.

TEST-TAKING HINT: PKU is a genetic disease that is characterized by the absence of the enzyme needed to metabolize phenylalanine, an essential amino acid. When clients with PKU consume phenylalanine, a metabolite that affects cognitive centers in the brain is created in the body. If a pregnant woman who has PKU were to eat foods high in phenylalanine, her baby would become severely developmentally disabled. Foods that are high in phenylalanine are those that are high in protein such as meat, fish, poultry, dairy, soy, legumes (dried beans), or nuts.

23. **Answers 1, 2, and 4 are correct.**
 1. **The BMI of 17 is of concern. This client is entering her pregnancy underweight.**
 2. **The rubella titer results should be reported to the nurse midwife.**
 3. This blood pressure is normal.
 4. **The hematocrit is below normal.**
 5. This hemoglobin is normal.

TEST-TAKING HINT: Weight gain monitoring is important for assuring healthy outcomes for the woman and her fetus during the pregnancy and in the future. Women who enter their pregnancies underweight, that is with a BMI less than 18.5 kg/m^2, are encouraged to gain slightly more—28 to 40 lb—during their pregnancies than are women of normal weight who are encouraged to gain between 25 and 35 lb (ACOG, 2013a). A rubella titer of 1:8 IU/mL or less indicates that the woman is non-immune to rubella because the ratio of IgG antibody to rubella is low. As a result, if she is exposed, she is at risk of developing the disease. It is generally accepted that a rubella titer of 1:10 IU/mL or greater indicates that an adequate supply of antibodies is present to provide immunity to rubella. Because a woman is at high risk of becoming anemic during her pregnancy, it is important to identify any woman who enters her pregnancy with a hematocrit that is below normal.

24. 1. The cervix should be long and thick.
 2. **The primary healthcare provider would expect to palpate an enlarged ovary.**
 3. The cervical mucus should be thin.
 4. The vaginal wall should be bluish in color.

TEST-TAKING HINT: The cervix should be long and thick to retain the pregnancy in the uterine cavity. The cervical mucus is thin and the vaginal wall is bluish in color as a result of elevated estrogen levels. The ovary is enlarged because the corpus luteum is still functioning to support the embryo.

25. **Answers 1 and 5 are correct.**
 1. **Women must fast for a minimum of 8 hours and a maximum of 16 hours prior to the test.**
 2. No urine test is performed.
 3. The client will be given 100 grams of glucose in a liquid form upon arrival at the laboratory.
 4. The 100-gram OGTT is a fasting test. Women should neither eat nor drink prior to arriving at the laboratory.
 5. **Smoking on the morning of the test can alter the results.**

TEST-TAKING HINT: There are two approaches to the oral glucose tolerance test (OGTT). In the United States, the American College of Obstetricians and Gynecologists (ACOG) recommends a two-step approach. The first step uses a 50-gram, glucose solution for the initial 1-hour *screening* test, which does not require fasting. If the results are abnormal, the client returns for a *diagnostic* fasting test using a 100-gram glucose solution for the OGTT. The second approach is a one-step method used primarily in Europe and recommended by the American Diabetes Association (ADA, 2021b, pp. S201, 202). This is a 2-hour fasting test using a 75-gram solution of glucose. Preparation for the test requires an overnight fast, as with the 100-gram diagnostic test. The test taker is advised to review the diagnostic blood glucose values for both the 50-gram and 100-gram tests. They can be accessed in the appendix.

The reason for the testing is that human placental lactogen (hPL) is an insulin antagonist, meaning it works against insulin and contributes to insulin resistance. At approximately 24 weeks' gestation, hPL levels can adversely alter a pregnant woman's glucose utilization. In normal pregnancy, there must be an approximate 200% to 250% increase in insulin secretion to maintain euglycemia in the mother (Catalano, et al., 1999) as shown in figure 1 in the appendix. The OGTT is performed to determine whether a woman has developed gestational diabetes, meaning her pancreas cannot keep up with the pregnancy demands for insulin. See "Gestational Diabetes" in the appendix for an allegorical

telling of diabetes in pregnancy and for additional information on this condition.

26. **Answers 2 and 4 are correct.**
    1. It is common for primigravid women not to feel fetal movement until 19 to 20 weeks' gestation.
    2. **The fundal height at 24 weeks should be 4 cm above the umbilicus, 24 cm from the top of the pubic bone. The fundal height at the level of the umbilicus is expected at 20 weeks' gestation.**
    3. Excessive salivation, called ptyalism, is an expected finding in pregnancy.
    4. **The woman may be going into preterm labor. Reports of uterine contractions must always be taken seriously.**
    5. Hemorrhoids are commonly seen in pregnant women.

TEST-TAKING HINT: It is important for the nurse to know the timing of key pregnancy changes as well as abnormal prenatal findings. The mother should feel fetal movement by 20 weeks' gestation, so the first client is not unusual. Primigravid women often feel fetal movement later than multigravid women. Ptyalism is not uncommon. If preterm labor is expected, the client may need hospitalization and medications to stop the labor and/or to prepare the fetal lungs for life outside the womb. Antenatal corticosteroids can help to accelerate fetal lung development. The second client with a lower-than-expected fundal height measurement is of concern. The fetus could be experiencing intrauterine growth restriction (IUGR). A baby delivered at 34 weeks' gestation is at high risk for neonatal complications, primarily respiratory issues due to generally low levels of lung surfactant at this gestational age. Premature neonates are often treated with surfactant. Surfactant reduces surface tension or "stickiness" within the alveoli, which prevents their collapse after exhalation (Nkadi et al., 2009). This makes breathing easier and more effective for the premature neonate.

27. 1. A positive pregnancy test will not necessarily promote fathers' interests in their partners' pregnancies.
    2. Most fathers are very involved with their partners' pregnancies well before childbirth education classes begin.
    3. **Hearing the fetal heartbeat often increases fathers' interests in their partners' pregnancies.**
    4. Meeting the healthcare practitioner is unlikely to promote fathers' interests in their partners' pregnancies.

TEST-TAKING HINT: Women who are in the first few weeks of pregnancy often experience a number of physical complaints—nausea and vomiting, fatigue, breast tenderness, and urinary frequency so the pregnancy is very "real" to them. Prospective fathers whose partners experience these complaints are often not very interested in the pregnancies. When the baby becomes "real" to them as well, with a positive heartbeat or fetal movement, the fathers often become very excited.

28. 1. Ballottement is not related to the mucous plug.
    2. **This is the definition of ballottement.**
    3. Palpating fetal parts is not related to ballottement.
    4. Fetal position is not related to ballottement.

TEST-TAKING HINT: Although this question discusses nurse–client interaction, it is simply a definition question. The test taker is being asked to identify the definition of the word "ballottement." While floating in the amniotic fluid, the fetus bounces away like a balloon when the head is gently pushed during the vaginal examination.

29. 1. Nausea is commonly seen in the first trimester but should have resolved by the time the second trimester begins.
    2. Dyspnea is commonly seen in the third trimester, not the second trimester.
    3. Urinary frequency is commonly seen in the first trimester and late in the third trimester, but it is rarely seen in the second trimester.
    4. **Leg cramping is often a complaint of clients in the second trimester.**

TEST-TAKING HINT: Although most women feel well during the second trimester, leg cramps can occur, especially at night, interrupting one's sleep. Experts are unsure what causes the cramps to occur. Sometimes changes in diet can help reduce the frequency or severity. The client's healthcare provider can sometimes help with suggestions for dietary changes. Urinary frequency and dyspnea are not commonly seen because the baby is not large enough to cause significant impact on bladder capacity and lung expansion.

30. 1. Estrogen levels are not related to glucose metabolism.
    2. Progesterone levels are unrelated to glucose metabolism.
    3. **Human placental lactogen is an insulin antagonist.**
    4. Human chorionic gonadotropin levels are unrelated to glucose metabolisms.

TEST-TAKING HINT: As explained in the answers to question #25 above, the hormone hPL is produced by the placenta. As the placenta grows,

the hormone levels rise, allowing for an increase in the mother's blood sugar. Excess glucose in her blood is available to cross into the fetal blood by facilitated diffusion to meet fetal metabolic needs. If performed earlier than 24 weeks' gestation, the OGTT may result in a false-negative result. A false negative test would imply there was adequate insulin production to maintain normal maternal glucose levels in spite of increased maternal insulin resistance. The danger of a false negative would be untreated gestational diabetes. The resultant hyperglycemia would put the fetus at risk of macrosomia and the mother at risk of an induction and cesarean section among other things. In the future, both the mother and the baby could be at risk of type 2 diabetes and other serious conditions (Farrar, 2016).

31. 1. The majority of the organ systems are developed before the end of the first trimester. This client is in her second trimester.
2. There are a number of over-the-counter medications that should be taken with care during pregnancy.
3. The physician will prescribe a medication that is safe to take during pregnancy.
4. Rectal medications are rarely necessary for headaches. Many medications administered rectally do enter the blood stream.

TEST-TAKING HINT: It is important for pregnant women to contact their primary healthcare providers to find out which medications and herbs are safe to take during pregnancy and which medications must be avoided. All medications are reviewed for their effects on the pregnancy. Although medications were once given a "pregnancy category" of A, B, C, D, or X, that no longer is true. Rather, strict guidelines have been developed to standardize pregnancy information included on medication labels. Drugs that cause structural defects are called teratogens, meaning they cause malformations of the embryo.

32. 1. This is not enough weight gain.
2. This is average weight gain. The woman would be expected to weigh 131 to 132 lb. At this stage of pregnancy, the woman is expected to gain about 0.8 to 1 lb a week.
3. This is more than average weight gain.
4. This is way more than average weight gain.

TEST-TAKING HINT: The incremental weight gain of a client is an important means of assessing the growth and development of the fetus. The nurse would expect that during the second and third trimesters, the woman should gain approximately 0.8 to 1 lb per week.

33. 1. Although breast cancer is hormonally driven, it is rare to see its development during pregnancy.
2. Nodular breast tissue is normal in pregnancy. The client is likely feeling these normal changes during her self breast exam.
3. The woman is not exhibiting psychotic behavior.
4. Anxiety attacks are not common during pregnancy.

TEST-TAKING HINT: The high levels of estrogen and progesterone seen in pregnancy result in a number of changes. The hypertrophy and hyperplasia of the breast tissue, in preparation for neonatal lactation, are two of the changes.

34. 1. An evaluation of the client's exercise schedule should be performed.
2. Goodell's sign is a physiological finding—a softened cervix.
3. Hegar's sign is a physiological finding—a softened uterine isthmus.
4. Leg cramps are likely related to the woman's level of exercise, not her diet.

TEST-TAKING HINT: Leg cramps, which are very painful, are most likely related to the weight of the developing fetus in conjunction with circulatory changes in the extremities. Regular exercise—for example, walking accompanied by stretching of the extremities—can help to reduce the incidence of leg cramps. Strenuous exercise, however, as some professional athletes may wish to do, can result in fetal compromise (Salvesen et al., 2012).

35. 1. The Kegel exercises are done to promote the muscle tone of the perineal muscles.
2. The pelvic tilt is an exercise that can reduce backache pain.
3. Leg lifts will not help to reduce backache pain.
4. Crunches will not help to reduce backache pain.

TEST-TAKING HINT: Pelvic tilt exercises help to reduce backache pain. The client is taught to get into a crawling position on her hands and knees. She is then taught to force her back out while tucking her head and buttocks under (like an angry cat) and holding that position for a few seconds, followed by holding the alternate

position for a few seconds, lifting her head toward the ceiling while bringing her abdomen toward the floor. These positions should be alternated repeatedly for about 5 minutes. The exercises are very relaxing while also improving the muscle tone of the lower back.

36. 1. Although some women do have difficulty breastfeeding, many women with inverted nipples are able to breastfeed with little to no problem.
2. The client should be referred to a lactation consultant.
3. There is no need to telephone the labor unit. However, it would be appropriate to document the finding on the client's prenatal record.
4. It is not recommended that exercises be done to evert the nipples.

TEST-TAKING HINT: Breast manipulation can bring on contractions since it can stimulate endogenous oxytocin production. Lactation consultants are breastfeeding specialists who can assist women with preparing for breastfeeding during pregnancy and while breastfeeding the baby after the birth.

37. 1. The blood pressure should not elevate during pregnancy. This change should be reported to the healthcare practitioner.
2. An increase in the respiratory rate is expected.
3. An increase in the heart rate is expected.
4. A slight increase in temperature is expected.

TEST-TAKING HINT: The client's blood pressure generally drops slightly during the second trimester and returns to the original reading in the third trimester. For this client, a blood pressure of 140/90 in the third trimester could signal pre-eclampsia. The basal metabolic rate of the woman increases during pregnancy. As a result the nurse would expect to observe a respiratory rate of 20 to 24 rpm. High levels of progesterone in the body result in a decrease in the contractility of the smooth musculature throughout the body. This results in an increase in the pulse rate. In addition, progesterone is thermogenic, resulting in a slight rise in the woman's core body temperature.

38. 1. Evening primrose does not affect back strain.
2. Evening primrose does not affect lactation.
3. Evening primrose converts to a prostaglandin substance in the body. Prostaglandins are responsible for readying the cervix for dilation.
4. Evening primrose does not affect the development of hemorrhoids.

TEST-TAKING HINT: Some nurse midwives recommend complementary therapies during pregnancy as well as during labor and delivery. For clients seeking to use natural means for maintaining a healthy pregnancy and for stimulating labor, evening primrose is a suggested intervention for cervical ripening. However, it should be used only after consultation with the primary healthcare provider.

39. 1. Evening primrose has been shown to cause skin rash in some women.
2. Evening primrose has not been shown to cause pedal edema.
3. Evening primrose has not been shown to cause blurred vision.
4. Evening primrose has not been shown to cause tinnitus.

TEST-TAKING HINT: Even though evening primrose is a "natural" substance, it can cause side effects in some clients. The most common side effect seen from the oil is a skin rash. Headaches and nausea have also been seen.

40. 1. It is unlikely that the client has a galactocele.
2. The woman should not pump her breasts during pregnancy.
3. A breast infection is not likely at this time. Colostrum is normally seen at this time and is a reassuring sign that the breasts are preparing to make milk for the baby.
4. It is normal for colostrum to be expressed late in pregnancy. It can be a number of colors, including whitish, yellowish, reddish, and brownish.

TEST-TAKING HINT: Even though colostrum is present in the breasts in the latter part of the third trimester, it is important for women not to pump their breasts. Oxytocin, the hormone that promotes the ejection of milk during lactation, is the hormone of labor. Pumping of the breasts, therefore, could stimulate the uterus to contract.

41. 1. There is nothing in the question to suggest hypertension.
2. The fundal height is the likely cause of the woman's dyspnea.
3. There is nothing in the question to suggest the woman has hydramnios.
4. There is nothing in the question to suggest that the woman has congestive heart failure.

TEST-TAKING HINT: A client should be encouraged not to lie flat on her back. The uterus lies on the aorta and vena cava like a bowling ball and

can block flow to and from the legs and the uterus. As the uterus enlarges, other organs are also affected by the uterine size and weight. At 36 weeks, the fundus is at the level of the xiphoid process. The diaphragm is elevated and the lungs are displaced. As a result, when a client lies flat she has difficulty breathing. Most women use multiple pillows at night for sleep. Whenever caring for a pregnant woman, the nurse should offer to elevate the head of the bed, or to position the client comfortably on her side with pillows between the knees to maintain spinal alignment.

42. Answers 1, 2, and 3 are correct.
1. **Urinary frequency is seen once lightening, or the descent of the fetus into the pelvis, has occurred.**
2. **Heartburn is a common complaint of pregnant women.**
3. **Backaches are common complaints of pregnant women.**
4. Persistent headache should not be seen in pregnant women.
5. Pregnant women should not complain of blurred vision.

TEST-TAKING HINT: This question is asking the nurse to differentiate between complaints that are expected during the third trimester and those that are abnormal. Heartburn and backaches are expected complaints. In addition, once lightening has occurred, frequent urination also returns. In each of the three cases, the signs do not indicate pathology. Both persistent headache and blurred vision, however, are signs that the woman may have developed pre-eclampsia, a serious complication of pregnancy. If these symptoms develop, the client should be advised to report them to the healthcare practitioner.

43.
1. Telling the client she will know when labor starts, ignores and dismisses the client's concerns as unimportant.
2. **This is a true statement. Labor contractions often begin in the back. The pain comes and goes rhythmically.**
3. Although active labor is usually more uncomfortable than the normal aches and pains of pregnancy, that is not necessarily true of prodromal labor or the latent phase of labor.
4. The nurse is making an assumption here. Coming to the hospital "too early" may not be the client's concern at all.

TEST-TAKING HINT: Labor contractions often begin in a woman's back, feeling much like a backache. Some clients describe it as the recurring sensation of a hot, metal belt being tightened from the lower back to the front, below the uterus. Unlike pregnancy aches and pains, labor contractions come and go rhythmically, increasing in strength and regularity. The client should be advised to attend to any pains that come and go and to time them from the start of one to the start of the next one. She should also include the duration of each contraction. Her body might be at the start of the labor process.

44.
1. **Anemia is an expected finding.**
2. The client should not be thrombocytopenic. Although some women do develop idiopathic thrombocytopenia of pregnancy, this is a complication of pregnancy.
3. The nurse would not expect to see polycythemia.
4. The nurse would not expect to see hyperbilirubinemia.

TEST-TAKING HINT: By the end of the second trimester, the blood supply of the woman increases by approximately 50%. This increase is a normal preparation by the body for blood loss during the delivery, which can be around 500 mL with a vaginal birth (Aguree & Gernand, 2019). Plasma volume expansion is greater than red blood cell (RBC) mass increase, resulting in hemodilution. Because the hematocrit measurement is the percent of red blood cells in a drop of blood, it follows that if that drop of blood has more plasma than red blood cells, the percentage will be lower. A similar thing happens with the hemoglobin, which is measured as the number of milligrams per deciliter. Blood with a higher amount of plasma will show a lower number of milligrams of hemoglobin per deciliter. Because of these lower numbers, clients develop what is commonly called "physiologic anemia of pregnancy" even though their anemia is not related to poor nutrition. A hematocrit of 32% is considered normal for a pregnant woman. A hemoglobin level of 10.5 is within normal for a pregnant woman.

45.
1. Although the orthopneic position is a safe position for the client to be placed in, a prenatal examination cannot be performed in this position.
2. Although the lateral-recumbent position is a safe position for the client to be placed in, a prenatal examination cannot be performed in this position. In addition, the pregnant abdomen may not enable the client fully to attain this position.
3. Although the Sims position is a safe position for the client to be placed in, a prenatal examination cannot be performed in this position, and the pregnant abdomen may not enable the client fully to attain this position.

4. **The client should be placed in a low, semi-Fowler's position, about 15 degrees.**

TEST-TAKING HINT: Because of the growth of the uterus, it is very difficult for women in the third trimester to breathe in the supine position. In addition, the weight of the uterus on the aorta and vena cava can reduce blood circulation to the legs and to the uterus. During the prenatal visit, the baby's heartbeat will be monitored and the fundal height will be assessed. Both of these procedures can safely be performed in the low, semi-Fowler's position.

46. Answers 2, 3, and 4 are correct.

1. Urine glucose is performed at each visit, not the blood glucose.
2. **The blood pressure is assessed at each prenatal visit.**
3. **The fetal heart rate is assessed at each prenatal visit by the doppler or fetoscope. The fetal heart is audible via Doppler many weeks before it is audible via fetoscope.**
4. **Urine protein is performed at each prenatal visit.**
5. Ultrasounds are performed only when needed.

TEST-TAKING HINT: The test taker must read the question carefully. Although urine glucose assessments are done at each visit, blood glucoses are assessed only intermittently during the pregnancy. Similarly, although ultrasound assessments may be ordered intermittently during a pregnancy, they are not usually performed at every prenatal visit.

47. Answers 1, 2, 3, and 5 are correct.

1. **Although annoying, leg cramps are not pathological.**
2. **Varicose veins are normal, although client teaching may be needed.**
3. **Hemorrhoids are normal, although client teaching may be needed.**
4. Fainting spells are not normal, although the client may feel faint when rising quickly from a lying position.
5. **Lordosis, or change in the curvature of the spine, is normal, although client teaching may be needed.**

TEST-TAKING HINT: There are a number of physical complaints that are "normal" during pregnancy. There are interventions, however, that can be taught to help to alleviate some of the discomforts. The nurse should be familiar with information the client needs regarding the physical complaints of pregnancy.

48. 1. The nurse would expect to note hypotension rather than hypertension.
2. **Dizziness is an expected finding.**
3. The nurse would expect to see dyspnea, not rales.
4. The nurse would not expect to see any skin changes.

TEST-TAKING HINT: Because the weight of the gravid uterus compresses the great vessels, the nurse would expect the client to become hypotensive and to complain of dizziness when lying supine. In addition, the fetal heart rate may drop. The blood supply to the head and other parts of the body, including the placenta, is diminished when the great vessels are compressed.

49. 1. It is appropriate to ask the client if she plans to breastfeed.
2. **It is inappropriate to ask the Muslim client about the name for the baby.**
3. It is appropriate to ask the client the name of her chosen pediatrician.
4. It is appropriate to ask the client how she feels about having an episiotomy.

TEST-TAKING HINT: Traditional Muslim couples may not tell anyone the baby's name until they have gone through the official naming ceremony, called *aqiqah*. Babies may not be named before a week of age. The parents need time to get to know their baby and decide on an appropriate name for them.

50. 1. The oral glucose tolerance test (OGTT) is performed at approximately 24 weeks' gestation.
2. Amniotic fluid volume assessment is part of the biophysical profile (BPP). The BPP is performed when the healthcare practitioner is concerned about the health and well-being of the fetus.
3. **Vaginal and rectal cultures are done at approximately 36 weeks' gestation.**
4. Karyotype analysis or chromosomal analysis, if performed, is done early in pregnancy.

TEST-TAKING HINT: Vaginal and rectal cultures are done to assess for the presence of group B streptococcal (GBS) bacteria in the woman's vagina and rectum. If the woman has GBS as part of her normal flora, she will be given IV antibiotics during labor to prevent vertical transmission to her baby at birth. GBS has been called "the baby killer" because many babies died in the past, before prenatal testing and antibiotic administration was standard of care.

51. 1. Unless nosebleeds are excessive, it is rare for them to lead to severe anemia.
2. Clients with nosebleeds rarely have temperature elevations.
3. This is an accurate statement. Hormonal changes in pregnancy make the nasal passages prone to bleeding.
4. Nosebleeds are an expected complication of pregnancy.

TEST-TAKING HINT: Estrogen, one of the important hormones of pregnancy, promotes vasocongestion of mucous membranes, including the small blood vessels in the nose. Due to the increase in blood circulation during pregnancy, these blood vessels are more prone to burst, causing a nosebleed.

52. **1. The woman implies that she and her husband are not having sex. There is no need to refrain from sexual intercourse during a normal pregnancy—so the woman and her husband could benefit from information on this topic.**
2. Some men do gain weight during pregnancy. This is viewed as a sympathetic response to the woman's weight gain.
3. Men often become much more concerned about the finances of the household during a woman's pregnancy.
4. The father is exhibiting a strong attachment to the unborn baby.

TEST-TAKING HINT: *Couvade* is the term given to a father's physiological responses to his partner's pregnancy. Men have been seen to exhibit a number of physical complaints/changes that simulate their partner's physical complaints/changes—for example, indigestion, weight gain, urinary frequency, and backache.

53. 1. The nurse would expect the hematocrit to drop with physiologic anemia of pregnancy.
2. The nurse would expect to see an elevated white blood cell count.
3. The nurse would not expect to see an abnormal potassium level.
4. The nurse would not expect to see an abnormal sodium level.

TEST-TAKING HINT: At the end of the third trimester and through to the early postpartum period, a normal leukocytosis, or rise in white blood cell count, is seen. This is a natural physiological change that protects the woman's body from the invasion of pathogens during the birth process. The nurse should rely on a temperature elevation to suggest whether or not the woman has an infection.

54. 1. Clients at 35 weeks' gestation should not complain of nausea and vomiting.
2. Clients at 35 weeks' gestation should not be ambivalent about their pregnancies.
3. At 35 weeks, the fundus should be 35 cm above the pubic bone.
4. Although edema is a normal finding in the third trimester, pitting edema is not a normal finding.

TEST-TAKING HINT: It is essential that the nurse differentiate between normal and abnormal findings at various points during the pregnancy—for example, nausea and vomiting are normal during the first trimester but not during the second or third trimester. The fundal height measurement is also important to remember. The measurements are approximately the same number of centimeters above the symphysis pubis as the number of weeks of fetal gestation. For example, at 24 weeks' gestation, the height is usually 24 cm above the symphysis. At 35 weeks' gestation, the height is usually 35 cm above the symphysis pubis, and so on. Edema can be a normal finding at 35 weeks, although pitting edema is not normal.

55. 1. Unless a woman is at high risk for preterm labor, there is no reason to refrain from making love during pregnancy. Therefore, this is an inappropriate statement. Drinking water will not change anything.
2. This is an accurate statement. An orgasm does not generally lead to preterm labor.
3. Unless a woman is at high risk for preterm labor, this is an inappropriate statement. She does not need to be seen by the primary healthcare provider.
4. This is an inappropriate statement. Neither the pregnancy or the fetus is at risk. A fetal kick count is unnecessary.

TEST-TAKING HINT: There is no contraindication to intercourse or to orgasm during pregnancy, unless it has been determined that a client is at high risk for preterm labor. Until late in pregnancy, there are very few oxytocin receptor sites on the uterine body. The woman will, therefore, not go into labor as a result of an orgasm during sexual relations.

56. 1. Although the tour of the facility is important, this should not be the couple's first step.
2. It is best that a couple first develop a birth plan.
3. Although appointments should be made, this should not be the couple's first step.

4. Although the couple may wish to research the healthcare practitioner's malpractice history, this should not be the couple's first step.

TEST-TAKING HINT: A birth plan doesn't need to be official or final; it serves as a list of what's important to the woman and her partner during labor and delivery. It may change as she learns more about her options and about routine care throughout labor and after the delivery. It is important that a couple's needs and wants match their obstetrical care practitioner's philosophy of care. If, for example, the couple is interested in the possibility of having a water birth, it is important that the healthcare provider be willing to perform a water birth. If, however, the woman wants to be "completely pain-free," the healthcare provider must be willing to order pain medications throughout the labor and delivery. A birth plan will list the couple's many wishes and can guide the conversation.

57. 1. **Clients who experience ptyalism have an excess of saliva. They should be advised to be vigilant in the care of their teeth and gums. Ptyalism is often accompanied by gingivitis and nausea and vomiting.**
2. Ptyalism is not related to a change in blood pressure.
3. Ptyalism is not related to changes in the lower extremities.
4. Ptyalism is not related to the meat intake.

TEST-TAKING HINT: Ptyalism is related to the increase in vascular congestion of the mucous membranes from increased estrogen production. Women with increased salivation often also experience gingivitis, which is also related to estrogen production. In addition, ptyalism is seen in women with nausea and vomiting. Because of the caustic effects of gastric juices on the enamel of the teeth, the inflammation seen in the gums, and the increased salivation, it is essential that the pregnant woman take special care of her teeth during pregnancy, including regular visits to the dentist and/or the dental hygienist.

58. 1. **The woman should receive the influenza injection. The nasal spray, however, should not be administered to a pregnant woman.**
2. The mumps vaccine should not be administered to the pregnant client.
3. The rubella vaccine should not be administered to the pregnant client.
4. The varicella vaccine should not be administered to the pregnant client.

TEST-TAKING HINT: It is very important for pregnant women to be protected from the flu by receiving the inactivated influenza injection. The fetus will not be injured by the shot and the woman will be protected from the many sequelae that can develop from the flu. However, the nasal flu spray should not be administered to pregnant women because it contains live virus. It is contraindicated to vaccinate pregnant women with many other vaccines, including the measles-mumps-rubella (MMR) and the varicella vaccines. A pregnant woman must always check with her primary healthcare provider before receiving a vaccination of any kind.

59. 1. **The woman should stay out of rooms that are being renovated.**
2. The water should be tested for the presence of lead. If there is lead in the water, it is recommended that the water from the hot water tap not be consumed.
3. Unless mold has been found, there is no reason the client should refrain from entering the basement.
4. As long as she is feeling well, there is no reason the client should refrain from walking up the stairs.

TEST-TAKING HINT: Vintage houses often contain lead-based paint and water piping that has been soldered with lead-based solder. Lead, when ingested either through the respiratory tract or the GI tract, can cause permanent damage to the central nervous system of the unborn child. It is very important, therefore, that the woman not breathe in the air in rooms that have recently been sanded. The paint aerosolizes and the lead can be inhaled. In addition, lead leaches into hot water more readily than into cold, so water from the cold tap should be consumed—but only after the water has run through the pipes for a minimum of 2 minutes.

60. 1. An allergy to strawberries is not the likely reason.
2. Strawberries have not been shown to cause birth defects.
3. **The woman believes in old wives' tales.**
4. A previous poor pregnancy outcome is not the likely reason.

TEST-TAKING HINT: There are a number of old wives' tales that some pregnant women believe in and live by. One of the common tales relates to the ingestion of strawberries, that *Women who eat strawberries have babies with strawberry marks on their bodies.* Unless belief in old wives' tales has the potential to affect the health of the baby and/or mother, it is ill advised and unnecessary to argue with the mother about her beliefs.

61. 1. Unless a woman is at high risk for preterm labor, has been diagnosed with placenta previa, or has preterm rupture of the membranes, sexual intercourse is not contraindicated.
2. Breast fondling should be discouraged only if the client is at high risk for preterm labor.
3. With increasing size of the uterine body, the couple may need counseling regarding alternate options for sexual intimacy.
4. There is no contraindication for vaginal lubricant use in pregnancy. As a matter of fact, with the increased discharge experienced by many mothers, lubricants are often not needed.

TEST-TAKING HINT: Pregnancy lasts 10 lunar months (each lunar month is 4 weeks). It is essential that the nurse counsel clients on ways to maintain health and well-being in the many facets of their lives. Sexual intimacy is one of the important aspects of a married couple's life together. The couple can be counseled to use alternate positions, or discover other means to satisfy their needs for sexual expression during the pregnancy period.

62. 1. Linea nigra—the darkened area on the skin from the symphysis to the umbilicus—is a normal skin change seen in pregnancy.
2. Melasma—the "mask" of pregnancy—is a normal skin change seen in pregnancy.
3. Petechiae are pinpoint red or purple spots on the skin. They are seen in hemorrhagic conditions.
4. Spider nevi—benign radiating blood vessels—are normal skin changes seen in pregnancy.

TEST-TAKING HINT: There are many skin changes that occur normally during pregnancy. Most of the changes—such as linea nigra, melasma, and hyperpigmentation of the areolae—are related to an increase in the melanin-producing bodies of the skin as a result of stimulation by the female hormones estrogen and progesterone. The presence of petechiae is usually related to a pathological condition, such as thrombocytopenia.

63. 1. The estimated date of delivery is not May 30, 2022.
2. The estimated date of delivery is not June 20, 2022.
3. The estimated date of delivery is June 27, 2022.
4. The estimated date of delivery is not July 3, 2022.

TEST-TAKING HINT: Nagele's rule is a simple method used to calculate a client's estimated date of confinement (EDC) or estimated date of delivery (EDD) from the last normal menstrual period (LMP). Count back 3 months from the last menstrual period. For this client, whose period was September 20th, count back to June 20th and add 7 days, giving you June 27th. Since the baby will be born the next year, her due date is June 27th, 2022.

64. Answers 1, 4, and 5 are correct.
1. Heartburn is a common symptom.
2. It is inappropriate for a prospective father to engage in promiscuity.
3. Hypertension in a prospective father should be investigated.
4. Some fathers complain of abdominal bloating.
5. Some fathers complain of abdominal pain.

TEST-TAKING HINT: Heartburn, bloating, and abdominal pain are subjective complaints that significant others often experience during their partners' pregnancies. Those who experience couvade symptoms are exhibiting a strong affiliation between themselves and their partners. It is inappropriate and highly unusual for prospective partners to engage in illicit relationships and/or to show indifference toward their partners' pregnancies. They are generally fully engaged in the process. The expectant partner should be referred to their own primary healthcare provider for further investigation of hypertension, as it is not likely part of couvade syndrome. The significant other may have developed a pathological condition.

65. Answers 1, 2, 3, and 4 are correct.
1. Convulsions are a danger sign of pregnancy.
2. Double vision is a danger sign of pregnancy.
3. Epigastric pain is a danger sign of pregnancy.
4. Persistent vomiting is a danger sign of pregnancy.
5. Although polyuria may be a sign of diabetes or another illness, it is not highlighted as a danger sign of pregnancy.

TEST-TAKING HINT: The danger signs of pregnancy are signs or symptoms that can occur in an otherwise healthy pregnancy that are likely due to serious pregnancy complications. For example, double vision, epigastric pain, and blurred vision are symptoms of the hypertensive illnesses of pregnancy, and persistent vomiting is a symptom of hyperemesis gravidarum.

66. 1. This does not reflect an accurate picture.
2. This does not reflect an accurate picture.
3. This accurately reflects this woman's gravidity and parity—G5 P1122.
4. This does not reflect an accurate picture.

TEST-TAKING HINT: Gravidity refers to pregnancy and parity refers to the number of children previously born. Every time a woman is pregnant, it is counted as one gravida (G). The parity (P) history is divided into four criteria in a distinct order, which make up the acronym "TPAL," which may be helpful for the nurse to remember. The first number "T" refers to the number of term births or births at or greater than 38 weeks' gestation; the second number "P" represents the number of preterm births or births between 20 and 37 weeks' gestation; the third number "A" refers to abortions, whether spontaneous or therapeutic; and "L," referring to the fourth number, is the number of living children. The client in this question has been pregnant 5 times (G5); she gave birth to 1 daughter at term (T); 1 preterm son (P); had 2 abortions/miscarriages (A); and has 2 living children (L) for a parity of P1122. Her gravidity is the sum of the first 3 numbers of her pregnancy history (1 + 1 + 2 = 4), plus one for this pregnancy, making this client's gravidity G5. If this were her first pregnancy, she would be G1 P zero. If it were her second pregnancy and she had one child born at term and no other pregnancies, she would be G2 P1001. Note that a pregnancy with multiple fetuses counts as one pregnancy and one delivery. However, each living child is included for the "L" of living children.

67. 1. Tofu, legumes, and broccoli are excellent substitutes for the restricted foods.
2. Although corn, yams, and green beans are foods consistent with a vegan diet, they are not high either in protein or in iron.
3. Although potatoes, parsnips, and turnips are vegetables, they are not high either in protein or in iron.
4. These are examples of a vegan's restricted foods.

TEST-TAKING HINT: Vegans are vegetarians who eat absolutely no animal products. Since animal products are most clients' sources of protein, iron, and vitamin B12, it is necessary for vegans to be very careful to meet their increased needs by eating excellent sources of these nutrients. It is recommended that vegans meet with a registered dietitian early in their pregnancies to discuss diet choices.

68. 1. Although the client is meeting her daily fruit requirements, this is not the most important communication for the nurse to make.
2. Fruit juices are good sources of folic acid, but this is not the most important communication for the nurse to make.
3. It is recommended that pregnant clients eat whole fruits rather than consume large quantities of fruit juice. This is the most important statement for the nurse to make.
4. Although the client is exceeding the daily fruit requirement, this is not the most important communication for the nurse to make.

TEST-TAKING HINT: It is recommended that moderately active women of childbearing age consume the equivalent of at least 2 cups of fruit per day. Approximately 8 oz of fruit juice equals 1 cup of fruit. Fruit juices, however, are rarely made of 100% juice and almost always contain added sugar. This can put added strain on the woman's pancreas to release insulin, even if she does not have gestational diabetes. In addition, the client is not receiving the benefit of the fiber that is contained in the whole fruit. The nurse should compliment the client on her fruit intake but encourage her to consume whole fruits rather than large quantities of juice.

69. 1. Supplementation of vitamin C has not been shown to be harmful during pregnancy.
2. Vitamin D supplementation can be harmful during pregnancy.
3. Supplementation of the B vitamins has not been shown to be harmful during pregnancy.
4. Supplementation of the B vitamins has not been shown to be harmful during pregnancy.

TEST-TAKING HINT: The water-soluble vitamins, if consumed in large quantities, have not been shown to be harmful during pregnancy. The body eliminates the excess quantities through the urine and stool. However, the fat-soluble vitamins—vitamins A, D, E, and K—can build up in the body. Vitamins A and D have been shown to be teratogenic to the fetus in megadoses.

70. 1. Vitamin B1 (thiamine) does not need to be supplemented.
2. Vitamin B2, (niacin), does not need to be supplemented.
3. Vitamin B6, pyridoxine, does not need to be supplemented.
4. Vitamin B12 (cobalamin) should be supplemented.

TEST-TAKING HINT: Vitamin B12 (cobalamin) is found almost exclusively in animal products—meat, dairy, eggs. Since vegans do not consume animal products and the vitamin is not in most nonanimal sources, it is strongly recommended

that vegans supplement that vitamin. Those who take in too little of the vitamin are susceptible to anemia and nervous system disorders. In addition, the vitamin is especially important during pregnancy since it is essential for DNA synthesis.

71. 1. Pasta is a low-fiber food.
2. Rice is a low-fiber food.
3. Dairy products are low-fiber foods.
4. Celery is an excellent food to reverse constipation. It is a high-fiber food.

TEST-TAKING HINT: Most women complain of constipation during pregnancy. Progesterone, a muscle relaxant, is responsible for a slowing of the digestive system. It is important, therefore, to recommend foods to pregnant clients that will help to alleviate the problem. Foods high in fiber, such as fresh fruits and vegetables, are excellent suggestions.

72. 1. Turnip greens are calcium rich.
2. Green beans are not high in calcium.
3. Cantaloupes are not high in calcium.
4. Nectarines are not high in calcium.

TEST-TAKING HINT: There are a number of women who, for one reason or another, do not consume large quantities of dairy products. The nurse must be prepared to suggest alternate sources since dairy products are the best sources for calcium intake. Any of the dark green, leafy vegetables such as kale, spinach, collards, and turnip greens are excellent sources as are small fish that are eaten with the bones such as sardines.

73. 1. This is an accurate statement. A serving of meat—typically a 2 to 3 oz serving—is approximately equal to a deck of cards.
2. A paperback book is too large.
3. A clenched fist is too large.
4. A large tomato is too large.

TEST-TAKING HINT: The dietary recommendation of the protein group for moderately active women of childbearing age is the equivalent of 5 ½ oz of lean meat, fish, or fowl per day. A 1 oz equivalent is defined as 1 oz of meat, fish, or poultry or one egg. The average American diet well exceeds the recommended protein intake since most Americans consider a serving of meat to be much larger than a deck of cards. Additional and healthier sources of protein are peanut butter, nuts, or seeds and cooked beans or peas. It is recommended that 4 to 5 servings of these sources be consumed each week. It is also recommended that pregnant women eat at least 8 oz of seafood per week up to a maximum of 12 oz per week.

74. 1. 2 tbsp of peanut butter = a 2 oz nonmeat serving of protein.
2. 1 egg = a 1 oz nonmeat serving of protein.
3. 1 cup of cooked lima beans = four 1 oz nonmeat servings of protein.
4. 3 ounces of nuts = six 1 oz nonmeat servings of protein.

TEST-TAKING HINT: The nurse should refer to the U.S. Dietary Association information for up-to-date dietary recommendations. As more research information is forthcoming, dietary recommendations change. The current recommendations can be found at https://www.dietaryguidelines.gov/sites/default/files/2020-12/Dietary_Guidelines_for_Americans_2020-2025.pdf

75. Answers 2, 4, and 5 are correct.
1. 1 bagel = two or more 1 oz servings (depending on the size of the bagel).
2. 1 slice bread = one 1 oz serving.
3. 1 cup cooked pasta = two 1 oz servings.
4. 1 tortilla = one 1 oz serving.
5. 1 ounce dry cereal = one 1 oz serving.

TEST-TAKING HINT: The recommendation for moderately active women of childbearing age is to consume six to eight servings of grain each day. However, one sandwich equals two servings since each slice of bread equals one 1 oz serving. Also, it is important to counsel women to eat whole grain foods rather than processed grains. More nutrients as well as more fiber are obtained from whole grain foods. In addition, whole grain foods raise the blood sugar levels more slowly.

76. 1. Although herbals are natural substances, there are many herbals that are unsafe for consumption during pregnancy.
2. Both licorice and cat's claw should be avoided during pregnancy. There is evidence that licorice may increase the incidence of preterm labor, and cat's claw has been used to prevent and to abort pregnancies.
3. There is not enough evidence to determine whether or not many herbals are safe in pregnancy.
4. Every woman should advise her primary healthcare provider of what she is consuming, including food, medicines, herbals, and all other substances.

TEST-TAKING HINT: Herbal medicines are not regulated by the Food and Drug Administration (FDA). There is some information on selected herbal medicines or botanicals at the National Institutes of Health Web site—http://nccam.nih.gov/health—but because research on pregnant

women is particularly sensitive there is very little definitive information on the safety of many of these products in pregnancy. No matter what is consumed by the mother, however, the primary healthcare provider should be consulted.

77. **1. Bologna should not be consumed during pregnancy unless it is thoroughly cooked.**
2. Cantaloupe is an excellent source of vitamins A and C.
3. Asparagus is an excellent source of vitamin K and folic acid.
4. Popcorn is an excellent source of fiber, although if loaded with butter and salt is not the most healthy fiber choice.

TEST-TAKING HINT: Because pregnant women are slightly immunocompromised, they are especially susceptible to certain diseases. Deli meats, unless heated to steaming hot, can cause listeriosis. Pregnant women should avoid these foods. Other foods that contain *Listeria monocytogenes* and should be avoided are unpasteurized milk, soft cheese, and undercooked meats. Other food-borne pathogens, for example, Campylobacter and Cryptosporidium, can also cause serious illness in pregnant women.

78. 1. Fish is a very healthy choice, but the recommendation is that the fish be well cooked.
2. Although pregnant women should not overeat salty foods, sushi should be avoided because it is raw, not because of its salt content.
3. All fish contain methylmercury, but there are some fish with such high levels that they should not be eaten at all; for example, swordfish, tilefish, king mackerel, and shark. The mercury level does not change when a fish is eaten cooked versus raw.
4. This is correct. It is recommended that during pregnancy the client eat only well-cooked fish.

TEST-TAKING HINT: Fish is an excellent source of omega-3 oil and protein, but during pregnancy fish should be well cooked to avoid ingestion of pathogens. It is recommended that pregnant women consume 8 to 12 oz of seafood per week. No more than 12 oz per week is recommended, however, to reduce the potential of consuming toxic levels of methylmercury.

79. 1. Raisins contain some iron but they are not the best source of iron.
2. Hamburger contains the most iron.
3. Broccoli contains some iron but it is not the best source of iron.
4. Molasses contains some iron but it is not the best source of iron.

TEST-TAKING HINT: Iron is present in most animal sources—seafood, meats, eggs—although it is not present in milk. There also is iron in vegetable sources, although not in the same concentration as in animal products. If the nurse is caring for a pregnant vegan or vegetarian, the nurse must counsel the client regarding non-animal sources of all nutrients.

80. 1. Hypothyroidism is not related to pica.
2. Iron-deficiency anemia is often seen in clients who engage in pica.
3. Hypercalcemia is not related to pica.
4. Overexposure to zinc is not related to pica.

TEST-TAKING HINT: Clients who engage in pica eat large quantities of nonfood items like ice, laundry starch, soap, and dirt. There are a number of problems related to pica, including teratogenesis related to eating foods harmful to the fetus. More commonly, the women fill up on items like ice instead of eating high-quality foods. This practice is thought to be related to iron deficiency.

81. 1. Replacing laundry starch with salt is not an appropriate substitute. High levels of salt can lead to elevated blood pressure and fluid retention.
2. Replacing ice with fruit juice popsicles is an excellent suggestion. Fruit juice, although high in sugar, does contain vitamins.
3. Replacing soap with cream cheese is not an appropriate substitute. Cream cheese has little to no nutritional benefit.
4. Replacing soil with uncooked pie crust is not an appropriate substitute. Uncooked pie crust is high in fat and flour. It provides little to no nutritional benefit.

TEST-TAKING HINT: Although the nurse might prefer that a client completely stop a behavior that the nurse deems unsafe or inappropriate, the client may disagree. The nurse, therefore, must attempt to provide a substitute for the client's behavior. Pica is a behavior that should be discouraged because of its potentially detrimental effects. If the client wishes to consume ice, an excellent alternative is ice pops, Italian ices, or iced fruit juice.

82. **1. Ginger has been shown to be a safe antiemetic agent for pregnant women.**
2. Sage has not been shown to reduce nausea and vomiting in pregnant women.
3. Cloves have not been shown to reduce nausea and vomiting in pregnant women.

4. Nutmeg has not been shown to reduce nausea and vomiting in pregnant women.

TEST-TAKING HINT: Morning sickness and daytime nausea and vomiting are common complaints of pregnant women during the first trimester. Ginger—consumed as ginger tea, ginger ale, and the like—has been shown to be a safe and an effective anti-nausea agent for many pregnant women.

83. 1. Barley and brown rice are not good vitamin C sources.
2. **Strawberries and potatoes are excellent sources of vitamin C, as are zucchini, blueberries, kiwi, green beans, and green peas.**
3. Buckwheat and lentils are not good vitamin C sources.
4. Wheat flour and figs are not good vitamin C sources.

TEST-TAKING HINT: The nurse must be prepared to answer basic nutrition questions related to the health of the pregnant woman. Even though citrus fruits are commonly thought of as the primary sources of vitamin C, the nurse should realize that virtually all fruits and vegetables contain the vitamin, while grains do not.

84. 1. Frozen yogurt, although relatively high in calories, is an excellent dairy source. Its intake should be encouraged.
2. Parmesan cheese is an excellent dairy source. Its intake should be encouraged.
3. **The intake of gorgonzola cheese should be discouraged during pregnancy.**
4. Chocolate milk, although relatively high in calories, is an excellent dairy source. Its intake should be encouraged if the client refuses to drink unflavored milk.

TEST-TAKING HINT: Any dairy product that is not pasteurized should be avoided. Gorgonzola cheese is one of these, a soft cheese. Soft cheeses often harbor *Listeria monocytogenes*, the organism that causes listeriosis. Pregnant women are at high risk of developing this infection because they are slightly immunosuppressed. The adult disease can assume many forms, including meningitis, pneumonia, and sepsis. Pregnant women who develop the disease often deliver stillborn babies or babies who are at risk of dying postdelivery from fulminant disease.

85. **Answers 2, 3, 4, and 5 are correct.**
1. The umbilical cord, not the amniotic fluid, delivers nutrition to the developing fetus.
2. **Amniotic fluid does cushion the fetus from injury.**
3. **Amniotic fluid enables the fetus's limbs and body to move freely so that the baby can grow unencumbered.**
4. **The amniotic fluid is maintained at the mother's body temperature, providing the fetus with a neutral thermal environment.**
5. **The fetus does swallow the amniotic fluid while in utero.**

TEST-TAKING HINT: For the first 16 weeks of the pregnancy, most of the amniotic fluid consists of maternal plasma which passes through the placenta into the gestational sac (Beall et al., 2007). Once the fetal kidney begins working at around 16 weeks gestation, fetal urine becomes the primary source, although the fetal lungs also contribute a small amount of fluid (Brace et al., 2018). In addition to the functions noted in the answers above, the baby practices "breathing" as the amniotic fluid moves in and out of the lungs in preparation for breathing air in the extrauterine environment and "drinks" the amniotic fluid in preparation for extrauterine feeding.

86. 1. **This statement is true. Organogenesis begins prior to the missed menstrual period.**
2. Insurance companies do not require that a woman be preapproved to become pregnant.
3. This statement is untrue. Only women with specific physical complications may be counseled to limit the numbers of pregnancies that they should carry.
4. This statement is untrue. The cardiovascular system is stressed during each pregnancy.

TEST-TAKING HINT: The test taker may be unfamiliar with the term "organogenesis." To answer the question correctly, it is essential that the test taker be able to decipher the definition. When the word is broken down into its parts, the meaning is clear. "Organo" means "organ" and "genesis" means "origin." The definition of the term, therefore, is origin, or development, of the organ systems.

87. **Answers 1, 2, 3, and 5 are correct.**
1. **Although not yet clearly visible on ultrasound, the genitalia are formed by the end of the first trimester.**
2. **The heart is formed by the end of the first trimester.**
3. **The fingers are formed by the end of the first trimester.**
4. The alveoli will not be formed until well into the second trimester.
5. **The kidneys are formed by the end of the first trimester.**

TEST-TAKING HINT: The test taker should be familiar with the basic developmental changes that occur during the three trimesters. In addition, the test taker should be able to develop a basic timeline of developmental milestones that occur during the pregnancy. By the conclusion of the first trimester, all major organs are completely formed, but the maturation of the organ systems must still occur throughout the subsequent trimesters.

88. 1. The foramen ovale is a hole between the atria.
2. The umbilical vein carries oxygen-rich blood.
3. The right atrium does contain both oxygen-rich and oxygen-poor blood.
4. The ductus venosus lies between the umbilical vein and the inferior vena cava, not between the aorta and the pulmonary artery.

TEST-TAKING HINT: The test taker should have an understanding of fetal circulation. One principle to remember when studying the circulation of the fetus is that the majority of fetal blood bypasses the lungs since the baby is receiving oxygen-rich blood directly from the placenta via the umbilical vein. The location of the three ducts—ductus venosus, formen ovale, ductus arteriosus—enables the blood to bypass the lungs. For more information on fetal circulation, see the appendix.

89. **1. This is a true statement. In the morula stage, about 2 to 4 days after fertilization, the fertilized egg has not yet implanted in the uterus.**
2. Lung development occurs much later than the morular stage.
3. The sex of the fetus is identified much later than the morular stage.
4. The fetal eyelids unfuse much later than the morular stage.

TEST-TAKING HINT: The morula is the undifferentiated ball of cells that migrates down the fallopian tube toward the uterine body. The morular stage lasts from about the 2nd to the 4th day after fertilization.

90. 1. This is true of monozygotic twins; they develop from the same ovum, or egg.
2. This is a true statement. Dizygotic twins result from two mature ova that are fertilized independently.
3. Monozygotic twins share the same placenta and have a common chorion.
4. Monozygotic twins have the same sex and blood type.

TEST-TAKING HINT: The best way for the nurse to differentiate between monozygotic twinning and dizygotic twinning is to remember the meaning of the prefixes to the two words. "Mono" means "one." Monozygotic twins, therefore, originate from one fertilized ovum. The babies have the same DNA; therefore, they are the same sex. They share a placenta and chorion. "Di" means "two." Dizygotic twins arise from two separately fertilized eggs. Their genetic relationship is the same as if they were siblings born from different pregnancies. They may be of differing sexes.

91. 1. The fetal heart begins to beat during the first trimester, not when quickening is detected at 16 to 20 weeks.
2. Lanugo does cover the fetal body at approximately 20 weeks' gestation.
3. The kidneys secrete urine by about week 12, before quickening is detected. Amniotic fluid is composed predominantly of fetal urine.
4. Fingernails begin to form at about week 10 but do not completely cover the tips of the fingers until mid third trimester.

TEST-TAKING HINT: Although the nurse need not memorize all fetal developmental changes, it is important to have an understanding of major periods of development. For example, organogenesis occurs during the first trimester with all of the major organs functioning at a primitive level by week 12.

92. 1. The client should be assured that it is unlikely that the fetus was affected.
2. This statement is true.
3. It is inappropriate for the nurse to suggest that the client seek an abortion.
4. The client should be assured that it is unlikely that the fetus was affected.

TEST-TAKING HINT: The 2-week period between ovulation and implantation is often called "the all or nothing period." During that time, the fertilized egg/embryo is floating freely in the client's fallopian tubes toward the uterine body. The mother is not supplying the embryo with nutrients at this time. Rather, the embryo is self-sufficient. If a teratogen is ingested or an abdominal x-ray is taken during this time, the embryo is completely spared.

93. **1. Surfactant is usually forming in the fetal lungs by the 36th week.**
2. The eyes open and close at about 28 weeks.
3. Fetal respiratory movements begin at about 24 weeks.
4. The spinal column is completely formed well before the end of the first trimester.

TEST-TAKING HINT: The test taker should realize that this question is asking two things. First, what stage of pregnancy is the woman in when the fundal height is at the xiphoid process? Second, what other change or process is likely to be occurring at 36 weeks? The spinal column is completely formed by the end of the first trimester, fetal respiratory movements begin at about 24 weeks, and the eyes open and close at about 28 weeks. Surfactant, which is essential for mature lung function, is forming in the fetal lungs at about 36 weeks. It is important for the nurse to realize that babies who are born preterm are at high risk for a number of reasons, including lack of surfactant, lack of iron stores to sustain them during the early months of life, and lack of brown adipose tissue needed for thermoregulation.

94. The correct order is 3, 1, 2, 4.
   3. The blastocyst is developed about 6 days after fertilization and before implantation in the uterus has occurred.
   1. The four-chambered heart is formed during the early part of the first trimester.
   2. Vernix caseosa is present during the latter half of pregnancy.
   4. The testes descend in the scrotal sac about mid third trimester.

TEST-TAKING HINT: Before putting these items into chronological order, the test taker should carefully analyze each choice. The blastocyst is developed by about day 6 after fertilization. The egg has yet to implant into the uterine body at this point. The fetal heart develops during the early part of the first trimester, but after implantation. Vernix is present during the entire latter half of the pregnancy to protect the skin of the fetus. It appears, therefore, at about week 20. And, finally, the testes do not descend into the scrotal sac until the middle of the third trimester. An examination of the testes of male preterm babies shows the testes are most often undescended.

95.
1. Fingernails would likely be quite long.
2. Eyelashes would be present.
3. **Because this baby is post-term, lanugo would likely not be present.**
4. Milia would be present.

TEST-TAKING HINT: Lanugo is a fine hair that covers the body of the fetus. It begins to disappear at about 38 weeks and very likely has completely vanished by 41 weeks' gestation.

96.
1. 15 weeks is too early for quickening. At 15 weeks, the fetus would not have lanugo.
2. **This fetus is about 22 weeks' gestation. Quickening occurs by week 20. It generally is felt first, between weeks 16 and 18. Nails start to develop in the first trimester, and lanugo starts to develop at about 20 weeks, but eyes remain fused until about 29 weeks.**
3. The eyes are unfused by 29 weeks' gestation so the gestation is shorter than that.
4. The eyes are unfused by 29 weeks' gestation so the gestation is shorter than that.

TEST-TAKING HINT: This is an application question that requires the test taker to take things apart and put them back together again. Each of the signs is unique and relates to a specific period in fetal development. After an analysis, the only response that is plausible is choice 2.

97.
1. This response is incorrect. The circulatory systems are never connected.
2. This response is incorrect. The blood never mixes.
3. This response is incorrect. The systems are never connected.
4. **The blood supplies are completely separate.**

TEST-TAKING HINT: It is important to understand the relationship between the maternal vascular system and the fetal system. There is a maternal side to the placenta and a fetal side. By the time the placenta is fully functioning, at about 12 weeks' gestation, fetal blood vessels have burrowed into the thickened, decidual lining of the uterus and maternal vessels have burrowed into the chorionic layer. The vessels, therefore, lie next to each other, but do not join. Gases and nutrients move across the membranes of the vessels by osmosis, to provide the baby with needed substances and for the mother to dispose of metabolic fetal waste products such as carbon dioxide. In that way, the placenta serves as the "fetal lung." For more information on placental functioning, and fetal circulation, see the appendix.

98.
1. **This statement is correct. The maternal mortality rate is the number of deaths of women as a result of the childbearing period per 100,000 live births.**
2. This statement is incorrect. The maternal mortality rate is not calculated by the number of women of childbearing age in the country.

3. This statement is incorrect. The maternal mortality rate is not calculated by the number of pregnancies in the country.
4. This statement is incorrect. The maternal mortality rate is not calculated by the number of women in the country.

TEST-TAKING HINT: One important indicator of the quality of health care in a country is its maternal mortality rate. The rate in the United States is very low as compared to many other countries in the world and yet well above other countries. Although still much too high in total around the world, the rate is declining, especially in many developing countries.

99. 1. Rotavirus is administered to infants at 2, 4, and 6 months of age. It protects infants from a serious diarrheal illness.
2. This statement is correct. The Centers for Disease Control and Prevention (CDC) recommends the administration of the Tdap vaccine to all pregnant women during the third trimester to provide their neonates with passive immunity to whooping cough.
3. The human papillomavirus vaccine is not administered during pregnancy. The CDC recommends its administration to boys and girls beginning at 11 years of age.
4. The varicella vaccine is never administered during pregnancy. The CDC recommends its administration at the beginning of the second year of a child's life.

TEST-TAKING HINT: Neonates are especially at high risk for pertussis (whooping cough). They do not begin receiving the vaccine until they are 2 months of age. To protect them from the disease, the CDC recommends that all pregnant women receive the Tdap vaccine in their third trimester and for all family members who will have close contact with the baby to have received the vaccine within the last 10 years (CDC, n.d.-f).

100. Answers 2 and 3 are correct.
1. Women should be counseled to consume well done meat throughout their pregnancies. They should avoid eating rare meat.
2. This statement is true. Throughout their pregnancies, women should avoid traveling to locations where the Zika virus is endemic.
3. This statement is true. Women should engage in a daily exercise program throughout their pregnancies.
4. Women should be counseled to consume no alcohol throughout their pregnancies.

TEST-TAKING HINT: Some mothers who contracted the Zika virus during their pregnancies have delivered babies with small heads and brains, a syndrome called microcephaly. To reduce the potential of mothers being exposed to the virus, the Centers for Disease Control and Prevention (CDC) recommends that any woman who is pregnant or who is planning to become pregnant should not travel to a Zika endemic region. In addition, because the virus can be transmitted via sexual contact, the women's partners should also refrain from traveling to those regions.

5 Low Risk Intrapartum

This chapter covers uncomplicated labor and delivery, also referred to as "normal birth." In 1997, the World Health Organization (WHO) defined normal birth as "spontaneous in onset, low-risk at the start of labor and remaining so throughout labor and delivery. The infant is born spontaneously in the vertex position between 37 and 42 completed weeks of pregnancy. After birth, mother and infant are in good condition" (WHO, 1997, p. 121). That definition still stands.

Pregnancy is a uniquely feminine task, and the culmination of childbirth is a pivotal event in a woman's life. The intrapartum phase covers the onset of labor through childbirth and ends with delivery of the placenta. Throughout labor, the nurse monitors the intricate interplay of the classic 3 P's of labor: (1) the powers, (2) the passenger, and (3) the passage. If these three elements do not work together smoothly, a cesarean is often necessary.

Every woman desires a positive childbirth experience, described once again by WHO as "one that fulfils or exceeds a woman's prior personal and sociocultural beliefs and expectations, including giving birth to a healthy baby in a clinically and psychologically safe environment with continuity of practical and emotional support from a birth companion(s) and kind, technically competent clinical staff. It is based on the premise that most women want a physiological labour and birth, and to have a sense of personal achievement and control through involvement in decision-making, even when medical interventions are needed or wanted" (WHO, 2018, p. 1).

Nursing care during childbirth begins when the pregnant woman presents to the labor unit with her partner and often other family members. It has often been said that the labor and delivery nurse has two patients: one that is seen, and one whose needs can be interpreted only by listening to its heart rate. When the birthing process ends, there is an additional member of the family who was previously unseen. It is a distinct privilege to support women and their babies through the almost magical process of childbirth, when another human enters the world.

In spite of the excitement around labor and delivery, the intrinsic experience for both mother and fetus is painful and challenging and deserves our respect. It's no wonder the baby cries after birth. What a journey it has just completed. It might come as no surprise that, for the fetus, the process of labor has been referred to by some as *traumatic* (Basaldella et al., 2011 as cited in Irland, 2018). Apparently, the fetus is not just smoothly pressed "down and out." Driven by a fierce, primal urge to empty itself, the uterus acts more like a screwdriver on the fetus. Uterine contractions compel a sort of torque, or twisting motion on the fetus in response to a brief delay in electrical impulses from one side of the uterus to the other (Miftahof & Nam, 2011). This repeated force of up to 50 mm Hg or more, as measured by an intrauterine pressure catheter, often continues every 2 to 3 minutes for several hours (Irland, 2018). Using Cornell University's online calculator, the force of 50 mm Hg can be converted to 0.96 psi, or nearly 1 pound per square inch (Cornell University, 2000). It is no wonder that labor is painful and challenging for both mother and fetus, and why the position of the fetus is so important as it is propelled through the pelvis. When a fetus is in the posterior position, the bony back of the fetal *head*, rather than the soft face, is pressed against the mother's spine with the force of 1 pound per square inch with each contraction. Clearly, the newborn baby needs snuggling and gentleness after all of this.

Fetal evaluations in labor include fetal heart rate, fetal position, and fetal descent. The nurse is advised to review drawings and information on fetal positioning and descent while working through this chapter.

The nurse must be familiar not only with the many physiological needs of the woman in labor but also of the psychosocial needs of the woman and her family. In addition, the nurse must be prepared to assist the mother with her needs for pain relief in the manner that is most appropriate, keeping her cultural, spiritual, and emotional needs in the mix. Interventions must be medically indicated and supported by sound evidence.

In spite of its fierceness, birthing is a natural process. Of the approximately 140 million births that occur annually around the world, the majority are accomplished by women without risk to themselves or their babies throughout labor and delivery (WHO, 2018). However, the astute nurse understands that complications may arise. Some can be reduced. The nurse is the sentinel on guard to carefully monitor both the mother's and the baby's physiological responses. The nurse is always alert to signals that the labor is moving outside the realm of "normal" so that appropriate and timely interventions can support a positive childbirth experience.

Overall, nurses and other healthcare providers must protect "physiologic birth" (Adams, et al., 2016)—the process of allowing and supporting one's body to labor innately under its own power. This is done by ensuring a quiet and private environment, routinely promoting comfort and labor progress through rest, hydration, positioning, comfort measures, and encouragement. Finally, once the baby is born, the nurse must ensure that mothers and babies are not separated or disturbed by routine tasks that could wait until later.

KEYWORDS

The following words include English vocabulary, nursing/medical terminology, concepts, principles, or information relevant to content specifically addressed in the chapter or associated with topics presented in it. English dictionaries, your nursing textbooks, and medical dictionaries such as *Taber's Cyclopedic Medical Dictionary* are resources that can be used to expand your knowledge and understanding of these words and related information.

Acceleration of fetal heart rate
Active phase (phase 2) of the first stage of labor
Attitude
The Bradley Method®
Cardinal movements of labor
- Flexion
- Descent
- Internal rotation
- Extension
- External rotation (restitution)
- Expulsion

Category I fetal heart rate
Category II fetal heart rate
Category III fetal heart rate
Childbirth education
Contraction
Delivery
Dilation (dilatation)
Doula
Duration
Early deceleration
Effacement
Effleurage
Electronic fetal monitoring
Engagement
Epidural
Fetal heart rate
Fetal hemoglobin (Hb F)
Frequency
Intensity
Labor
Lamaze®
Late deceleration
Latent phase (phase 1) of the first stage of labor
Leopold maneuvers
Lie
Mentum
Midwife
Nitrous oxide
Pelvic measurements
Pelvic rock
Placenta
Position
Presentation
- Occipital
- Mentum
- Sacral
- Scapular

Precipitous delivery
Regional anesthesia
Stage 1 of labor (cervical change to 10 centimeters dilation)
Stage 2 of labor (full dilation to birth of the baby)

Stage 3 of labor (birth of the baby to birth of the placenta)
Station
Surrogate
Transition (phase 3) of the first stage of labor
Vaginal introitus
Variability
Variable deceleration

QUESTIONS

CASE STUDY: *The first six questions below are part of an evolving case study. All six questions follow the Next Generation NCLEX© question format of six steps:*

1. Recognize cues—What matters most?
2. Analyze cues—What could it mean?
3. Prioritize hypotheses—Where do I start?
4. Generate solutions—What can I do?
5. Take action—What will I do?
6. Evaluate outcomes—Did it help?

(National Council of State Boards of Nursing [NCSBN], 2020). For more information on the Next Generation NCLEX (NGN) question formats, see NGN quarterly newsletters at https://www.ncsbn.org.
NCLEX questions assume the nurse has a provider's order for listed interventions, unless noted otherwise.

0600: A 22-year-old pregnant client enters the labor unit. Her husband states she is in labor. She is grimacing and bending over, holding her stomach and saying, "I can't do this anymore!" The triage nurse accompanies the client and her husband to a triage room, where the client prepares for the exam.

In reviewing the patient's history and physical in the electronic medical record, the nurse notes that the client is G3 P2002 at 39 weeks gestation. Obstetrical history indicates her previous babies have weighed 8 lbs (3,628 grams) and 9 lbs 12 oz (4,422 grams). She had a mild shoulder dystocia with the delivery of her second child. Her recent group B-strep (GBS) culture was positive. She has gained 40 lbs with this pregnancy and has reported no problems. Her medical history indicates asthma and anxiety. She has no known drug allergies.

The client's cervical exam is 6 cm, 100% effaced, +1 (plus one) station with bloody show. Vital signs are T 100.4° F (38.0° C), P 88, R 20, BP 135/82. The fetal heart rate tracing is shown below.

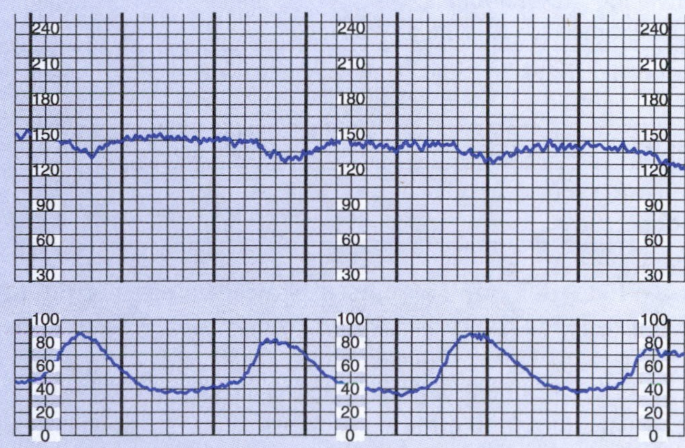

1. **Recognize cues. What matters most?** It is now 0630 and the client has been monitored for 30 minutes. From the admission findings above, select the nurse's top four findings of concern:

Admission Exam Findings
1. Vital signs
2. Fetal heart rate pattern
3. Group B strep status
4. Obstetrical history
5. Cervical exam findings
6. Medical history findings

2. **Analyze cues. What could it mean?** What can the nurse anticipate might happen? **Select all that apply.**
   1. Patient's bag of waters might break.
   2. Patient could develop chorioamnionitis.
   3. Patient could deliver after just 1 dose of antibiotics.
   4. Fetal heart rate (FHR) will show late decelerations.
   5. Patient will request an epidural.

3. **Prioritize hypotheses. Where do I start?** Which of the following is most likely occurring based on the nurse's assessments? **Select all that apply.**
   1. The client is developing chorioamnionitis.
   2. The client has an abruptio placenta.
   3. The client is experiencing a normal labor pattern.
   4. The client has pre-eclampsia.
   5. The fetus has cephalopelvic disproportion.

4. **Generate solutions. What can I do?** The nurse is planning care for the client. The nurse-midwife does not use standing orders and has requested that the nurse call her to request an order for each medication needed during labor. For each potential nursing intervention, place a checkmark in one appropriate box to indicate whether it is *Indicated*, *Nonessential*, or *Contraindicated*.

Potential Intervention	Indicated (a)	Nonessential (b)	Contraindicated (c)
1. Provide oxygen by re-breather mask			
2. Insert indwelling catheter and send urine specimen to lab			
3. Request an order for IV penicillin			
4. Place a fetal scalp electrode			
5. Request an order for acetaminophen			

5. **Take action. What will I do?** The nurse has received orders from the nurse-midwife. **Which order is the most urgent to complete? Select one.**
   1. Notify anesthesia for epidural placement.
   2. Administer Acetaminophen 650 mg po Q 4 hours, prn.
   3. Administer Penicillin G 5.0 million units intravenously now, followed by 2.5 million units intravenously every 4 hours until delivery.
   4. Insert indwelling urinary catheter.

6. Evaluate outcomes. Did it help?
0800: The client is resting comfortably with an epidural in place. The nurse has administered acetaminophen and penicillin and has assisted the client to change positions every 30 minutes. Which of the following findings indicate positive outcomes related to nursing actions? **Select all that apply.**
1. Maternal vital signs: T 99° F (37.2° C), RR 18, Pulse 80.
2. FHR 145 bpm with variable decelerations and moderate variability.
3. Contractions every 2 minutes, 60 second duration.
4. Cervical exam: 10 cm, 100% effaced, +3 (plus three) station.
5. Penicillin has been administered.

7. A client enters the labor and delivery suite stating that she thinks she is in labor. Which of the following information about the woman should the nurse gather from the woman's prenatal record when planning nursing care? **Select all that apply.**
   1. Weight gain.
   2. Ethnicity and religion.
   3. Age.
   4. Type of insurance.
   5. Gravidity and parity.

8. A woman who states that she "thinks" she is in labor enters the labor suite. Which of the following assessments will provide the nurse with the most valuable information regarding the client's labor status?
   1. Leopold maneuvers.
   2. Fundal tone.
   3. Fetal heart rate assessment.
   4. Cervical examination.

9. A laboring client with an obstetrical history of G2 P1001, was admitted 1 hour ago at 4 cm dilated and 50% effaced. She was talkative and excited at that time. During the past 10 minutes she has become serious, closing her eyes and breathing shallowly with each contraction. Which of the following is an accurate nursing assessment of the situation?
   1. The client is at risk of having a seizure.
   2. The client is exhibiting an expected behavior for labor.
   3. The client is becoming hypoxic and hypercapnic.
   4. The client needs her alpha-fetoprotein levels checked.

10. A woman has just arrived at the labor and delivery suite. Before reporting the client's arrival to her primary healthcare practitioner, which of the following assessments should the nurse perform? **Select all that apply.**
    1. Fetal heart rate.
    2. Contraction pattern.
    3. Urinalysis.
    4. Vital signs.
    5. Biophysical profile.

11. While performing Leopold maneuvers on a woman in labor, the nurse palpates a hard round mass in the fundal area, a flat surface on the left side, small objects on the right side, and a soft round mass just above the symphysis. Which of the following is a reasonable conclusion by the nurse?
    1. The fetal position is transverse.
    2. The fetal presentation is vertex.
    3. The fetal lie is vertical.
    4. The fetal attitude is flexed.

12. At which time/s during the latent phase of labor should the nurse assess the fetal heart rate pattern of a low-risk woman with an obstetrical history of G1 P0000? **Select all that apply.**
    1. With vaginal examinations.
    2. Before administration of analgesics.
    3. Periodically throughout several contractions.
    4. Every 10 minutes.
    5. Before ambulating.

13. The nurse is assessing the fetal station during a vaginal examination. Which of the following structures should the nurse palpate?
    1. Sacral promontory.
    2. Ischial spines.
    3. Cervix.
    4. Symphysis pubis.

14. The labor and delivery nurse performs Leopold maneuvers. A soft round mass is felt in the fundal region. A flat object is noted on the client's left and small objects are noted on the right of the uterus (the client's right). A hard round mass is noted above the symphysis. Which of the following positions is consistent with these findings?
    1. Left occipital anterior (LOA).
    2. Left sacral posterior (LSP).
    3. Right mentum anterior (RMA).
    4. Right sacral posterior (RSP).

15. A nurse is caring for a laboring woman who is in transition. She does not have an epidural for pain control. Which of the following signs/symptoms would indicate that the woman is progressing into the second stage of labor? **Select all that apply.**
    1. Bulging perineum.
    2. Increased bloody show.
    3. Spontaneous rupture of the membranes.
    4. Uncontrollable urge to push.
    5. Inability to breathe through contractions.

16. During a vaginal examination, the nurse palpates fetal buttocks that are in the left posterior position and are 1 cm above the ischial spines. Which of the following is consistent with this assessment?
    1. LOA, −1 station.
    2. LSP, −1 station.
    3. Left mentum posterior (LMP), +1 station.
    4. Left sacral anterior (LSA), +1 station.

17. The nurse enters a laboring client's room. The client is complaining of intense back pain with each contraction. The nurse concludes that the fetus is likely in which of the following positions?
    1. Mentum anterior.
    2. Sacrum posterior.
    3. Occiput posterior.
    4. Scapula anterior.

18. When performing Leopold maneuvers, the nurse notes that the fetus is in the left occiput anterior (LOA) position. Which is the best position for the nurse to place a fetoscope to hear the fetal heart rate?
    1. Left upper quadrant.
    2. Right upper quadrant.
    3. Left lower quadrant.
    4. Right lower quadrant.

19. On examination of a full-term primiparous client, a labor nurse notes: active labor, right occiput anterior (ROA) position, 10 cm dilated, and +3 station (using a 5-cm scale). Which of the following should the nurse report to the physician?
   1. Descent is progressing well.
   2. Fetal head is not yet engaged.
   3. Vaginal delivery is imminent.
   4. External rotation is complete.

20. One hour ago, a multiparous client was examined with the following results: 8 cm, 90% effaced, and +1 station. She does not have an epidural and is now pushing involuntarily with contractions. The fetal head is seen at the vaginal introitus. The nurse concludes that the client is now:
   1. 9 cm dilated, 90% effaced, and +2 station.
   2. 9 cm dilated, 90% effaced, and +3 station.
   3. 10 cm dilated, 90% effaced, and +4 station.
   4. 10 cm dilated, 100% effaced, and +5 station.

21. The nurse is caring for a nulliparous client who attended Lamaze childbirth education classes. Which of the following techniques should the nurse include in her plan of care? **Select all that apply.**
   1. Hypnotic suggestion.
   2. Rhythmic chanting.
   3. Muscle relaxation.
   4. Pelvic rocking.
   5. Abdominal massage.

22. The nurse knows that which of the following responses is the primary rationale for the information taught in childbirth education classes?
   1. Mothers who are performing breathing exercises during labor refrain from yelling.
   2. Breathing and relaxation exercises are less exhausting than crying and moaning.
   3. Knowledge learned at childbirth education classes helps to break the fear-tension-pain cycle.
   4. Childbirth education classes help to promote positive maternal–newborn bonding.

23. The Lamaze childbirth educator is teaching a class of expectant couples the breathing technique that is most appropriate during the second stage of labor. Which of the following techniques is the nurse teaching the women to do?
   1. Alternately pant and blow.
   2. Take rhythmic, shallow breaths.
   3. Push down with an open glottis.
   4. Do slow chest breathing.

24. A nurse is teaching childbirth education classes to a group of pregnant teens. Which of the following strategies would promote learning by the young women?
   1. Avoiding the discussion of uncomfortable procedures like vaginal examinations and blood tests.
   2. Focusing the discussion on baby care rather than on labor and delivery.
   3. Utilizing visual aids like movies and posters during the classes.
   4. Having the classes at a location other than high school to reduce their embarrassment.

25. A client who is 7 cm dilated and 100% effaced is breathing at a rate of 50 breaths per minute during contractions. Immediately after a contraction, she complains of tingling in her fingers and some light-headedness. Which of the following actions should the nurse take at this time?
   1. Assess the blood pressure.
   2. Have the woman breathe into a bag.
   3. Turn the woman onto her side.
   4. Check the fetal heart rate.

26. A nurse is teaching a class of expectant couples the most therapeutic Lamaze breathing technique for the latent phase of labor. Which of the following techniques is the nurse teaching?
    1. Alternately panting and blowing.
    2. Rapid, deep breathing.
    3. Grunting and pushing with contractions.
    4. Slow chest breathing.

27. A woman with an obstetrical history of G2 P0101, is 5 cm dilated and 75% effaced. She is doing first-level Lamaze breathing with contractions. The nurse detects that the woman's shoulder and face muscles are beginning to tense during the contractions. Which of the following interventions should the nurse perform first?
    1. Encourage the woman to have an epidural.
    2. Encourage the woman to accept intravenous analgesia.
    3. Encourage the woman to change her position.
    4. Encourage the woman to perform the next level breathing.

28. In addition to breathing with contractions, the nurse should encourage women in the first stage of labor to perform which of the following therapeutic actions?
    1. Lying in the lithotomy position.
    2. Performing effleurage.
    3. Practicing Kegel exercises.
    4. Pushing with each contraction.

29. A client is in the second stage of labor. She falls asleep immediately after a contraction. Which of the following actions should the nurse perform at this time?
    1. Awaken the woman and remind her to push.
    2. Cover the woman's perineum with a sheet.
    3. Assess the woman's blood pressure and pulse.
    4. Administer oxygen to the woman via face mask.

30. A client with an obstetrical history of G3 P2002 was examined 5 minutes ago. Her cervix was 8 cm dilated and 100% effaced. She now states that she needs to move her bowels. Which of the following actions should the nurse perform first?
    1. Offer the client the bedpan.
    2. Evaluate the progress of labor.
    3. Notify the physician.
    4. Encourage the patient to push.

31. The nurse auscultates a fetal heart rate of 150 beats per minute (bpm) on a client in early labor. Which of the following actions by the nurse is appropriate?
    1. Inform the mother that the rate is normal.
    2. Reassess in 5 minutes to verify the results.
    3. Immediately report the rate to the healthcare practitioner.
    4. Place the client on her left side and apply oxygen by face mask.

32. While caring for a client in the transition phase of labor, the nurse notes that the fetal monitor tracing shows moderate variability with a baseline of 140 bpm. What should the nurse do?
    1. Provide caring labor support.
    2. Administer oxygen via face mask.
    3. Change the client's position.
    4. Speed up the client's intravenous fluids.

33. While evaluating the fetal heart rate (FHR) monitor tracing on a client in labor, the nurse notes that there are decelerations present. Which of the following assessments must the nurse make at this time?
    1. The relationship between the decelerations and the labor contractions.
    2. The maternal blood pressure.
    3. The gestational age of the fetus.
    4. The placement of the fetal heart rate transducer in relation to the fetal position.

34. A client is complaining of severe back labor. Which of the following nursing interventions would be most effective?
 1. Assist mother with childbirth breathing.
 2. Encourage mother to have an epidural.
 3. Provide direct sacral pressure.
 4. Move the woman to a hydrotherapy tub.

35. An obstetrician is performing an amniotomy on a laboring woman in transition. Which of the following assessments must the nurse make throughout the procedure?
 1. Maternal blood pressure.
 2. Maternal pulse.
 3. Fetal heart rate.
 4. Fetal fibronectin level.

36. A nurse has just performed Leopold's maneuvers on a client in labor. The nurse palpates the baby's buttocks as the presenting part and determines they are facing the mother's right side. Where should the nurse place the external fetal heartrate transducer?
 1. Left upper quadrant (LUQ).
 2. Left lower quadrant (LLQ).
 3. Right upper quadrant (RUQ).
 4. Right lower quadrant (RLQ).

37. Upon examination, a nurse notes that a woman is 10 cm dilated, 100% effaced, and −3 station. Which of the following actions should the nurse consider during the next contraction?
 1. Encourage the woman to push.
 2. Provide firm fundal pressure.
 3. Move the client into a squat.
 4. Monitor for signs of rectal pressure.

38. A woman has decided to hire a doula to work with her during labor and delivery. Which of the following actions would be appropriate for the nurse to delegate to the doula? **Select all that apply.**
 1. Give the woman a back rub.
 2. Assist the woman with her breathing.
 3. Assess the fetal heart rate.
 4. Check the woman's blood pressure.
 5. Regulate the woman's intravenous infusion rate.

39. The nurse is assessing a client who states, "I think I'm in labor." Which of the following findings would positively confirm the client's belief?
 1. She is contracting q 5 min × 60 sec.
 2. Her cervix has dilated from 2 to 4 cm.
 3. Her membranes have ruptured.
 4. The fetal head is engaged.

40. The childbirth education nurse is evaluating the learning of four women at term, regarding when they should go to the hospital. The nurse determines that the teaching was successful when a client makes which of the following statements? **Select all that apply.**
 1. The client who says, "If I feel a pain in my back and lower abdomen every 5 minutes."
 2. The client who says, "When I feel a gush of clear fluid from my vagina."
 3. The client who says, "When I go to the bathroom and see the mucous plug on the toilet tissue."
 4. The client who says, "If I ever notice a greenish discharge from my vagina."
 5. The client who says, "When I have felt cramping in my abdomen for 4 hours or more."

41. A woman at 38 weeks' gestation calls her obstetrical provider's advice nurse and reports, "I just saw pink streaks on the toilet tissue when I went to the bathroom. I'm bleeding." Which of the following responses should the nurse make first?
   1. "Does it burn when you void?"
   2. "You sound frightened."
   3. "That is just the mucous plug."
   4. "How much blood is there?"

42. A pregnant client at term called the labor suite at 1900, questioning whether she was in labor. The nurse determined that the client was likely in labor after the client stated:
   1. "At 5:00 p.m., the contractions were about 5 minutes apart. Now they're about 7 minutes apart."
   2. "I took a walk at 5:00 p.m., and now I talk through my contractions easier than I could then."
   3. "I took a shower about a half hour ago. The contractions hurt more than they did before."
   4. "I had some tightening in my belly late this afternoon, and I still feel it after waking up from my nap."

43. A nurse describes a client's contraction pattern as: frequency every 3 minutes and duration of 60 seconds. Which of the following responses corresponds to this description?
   1. Contractions lasting 60 seconds followed by a 1-minute rest period.
   2. Contractions lasting 120 seconds followed by a 2-minute rest period.
   3. Contractions lasting 2 minutes followed by a 60-second rest period.
   4. Contractions lasting 1 minute followed by a 120-second rest period.

44. A nurse determines that a client is carrying a fetus in the vertical lie. The nurse's judgment should be questioned if the fetal presenting part is which of the following?
   1. Sacrum.
   2. Occiput.
   3. Mentum.
   4. Scapula.

45. A nurse is educating a pregnant woman regarding the moves a fetus makes during the birthing process. Please place the following cardinal movements of labor in order:
   1. Descent.
   2. Expulsion.
   3. Extension.
   4. External rotation.
   5. Internal rotation.

46. The nurse sees the fetal head at the vaginal introitus when a woman pushes. The nurse, interpreting this finding, tells the client, "You are pushing very well." In addition, the nurse could also state which of the following?
   1. "The baby's head is engaged."
   2. "The baby is floating."
   3. "The baby is at the ischial spines."
   4. "The baby's head is almost crowning."

47. A midwife advises a mother that her obstetric conjugate is of average size. How should the nurse interpret that information for the mother?
   1. The anterior to posterior diameter of the pelvis will accommodate a fetus with an average-sized head.
   2. The fetal head is flexed so that it is of average diameter.
   3. The mother's cervix is of average dilation for the start of labor.
   4. The distance between the mother's physiological retraction ring and the fetal head is of average dimensions.

48. The frequency of the contractions seen on the monitor tracing below is every ___ minutes.

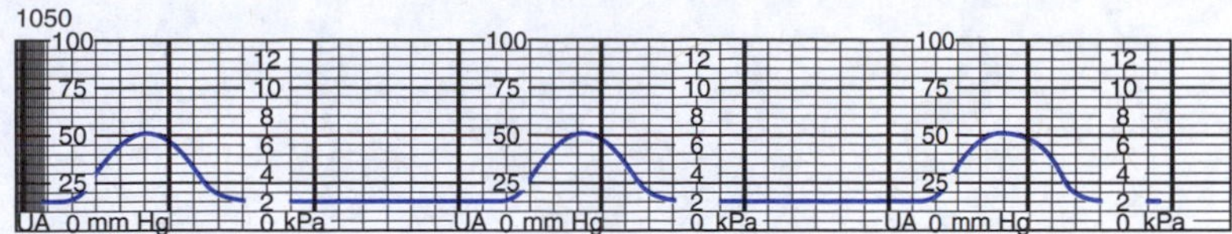

49. The duration of the contractions seen on the monitor tracing below is ____ seconds.

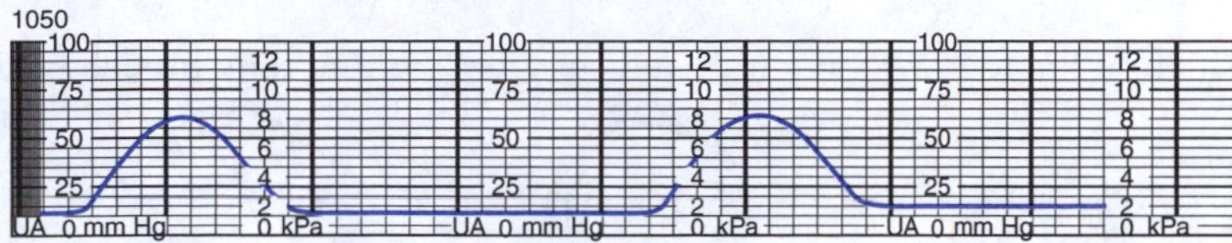

50. Which of the following frequency and duration assessments is consistent with the pattern shown below?

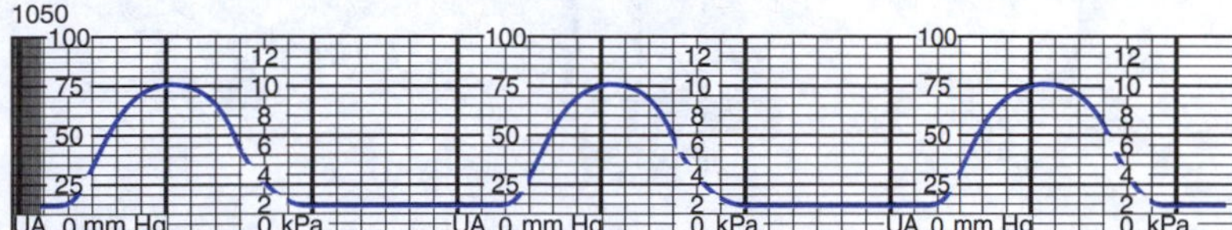

1. q 2 min × 60 sec.
2. q 2 min × 90 sec.
3. q 3 min × 60 sec.
4. q 3 min × 90 sec.

51. A woman who is in active labor is told by her obstetrician, "Your baby's head is flexed." When she asks the nurse what that means, what should the nurse say?

1. The baby is in the breech position.
2. The baby is in the horizontal lie.
3. The baby's presenting part is engaged.
4. The baby's chin is resting on its chest.

52. An ultrasound report states, "The fetal head has entered the pelvic inlet." How should the nurse interpret this statement?

1. The fetus is full term.
2. The fetal head has entered the true pelvis.
3. The fetal lie is horizontal.
4. The fetus is in an extended attitude.

53. Which of the following pictures depicts a fetus in the ROP position?

1.

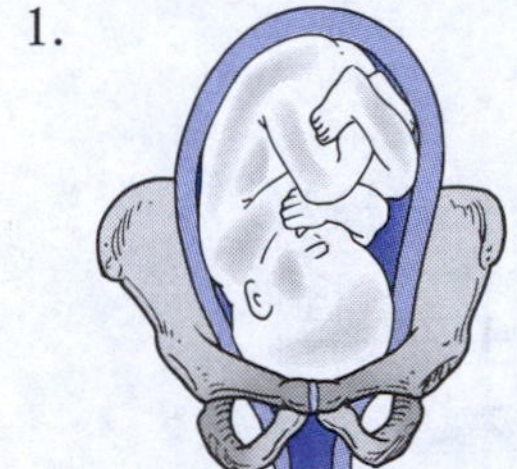

2.

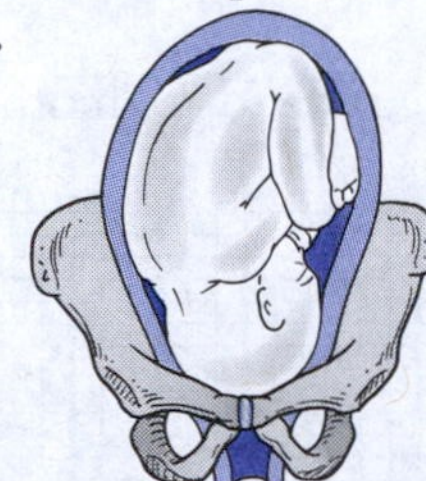

3.

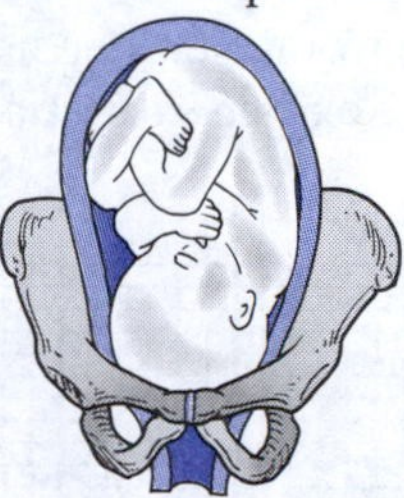

4.

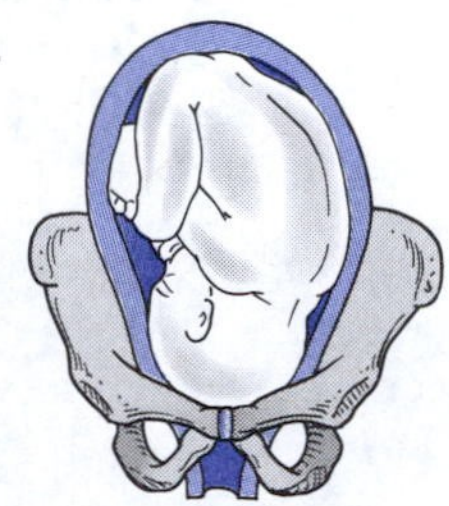

54. Which of the following pictures depicts a fetus in the LSA position?

1. 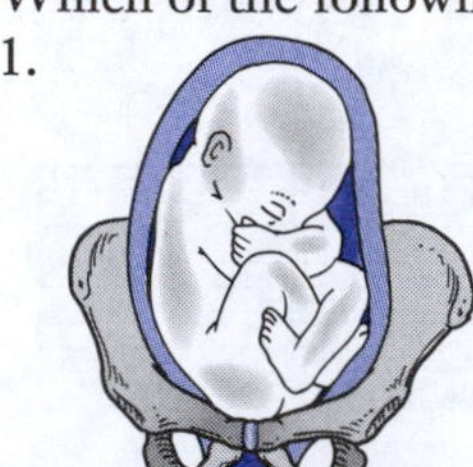
2. 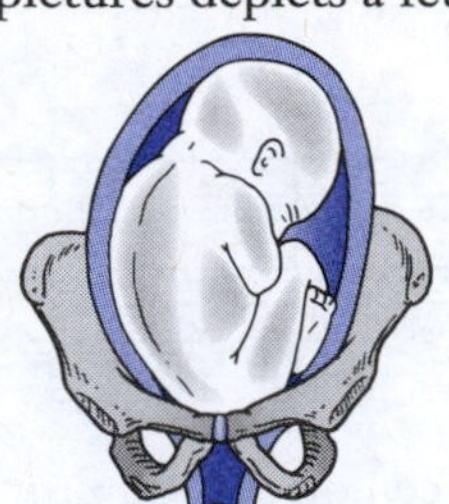
3. 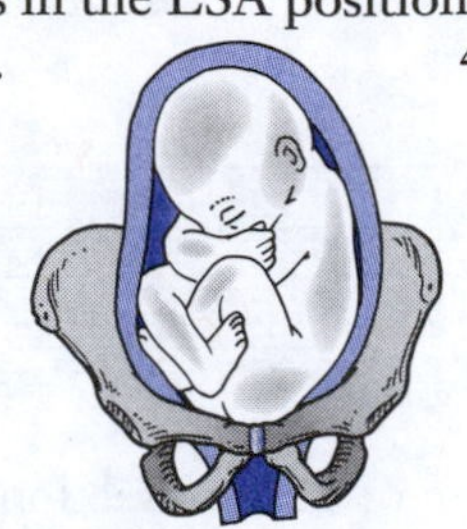
4. 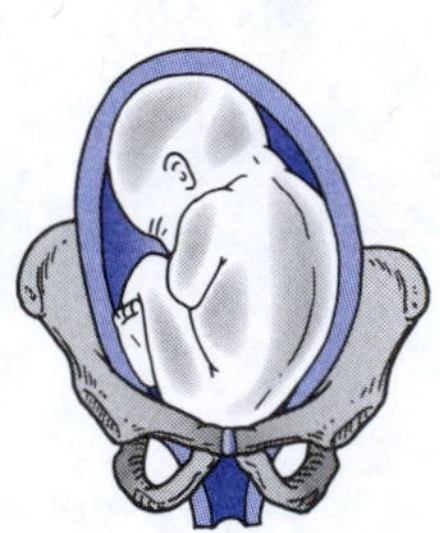

55. Which of the following pictures depicts a fetus in the frank breech position?

1. 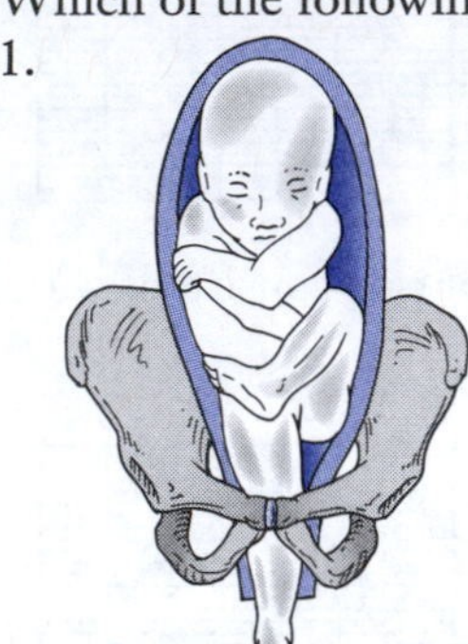
2. 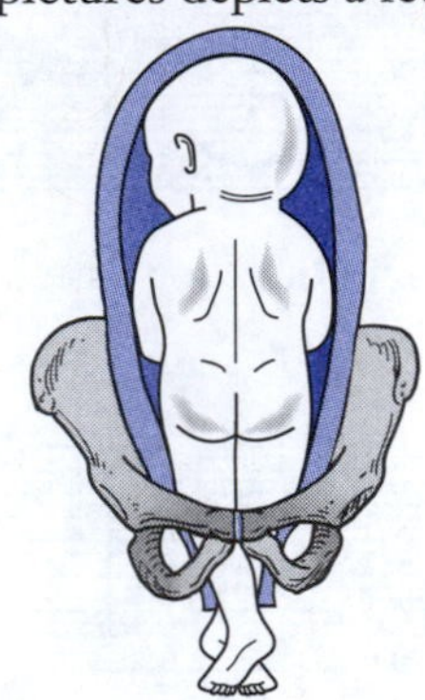
3. 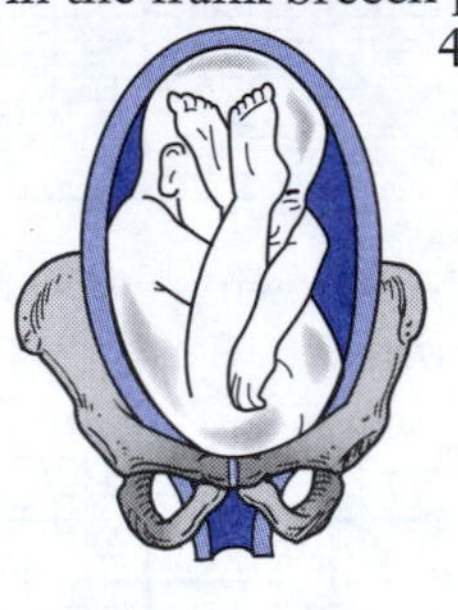
4. 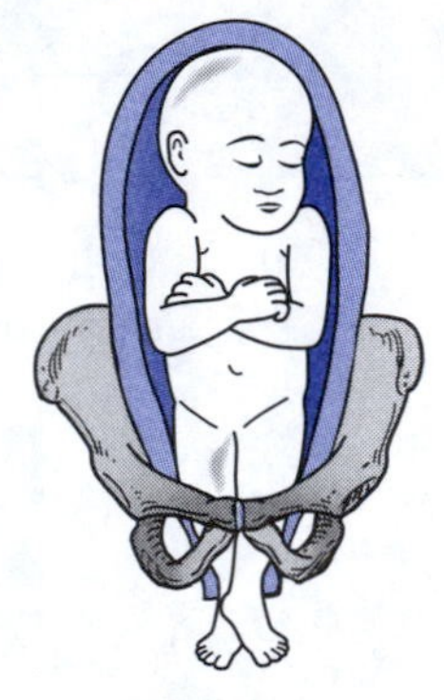

56. During delivery, the nurse notes that the baby's head has just been delivered. The nurse notes that the baby has just completed which of the following cardinal moves of labor?
1. Flexion.
2. Internal rotation.
3. Extension.
4. External rotation.

57. The nurse wishes to assess the variability of the fetal heart rate. Which of the following actions must the nurse perform at this time?
1. Place the client in the lateral recumbent position.
2. Carefully analyze the baseline data on the monitor tracing.
3. Administer oxygen to the mother via face mask.
4. Ask the mother to indicate when she feels fetal movement.

58. The nurse is interpreting the fetal monitor tracing below. Which of the following actions should the nurse take at this time?
1. Provide caring labor support.
2. Administer oxygen via tight-fitting face mask.
3. Turn the woman on her side.
4. Apply the oxygen saturation electrode to the mother.

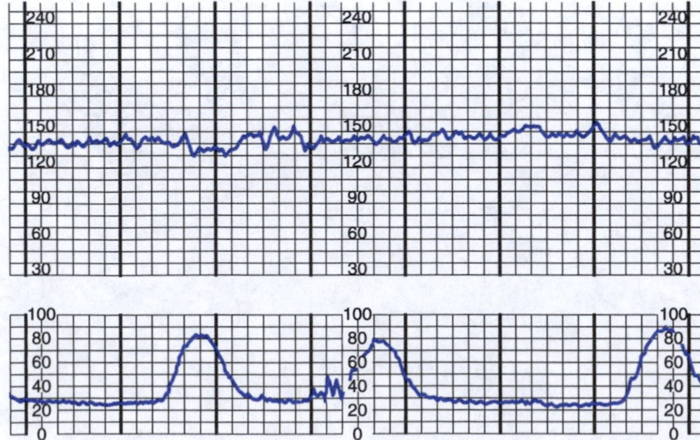

59. After analyzing an internal fetal monitor tracing, the nurse concludes that there is moderate variability. Which of the following interpretations should the nurse make in relation to this finding?
   1. The fetus is becoming hypoxic.
   2. The fetus is becoming alkalotic.
   3. The fetus is in the middle of a sleep cycle.
   4. The fetus has a healthy nervous system.

60. When would the nurse expect to see the fetal monitor tracing shown below?
   1. During the first stage of labor.
   2. During an epidural insertion.
   3. During the second stage of labor.
   4. During delivery of the placenta.

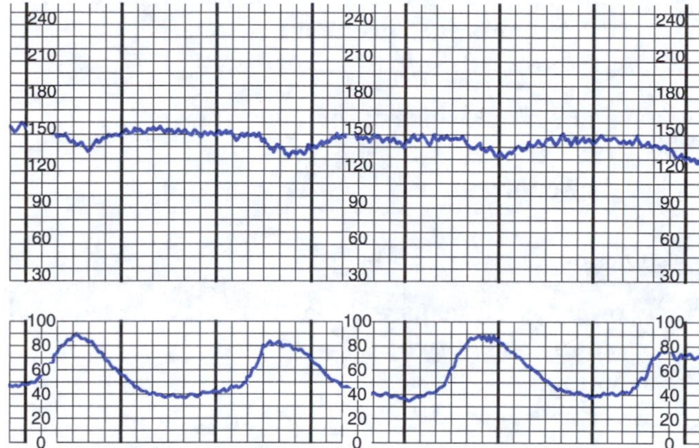

61. When would the nurse expect to see the fetal heart rate changes noted on the fetal monitor tracing shown below?
   1. During fetal movement.
   2. After the administration of analgesics.
   3. When the fetus is acidotic.
   4. With poor placental perfusion.

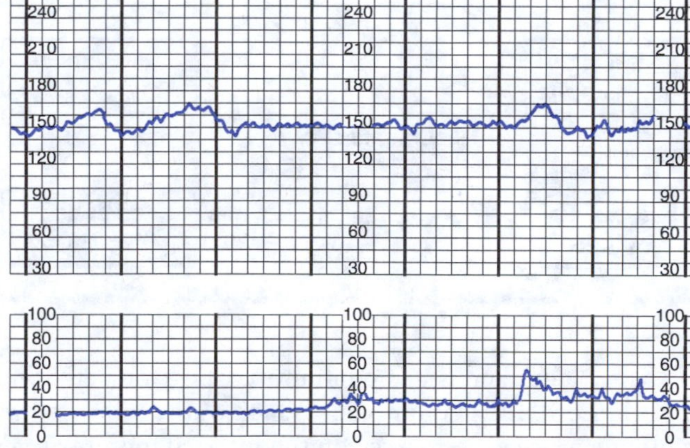

CASE STUDY: Questions 62–64 are part of a case study. This is based on a bowtie question format that nursing graduates may see in the Next Generation NCLEX© exam (NCSBN, 2021). On the computerized test, the test taker will drag the appropriate answer into the appropriate box. Note that the first answer applies to the center box, with answers to question 2 in the boxes on the left, and answers to question 3 in the boxes on the right. For the purposes of this book, the test taker can select the correct answers as in any multiple-choice question. The bowtie diagram is given to provide familiarity with the format.

A nurse assumes care of a client with an obstetrical history of G2 P1001. The nurse going off shift reports that the client is completely dilated and has been pushing for 1 hour with open glottis pushing. The client is 42 weeks pregnant and the provider estimates the fetal weight to be 9 lbs (4,082 grams). When the client started pushing, her vaginal exam was 10 cm, 100% effaced, 0 station. The oncoming nurse rechecks her now, and finds a swollen cervical anterior lip, 90% effaced, +1 station.

62. The nurse is concerned about which of the following?
1. Fetal malpresentation.
2. Cephalopelvic disproportion.
3. Tachysystole.
4. Uterine dysfunction.

63. Which of the following assessments will the nurse make to reduce the risk of the identified complication? **Select two.**
1. Confirm fetal position.
2. Confirm contraction frequency.
3. Assess fetal heart rate.
4. Monitor fetal descent.

64. Which interventions should the nurse recommend to the client as a way to reduce the risk of the identified complication? **Select two.**
1. Closed glottis pushing.
2. Uterine effleurage.
3. Change positions.
4. Stop pushing.

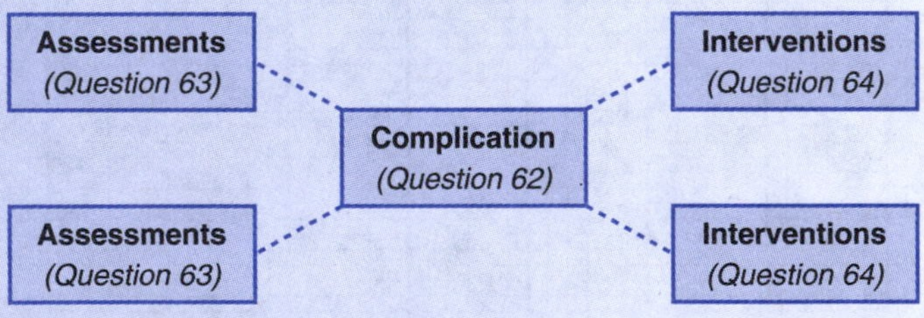

65. A woman is in active labor and is being monitored electronically. She has just received fentanyl citrate 50 mcg IV for pain. Which of the following fetal heart rate responses would the nurse expect to see on the internal monitor tracing?
1. Variable decelerations.
2. Late decelerations.
3. Decreased variability.
4. Transient accelerations.

66. A woman is in the second stage of labor with a strong urge to push. Which of the following actions by the nurse is appropriate at this time?
1. Assess the fetal heart rate at least every 5 minutes during and after the contraction.
2. Encourage the woman to hold her breath and push during contractions.
3. Assess the pulse and respirations of the mother every 5 minutes.
4. Position the woman on her back with her knees on her chest.

67. A nurse is coaching a woman who is in the second stage of labor. Which of the following should the nurse encourage the woman to do?
1. Hold her breath for 20 seconds during every contraction.
2. Blow out forcefully during every contraction.
3. Push between contractions until the fetal head is visible.
4. Take a cleansing breath before bearing down.

68. A primigravida is pushing with contractions. The nurse notes that the woman's perineum is beginning to bulge and that there is an increase in bloody show. Which of the following actions by the nurse is appropriate at this time?
1. Report the findings to the woman's healthcare practitioner.
2. Immediately assess the woman's pulse and blood pressure.
3. Continue to provide encouragement during each contraction.
4. Place the client on her side with oxygen via face mask.

69. A multipara with a fetus in the LOA position at +3 station has had no pain medication during her labor. She is now in second stage. She states that her pain is 6 on a 10-point scale and that she wants an epidural. Which of the following responses by the nurse is appropriate?
1. "Epidurals do not work well when the pain level is above level 5."
2. "I will contact the doctor to get an order for an epidural right away."
3. "The baby is going to be born very soon. It is really too late for an epidural."
4. "I will check the fetal heart rate. You can have an epidural if it is over 120."

70. A pregnant woman is discussing possible delivery options with a labor nurse. Which of the following client responses indicate that the woman understood the information? **Select all that apply.**
1. When the client states, "I am glad that deliveries can take place in a variety of places, including in the labor bed."
2. When the client says, "I heard that for doctors to deliver babies safely, it is essential that I lie on my back with my legs up."
3. When the client states, "I understand that if the fetus needs to turn during labor, I may end up delivering the baby on my hands and knees."
4. When the client says, "During difficult deliveries it is sometimes necessary to put a woman's legs up in stirrups."
5. When the client states, "I heard that midwives often deliver their patients either in the side-lying or squatting position."

71. During the third stage of labor, the following physiological changes occur. Please place the changes in chronological order.
1. Hematoma forms behind the placenta.
2. Membranes separate from the uterine wall.
3. The uterus contracts.
4. The uterine surface area dramatically decreases.

72. A woman had a baby by spontaneous vaginal delivery 10 minutes ago. The nurse notes that a gush of blood was just expelled from the vagina and the umbilical cord lengthened. What should the nurse conclude?
1. The woman has an internal laceration.
2. The woman is about to deliver the placenta.
3. The woman has an atonic uterus.
4. The woman is ready to expel the cord bloods.

73. A client is in the third stage of labor. Which of the following assessments should the nurse make/observe for? **Select all that apply.**
1. Lengthening of the umbilical cord.
2. Fetal heart rate assessment after each contraction.
3. Uterus rising in the abdomen and feeling globular.
4. Rapid cervical dilation to 10 centimeters.
5. Maternal complaints of intense rectal pressure.

74. A woman is in the transition phase of labor. Which of the following comments should the nurse expect to hear?
 1. "I am so excited to be in labor."
 2. "I can't stand this pain any longer!"
 3. "I need ice chips because I'm so hot."
 4. "I have to push the baby out right now!"

75. A client in labor is talkative and happy. How many centimeters dilated would a maternity nurse suspect that the client is at this time?
 1. 2 cm.
 2. 4 cm.
 3. 8 cm.
 4. 10 cm.

76. A nurse is assessing the vital signs of a client in labor at the peak of a contraction. Which of the following findings would the nurse expect to see?
 1. Decreased pulse rate.
 2. Hypertension.
 3. Hyperthermia.
 4. Decreased respiratory rate.

77. A woman with an obstetrical history of G1 P0000 at 40 weeks' gestation enters the labor suite stating that she is in labor. Upon examination the nurse finds that the woman is 2 cm dilated, 25% effaced, contracting every 12 minutes × 30 seconds. Fetal heart rate is 140 bpm with moderate variability and accelerations. What should the nurse conclude when reporting the findings to the primary healthcare practitioner?
 1. The woman is at high risk and should be placed on tocolytics.
 2. The woman is in latent labor and could be sent home.
 3. The woman is at high risk and could be induced.
 4. The woman is in active labor and should be admitted to the unit.

78. A nurse concludes that a woman is in the latent phase of labor. Which of the following signs/symptoms would lead a nurse to that conclusion?
 1. The woman talks and laughs during contractions.
 2. The woman complains about severe back labor.
 3. The woman performs effleurage during a contraction.
 4. The woman asks to go to the bathroom to defecate.

79. On vaginal examination, it is noted that a woman with a well-functioning epidural is in the second stage of labor, but feels no urge to push. The fetus is at zero station and the baseline fetal heart rate is 130 bpm with no decelerations. Which of the following nursing actions is appropriate at this time?
 1. Coach the woman to hold her breath while pushing 3 to 4 times with each contraction.
 2. Administer oxygen via face mask at 8 to 10 liters per minute.
 3. Allow the mother to labor down.
 4. Place the woman on her side and assess her oxygen saturation.

80. A nurse is preparing to assist an anesthesia provider who is setting up for insertion of an epidural catheter. Which of the following positions should the nurse anticipate the provider might request the client to assume? **Select all that apply.**
 1. Fetal position.
 2. Lithotomy position.
 3. Trendelenburg position.
 4. Sitting position.

81. Which of the following actions would the nurse expect to perform before a woman is to have regional anesthesia? **Select all that apply.**
1. Assess fetal heart rate.
2. Infuse 500–1,000 mL of Ringer's lactate solution.
3. Place the woman in the Trendelenburg position.
4. Monitor blood pressure every 5 minutes for 15 minutes.
5. Have the woman empty her bladder.

82. Immediately following administration of epidural anesthesia, the nurse must monitor the mother for which of the following side effects?
1. Paresthesias in her feet and legs.
2. Drop in blood pressure.
3. Increase in central venous pressure.
4. Fetal heart rate accelerations.

83. A client with an obstetrical history of G2 P1001, is 5 cm dilated and 90% effaced. She has just received an epidural. Which of the following actions is important for the nurse to take at this time?
1. Assess the woman's temperature.
2. Place a wedge under the woman's side.
3. Place a blanket roll under the woman's feet.
4. Assess the woman's pedal pulses.

84. The nurse-midwife is performing a fetal scalp stimulation test. Which of the following fetal responses would the nurse expect to see?
1. Spontaneous fetal movement.
2. Fetal heart rate acceleration.
3. Increase in fetal heart rate variability.
4. Resolution of late decelerations.

85. Which of the following nonpharmacological interventions recommended by nurse-midwives may help a client at full term to go into labor? **Select all that apply.**
1. Engage in sexual intercourse.
2. Ingest evening primrose oil.
3. Perform yoga exercises.
4. Eat raw spinach.
5. Massage the breast and nipples.

86. To decrease the possibility of a perineal laceration during delivery, the nurse performs which of the following interventions prior to the delivery?
1. Assists the woman into a squatting position.
2. Advises the woman to push only when she feels the urge.
3. Encourages the woman to push slowly and steadily.
4. Massages the perineum with mineral oil.

87. The physician writes the following order for a newly admitted client in labor: Lactated Ringer's solution, 1000 mL IV at 150 mL/hr. The IV tubing states that the drop factor is 10 gtt/mL. **Please calculate the drip rate to the nearest whole.**

_______ gtt/min

88. The primary healthcare provider orders the following medication for a laboring client: Butorphanol Tartrate 0.5 mg IV STAT for pain. The drug is on hand in the following concentration: Butorphanol Tartrate 2 mg/mL. How many mL of medication will the nurse administer? **Calculate to the nearest hundredth.**

_______ mL

89. The nurse is performing a vaginal examination on a client in labor. The client is found to be 5 cm dilated, 90% effaced, and –2 station. Which of the following has the nurse palpated?
1. Thin cervix.
2. Bulging fetal membranes.
3. Head at the pelvic outlet.
4. Closed cervix.

90. It is 1600. A laboring client with an obstetrical history of G1 P0000 who is 3 cm dilated, asks the nurse when the dinner tray will be served. The nurse replies:
1. "Laboring clients are never allowed to eat."
2. "Believe me, you will not want to eat by the time it is the dinner hour. Most women throw up, you know."
3. "The dinner tray should arrive in an hour or two."
4. "A heavy meal is discouraged. I can get clear fluids for you whenever you would like them, though."

91. In response to a patient's request, the nurse asks the patient's primary healthcare provider for medication to relieve the pain of labor. The healthcare provider orders self-administered inhaled nitrous oxide (N2O) in a N2O 50% / O2 50% mixture for the client. Which of the following common side effects should the nurse carefully monitor the client for? **Select all that apply.**
1. Nausea.
2. Hypotension.
3. Dehydration.
4. Light-headedness.
5. Late decelerations on the fetal heart rate tracing.

92. Between contractions, a client in the active phase of labor states, "Not only do these contractions really hurt me, but what are they doing to my baby? I am so scared and I can't stop thinking about how my baby might be hurting, too." The patient requests medication to reduce her pain. It would be most appropriate for the nurse to suggest and discuss which of the following labor pain-relieving methods with the client before requesting an order?
1. Epidural.
2. Nitrous oxide.
3. Narcotic analgesic.
4. Spinal.

ANSWERS AND RATIONALES

The correct answer number and rationale for why it is the correct answer are given in **boldface blue type.** Rationales for why the other possible answer options are incorrect also are given, but they are not in boldface type.

1. **Recognize cues. What matters most? Answers 1, 3, 4, and 5 are correct.**
   1. **Her temperature is 100.4° F (38° C), which meets criteria for a maternal fever (Ashwal et al., 2018).**
   2. The fetal heart rate pattern is reassuring, with moderate variability and early decelerations, which are benign.
   3. **The Group B strep status was positive. As a result, she will need an order for penicillin to be started and administered every 4 hours before the birth.**
   4. **Her obstetrical history of a previous shoulder dystocia must be kept in mind in case this baby is around the same size. A weight gain of 40 lb may indicate another large baby and another shoulder dystocia is possible.**
   5. **Since she's a multipara at 6 cm, +1 station and 100% effaced, she's entering the active phase of labor and she could be pushing and delivering soon. The order for penicillin must be obtained and started stat.**
   6. There is no indication in the question that either her asthma or her anxiety are issues of concern at this time.

TEST-TAKING HINT: Conditions that can affect survival, the first or widest level on Maslow's hierarchy of needs, must be considered first. The mother's positive Group B strep culture puts both her and the fetus at high risk for infection. Her fever puts the fetus at risk for tachycardia if the fever is untreated. All pregnant patients are tested for Group B strep at around 36 weeks' gestation. It is the standard of care that women whose prenatal Group B strep test was positive will receive at least one dose of antibiotics, 4 hours before delivery if possible. The preference is for the woman to receive at least 2 doses before delivery. This assures that the fetus will receive some coverage before birth. Penicillin G 5 million units IV is recommended by the Centers for Disease Control and Prevention (CDC) for the first dose, followed by 2.5 million units IV every 4 hours until delivery. If the woman is allergic to penicillin, other antibiotic options are suggested (Verani et al., 2010). A difficult delivery with prolonged shoulder dystocia can negatively affect the baby's oxygenation. The client's multiparity adds a ticking clock, since some interventions must be performed before the birth to promote the best outcome.

2. **Analyze cues. What could it mean? Answers 1, 2, 3, and 5 are correct.**
   1. **If a woman's bag of waters has not broken before labor begins, it often breaks spontaneously in active labor, especially at 6 cm dilation, as the fetus is pushed more deeply into the birth canal.**
   2. **The client's temperature could rise even higher, related to chorioamnionitis as a result of the GBS positive status.**
   3. **Since this patient is a multipara at 6 cm, she will most likely deliver before the next 4 hours have passed and will not likely receive 2 doses of penicillin, which is recommended. The average length of active labor after 6 cm for a multipara is less than 2 hours, and the average pushing stage for a multipara is 20 minutes (Zhang et al., 2010). If her progress continues to be average, she could have her baby in her arms within 2.5 hours. The newborn will require close monitoring for any symptoms of sepsis.**
   4. The FHR is not of concern at this time. It shows moderate variability and early decelerations, which are benign. There is nothing to indicate it will change for the worse. Late decelerations are not expected in this client's case. If the client develops a rising fever, the FHR could show fetal tachycardia.
   5. **The client's statement, "I can't do this anymore!" makes it likely she will ask for an epidural.**

TEST-TAKING HINT: Sometimes the slow changes in labor progression can be worrisome. In this situation, rupture of the membranes indicates labor progression, which is good, but it also increases the risk of infection for both mother and baby. It introduces a time constraint. Because IV antibiotics are given every 4 hours in labor and she is likely to deliver within 2.5 hours, she will likely receive just one dose of antibiotics before the birth, not the recommended two doses. The risk of chorioamnionitis increases with the number of

vaginal examinations she has, as the bacteria in her vagina is pushed toward the cervix and the bag of waters during the exams. Once the bag of waters breaks, the risk of infection increases. If the client's fever is lowered with a dose of acetaminophen, that will reduce the likelihood of fetal tachycardia. Not all clients who say "I can't take this anymore" actually want an epidural, but most do. If the client is serious about wanting an epidural, she must make her decision immediately, since she is at the threshold of active labor at 6 cm dilation. She will need an IV fluid bolus before the epidural insertion; that could delay the start of the epidural insertion by around 30 minutes. At that point, it might be time to push, which could be too late to be effective. The nurse may have a series of competing priorities. They must be taken in the order of importance for maintaining client and fetal safety. The nurse must consider timing of the intervention and time constraints, as well as immediate interventions needed to promote safety of both the mother and baby.

3. Prioritize hypotheses. Where do I start? Answers 1 and 3 are correct.
   1. The client's temperature of 100.4° F (38° C) indicates she has a fever. Her positive Group B strep test makes it more likely she is developing chorioamnionitis, even though her bag of waters is not broken.
   2. There is nothing to suggest abruptio placenta in spite of her behavior.
   3. She is showing signs of a normal labor pattern. In fact, dilation of 6 centimeters and +1 station on admission is very favorable.
   4. There is nothing to indicate pre-eclampsia.
   5. There are no signs of cephalopelvic disproportion. In fact, her cervical exam with the fetus at +1 station would contradict that possibility. The fetus is fitting through the pelvis nicely.

TEST-TAKING HINTS: The nurse sorts through all the possibilities and narrows them down to the most likely hypothesis that she will focus on first. In this case, the most serious risk for the client is developing chorioamnionitis. The client's normal labor pattern, which suggests a fairly short window of time before the birth, signals the nurse that interventions to treat the possible chorioamnionitis must be completed as soon as possible. In that way, both of these hypotheses are connected.

4. Generate Solutions. What can I do? Answers 1(b), 2(c), 3(a), 4(c), and 5(a) are correct.

Potential Intervention	Indicated (a)	Nonessential (b)	Contraindicated (c)
1. Provide oxygen by re-breather mask		X	
2. Insert indwelling catheter and send urine specimen to lab			X
3. Request an order for IV penicillin	X		
4. Place a fetal scalp electrode			X
5. Request an order for acetaminophen	X		

1(b) There is no concern with the FHR, making oxygen by mask nonessential.

2(c) Insertion of an indwelling catheter is invasive and increases the risk of infection. It is contraindicated at this time. A urine culture does not need to be sent to the lab. Although some patients benefit from an indwelling catheter after an epidural is inserted, that is primarily indicated if the client is unable to void spontaneously and when several hours of labor are anticipated. In contrast, this client does not yet have an epidural in place. Once she does, she will likely deliver within 2 hours of the epidural insertion, making an indwelling catheter unnecessary.

3(a) The client has no known drug allergies, and penicillin G is the gold standard for Group B strep prophylaxis. A request for an order is indicated and should be one of the first tasks the nurse completes, since the client is a multipara at 6 cm.

4(c) This is strongly contraindicated. Not only is the FHR tracing reassuring without a pattern of concern, but more importantly, the application of a fetal scalp electrode makes fetal infection with Group B strep more likely. It breaks the skin on the fetal scalp, creating a portal for infection. It should be avoided at all costs in patients with infection of any kind, unless the benefit is higher than the risk.

5(a) A provider's order for acetaminophen is indicated since the client has a fever.

TEST-TAKING HINTS: The nurse's interventions and the client needs should be considered in light of the GBS infection identified in step 3—"prioritize hypotheses."

5. Take action. What will I do?
   1. The case study doesn't indicate that the client wants an epidural.
   2. The client has a low-grade fever, and will need acetaminophen, but because the FHR is not yet showing tachycardia, treating the Group B strep is the most important step at this time.
   3. **Administration of penicillin is the most urgent treatment at this time because of the client's multiparity and dilation and the benefit of medication administration to both mother and baby if given as early as possible in labor.**
   4. The client does not need and should not receive an indwelling catheter at this time.

TEST-TAKING HINT: This question asks what is the most urgent order to complete, in order to assess the test taker's ability to prioritize. The correct answer is the one that treats the biggest threat to the client and her baby—the positive GBS status. In actual practice, the nurse might not have the penicillin on the unit and might need to wait for the penicillin to be sent from the pharmacy. In that case, the nurse would move to the next important treatment, reducing the client's fever. If the acetaminophen is readily available, that might end up being the medication the nurse administers first. Because processes may vary between hospitals, the question does not ask which medication the nurse will administer first; it asks what order is the most urgent to complete. For further information on testing and treating Group B Strep, see https://www.cdc.gov/mmwr/pdf/rr/rr5910.pdf.

6. Evaluate outcomes—Did it help? Answers 1 and 4 are correct.
   1. **The client's temperature is down following the acetaminophen administration.**
   2. The FHR is unrelated to nursing actions. The variable decelerations are likely an indication of normal labor progress as the fetus descends. Although the nurse's actions of assisting the client to turn every 30 minutes may have contributed to fetal descent, the nurse's actions did not cause the variable decelerations. The decelerations are not unexpected and must continue to be assessed. They indicate the fetus is experiencing periods of hypoxemia (low oxygen available in the blood) as a result of cord compression.
   3. The contractions are unrelated to nursing actions, but they could indicate the beginning of second stage labor as the uterus gets serious about pushing the fetus out and resting.
   4. **Position changes throughout labor can contribute to fetal descent and cervical dilation as the slippery fetus rotates in response to uterine forces. This is a positive response to nursing actions. Because of the epidural, the client may not feel a rectal urge to push. Instead, the client may report a sensation of discomfort in the front, below the pubic bone.**
   5. The administration of penicillin is an action, not an outcome.

TEST-TAKING HINTS: There is a discrete difference between *actions* the nurse completes, and measureable client *outcomes* that occur as a likely result of nursing actions. In this case, the client's temperature has been reduced (an *outcome*) as a result of the nurse's action of administering of acetaminophen. The nurse's diligent attention to client position changes (an *action*) has likely contributed to the cervical exam changes and fetal descent (an *outcome*).

7. Answers 1, 2, 3, and 5 are correct.
   1. **The nurse should check the client's weight gain reported in her prenatal record. This will guide how the nurse plans for delivery and newborn care.**
   2. **The client's ethnicity and religion should be noted. This allows the nurse to proceed in a culturally sensitive manner.**
   3. **The client's age should be noted. Clients over age 35 (advanced maternal age) are at risk for prolonged labor and postpartum bleeding.**

4. The type of insurance the woman has is not relevant to the nurse.
5. **The client's gravidity and parity—how many times she has been pregnant and how many times she has given birth—should also be noted as a guide for the anticipated length of labor and client teaching that may be necessary.**

TEST-TAKING HINT: The prenatal record is a summary of the woman's history from the time she started prenatal care until the record was sent to the labor unit by the provider's office (usually at 36 weeks' gestation or later if prenatal records are sent on paper). Virtually all of the physical and psychosocial information relating to this woman is pertinent to the care by the nurse. For example, the nurse may need to change some aspects of care in relation to the woman's ethnicity and religion, her age, and so on. If a woman has gained very little weight during her pregnancy, the baby may be small-for-gestational age (SGA). This will be important for newborn care after the delivery. If the woman has gained a fair amount of weight, the baby might be large, leading to a difficult delivery or shoulder dystocia, and the nurse should be prepared for that event. The woman's type of insurance makes no difference to the care the woman receives and should be of no concern to the nurse in planning labor care.

8. 1. Leopold maneuvers, although performed on a woman in labor, assess for fetal position, not the progress of labor.
   2. Fundal tone assesses for the presence and duration of uterine contractions, but this is not the most valuable information.
   3. Assessment of the fetal heart rate is critically important in relation to fetal well-being, but it will not determine the progress of labor.
   4. **A vaginal examination of the cervix will provide the nurse with the best information about the status of labor.**

TEST-TAKING HINT: Each of the assessments listed is performed on a woman who enters the labor suite for assessment. However, the only assessment that will determine whether or not a woman is in true labor is a vaginal examination of the cervix in combination with fetal descent and rotation. Only when there is cervical change—dilation and/or effacement—accompanied by fetal descent and/or rotation is it determined that a woman is in true labor.

9. 1. There is no indication that this client is about to have a seizure.
   2. **The woman is showing expected signs of the active phase of labor.**
   3. There is no indication that this woman is showing signs of hypoxia and/or hypercapnia.
   4. The alpha-fetoprotein assessment is a test to screen for Down's syndrome and neural tube defects in the fetus. It is done during pregnancy.

TEST-TAKING HINT: The nurse must be familiar with the different phases of the first stage of labor: latent, active, and transition. The multiparous woman in the scenario entered the labor suite in the latent phase of labor when being talkative and excited is normal. After 1 hour she has progressed into the active phase of labor, generally around 6 cm, in which being serious and breathing shallowly with contractions are expected behaviors. Her obstetrical history of G2 P1001 indicates this is her second pregnancy. As such, the nurse must anticipate that cervical dilation may occur more quickly than if this were her first childbirth experience.

10. **Answers 1, 2, and 4 are correct.**
   1. **The nurse should assess the fetal heart rate before reporting the client's status to the healthcare provider.**
   2. **The nurse should assess the contraction pattern before reporting the client's status.**
   3. A complete urinalysis is not generally indicated, but this depends on the client's medical history. This can be obtained once the patient is admitted, unless the client reports symptoms that require immediate testing. Some standard orders include a limited urine sample for the presence of protein, but this also can wait.
   4. **The nurse should assess the woman's vital signs before reporting her status.**
   5. A biophysical profile is performed only if ordered by a healthcare practitioner.

TEST-TAKING HINT: The fetal heart rate, contraction pattern, and maternal vital signs should all be assessed to provide the healthcare practitioner with a picture of the health status of the mother and fetus. In most hospitals, the nurse must also do a vaginal examination to assess for cervical change unless contraindicated.

11. 1. With the palpation findings of a hard round mass in the fundal area and soft round mass above the symphysis, the nurse can conclude that the fetal position is not transverse.
   2. The findings on palpation also indicate that the presentation is not vertex.
   3. **With the findings of a hard round mass in the fundal area and soft round mass**

above the symphysis, the nurse can conclude that the fetal lie is vertical, with the fetus in the breech position.

4. The attitude is difficult to determine when performing Leopold maneuvers.

TEST-TAKING HINT: Many obstetric assessments rely on the healthcare provider's sense of touch, combined with creating a "picture" in the mind and interpreting the findings. Leopold maneuvers require this practice. The nurse palpates specific areas of the pregnant abdomen and then must imagine "seeing" the fetal head, small parts (fists and feet), and back, to translate what is being palpated. For example, in the scenario presented, the nurse palpates a hard round mass in the fundal area of the uterus and must interpret that as the fetal head. Having done that, the nurse palpates a flat surface on the client's left side and imagines that as the fetal back. "Small objects on the right side" are interpreted to be fetal hands and feet. The soft, round mass above the symphysis is then easily interpreted as the fetal buttocks. With these findings and interpretations, the nurse will then conclude that the fetal lie is vertical, but the baby is breech.

12. Answers 1, 2, 3, and 5 are correct.

1. **The nurse should assess the fetal heart rate with all vaginal examinations.**
2. **The nurse should assess the fetal heart rate before giving the mother any analgesics.**
3. **The fetal heart rate should be assessed periodically at the end of a contraction.**
4. The fetal heart rate pattern should be assessed at least every hour during the latent phase of a low-risk labor. It is not standard protocol to assess every 10 minutes during this labor phase.
5. **The nurse should assess the fetal heart rate before the woman ambulates.**

TEST-TAKING HINT: The most important part of this question is the phase of labor, the latent phase. Fetal stress is generally minimal in this phase. As such, the recommendation is to assess the fetal heart rate for a short period of time every hour, and additionally during the times indicated here. As labor becomes active, fetal heart rate monitoring is done to detect changes in the normal heart rate patterns that validate the well-being of a fetus during labor, or suggest that the fetus is not doing well and interventions are necessary. The fetal heart rate pattern should, therefore, be assessed whenever maternal factors could affect the fetus or the circulation through the umbilical cord. With the vaginal examinations, the fetal heart rate may accelerate, indicating fetal well-being. The fetal heart rate may slow down a bit and show minimal variability after analgesics are given, so the nurse will want to have a reassuring baseline fetal heart rate for comparison. The fetal heart rate may show a deceleration from the beginning of a contraction, through the peak, and after the contraction has ended. Each of these patterns indicates fetal status, which guides nursing interventions. Finally, it is important to confirm fetal well-being before the client gets out of bed to ambulate without telemetry, as the fetus will not be monitored during that time.

13. 1. Palpating the sacral promontory assesses the obstetric conjugate, not the fetal station.

2. **Station is assessed by palpating the ischial spines.**
3. Palpating the cervix assesses dilation and effacement, not fetal station.
4. Palpating the symphysis pubis assesses the obstetric conjugate, not the fetal station.

TEST-TAKING HINT: The nurse must be thoroughly familiar with the anatomy of the female reproductive system and the measurements taken during pregnancy and labor. Station is determined by creating an imaginary line between the ischial spines. The descent of the presenting part of the fetus is then compared with the level of that "line." This is a difficult assessment to make, and is uncomfortable for the patient. A nurse new to obstetrics might require some time to master the assessment. It is still possible to *estimate* station without feeling the ischial spines.

14. 1. The nurse's findings upon performing Leopold maneuvers indicate that the fetus is in the left occiput anterior (LOA) position, the best position for birth. The fetal back is felt on the mother's left side (L), the back of the baby's head, the occiput (O) is toward the anterior, or front of the mother (A) and the small parts (hands and feet) are felt on her right side. The soft, round buttocks are felt in the fundal region, and the head is felt above her symphysis as a hard, round mass.

2. The findings after the nurse performs Leopold maneuvers do not indicate that the fetus is in the left sacral posterior (LSP) position; in that position, the fetal back is on the mother's left side (L); the fetal buttocks (S or sacrum) are tilted posteriorly (P)

toward the bed and the mother's back; a hard round mass is felt in the fundal region, and a soft round mass is felt above the symphysis.

3. The findings after the nurse performs Leopold maneuvers do not indicate that the fetus is in the right mentum anterior (RMA) position; in that position, the fetal chin (M or mentum) is to the mother's right (R), presenting. The baby's head is not flexed. Instead, it is tilted back, as though looking at the sun, and faces the front of the mother, anteriorly (A). Small objects are felt on the right of the mother's abdomen with a flat area felt on the mother's left side.
4. The findings after the nurse performs Leopold maneuvers do not indicate that the fetus is in the right sacral posterior (RSP) position; in that position, the fetus's sacrum (S) is facing the mother's back on the right, posteriorly (RP) and a hard round mass is felt in the fundal region while a soft round mass is felt above the symphysis.

TEST-TAKING HINT: The test taker must review fetal positioning. This is an especially difficult concept to understand. The best way to learn the three-dimensional concept of fetal position is to look at the pictures in a text. Using a doll, the nurse or test taker can then imitate the pictures by placing the doll into each of the positions.

Remember that the word "left" or "right" indicates which side of the mother's abdomen the presenting part is facing. "LO" indicates that the *occiput* (O), the back of the fetal head (and thus, the fetal back) is on the mother's *left* (L) side. "LS" indicates the *sacrum* (S), or buttocks are on the mother's *left* (L) side; "RS" means the *sacrum* (S) or buttocks are on the mother's *right* (R). "RM" means the *mentum* (M), or chin, is on the mother's *right* (R). The third letter tells us whether the "O" (occiput), "S" (sacrum) or "M" (chin, or mentum) is located down toward the bed (P, posterior) or up toward the mother's belly (A, anterior). As such, RMA indicates the mentum or chin is on the mother's right, and is up, facing her belly. RMP indicates the chin is down, toward the bed.

15. Answers 2, 4, and 5 are correct.

1. A bulging perineum does not occur until shortly before delivery, at the end of the second stage, not upon entering this stage.
2. **The bloody show increases as a woman enters the second stage of labor.**
3. The amniotic sac can rupture at any time.
4. **With a fully dilated cervix and bulging perineum, laboring women usually feel a strong urge to push.**
5. **The client's ability to work with her body's demands can change throughout the stages of labor. Often, the intensity of the contractions and the sensation of the fetus moving through the birth canal and stretching the tissues causes the client to cry out. Some scream; many push involuntarily.**

TEST-TAKING HINT: It is important to note that there are three *stages* of labor and three *phases* of the first stage of labor. The three *phases* of the first *stage* of labor—latent, active, and transition—are related to changes in cervical dilation, fetal descent, and maternal behaviors. The three stages of labor are defined by specific labor progressions—cervical change to full dilation (stage 1), full dilation to birth of the baby (stage 2, pushing), birth of the baby to birth of the placenta (stage 3).

16. 1. The LOA position refers to a fetus whose occiput (O) is facing toward the mother's left side (L) and is in an anterior position toward the mother's belly (A). The presenting part is at −1 (minus one) station, meaning it is 1 cm above the ischial spines and not yet engaged.
2. **The LSP position is the correct answer. The fetal sacrum (S) is presenting and is toward the mother's left side (L). The sacrum is tilted to the mother's back posteriorly (P). The baby is breech. The buttocks are at –1 station, meaning they are 1 cm above the ischial spines.**
3. The LMP position refers to a fetus whose chin (M or mentum) is facing toward the mother's left (L) side. This is also called a face presentation. The fetal chin is down toward the bed, and the mother's spine (P, posterior). In a face presentation, the baby's chin, not the occiput, is the point of reference. So, it may seem like the reverse of LOP where the baby's back is along the mother's left side. In LMP, the baby's *chin* is toward the mother's left side, meaning the back is toward the mother's right. A presenting part at plus one (+1) station is 1 cm below the ischial spines, toward the vaginal opening.
4. The LSA position refers to a fetus whose buttocks (S) are facing toward the mother's left side (L) anteriorly (A, toward her belly) and a presenting part at +1 station is 1 cm below the ischial spines.

TEST-TAKING HINT: An understanding of the definition of "station" easily eliminates two of the four responses in this question. When the

presenting part of the fetus is at zero (0) station, the part is at the same level as an imaginary line between the mother's ischial spines. The baby is engaged. When the presenting part is above the spines and has not yet entered the birth canal, the station is referred to as minus (−) one, minus two, and so on. When the presenting part has moved past the spines (deeper into the birth canal) toward the opening of the vagina, the station is defined as plus (+) one, plus two, and so on. Because the question states that the nurse palpated the buttocks above the spines, the station is in the minus category. This effectively eliminates the two answer options that include a plus 1 or positive station, since a location of 1 cm *above* the ischial spines is a minus one (−1) station.

17. 1. A fetus in the mentum anterior position is unlikely to elicit severe back pain in the mother.
2. A fetus in the sacral posterior position is unlikely to elicit severe back pain in the mother.
3. When a fetus is in the occiput posterior position, mothers frequently complain of severe back pain.
4. A fetus in the scapula anterior position is in a shoulder presentation and is unlikely to elicit severe back pain in the mother.

TEST-TAKING HINT: A fetus in the occiput posterior (OP) position is lying with the back of its skull toward the mother's spine. The baby's head is pressed against the mother's coccyx with each contraction. This is very painful. With the mother lying in bed, the baby's face is toward the ceiling, or "face up."

18. 1. The left upper quadrant would be the appropriate location for a fetoscope, to hear the fetal heart rate if the baby were breech, in the LSA position, not the LOA position.
2. The right upper quadrant would be appropriate if the baby were breech, in the right sacral anterior (RSA) position.
3. The fetoscope should be placed in the left lower quadrant for a fetus positioned in the LOA position as described in the question. This positions the fetoscope to record the fetal heart rate through the fetal back, which is recommended.
4. The right lower quadrant would be appropriate if the baby were in the ROA position.

TEST-TAKING HINT: The fetal heart rate is best heard through the fetal back. Because the Leopold maneuvers have indicated the baby is LOA, the fetal back (and, hence, the fetal heart rate) is in the left lower quadrant.

19. 1. Descent is progressing well. The presenting part is 3 centimeters below the ischial spines, well into the birth canal.
2. The fetal head is well past engagement. Engagement is defined as 0 station.
3. Because the client is a primipara, delivery is not likely to be imminent.
4. External rotation does not occur until after delivery of the fetal head.

TEST-TAKING HINT: This question includes a number of concepts. Descent and station are discussed in answer options 1 and 2. Length of second stage, which is related to the fact that the woman is a primigravida, is discussed in choice 3. And one of the cardinal moves of labor—external rotation—is included in choice 4. The test taker must be prepared to answer questions that are complex and that include diverse information. In a 10 cm dilated primiparous client with a baby at +3 station, vaginal delivery is not imminent, but the fetal head is well past engagement and descent is progressing well. External rotation has not yet occurred because the baby's head has not yet been born. Fetal station may be reported using a 3-cm scale or a 5-cm scale. It is a subjective measurement. In this question, the scale is a 5-cm scale. If one were using a 3-cm scale, the birth would be imminent.

20. 1. This client is still in stage 1 (the cervix is not fully effaced or fully dilated). The fetal head would not be visible at the introitus.
2. This client is still in stage 1 (the cervix is not fully effaced or fully dilated), but the station is low. Still, the fetal head would not be visible at the introitus.
3. Although this client is fully dilated, the cervix is not fully effaced, and the baby has not descended far enough for delivery or to be visible at the introitus.
4. The cervix is fully dilated and fully effaced and the baby is low enough to be seen at the vaginal introitus.

TEST-TAKING HINT: To answer this question, the test taker must methodically evaluate each of the given responses. Once the nurse determines that a woman is not yet fully dilated or effaced, it can be determined that the woman is still in stage 1 of labor. The fetal head would not be at the introitus if a client is still in stage 1 of labor. This eliminates answers 1 and 2. Choice 3 does show a woman who is fully dilated but whose cervix is not yet fully effaced. Because 100% effacement

occurs before a cervix dilates to 10 cm, this answer is also unlikely. Only choice 4 meets all criteria posed in the question.

21. Answers 3, 4, and 5 are correct.

1. Hypnotic suggestion is usually not included in childbirth education based on the Lamaze method.
2. Rhythmic chanting is usually not included in childbirth education based on the Lamaze method.
3. **Muscle relaxation is an integral part of Lamaze childbirth education.**
4. **Pelvic rocking is taught in Lamaze classes as a way of easing back pain during pregnancy and labor.**
5. **Abdominal massage, called effleurage, is also an integral part of Lamaze childbirth education.**

TEST-TAKING HINT: The test taker may have expected to find breathing techniques included in the question related to Lamaze childbirth education. Although breathing techniques are taught, there are a number of other techniques and principles that couples learn in Lamaze classes. The test taker should be familiar with all aspects of childbirth education.

22.

1. Childbirth educators are not concerned with the possible verbalizations that laboring women might make.
2. Breathing exercises can be quite tiring. Simply being in labor is tiring. The goal of childbirth education, however, is not related to minimizing the energy demands of labor.
3. **Some of the techniques learned at childbirth education classes are meant to break the fear-tension-pain cycle.**
4. Although childbirth educators discuss maternal–newborn bonding, it is not a priority goal of childbirth education classes.

TEST-TAKING HINT: Most women are anxious when they come to the hospital in labor. As the labor contractions become stronger, the client may tense her muscles, causing the pain to be worse and causing her more fear. This can become a vicious cycle of increasing pain and fear, which may delay labor progress, raise the mother's blood pressure, and negatively impact the fetus. The information and skills learned at childbirth education classes are designed to break the cycle and to help the woman work with her body in giving birth. This promotes physiologic birth.

23.

1. The alternate pant-blow technique is used during stage 1 of labor.
2. Rhythmic, shallow breaths are used during stage 1 of labor.
3. **Open glottal pushing is recommended by many midwives during the second stage of labor.**
4. Slow chest breathing is used during stage 1.

TEST-TAKING HINT: This client is in second stage, the pushing stage of labor. Answers 1, 2, and 4 are not appropriate for second stage. Whether or not the test taker has seen open glottis pushing, answer 3 is the only possible answer because it speaks to pushing. In second stage, the woman will change from using breathing techniques that help during first stage contractions, to pushing with the contractions to promote fetal descent. Open glottal pushing is recommended by many providers because pushing against a closed glottis can decrease the mother's oxygen saturation. However, some providers prefer that their patients use closed glottis pushing which is sometimes more effective in moving the baby down. In any case, pushing is the task of second stage labor.

24.

1. It is important to include all relevant information in the childbirth class.
2. Baby care should be included, but it is also important to include information about labor and delivery.
3. **Using visual aids can help to foster learning in teens as well as adults.**
4. Having the classes conveniently located in the school setting often enhances teens' attendance.

TEST-TAKING HINT: Because of their classroom experiences, adolescents are accustomed to learning in groups. The school setting is comfortable for them and, because of its location and its familiarity, is an ideal setting for childbirth education programs. In addition, educators often use visual aids to promote learning. Movies are especially effective in conveying information.

25.

1. Although this client is light-headed, her problem is unlikely related to her blood pressure.
2. **This client is showing signs of hyperventilation. The symptoms will likely subside if she re-breathes her exhalations for a few minutes.**
3. It is unnecessary for this client to be moved to her side.
4. The baby is not in jeopardy at this time.

TEST-TAKING HINT: It is essential that the test taker attend to the specific clues in the question and not assume that other issues may be occurring. This client is light-headed as a result of hyperventilating during contractions. Hyperventilation, which can result from breathing too rapidly, is characterized by tingling

and light-headedness. By re-breathing some of the carbon dioxide she is blowing off, she can re-balance her oxygen/carbon dioxide levels, which should correct the problem. This can be done by covering her mouth with her hand, or a paper sack for a short period of time.

26. 1. The pant-blow breathing technique is usually used during the transition phase of labor.
2. Rapid, deep breathing is rarely used in labor.
3. Grunting and pushing, characteristic of open glottal pushing, is the method that women instinctively use during the second stage of labor. It is also the safest method of pushing.
4. Most women find slow chest breathing effective during the latent phase, as it helps with relaxation.

TEST-TAKING HINT: Because the latent phase is the first and longest phase of stage one, the contractions are usually mild and they rarely last longer than 30 seconds. A slow chest breathing technique, therefore, is effective and does not tire the woman out for the remainder of her labor. It is important to note that women who have learned the Bradley method of childbirth are encouraged to perform relaxed breathing throughout labor.

27. 1. It is inappropriate to encourage her to have an epidural as the next step at this time.
2. It is inappropriate to encourage her to have an IV analgesic at this time.
3. A change of position might help but will probably not be completely effective.
4. This woman is in the active phase of labor. The first phase breathing is probably no longer effective. Encouraging her to shift to the next level of breathing is appropriate at this time.

TEST-TAKING HINT: If a woman has learned Lamaze breathing, it is important to support her actions. Encouraging her to take pain-relieving medications may undermine her resolve and make her feel like she has failed. The initial response by the nurse should be to support her by encouraging her to use the breathing techniques she has prepared to use, guiding her to use them appropriately and effectively.

28. 1. The lithotomy position is not physiologically supportive of labor and birth.
2. Effleurage is a light massage that can soothe the mother during labor.
3. Practicing Kegel exercises can help to build up the muscles of the perineum after the birth, but will not help the woman to work with her labor.
4. Pushing is not performed until the second stage of labor.

TEST-TAKING HINT: There are a number of actions that women can take to support their breathing during labor. Walking, swaying, and rocking can all help during the process. Effleurage, the light massaging of the abdomen or thighs, is often soothing for laboring women.

29. 1. The woman should not push until the next contraction. She should be allowed to sleep at this time.
2. The woman's privacy should be maintained while she is resting.
3. The woman is in no apparent distress. Vital sign assessment is not indicated.
4. The woman is in no apparent distress. Oxygen is not indicated.

TEST-TAKING HINT: Because the woman is in second stage, she is pushing with contractions. If she is very tired, she is likely to fall asleep immediately following a contraction. It is important for the nurse to maintain the woman's privacy by covering her perineum with a sheet between contractions. This also prevents the vaginal mucosa from drying out.

30. 1. This client has probably moved into the second stage of labor. Providing a bedpan is not the first action.
2. The nurse should first assess the progress of labor to see if the client has moved into the second stage of labor.
3. It is too early to notify the physician.
4. It is too early to advise the mother to push.

TEST-TAKING HINT: This is the client's third baby. The average length of transition in clients who are multiparas is 10 minutes. This client is therefore likely to have moved into the second stage of labor. As the fetus moves deeper into the birth canal, one of the first sensations the mother feels is that she needs to move her bowels. The nurse's first action when this sensation is reported, therefore, is to assess the progress of labor. If the client is in second stage, the provider will be notified. Since this patient is a multipara, the second stage is not likely to last very long, so the nurse must assess fetal station and determine whether the client should be encouraged to push with the contractions, or should pant through contractions to allow fetal descent to happen with the power of the contractions until the provider arrives. The risk of encouraging a multiparous patient to push before the provider arrives is that the baby might descend rapidly and be delivered by the nurse. However, the nurse should never hold the client's knees together to prevent the

fetus from being born. If the client is not yet in second stage, she should continue breathing with her contractions.

31. 1. **This is the correct response. A fetal heart rate of 150 bpm is normal.**
    2. This woman is in early labor. The fetal heart rate does not need to be assessed every 5 minutes.
    3. The rate is normal. There is no need to report the rate to the healthcare practitioner.
    4. The rate is normal. There is no need to institute emergency measures.

TEST-TAKING HINT: It is essential to know the normal physiological responses of women and their fetuses in labor. The normal fetal heart rate is 110 to 160 bpm. Therefore, a rate of 150 is within normal limits. No further action is needed at this time.

32. 1. **The tracing is showing a normal fetal heart rate tracing. No intervention is needed.**
    2. There is no need to administer oxygen at this time. The tracing is normal.
    3. If the client is comfortable, there is no need to change her position.
    4. There is no need to speed up the intravenous fluids at this time.

TEST-TAKING HINT: The baseline fetal heart rate variability is the most important fetal heart rate assessment that the nurse makes. If the baby's heart rate shows moderate variability, this is a reassuring, Category 1 tracing and the nurse can assume that the baby is not hypoxic or acidotic. In addition, the fetal heart rate of 140 bpm is within the normal range of 110–160.

33. 1. **The relationship between the decelerations and the contractions will determine the type of deceleration pattern.**
    2. The maternal blood pressure is not related to the scenario in the question.
    3. Although some fetuses are at higher risk for fetal intolerance of labor, the nurse must first determine which type of deceleration is present.
    4. If the nurse is able to identify that a deceleration is present, the transducer placement is adequate.

TEST-TAKING HINT: The nurse must understand the physiology of fetal heart rate deceleration patterns and appropriate interventions associated with each type. Decelerations are defined by their relationship to the contraction pattern. It is essential that the nurse determine which of the three types of decelerations is present, as they give a clue to the fetal experience during labor. Early decelerations mirror contractions and are benign. Late decelerations begin "late" in the contraction, at the peak, and often return to baseline well after contractions are over. They are often seen with clients who have pre-eclampsia or diabetes, and indicate poor placental function and fetal hypoxemia. Variable decelerations can occur at any time and are often unrelated to contractions. They indicate umbilical cord occlusion. If the nurse remembers that blood flow from the fetus through the umbilical arteries to the placenta and back again to the fetus through the umbilical vein is a closed system powered by the fetal heart, it makes sense that when the umbilical cord is temporarily occluded and blood flow cannot pass through it, the fetal heart slows down in response to the blockage. For more information on fetal blood circulation, see the appendix.

34. 1. Breathing will help with contraction pain but is not as effective when a client is experiencing back labor.
    2. It is inappropriate to automatically encourage mothers to have anesthesia or analgesia in labor. There are other methods of providing pain relief.
    3. **When direct sacral pressure is applied, the nurse is providing a counteraction to the pressure being exerted by the fetal head.**
    4. Hydrotherapy is very soothing but will not provide direct relief.

TEST-TAKING HINT: Whenever a laboring woman complains of severe back labor, it is very likely that the baby is lying in the occiput posterior position. Every time the woman has a contraction, the fetal head is pushed into the mother's coccyx. Bone presses on bone. When direct pressure is applied to the sacral area, the nurse is providing counteraction to the pressure being exerted by the fetal head. Laboring clients have reported that this helps to reduce the back pain. Other positions and maneuvers are also helpful but are not discussed here.

35. 1. The maternal blood pressure is not the priority assessment after an amniotomy.
    2. The maternal pulse is not the priority assessment after an amniotomy.
    3. **It is essential to assess the fetal heart rate throughout and especially, immediately after an amniotomy to assess for possible umbilical cord prolapse reflected in variable or prolonged decelerations.**

4. Fetal fibronectin is assessed during pregnancy. It is not assessed once a woman enters labor.

TEST-TAKING HINT: Amniotomy, as the word implies, is the artificial rupture of the amniotic sac. During the procedure, especially when the cervix is dilated wider than the diameter of the umbilical cord and the fetal head is not tight against the cervix, there is a risk that the umbilical cord may become compressed by the baby's head within the uterus, or that a loop of cord may be carried out by the gush of water through the cervix and prolapse into the birth canal, causing cord occlusion and decelerations. Because there is no direct way to assess cord compression within the uterus, the nurse must assess the fetal heart rate for any adverse changes that may suggest cord compression.

36. 1. Because the baby's back is facing the mother's right side, the fetal monitor should not be placed in the LUQ on the mother's left side.

2. Because the baby's back is facing the mother's right side, the fetal monitor should not be placed LLQ on the mother's left side.

3. Because the baby's back is facing the mother's right side and the sacrum is presenting, the fetal monitor should be placed in her RUQ, on her right side.

4. The monitor electrode should have been placed in the RLQ if the nurse had assessed a vertex presentation.

TEST-TAKING HINT: Answers 1 and 2 can be easily eliminated with this question because they indicate the baby's buttocks, and therefore its back, is on the mother's left side. The best location for the fetal monitor is against the fetal back, at the level of the fetal heart. Although the question does not tell the test taker whether the sacrum is facing anteriorly (toward the mother's belly) or posteriorly (toward the mother's spine), it does provide the information that the sacrum is felt toward the mother's right. Because this baby is in the breech position with its back toward the mother's right side, the best location for the fetal monitor is in the RUQ, at the level of the fetal heart.

37. 1. This client is fully dilated and effaced, but the baby is not yet engaged. Until the baby descends and stimulates rectal pressure, it is inappropriate for the client to begin to push.

2. Fundal pressure is inappropriate.

3. Many women push in the squatting position, but it is too early to push at this time.

4. Monitoring for rectal pressure is appropriate at this time.

TEST-TAKING HINT: The nurse must interpret each piece of information about this cervical exam in order to answer this question correctly: dilation, effacement, and station. The primary concern with this client is that although she is 10 cm dilated and 100% effaced, the fetus is at minus 3 (−3) station. One would expect the fetus to be at 0 or plus 1 (+1) station or more at this point. A fetus at minus 3 station at the start of second stage suggests cephalopelvic disproportion—a fetus that is too large to fit into the pelvic inlet. Although the nurse may see in practice that women are encouraged to begin to push as soon as they become fully dilated, it is best practice to wait until the fetus is engaged (at zero station or lower), or until the client exhibits signs of rectal pressure. Pushing when the fetus is not yet engaged may result in an overly fatigued woman or, more significantly, a prolapsed cord.

38. Answers 1 and 2 are correct.

1. An appropriate action by the doula is giving the woman a back massage.

2. An appropriate action by the doula is to assist the laboring woman with her breathing.

3. The nurse, not the doula, should assess the fetal heart rate.

4. The nurse, not the doula, should assess the blood pressure.

5. The nurse, not the doula, should regulate the IV.

TEST-TAKING HINT: The test taker can deduce the answers to this question by knowing the following: Questions 3 and 4 involve physiological assessments and question 5 involves a nursing intervention. Only two of the responses, numbers 1 and 2, deal with providing supportive care—the role of the doula.

39. 1. Women may contract without being in true labor.

2. Once the cervix begins to both efface and dilate, a client is in true labor.

3. Membranes can rupture before true labor begins.

4. Engagement can occur before true labor begins.

TEST-TAKING HINT: Although laboring women experience contractions, contractions alone are not an indicator of true labor. Only when the cervix thins and dilates is the client in true labor. False labor contractions are usually irregular and mild, but, in some situations, they can appear to be regular and can be quite uncomfortable in spite of not causing any change in the cervix.

40. **Answers 1, 2, and 4 are correct.**

1. **True labor contractions often begin in the back and, when the frequency of the contractions is regularly q 5 minutes or less and increasing in intensity, it is usually appropriate for the client to proceed to the hospital.**
2. **Even if the woman is not having labor contractions, rupture of membranes is a reason to go to the hospital to be assessed.**
3. Expelling the mucous plug is not sufficient reason to go to the hospital to be assessed.
4. **Greenish liquid is likely meconium-stained fluid. The client needs to be assessed in the hospital.**
5. The latent phase of labor can last up to a full day. In addition, Braxton Hicks contractions can last for quite a while. Even though a woman may feel cramping for 4 hours or more, she may not be in true labor.

TEST-TAKING HINT: The mucous plug protects the uterine cavity from bacterial invasion. It is expelled before or during the early phase of labor. In fact, it may be hours, days, or even a week after the mucous plug is expelled before true labor begins. During that time, a replacement mucous plug may form.

41. 1. Blood in the urine could indicate that the client has a urinary tract infection. First, however, the nurse should acknowledge the client's concerns.

2. **The nurse is using reflection to acknowledge the client's concerns.**
3. Although the woman might also have expelled her mucous plug, this response ignores the fact that the client is frightened by what she has seen.
4. The nurse will want to clarify that the woman isn't actually bleeding, but the question should follow an acknowledgment of the woman's concerns.

TEST-TAKING HINT: Pregnant women are very protective of themselves and of the babies they are carrying. Any time a change that might portend a problem occurs, a pregnant woman is likely to become concerned and frightened. Certainly, seeing any kind of blood loss from the vagina can be scary. The nurse must acknowledge that fear before asking other questions or making other comments. In addition, the advice nurse must have provider-approved, written protocols for advice in response to common questions. If a client's question is not on the list, the provider must be informed of the question and a personalized answer must be obtained for the client.

42. 1. The frequency of labor contractions has decreased. If the client was in true labor, the frequency would increase.

2. Labor contractions increase in intensity. They do not become milder.
3. **This response indicates that the labor contractions are increasing in intensity.**
4. This client has slept through the "tightening" and there is no increase in intensity. It is unlikely that she is in true labor.

TEST-TAKING HINT: The test taker should review the labor contraction definitions of frequency, duration, and intensity. As labor progresses, there is an increase in the frequency, duration, and intensity of the contractions. The nurse notes the change in intensity when he or she palpates the fundus of the uterus, and the client subjectively complains of increasing pain.

43. 1. The frequency and duration of this contraction pattern is every 2 minutes lasting 60 seconds. Contraction frequency is measured from the start of one contraction to the start of the next one. In this case, there are 120 seconds (2 minutes) from the start of one contraction to the start of the next one: a 60-second contraction, followed by a 60-second rest period, then the start of another contraction, meaning the contractions are coming every 2 minutes.

2. The frequency and duration of this contraction pattern is very dangerous for the fetus because of the duration of each contractions. The contractions show a duration of 2 minutes (120 seconds) followed by 2 minutes of rest, meaning they are coming every 4 minutes.
3. The frequency and duration of this contraction pattern is even more dangerous for the fetus. Once again, each contraction has a duration of 2 minutes, followed by a rest period of 1 minute. The contractions are coming every 3 minutes, with a duration of 2 minutes, which is too long.
4. **The frequency and duration of this contraction pattern is 60 second contractions every 3 minutes. The contraction begins, and ends after 60 seconds, followed by a 2-minute rest period before the start of the next contraction, making it a contraction frequency of every 3 minutes. This is ideal.**

TEST-TAKING HINT: To answer this question, the test taker must recall that contraction frequency is counted in minutes; duration is counted in seconds. Contraction frequency includes each

contraction and the rest period that follows. As such, contraction frequency is timed from the start of one contraction to the start of the next. By converting the contraction duration from seconds into minutes, the test taker can easily see that the correct answer is one in which both the contraction and the rest period are no more than 3 minutes long. Answer 1 adds up to a 2-minute pattern (1 minute contraction, 1 minute rest), so it is not an option. Answer 2 adds up to 4 minutes (2-minute contraction, 2-minute rest), so it also isn't right. Answer 3 adds up to a 3-minute frequency, but the contractions are 2 minutes long, not 1 minute. Answer 4 adds up to a 3-minute frequency with a 1-minute contraction. This is the correct answer.

44. 1. A fetus in a sacral presentation is in a vertical (up-and-down) lie.
2. A fetus in an occipital presentation is in a vertical (up-and-down) lie.
3. A fetus in a mentum presentation is in a vertical (up-and-down) lie.
4. A fetus in a scapular (shoulder) presentation is in a horizontal lie.

TEST-TAKING HINT: Lie is concerned with the relationship between the fetal spine and the maternal spine. When the spines are parallel, the lie is vertical (or longitudinal, up-and-down). When the spines are perpendicular, the lie is horizontal (or transverse). It is physiologically impossible for a baby in the horizontal lie to be delivered vaginally.

45. The correct order of the movements listed is: 1, 5, 3, 4, 2.
1. Descent.
5. Internal rotation.
3. Extension.
4. External rotation.
2. Expulsion.

TEST-TAKING HINT: The best labor nurses understand and visualize the cardinal movements of labor in order to assist with fetal descent through maternal positioning during labor. Descent occurs initially as the fetus enters the pelvis and becomes engaged, or fixed in the pelvis. Descent continues throughout labor until the birth. In order to descend effectively, the fetus must accomplish adequate flexion. If the fetus does not flex its chin to the chest, it may not be able to fit through the bony pelvis. The fetal head should be in normal alignment with the shoulders, one ear down toward the bed, one ear up toward the mother's belly. Once the fetus is flexed and engaged, contractions continue to force it through the pelvis.

Internal rotation is the next cardinal movement. While the fetal body remains in position, the shape of the pelvic outlet rotates the fetal head from its normal alignment, to the side, so it is "looking" over its lower shoulder, with the back of its head just below the mother's pubic bone. It is now facing down, toward her spine. This is optimum. The fetus maintains this position until external rotation.

Extension occurs before external rotation. As the fetus approaches the vaginal opening, a portion of the back of its head is pressed under the mother's pubic bone. The fetal head follows the shape of the pelvic outlet which is now an oval shape from front-to-back, instead of from right-to-left at the inlet. The fetal head extends upward as it moves under and past the pubic bone. The fetal head is delivered, facing down. In that moment, one can see external rotation as the baby's head moves back into alignment with the shoulders.

Expulsion, the delivery of the baby's body, follows in quick succession as the baby's shoulders form an oblique angle and shoulders slide under the pubic bone, followed by the baby's body. The baby is born.

46. 1. Engagement is equal to 0 station. This fetus is more like +4 station, well past 0 station.
2. A baby who is floating is in a minus station.
3. When the presenting part is at the ischial spines, the baby is engaged or at 0 station.
4. The baby's head is almost crowning.

TEST-TAKING HINT: A baby is crowning when the mother's perineal tissues are stretched around the fetal head at approximately the same location where a crown would sit. The station at this time is beyond +5 station (or 5 cm past the ischial spines). Many providers are more familiar with a calculated +3 measurement instead. If using that measurement, this baby would be beyond +3 station.

47. 1. The obstetric conjugate is the shortest anterior to posterior diameter of the pelvis. When it is of average size, it will accommodate an average-sized fetal head.
2. When the fetal head is flexed, the diameter of the head is minimized. This is not, however, the obstetric conjugate. The obstetric conjugate refers to the maternal pelvis, not the fetus.
3. Although 6 cm is the accepted start of *active* labor, there is no average dilation for the beginning of labor.
4. The physiological retraction ring is the area of the uterus that forms as a result of cervical effacement. It is not related to the obstetric conjugate.

TEST-TAKING HINT: The obstetric conjugate is measured by the healthcare practitioner to estimate the potential for the fetal head to fit through the anterior-posterior diameter of the maternal pelvis. It is the internal distance between the sacral promontory (the bottom of the pelvis) and the symphysis pubis (the upper part of the pelvis).

48. Every 3 minutes.

TEST-TAKING HINT: There are two things to remember when assessing contraction frequency: (1) Frequency is defined as the time from the *beginning* of one contraction to the *beginning* of the next contraction; (2) frequency is always expressed in minutes, not seconds. (Duration is expressed in seconds).

49. 90 seconds.

TEST-TAKING HINT: There are two things to remember when assessing duration: (1) duration of a contraction is measured from the beginning of the increment—the rise where the contraction begins to curve upward from baseline—to the end of the decrement—when the contraction returns to baseline; (2) duration is always written in seconds, not minutes. Each vertical column on the monitor strip represents 10 seconds. Each bold, vertical line represents 60 seconds. Each of these contractions covers the space of approximately 9 vertical columns, or 90 seconds.

50. 1. This is not correct. The contraction pattern is q 3 min × 90 sec.
2. This is not correct. The contraction pattern is q 3 min × 90 sec.
3. This is not correct. The contraction pattern is q 3 min × 90 sec.
4. **This is correct. The contraction pattern is q 3 min × 90 sec.**

TEST-TAKING HINT: Contraction frequency is an approximation, not a precise measurement. It includes the duration of a contraction and the rest period that follows. Frequency is important. It confirms that the uterus has an adequate rest period between contractions in order to provide oxygen to the placenta to refresh the fetal oxygen reserves.

There are two ways to determine frequency. First, the long way: place your pencil at the beginning of the increment, or rise of the first contraction and the beginning of the increment of the next contraction. Count the number of 10-second columns. There are 18 columns, which equals 180 seconds. Convert the 180 seconds into minutes (divide by 60) to get a frequency of 3 minutes. This is the contraction frequency.

A more efficient way is to use the dark, vertical lines which indicate one minute, or 60 seconds. Note how many of these 60-second time periods are included in the time from the start of one contraction to the start of the next one. This is the frequency. Note that one or two 10-second columns may be outside of the dark vertical lines before the next contraction's rise, but because the vertical columns indicate seconds, and contraction frequency is recorded in minutes, they do not need to be included in the frequency. In other words, one does not chart frequency in both minutes and seconds (i.e., 2 minutes, 50 seconds, and so forth). One could round that up to be 3 minutes.

To determine contraction duration, place your pencil at the beginning of the increment (the rise from the baseline) of the first contraction and at the end of the decrement (the return to baseline) of the same contraction. Count the number of vertical, 10-second columns between the rise and fall of the contraction. You will count 9 columns. Each vertical column is 10 seconds, so multiply 9 by 10 seconds, giving a 90-second duration. This is the duration and it should be recorded in seconds.

51. 1. A baby in the breech presentation may or may not be in the flexed attitude.
2. A baby in the horizontal lie may or may not be in the flexed attitude.
3. Engagement is unrelated to attitude.
4. **When the baby's chin is on its chest, the baby is in the flexed attitude.**

TEST-TAKING HINT: The diameter of the fetal head is dependent upon whether or not the head is flexed with the chin on the chest or extended with the chin elevated. When the baby is in the flexed attitude with the chin on the chest, the diameter of the fetal head entering the pelvis averages 9.5 cm (the suboccipitobregmatic diameter), whereas if the baby is in the extended attitude, with the chin elevated, the diameter of the fetal head entering the pelvis can be as large as 13.5 cm (the occipitomental diameter). For the fetal head to pass through the mother's pelvis, therefore, it is best for the head to be in the flexed attitude. The nurse can reassure the client that her baby is in the optimum position for labor and birth.

52. 1. A full-term baby may still have to enter the pelvic inlet.
2. **The true pelvis is the bowl-shaped opening between the pelvic inlet and the pelvic outlet.**
3. The baby is physiologically unable to enter the true pelvis when in a horizontal lie.
4. The attitude of the baby is not discussed in the ultrasound statement.

TEST-TAKING HINT: When the largest part of the fetal head, the biparietal diameter, is at a level below the plane of the pelvic inlet, the fetal head is engaged. This is positive confirmation of clinical adequacy of the fetal head to fit through the pelvis.

53. 1. **This is a picture of a fetus in the right occiput posterior (ROP) position.**
2. This is a picture of a fetus in the right occiput anterior (ROA) position.
3. This is a picture of a fetus in the left occiput posterior (LOP) position.
4. This is a picture of a fetus in the left occiput anterior (LOA) position.

TEST-TAKING HINT: When determining the position of a fetus, it is very important to consider the posture of the fetal presenting part in relation to the left and/or right side of the maternal body and not in relation to the left and/or right side of the test taker's body. Only two of these diagrams, answers 1 and 2, show the fetal back toward the mother's right side. The test taker can automatically eliminate answers 3 and 4. Of the two remaining answers, #2 shows the fetal head in an anterior position toward the mother's belly. Answer #1 shows the fetal head facing posteriorly, toward the mother's spine, so that is the correct answer, ROP: right occiput posterior.

54. 1. This is a picture of a fetus in the right sacral posterior (RSP) position.
2. This is a picture of a fetus in the right sacral anterior (RSA) position.
3. This is a picture of a fetus in the left sacral posterior (LSP) position.
4. **This is a picture of a fetus in the left sacral anterior (LSA) position.**

TEST-TAKING HINT: Only two of these diagrams apply to the question. The LSA position means the fetal back is facing the mother's left side (L). Answers 1 and 2 show the fetus facing the mother's right side, so those two can be eliminated immediately. All the fetuses are in the breech position, as indicated by the sacrum being the presenting part (S). Finally, the test taker is asked to identify the LSA position, so the choice must be the fetus whose sacrum is facing the mother's belly anteriorly (A). Answer 4 is the only one that shows that.

55. 1. This is a picture of a fetus in the single footling breech position.
2. This is a picture of a fetus in the double footling breech position.
3. **This is a picture of a fetus in the frank breech position.**
4. This is a picture of a fetus in the double footling breech position.

TEST-TAKING HINT: There are three main breech positions: frank, where the buttocks present and both feet are located adjacent to the fetal head; single footling, when one leg is extended through the cervix and vagina while the remaining leg is bent; and double footling, when both legs are extended through the cervix and vagina. It is likely that a woman carrying a breech in any position will have a cesarean section.

56. 1. Flexion is one of the first of the cardinal moves of labor.
2. Internal rotation occurs while the baby is still in utero.
3. **During extension, the baby's head is born.**
4. The baby rotates externally after the birth of the head.

TEST-TAKING HINT: The baby must move through the cardinal movements of labor in order to fit through the pelvis. During extension, the baby's head follows the upward curve of the pelvis, which forces its head under the pubic bone and up, through the vaginal opening. External rotation occurs once the fetal head is freed from the birth canal, just before, or in tandem with, expulsion as the fetal head re-aligns itself with its shoulders.

57. 1. When assessing the variability of the fetal heart rate, the mother can be in any position.
2. **The variability of the fetal heart rate is determined by analyzing the fluctuations of the baseline rate.**
3. Only after assessing a fetal monitor tracing that indicated fetal hypoxemia would the nurse administer oxygen.
4. Variability is unrelated to fetal movement.

TEST-TAKING HINT: There are many important principles related to electronic fetal heart rate monitoring. Variability is the most important feature of the baseline data. The classic National Certification Corporation (NCC) monograph (Simpson, 2016) describes variability as "determined in a 10-minute window, excluding accelerations and decelerations." It is described as "[f]luctuations in the baseline FHR that are irregular in amplitude and frequency and are visually quantified as the amplitude of the peak-to-trough in bpm" (p. 2). The "peak-to-trough" is also referred to as a "cycle." It is the repetitive up and down undulation of the fetal heart rate, also called the "bandwidth" of the baseline. It occurs as a result of the opposing activity of the sympathetic and parasympathetic nervous systems. As such, it reflects the well-being of the fetal autonomic nervous system. If the fetus is

sleeping, is acidotic, or if the mother has received opiates for pain, this bandwidth will show a reduction in baseline fetal heart rate variability on the fetal monitor (Preti & Chandraharan, 2018). When the fetal heart rate variability is adequate, therefore, the nurse can conclude that the baby's autonomic nervous system is well.

58. 1. **Because the variability is moderate (6 to 25 bpm from peak to trough), the nurse can conclude that the baby is well oxygenated. Regular, supportive care is indicated.**
2. Because the variability is moderate (6 to 25 bpm **from peak to trough**), there is no need for the mother to receive oxygen.
3. Because the variability is moderate (6 to 25 bpm **from peak to trough**), there is no need to move the mother to another position to improve the fetal heart rate.
4. Because the variability is moderate (6 to 25 bpm **from peak to trough**), there is no need to measure the mother's oxygen saturation.

TEST-TAKING HINT: A tracing that shows moderate variability—that is, 6 to 25 bpm in amplitude—indicates adequate variability and this, in turn, indicates normal pH and oxygenation of the fetus at that time.

59. 1. Moderate variability is indicative of fetal health, not of hypoxia.
2. A change in variability can reflect fetal acidosis, not alkalosis. In this situation, there is no indication of acidosis.
3. During sleep cycles, fetal heart rate variability may decrease.
4. **Moderate variability is indicative of fetal health and well-being.**

TEST-TAKING HINT: It is important for the nurse to be familiar with situations that can change the fetal heart rate variability. Normal situations that can decrease the variability include fetal sleep, administration of central nervous system depressant medications, and prematurity. A normal situation that can increase the variability is fetal activity.

60. 1. **Early decelerations are generally seen during the first stage of labor.**
2. Epidural insertion is not associated with early decelerations.
3. Early decelerations are not generally seen during the second stage of labor.
4. By the time the placenta is being delivered, the baby is already born.

TEST-TAKING HINT: Early decelerations are common decelerations in the first stage of labor and are considered benign (Choe et al., 2020). No interventions are necessary. They are recognized as shallow, spoon-shaped dips in the fetal heart rate that mirror the contraction; that is, unlike a late deceleration, the fetal heart rate with an early deceleration begins when the contraction begins and returns to the baseline by the time the contraction ends. Early decelerations are noted during the first stage of labor, generally between 3 and 7 cm dilation due to compression of the fetal head. The literature indicates that early decelerations represent an autonomic response to vagal stimulation as the fetal head is compressed during a uterine contraction (Choe et al., 2020).

61. 1. **The fetal heart rate normally accelerates during fetal movement.**
2. When analgesics are administered, the fetal heart rate variability drops and accelerations are rarely seen.
3. When a fetus is acidotic, the fetal heart rate variability drops and accelerations are rarely seen.
4. With poor placental perfusion, the fetal heart rate variability drops and accelerations are rarely seen.

TEST-TAKING HINT: Fetal heart rate accelerations, defined as a rise in the fetal heart rate above baseline of at least 15 bpm and that lasts a minimum of 15 seconds, are a sign of fetal well-being. When the baby is healthy and well-oxygenated, they are almost always noted during periods of fetal movement. Similar to what occurs in a runner, with increased movement, the fetal heart rate speeds up to accommodate increasing energy needs.

62. 1. **The nurse is concerned about fetal malpresentation, specifically an occiput posterior position. This position often results in a swollen anterior lip of the cervix.**
2. The fetus has descended from 0 station to +1 station, so cephalopelvic disproportion is not a concern at this point.
3. Tachysystole (more than 5 contractions in 10 minutes averaged over 30 minutes) does not contribute to anterior lip and is not a factor in this case study.
4. Uterine dysfunction does not contribute to anterior lip and is not a factor in this case study.

TEST-TAKING HINTS: The nurse must recognize factors that indicate where interventions are indicated. In this situation, the fetus has descended from 0 station to +1 station, so cephalopelvic disproportion is not likely at this point. Because cervical effacement has

decreased, indicating the cervix is swelling, fetal malpresentation is a more likely factor. Factors associated with cervical swelling include fetal malpresentation in the occiput posterior position. In the occiput posterior position, the fetal head is positioned face-up instead of face-down, so that it rams the cervix with each contraction, instead of sliding through it. The nurse must confirm her hypothesis if possible, and intervene to promote further fetal descent past the cervix, if possible.

63. Answers 1 and 4 are correct.

1. **The oncoming nurse should confirm the fetal presentation to determine if fetal malpresentation is a factor in the anterior lip.**
2. Contraction frequency is not an issue in this case study and does not relate to fetal malpresentation.
3. The fetal heart rate is important to monitor, but it does not relate to fetal malpresentation in this case study.
4. **Fetal descent will assist the nurse in evaluating whether or not the recommended interventions are effective. Fetal descent is often slower with an occiput *posterior* position. If the fetus rotates to an occiput *anterior* position, fetal descent will be more rapid.**

TEST-TAKING HINTS: The answers to this question must relate directly to the answer and hypothesis in the previous question.

64. Answers 3 and 4 are correct.

1. The client's method of pushing is unrelated to the development of an anterior cervical lip.
2. Uterine effleurage is unrelated to the development of an anterior cervical lip.
3. **A number of interventions are appropriate for rotating a fetus from the occiput posterior position to occiput anterior. These include frequent position changes of left to right, pushing on all fours, getting in the shower, squatting while pushing, or laboring in the tub. The client with an epidural will be limited in these options, of course, but can certainly turn from side to side.**
4. **If the client has an epidural, she will likely be able to stop pushing for up to 30 minutes to allow the fetal head to rotate and slip past the pubic bone and deeper into the pelvis.**

TEST-TAKING HINTS: Once again, the answers to this question must relate directly to the nurse's hypothesis in the first of these three case-study questions.

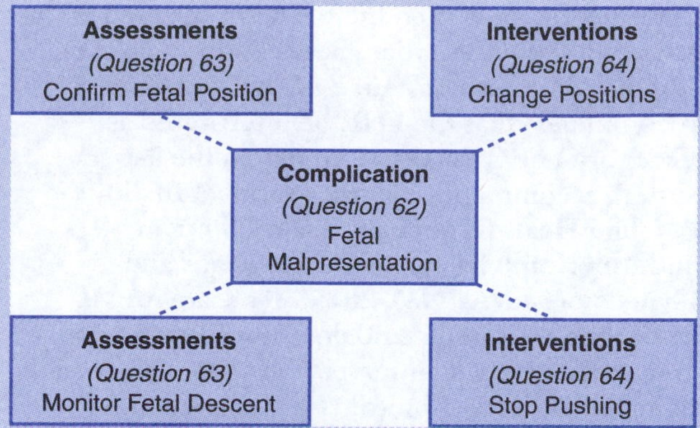

65.
1. The baby's heart rate should not exhibit variable decelerations as a response to maternal pain-relieving medication.
2. The baby's heart rate should not exhibit late decelerations after the mother is given an analgesic.
3. **Analgesics are central nervous system (CNS) depressants. The variability of the fetal heart rate, therefore, will be decreased.**
4. The baby's heart rate is unlikely to exhibit transient accelerations after the mother receives analgesics.

TEST-TAKING HINT: It is important for the nurse to remember the side effects of commonly-used medications. The analgesics used in labor are opiates. The CNS-depressant effect of the opiates is therapeutic for the mother who is in pain, but the baby is also affected by the medication, often exhibiting decreased heart rate variability.

66.
1. **The fetal heart rate should be assessed during and after a contraction, every 5 minutes during the second stage of labor.**
2. The woman should be encouraged to follow her body's urges during contractions, but it is not generally necessary to hold one's breath and push on command.
3. The pulse should be assessed, but it is unnecessary to do so every 5 minutes.
4. There is no specific pushing position that is required, but the woman should avoid lying flat on her back. Women may push while squatting, on hand and knees, or in a number of other positions.

TEST-TAKING HINT: Fetal heart rate surveillance is performed during labor to detect clinically significant fetal acidemia. The nurse must follow accepted standards of care and written protocols for intermittent auscultation (IA) as established by the birthing center or hospital. With IA, both

the mother's pulse and the FHR are counted at the same time to differentiate between the two. The American College of Nurse-Midwives (ACNM) recommends that the FHR be interpreted as Category I or Category II, based on the 3-tier system recommended by the National Institute of Child Health and Human Development and American College of Obstetricians and Gynecologists (ACNM, 2015). If a Category II FHR pattern is noted and does not resolve with appropriate nursing interventions, the placement of electronic fetal monitor (EFM) for further surveillance is recommended (ACNM, 2015). During second stage labor, the woman may push with an open glottis to prevent the vasovagal response. Research has shown that when women push without being coached, they often do not hold their breath to bear down, but instead grunt during the second stage. Often, however, the provider's recommendation is the one the client uses.

67\. 1. Holding the breath for 20 seconds during each contraction can stimulate the Valsalva maneuver, which can lead to a sudden drop in blood pressure and fainting.
2. One cannot push and blow out at the same time. This will not facilitate the delivery of the baby.
3. Pushing should be done only during contractions, not between contractions.
4. **By taking a cleansing breath before pushing, the woman is waiting until the contraction builds to its peak. Her pushes will be more effective at this point in the contraction.**

TEST-TAKING HINT: It is essential that the test taker read each question and the possible answer options carefully. If response 3 is read quickly, the test taker might mistakenly choose it as the correct response. Because the woman is being encouraged to push between contractions, however, the answer is incorrect.

This question may seem like a contradiction to the previous question. This is because expert opinions vary on the topic of pushing in second stage. The nurse must be open to coaching the client in the method agreed upon by the provider and the client. Women and providers who prefer a more natural approach may recommend undirected, open glottis pushing. Physicians often recommend a more traditional approach of directed pushing to a count of ten. With each contraction, the client will be coached to complete approximately three pushes, counting to ten through each of the three pushes, then rest until the next contraction. This approach may be encouraged if the fetal heart rate indicates that the fetus is showing signs of hypoxia and must be delivered shortly. If this approach is used, the pushing is more effective if the client takes a breath in and out "for herself" and then takes another one to hold "for the baby" while she pushes.

68\. 1. Bloody show and perineal bulging are normal findings. There is no need to notify the healthcare practitioner at this time.
2. Bloody show and perineal bulging are normal findings. The woman is not in need of immediate cardiovascular assessment.
3. **Because this is a normal finding, the nurse should continue to provide labor support and encouragement.**
4. Bloody show and perineal bulging are normal findings. There is no need to administer oxygen or to change the woman's position.

TEST-TAKING HINT: The bulging perineum is an indication that the baby is descending through the birth canal and the bloody show results from injury to the capillaries in the mother's cervix. Because this woman is a primigravida, she will likely need to push for a while longer, so it is not necessary to notify the healthcare provider until additional signs are noted, as long as the healthcare provider is readily available.

69\. 1. Epidurals are a form of regional anesthesia. They are used to obliterate pain.
2. It is inappropriate to encourage the woman to receive an epidural at this time.
3. **Because this woman is a multipara, the position is LOA, and the station is +3, this is an accurate statement.**
4. It is inappropriate to encourage the woman to receive an epidural at this time.

TEST-TAKING HINT: The average length of the second stage of labor for multiparous women is about 15 minutes, whereas the average time for an epidural to be inserted and to take effect is approximately 20 minutes. In addition, the fetus in the scenario has already descended to +3 station and is in the optimal position for delivery—LOA. It is very likely that this baby will be born after just a few more contractions. Although the nurse may wish to meet the client's requests, that is not always possible. The nurse must give the client a realistic assessment and encourage the client to continue pushing with her contractions.

70\. **Answers 1, 3, 4, and 5 are correct.**
1. **This statement is true. Depending on the provider's recommendations and experience, a birth may take place in a variety of locations and positions, including sitting on a stool in the shower,**

kneeling while holding onto the back of the labor bed, or even while standing.

2. The nurse should provide additional information to this client. Many deliveries are performed safely in positions other than the lithotomy position. Like the words "always" and "never," the word "essential" is the word that makes this response incorrect, because it allows no room for other options.
3. **If the fetus is in the posterior position, the woman may be encouraged to push while on her hands and knees. This may enable the baby to turn into the anterior position and the delivery may soon follow.**
4. **Many mothers deliver in their labor beds without stirrups. Some beds transform into delivery beds and some are regular hospital beds. Still others are double or queen-sized beds so that the client's support person can also relax in the bed. When forceps or other interventions are needed for a delivery, however, stirrups may be required. Nurses are encouraged not to do the work of stirrups by holding a client's legs, as this can injure the nurse's back.**
5. **Midwives deliver their clients in a variety of positions, including the side-lying, squatting, and lithotomy positions, as well as when the clients are on their hands and knees.**

TEST-TAKING HINT: Deliveries can be performed in a variety of positions, including lithotomy, squatting, and side-lying. They can also be completed in a variety of locations, including labor bed, delivery bed, shower, or in water. It is recommended that mothers consult with their primary healthcare provider early in the pregnancy regarding the provider's delivery practices, including birth positions. The mother's birth preference may influence her choice of caregiver.

71. The order of change during the third stage of labor is: 3, 4, 1, 2.

3. **The contraction of the uterus after delivery of the baby is the first step in the third stage of labor.**
4. **As the uterus contracts, its surface area decreases more and more.**
1. **A hematoma forms behind the placenta as the placenta separates from the uterine wall after the uterus has contracted and its surface area has decreased.**
2. **The membranes separate from the uterine wall after the placenta separates and begins to be expelled.**

TEST-TAKING HINT: Once the baby is born, the uterus contracts. When it does so, the surface area of the internal uterine wall decreases, forcing the placenta to begin to separate since it doesn't fit anymore. As the placenta separates, uterine bleeding forms a hematoma behind it, promoting further placental separation. Once the placenta separates and begins to be expelled, the membranes peel off the uterine wall and are delivered.

72. 1. Considering the signs, this is an unlikely reason.
2. **These are positive signs of placental separation and pending placental delivery.**
3. Considering the signs, an atonic uterus is an unlikely reason.
4. Cord bloods are obtained by the practitioner once the cord is cut. The clamp on the cord that is still attached to the placenta is released and blood is obtained from the cut cord.

TEST-TAKING HINT: Although they sound abnormal, the following are the normal signs of placental separation: The uterus rises in the abdomen and becomes globular, there is a gush of blood expelled from the vagina, and the umbilical cord lengthens as the placenta detaches from the uterus and moves toward the cervix. The placenta should be delivered between 5 and 30 minutes after the delivery of the baby to allow adequate contraction of the uterus and prevent silent build-up of blood behind the undelivered placenta.

73. Answers 1 and 3 are correct.

1. **Lengthening of the umbilical cord is a positive sign of placental separation.**
2. Once second stage is complete, the baby is no longer in utero.
3. **A globular uterus rising in the abdomen is a positive sign of placental separation.**
4. Dilation and effacement are complete before second stage begins.
5. Rectal pressure is usually a sign of fetal descent. Once the second stage is complete, the baby is no longer in utero.

TEST-TAKING HINT: It is essential that the nurse clearly differentiates between stage 1, stage 2, and stage 3 of labor. Stage 1, what is usually referred to as "labor," ends with full cervical dilation. At the end of stage 2, the baby is born. And at the conclusion of stage 3, the placenta is delivered.

74. 1. Excitement is consistent with a client in the latent phase of labor.
2. **"I can't stand the pain!" is a comment consistent with a client in the transition phase of stage 1.**
3. "I feel hot" is a comment that could be made at a variety of times during the labor.

4. "I need to push" is a comment consistent with a client in stage 2 labor.

TEST-TAKING HINT: The nurse must be familiar with not only the physiological changes that occur during each phase of labor but also with the maternal behaviors that are expected at each phase.

75. 1. The nurse would expect the woman to be 2 cm dilated.
2. At 4 cm, the woman is still not in the active phase of labor.
3. At 8 cm, the woman is in the transition phase of labor.
4. At 10 cm, the woman is in the second stage of labor.

TEST-TAKING HINT: In the latent phase of labor, clients are often very excited because the labor has finally begun. They frequently are very talkative and easily distracted from the discomfort of the contractions. It is important to remember that a patient may not move past 4 cm for several hours. Active labor is considered to begin at 6 cm dilation. At one time, if a client remained at 4 cm for at least 2 hours, she was diagnosed with "arrest of labor" and a cesarean section was performed. More recently, after researchers reviewed the original research on normal length of labor, and with a goal to prevent "the first cesarean section," it was determined that regardless of how long a woman's cervix was 4 cm dilated, more rapid dilation occurred after she reached 6 cm. As a result, the standard of care changed to use 6 cm as the start of active labor when making a decision for a primary cesarean section due to "arrest of labor" (Spong et al., 2012). The nurse should be familiar with the cervical changes that correlate with the various phases and stages of labor.

76. 1. With pain and increased energy needs, the pulse rate often increases.
2. The blood pressure rises dramatically.
3. Although the woman is working very hard, her temperature should remain normal.
4. With pain and increased energy needs, the respiratory rate often increases.

TEST-TAKING HINT: During contractions, the blood from the uterus is forced back into the maternal circulation like an auto-transfusion of 300 to 500 mL of blood (Burt & Durbridge, 2009). In response, there is an increase in cardiac output. The woman's blood pressure rises an average of 35 mm Hg systolic and 25 mm Hg diastolic. The blood pressure should never be assessed during a contraction because the reading will be a marked distortion of the woman's true blood pressure at rest.

77. 1. The woman is exhibiting no high-risk issues.
2. The woman is in latent labor. There is no need for her to be hospitalized at this time.
3. The woman is exhibiting no high-risk issues.
4. The woman is in early labor, not active phase.

TEST-TAKING HINT: The key facts to attend to in this question about a primigravida are the cervical dilation, the contraction pattern, and the fetal heart rate pattern. The woman is clearly in the latent phase because she is only 2 cm dilated, is 25% effaced, and is contracting infrequently q 12 minutes for just 30 seconds each time. The fetal heart rate is very reassuring with moderate variability and accelerations. The provider will no doubt send her home to labor in comfort since active labor is not likely to begin for several hours.

78. 1. Talking and laughing are characteristic behaviors of the latent phase.
2. Back labor can be experienced during any phase of labor.
3. Women in the latent phase often do perform effleurage, but it can also be performed during other phases of labor.
4. A woman in the latent phase might go to the bathroom but defecating is not indicative of the first phase of labor. It is more commonly seen at the start of second stage, as a signal to begin pushing.

TEST-TAKING HINT: Severe back labor is not common during the latent phase. Although effleurage is a massage that women are taught to use during the latent phase of labor, it is important to remember that some women find that effleurage works well for them during the active and transition phases of labor. Each client should be encouraged to use breathing techniques and other therapies that help them with their labors.

79. 1. It is recommended that women begin pushing once they are at 10 centimeters.
2. There is no indication for oxygen in this scenario.
3. The previous standard of "laboring down" is no longer recommended (American Academy of Obstetricians and Gynecologists [ACOG], 2019a).
4. There is no indication of maternal compromise in this scenario.

TEST-TAKING HINT: An epidural can reduce or completely eliminate the urge to push. It was once thought that if the woman begins pushing before she feels the urge to push, she may be too tired to push effectively once the fetus is lower in the birth

canal. It was common to recommend that women with an epidural who have no urge to push at 10 cm rest and wait for up to an hour or so, allowing the uterus to maneuver the fetus lower into the pelvis. This was referred to as "laboring down." However, in January of 2019, the ACOG released a committee opinion that there was no benefit for delaying the pushing stage (ACOG, 2019a). Morbidities such as increased risk of infection, hemorrhage, and neonatal acidemia were noted with delayed pushing (ACOG, 2019a). Women are now advised to begin pushing as soon as they are 10 cm dilated. The nurse can help facilitate fetal rotation and descent by recommending that the woman change positions about every 30 minutes, if possible.

80. Answers 1 and 4 are correct.
  1. The fetal position is preferred by some anesthesia providers.
  2. The lithotomy position is inappropriate.
  3. The Trendelenburg position is inappropriate.
  4. A sitting position is preferred by some anesthesia providers.

TEST-TAKING HINT: For the anesthesiologist to insert the epidural catheter into the epidural space, the woman must be placed in a position that curves the spinal column enough to widen the gap between the spines, facilitating easy entry of the needle. The woman may be asked to position herself "like an angry cat," or "like a shrimp," or a "letter C." This can be done in either the fetal position or while the client sits up on the side of her bed with her feet resting on a chair. In both of those positions, the woman's vertebrae separate, providing the anesthesiologist access to the epidural space.

81. Answers 1, 2, 4, and 5 are correct.
  1. Before a woman is given regional anesthesia, the nurse should assess the fetal heart rate to confirm fetal well-being.
  2. The nurse should receive an order to infuse Ringer's lactate before the woman is given regional anesthesia. The anesthesiologist will determine the amount of IV fluid the woman should receive, based on her medical condition. A woman with pre-eclampsia should be on fluid restrictions and generally just 500 mL of IV solution is ordered.
  3. It is not appropriate to place the woman in the Trendelenburg position.
  4. A baseline blood pressure is necessary, and successive blood pressures will be monitored frequently after the epidural insertion is completed, as ordered by the anesthesia provider.
  5. The nurse should ask the woman to empty her bladder. Because she may be unable to empty her bladder spontaneously after the epidural is inserted, this can prevent the immediate need for a catheterization after the epidural is in place.

TEST-TAKING HINT: Before any medication is administered during labor, whether analgesia or anesthesia, the fetal heart rate should be assessed to make sure that the baby is not already compromised. Before regional anesthesia administration, a bolus of fluid should be infused to increase the woman's vascular fluid volume. This will help to maintain her blood pressure after the epidural insertion. In addition, the woman's bladder should be emptied prior to the epidural insertion, because she will not have the sensation of a full bladder once the epidural is in place, and she may not be able to spontaneously void on her own. The nurse can begin the IV bolus as the woman ambulates to the bathroom to void and returns to her bed before the epidural. This can also assist with fetal descent. Baseline vital signs, including blood pressure, are important for trending purposes.

82.
  1. It is unlikely that the woman will experience adverse feelings in her lower extremities.
  2. Hypotension is a very common side effect of regional anesthesia.
  3. The epidural does not enter the circulatory system. It is placed in the "epidural space" outside of and parallel to the spinal cord.
  4. Fetal heart accelerations are positive signs. These are not adverse findings.

TEST-TAKING HINT: The nurse must be familiar with the side effects of all medications, whether or not the nurse administers them. If no other therapeutic interventions are performed, most women will show signs of hypotension after epidural administration. This is due to the action of medication, which blocks the sympathetic nervous system. In response, widespread arterial and venous vasodilation occurs, which causes a sort of hypovolemia and drops the client's blood pressure. The intravenous fluid bolus is meant to reduce this response by temporarily increasing the circulating fluid volume.

83.
  1. The temperature does not need to be assessed immediately after the epidural insertion.
  2. A wedge should be placed under one side of the woman to keep her off her back.

3. There is no indication that a blanket roll needs to be placed under the woman's feet at this time.
4. It is not necessary for the nurse to assess the pedal pulses at this time.

TEST-TAKING HINT: As indicated in the previous question, hypotension is the most common complication of epidural anesthesia in labor. This can be worsened by allowing the client to lie flat on her back. In that position, the vena cava and aorta are compressed by the pregnant uterus. When a wedge is placed under the woman's side—usually the right side, but any side will do—the uterus is tilted, relieving the pressure on the great vessels.

84. 1. Fetal movement is noted during labor, but it is not directly related to the fetal scalp stimulation test.
2. The fetal heart rate should accelerate in response to scalp stimulation.
3. The variability does not change in direct response to the fetal scalp stimulation test.
4. Late decelerations are related to uteroplacental insufficiency. The fetal scalp stimulation test will not affect a late deceleration pattern.

TEST-TAKING HINT: The fetal scalp stimulation test is performed by the healthcare provider or the nurse, when the fetal heart rate pattern is equivocal and there is uncertainty about fetal well-being. For example, if the fetal monitor tracing has shown minimal variability for close to an hour, the nurse or primary healthcare provider may perform the test. It is done by simply performing a vaginal exam and rubbing a finger over the fetal scalp to "tickle the fetal head" and elicit a response. If the fetal heart rate accelerates in response to the test, the response is interpreted as a positive sign of fetal well-being. It is important to note, however, that the scalp stimulation test is contraindicated while the fetal heart rate is showing signs of fetal stress such as during a deceleration.

85. Answers 1, 2, and 5 are correct.
1. Nurse-midwives sometimes recommend that women at full term engage in sexual intercourse to stimulate labor. Prostaglandins in the semen are thought to contribute to cervical ripening, similar to the action of misoprostol.
2. Ingesting primrose oil is also sometimes recommended. Primrose oil is believed to help ripen the cervix.
3. Exercise should be encouraged throughout pregnancy, but it is not used for induction.
4. Raw spinach is an excellent source of iron as well as a source of calcium and fiber. It is, however, not used for induction.
5. Nipple and breast massage is sometimes recommended to help induce labor by stimulating the release of oxytocin.

TEST-TAKING HINT: A test taker who is unfamiliar with nonpharmacological induction methods, can make some educated guesses by remembering that pharmacological medications for labor induction are prostaglandins and oxytocin. When a woman has an orgasm, she releases oxytocin. Nipple and breast massage also stimulate oxytocin production. Evening primrose oil contains a fatty acid that converts into a prostaglandin compound.

86. 1. Squatting is an alternate position for delivery, but it is not used to decrease perineal tearing.
2. Pushing the fetal head against the perineum is the cause of perineal tearing.
3. Pushing the fetal head against the perineum is the cause of perineal tearing.
4. Massaging of the perineum with mineral oil may help to reduce perineal tearing.

TEST-TAKING HINT: During the late pushing stage, as the fetal head descends, nurses and nurse-midwives may massage a woman's perineum to increase the elasticity of the tissue. Some may hold warm, moist cloths to the perineum as the fetal head crowns. Research is mixed on the benefits of perineal massage. Some studies have posited that massaging the perineum during second stage can cause swelling and resistance to stretching. Other studies suggest that perineal massage in the third trimester and perineal massage with warm compresses during pushing in labor make the tissue more elastic. Some researchers have found that as a result of perineal massage, the tissue is less inclined to tear during the delivery, and that it reduces the necessity for an episiotomy (Dekker, 2012).

87. 25 gtt/min

Standard method formula for drip rate calculations:

$$\frac{\text{Volume in mL}}{\text{Time in minutes}} \times \text{Drop factor}$$

$$\frac{150 \text{ mL}}{60 \text{ min}} \times \frac{10 \text{ gtt/mL}}{6} = 150$$

$$\frac{150}{6} = 25 \text{ gtt/min}$$

Dimensional analysis method formula:

Volume ordered	Drops	Time conversion	Volume conversion	= Infusion rate (gtt/min)
Time for infusion	per 1 mL	in minutes (if needed)	(if needed)	

150 mL	10 gtt	= 25 gtt/min
60 min	1 mL	

TEST-TAKING HINT: Although drip rates are used infrequently due to the more precise infusion provided by electronic pumps, the calculation process is still included in many nursing programs. Familiarity with the calculation can be helpful if the nurse delivers care in emergency situations when a pump is unavailable, or if the nurse is working in an undeveloped country. When the units for each of the numbers are included, the test taker will never make a mistake with drip rate calculations because, as can be seen above, the mLs are cancelled out and what remains is the required units, gtt/min. Drip rates are always calculated to the nearest whole number because it is impossible to administer a fraction of a drop.

88. 0.25 mL

Standard formula for calculating the volume of medication to be administered:

Known dosage : known volume = desired dosage : desired volume
2 mg : 1 mL = 0.5 mg : x mL
2 mg x = 0.5 mg
x = 0.25 mL

Dimensional analysis method for calculating the volume of medication to be administered:

Known volume	Desired dosage	= Desired volume
Known dosage		

1 mL	0.5 mg	= 0.25 mL
2 mg		

TEST-TAKING HINT: The examples provide the test taker with both a standard ratio and proportion method and a dimensional analysis method for solving the medication volume problem.

89. 1. **The cervix is thin.**
2. There is nothing in the scenario that suggests that the membranes are bulging.
3. At −2 station, the head is well above the ischial spines, not at the pelvic outlet.
4. The cervix is dilated 5 cm (or approximately 2 inches). The nurse would, therefore, not feel a closed cervix.

TEST-TAKING HINT: During pregnancy and early labor, the cervix is closed, long (about 4 cm, or 2 inches long), and thick. During the labor process, however, the cervix is pulled back and around the fetal head, changing shape and becoming paper thin as it dilates to 10 cm for a full-term fetus.

90. 1. Laboring clients are allowed to eat by some practitioners. Midwives are more likely to allow eating than physicians.
2. This is a very negative statement that does not answer the client's question.
3. It is unlikely that the woman will eat at established meal times. Plus, a regular diet is rarely given to laboring clients, even by midwives.
4. **This is the best response.**

TEST-TAKING HINT: Women are advised not to eat heavy meals during labor because there's a risk of vomiting and aspiration of stomach contents if an emergency arises that requires general anesthesia. Peristalsis slows dramatically during labor. Because of this, women rarely become hungry during labor, but they do need fluids and some nourishment. Clear fluids, including ice chips, popsicles, water, tea, and bouillon, are often allowed. Ultimately, though, it is the healthcare practitioner's decision about what and how much the client may consume. Nurse-midwives allow small meals more often than physicians do, especially in very early labor.

91. Answers 1 and 4 are correct.
1. **Both nausea and vomiting are side effects of nitrous oxide administration.**
2. When administered in a 50%/50% concentration, nitrous oxide has not been shown to cause hypotensive episodes.
3. Patients using N2O are not at high risk for dehydration.
4. **Patients often do exhibit light-headedness when using N2O.**
5. One important advantage of N2O over other labor pain-relieving methods is the fact that the fetus, and the baby after birth, rarely exhibit adverse responses to the medication.

TEST-TAKING HINT: Nitrous oxide is an important alternative to commonly used labor pain-relieving medications such as epidurals and intravenous analgesics. The fact that it is self-administered enables the mother to determine when she needs the medication and when she wants to stop taking the medication. Once the gas is no longer inhaled, it takes about 5 minutes for the woman

to no longer feel the effects of the gas (Likis et al., 2012).

92. 1. Although epidural anesthesia will relieve the client's pain, it will not act to reduce the client's fears.

2. During labor, inhaled nitrous oxide exerts both a pain-relieving action as well as an anxiety-reducing action.

3. Although a narcotic analgesic will reduce the client's pain, it will not act to reduce the client's fears.

4. Although used frequently for delivery, spinal anesthesia is rarely used during labor for two important reasons: (1) it paralyzes the patient, resulting in her inability to move until the medication is fully metabolized, and (2) once the medication is metabolized, if the client is still in pain, there is no way to readminister the medication.

TEST-TAKING HINT: When self-administered in a 50% N2O/50% O2 concentration, nitrous oxide has been shown to be an effective pain-relieving medication. Equally important is its anxiolytic action. For women who exhibit anxiety or fear during labor, nitrous oxide is an excellent pain-relieving option (Likis et al., 2012).

6 Normal Newborn

The experience of birth is thought to be very stressful for the neonate. It is an overwhelming cacophony of sound in addition to noxious, physical sensations. Compared to the buoyant, temperature-controlled and muted environment within the uterus, where the fetus never felt hunger or pain, at birth the newborn is thrust into a cold and noisy place. The dry towels on their skin must feel like sandpaper. Just as they begin to feel warm and drowsy at their mother's breast, their eyes are held open for placement of a cold gel, and their tender skin is pricked for the first time, by a needle. The diaper is a constant presence around their waist and legs. Their bowels move for the first time, perhaps feeling a bit like diarrhea.

Inside their bodies, physiological changes are required for survival, all of them driven by the need to obtain and maintain their own oxygenation. The baby's transition from the aquatic environment before birth to the air-breathing one outside the womb requires rapid, complex, and well-orchestrated steps. It is the responsibility of newborn care providers to understand these physiological changes in order to support the baby's transition to extrauterine life. Asphyxia alters the smooth transition and must be avoided at all costs.

Clamping of the umbilical cord leads to increased vascular resistance within the baby's circulatory system. The pressure within the left atrium increases and, with higher pressures in the left than in the right side of the heart, the flap across the foramen ovale begins to close. The lungs, which were moments ago filled with fluid, are now filled with air. Gas exchange begins in the lungs for the first time. Gas exchange is thought to be stabilized within 2 minutes of age (Morton & Brodsky, 2016). Improvement in the rate and regularity of the newborn heart rate is the best clinical indicator of adequate ventilation and gas exchange. Temperature stabilization is another sign of adequate circulation and oxygenation.

A successful transition also requires an increase in newborn metabolism and endocrine functions to support blood pressure and glucose levels. Each of these body systems affects the other. They must transition precisely and adequately to support newborn survival. Increased metabolism leads to newborn weight loss, which also must be monitored in the days that follow.

The newborn is not simply a tiny adult. Physical characteristics such as peripheral cyanosis, can be normal in a newborn, but not in an adult; shivering can be common in children and adults, but is not normal for a newborn. Seizures are sometimes mistaken as shivering in newborns. Because the nurse is at the bedside more often than the primary healthcare provider, the nurse is responsible for assessing and monitoring the newborn's transition. The nurse must note any deviations from normal, then intervene, and/or report these deviations to the primary healthcare provider as indicated.

Finally, because the nurse will not be going home with the baby and its parents, it is important that information about initial newborn care be shared with the parents in easily understandable language and in amounts they can remember. Some educators refer to this as "snack-sized" bits of knowledge to get them through at least the first week at home. It is best to focus on what is normal, balancing that with "danger signs." That immediate education, along with links or references for more, will give the parents a good start. The primary healthcare provider will add to the information as the baby grows.

Supporting baby humans and their families at the start of their lives together is one of the most satisfying ways to spend a day at work. It requires practiced, critical thinking and clinical judgment appropriate to each unique baby.

KEYWORDS

The following words include English vocabulary, nursing/medical terminology, concepts, principles, or information relevant to content specifically addressed in the chapter or associated with topics covered in this chapter. English dictionaries, your nursing textbooks, and medical dictionaries such as *Taber's Cyclopedic Medical Dictionary* are resources that can be used to expand your knowledge and understanding of these words and related information.

Anticipatory guidance
Apgar score
Babinski reflex
Bhutani nomogram
Bilirubin
Brown adipose tissue
Café au lait spot
Caput succedaneum
Cephalohematoma
Circumcision
Colic
Colostrum
Cryptorchidism
Dysplasia
En face
Epstein pearls
Erythema toxicum
Erythropoietin
Frenulum
Gomco clamp
Harlequin sign
Hepatitis B vaccine
Hypoglycemia
Hypothermia
Intracostal retractions
Jaundice
Kernicterus
Meconium
Milia
Mongolian spots
Moro reflex
Neonatal abduction
Neonatal feeding: breastfeeding and bottle feeding
Neonatal Galactorrhea (witch's milk)
Neonatal Infant Pain Scale (NIPS)
Neonatal mortality rate
Neonatal ophthalmic prophylaxis
Neonatal screening tests
Neonate
Ophthalmia neonatorum
Ortolani sign
Petechiae
Phytonadione (Vitamin K)
Plagiocephaly
Plastibell
Pseudomenses
Subconjunctival hemorrhages
Sudden infant death syndrome (SIDS)
Supernumerary nipples
Telangiectatic nevi
Tonic neck reflex
Transcutaneous bilirubin (TcB) measurement
Vernix caseosa

QUESTIONS

CASE STUDY: *The first six questions below are part of an evolving case study. All six questions follow the Next Generation NCLEX© question format of evaluating clinical judgment skills:*

1. Recognize cues—What matters most?
2. Analyze cues—What could it mean?
3. Prioritize hypotheses—Where do I start?
4. Generate solutions—What can I do?
5. Take action—What will I do?
6. Evaluate outcomes—Did it help?

(National Council of State Boards of Nursing, 2020). For more information on the Next Generation NCLEX (NGN) question formats, see NGN quarterly newsletters at https://www.ncsbn.org.
NCLEX questions assume the nurse has a provider's order for listed interventions, unless noted otherwise.

The nurse is caring for a client who is now G1 P1001. She delivered a 6 lb (2,721 gram) baby boy 48 hours ago at 39 weeks' gestation after a 24-hour oxytocin induction. The baby was in the occiput posterior position throughout labor and has a cephalohematoma. The baby was circumcised yesterday using a gomco clamp and has had two wet diapers since then. The mother is attempting to latch the baby to the breast using one hand to hold his head, but he is crying lustily and is not latching on. Seeing the nurse enter the room, the mother ends the breastfeeding attempt, wraps up the baby, and asks for a bottle of formula. "I can't do this," she says, "I have no milk and he's starving."

The nurse assesses the newborn. Vital signs are T 98° F (36.6° C), HR 100, R 20. The nurse notes the baby's face and shoulders have a slight tinge of yellow. The circumcision site is covered by white gauze.

1. **Recognize cues. What matters most?** Which of the following cues are of concern? **Select all that apply.**
   1. Breastfeeding issues.
   2. Jaundice.
   3. Baby's urinary output.
   4. Baby's vital signs.
   5. Circumcision site.
2. **Analyze cues. What could it mean?** What conditions relate to the assessments of concern? **Select all that apply.**
   1. Cephalohematoma.
   2. Small for gestational age.
   3. Circumcision method.
   4. Primiparity.
   5. Risk of increased red blood cell (RBC) hemolysis.
   6. Breastfeeding position.
3. **Prioritize hypotheses. Where do I start?** The nurse is creating the newborn's plan for care. Which two assessments are of priority and need further follow up?
   1. First assess **(Select one.)**
      a. Jaundice.
      b. Baby's stools.
      c. Newborn latch.
      d. Baby's weight.
   2. Followed by **(Select one.)**
      a. Jaundice.
      b. Baby's stools.
      c. Newborn latch.
      d. Baby's weight.
4. **Generate solutions. What can I do?** The nurse removes the baby's t-shirt and notes that the jaundice goes down to the baby's nipple line. The nurse notes meconium stool in the baby's diaper. Among other assessments, the nurse notes a 7% weight loss. Based on the information so far, what interventions or assessments are the most important to complete at this time? **Select all that apply.**
   1. Begin phototherapy.
   2. Promote breastfeeding success.
   3. Perform transcutaneous bilirubinometry.
   4. Check newborn blood glucose.

5. **Take action. What will I do?** The transcutaneous bilirubin measurement is 10 mg/dL (171 μmol/L). What is the most important action for the nurse to take next?
   1. Notify the primary healthcare provider.
   2. Begin phototherapy.
   3. Request an order for a cell blood count (CBC).
   4. Assist the mother with breastfeeding.

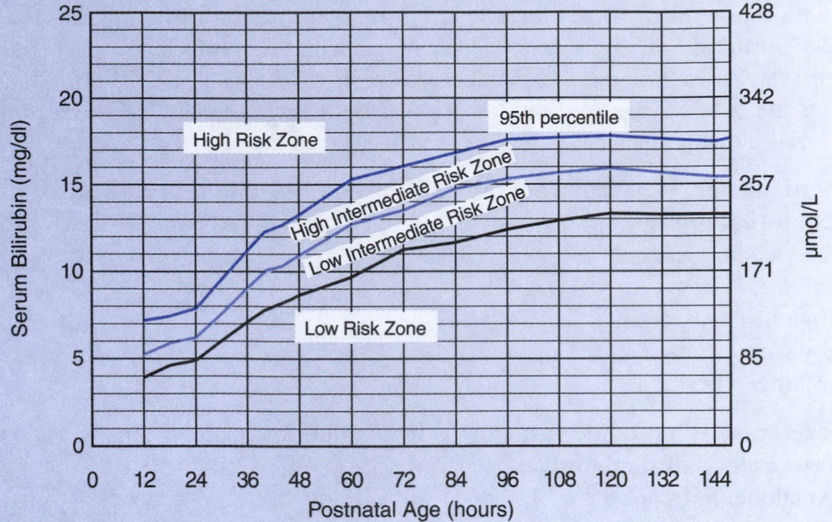

6. **Evaluate outcomes. Did it help?** The nurse assists the mother with breastfeeding, and suggests a position that does not put pressure on the baby's head. The baby breastfeeds for 10 minutes before falling asleep. Which of the following findings are reassuring? **Select all that apply.**
   1. Passage of a large, meconium stool.
   2. A drop of milk at the corner of the baby's mouth.
   3. Transcutaneous bilirubin (TcB) measurement of 10.
   4. Mother falls asleep with baby in her arms.

7. The nurse is discussing the neonatal blood screening test with a new mother. The nurse knows the teaching was successful when the mother states that the test screens for the presence in the newborn of which of the following diseases? **Select all that apply.**
   1. Hypothyroidism.
   2. Sickle cell disease.
   3. Galactosemia.
   4. Cerebral palsy.
   5. Cystic fibrosis.

8. The nursery nurse is careful to wear gloves when admitting neonates into the nursery. Which of the following is the scientific rationale for this action?
   1. Meconium is filled with enteric bacteria.
   2. Amniotic fluid may contain harmful viruses.
   3. The high alkalinity of fetal urine is caustic to the skin.
   4. The baby is at high risk for infection and must be protected.

9. A full-term newborn was just born and placed on the mother's chest. Which nursing intervention is important for the nurse to perform first?
   1. Remove wet blankets.
   2. Assess Apgar score.
   3. Insert eye prophylaxis.
   4. Elicit the Moro reflex.

10. To reduce the risk of hypoglycemia in a full-term newborn weighing 6 lbs 3 oz (2,900 grams), what should the nurse do?
    1. Maintain the infant's temperature above 97.7° F (36.5° C).
    2. Feed the infant glucose water every 3 hours until breastfeeding well.
    3. Assess blood glucose levels every 3 hours for the first 12 hours.
    4. Encourage the mother to breastfeed every 4 hours.

11. A mother asks the nurse to tell her about the responsiveness of neonates at birth. Which of the following answers is appropriate? **Select all that apply.**
    1. "Babies have a poorly developed sense of smell until they are 2 months old."
    2. "Babies respond to all forms of taste well, but they prefer to eat sweet things like breast milk."
    3. "Babies are especially sensitive to being touched and cuddled."
    4. "Babies are nearsighted with blurry vision until they are about 3 months of age."
    5. "Babies respond to many sounds, especially to the high-pitched tone of the female voice."

12. A mother who delivered one day ago, after a 3-hour labor and rapid, vaginal delivery, questions the nurse because her baby's face is "purple." Upon examination, the nurse notes petechiae over the scalp, forehead, and cheeks of the baby. The nurse's response should be based on which of the following?
    1. Petechiae are indicative of severe bacterial infections.
    2. Rapid deliveries can injure the neonatal presenting part.
    3. Petechiae are characteristic of the normal newborn rash.
    4. The injuries are a sign that the child has been abused.

13. A 2-day-old breastfeeding baby born via spontaneous vaginal delivery has just been weighed in the newborn nursery. The nurse determines that the baby has lost 3.5% of the birth weight. Which of the following nursing actions is appropriate?
    1. Do nothing because this is a normal weight loss.
    2. Notify the primary healthcare provider of the significant weight loss.
    3. Advise the mother to bottle feed the baby at the next feed.
    4. Assess the baby for hypoglycemia with a glucose monitor.

14. Four newborns are in the newborn nursery, none of whom is crying or in distress. Which of the babies should the nurse report to the primary healthcare provider?
    1. 16-hour-old baby who has yet to pass meconium.
    2. 16-hour-old baby whose blood glucose is 50 mg/dL (2.7 mmol/L).
    3. 2-day-old baby who is breathing irregularly at 70 breaths per minute.
    4. 2-day-old baby who is excreting a milky discharge from both nipples.

15. The primary healthcare provider has ordered phytonadione 0.5 mg IM for a newborn. The medication is available as 2 mg/mL. How many milliliters (mL) should the nurse administer to the baby? **Calculate to the nearest hundredth.**

    ____ mL

16. Which of the following actions should the nurse expect to see during a primary healthcare provider's evaluation of developmental dysplasia of the hip (DDH) in a newborn? **Select all that apply.**
    1. Grasp the baby's legs with the thumbs on the inner thighs and forefingers on the outer thighs.
    2. Gently adduct and abduct the baby's thighs.
    3. Palpate the trochanter during hip rotation.
    4. Place the baby in a fetal position.
    5. Compare the lengths of the baby's legs.

17. A nurse notes that a 6-hour-old neonate has cyanotic hands and feet. Which of the following actions by the nurse is appropriate?
1. Place the child in an isolette.
2. Administer oxygen.
3. Place the baby skin-to-skin with a parent.
4. Apply pulse oximeter.

18. A couple is asking the nurse whether or not their son should be circumcised. On which fact should the nurse's response be based?
1. Boys should be circumcised for them to establish a positive self-image.
2. Boys should not be circumcised because there is no medical rationale for the procedure.
3. Experts from the Centers for Disease Control and Prevention (CDC) argue that circumcision is desirable.
4. A statement from the American Academy of Pediatrics (AAP) asserts that circumcision is optional.

19. A baby boy is to be circumcised by the mother's obstetrician. Which of the following actions shows that the nurse is being a client advocate?
1. Before the procedure, the nurse prepares the sterile field for the physician.
2. The nurse refuses to unclothe the baby until the doctor orders something for pain.
3. The nurse holds the feeding immediately before the circumcision.
4. After the procedure, the nurse monitors the site for signs of bleeding.

20. Using the Neonatal Infant Pain Scale (NIPS), a nurse is assessing the pain response of a newborn who has just had a circumcision. The nurse is assessing a change in which of the following signs/symptoms? **Select all that apply.**
1. Heart rate.
2. Blood pressure.
3. Temperature.
4. Facial expression.
5. Breathing pattern.

21. A nurse is teaching a mother how to care for her 3-day-old son's circumcised penis. Which of the following actions demonstrates that the mother has learned the information?
1. The mother cleanses the glans with a cotton swab dipped in hydrogen peroxide.
2. The mother covers the glans with antifungal ointment after rinsing off any discharge.
3. The mother squeezes warm water from the wash cloth over the glans.
4. The mother replaces the dry sterile dressing at each diaper change.

22. Please put an "X" on the site where the nurse should administer phytonadione 0.5 mg IM to the neonate.

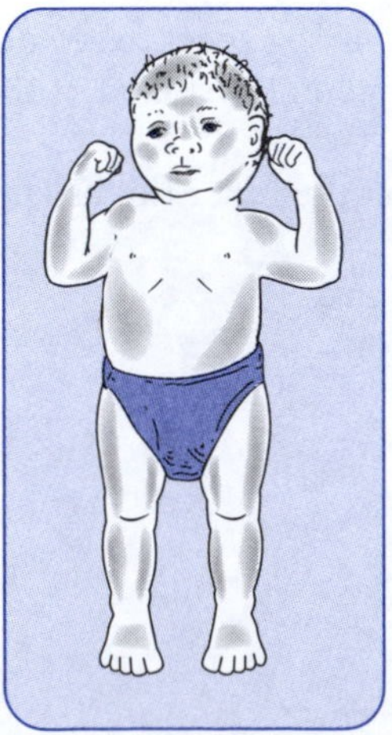

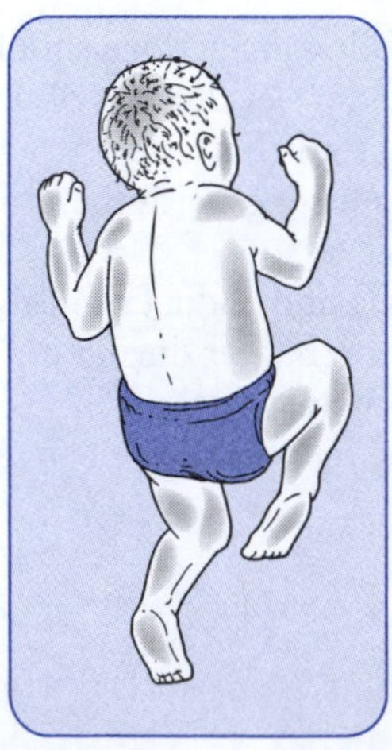

23. The nurse is teaching a mother about the baby's sutures and fontanelles. Please put an "X" on the fontanelle that will close at 6 to 8 weeks of age.

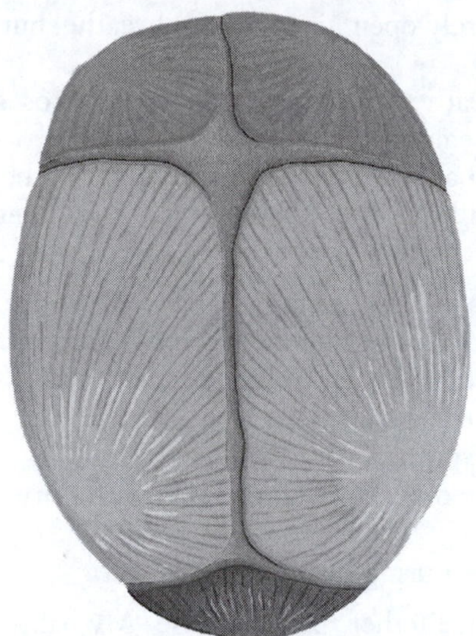

24. A neonate is being admitted to the well-baby nursery. Which one of the following findings should be reported to the primary healthcare provider?
    1. Umbilical cord with three vessels.
    2. Diamond-shaped anterior fontanelle.
    3. Cryptorchidism.
    4. Café au lait spot.

25. A female African American baby has been admitted into the nursery. Which of the following physiological findings would the nurse assess as normal? **Select all that apply.**
    1. Purple-colored patches on the buttocks.
    2. Bilateral whitish discharge from the breasts.
    3. Bloody discharge from the vagina.
    4. Sharply demarcated dark red area on the face.
    5. Deep hair-covered dimple at the base of the spine.

26. The nurse is assessing a newborn on admission to the newborn nursery. Which of the following findings should the nurse report to the primary healthcare provider?
    1. Intercostal retractions.
    2. Caput succedaneum.
    3. Epstein pearls.
    4. Harlequin sign.

27. Four babies have just been admitted into the newborn nursery. Which of the babies should the nurse assess first?
    1. Baby with a respiratory rate of 42, oxygen saturation 96%.
    2. Baby with Apgar 9/9, weight 10 lbs 3 oz (4,660 grams).
    3. Baby with temperature 98° F (36.7° C), length 21 inches.
    4. Baby with glucose 55 mg/dL (3.0 mmol/L), heart rate 121 bpm.

28. A neonate is in the active alert behavioral state. Which of the following would the nurse expect to see?
    1. Baby is showing signs of hunger and frustration.
    2. Baby is starting to whimper and cry.
    3. Baby is wide awake and attending to the mother's face.
    4. Baby is asleep and breathing rhythmically.

29. A mother asks whether or not she should be concerned that her baby never opens his mouth to breathe when his nose is so small. Which of the following is the nurse's best response?

1. "The baby does rarely open his mouth to breathe, but you can see that he isn't in any distress."
2. "Babies usually breathe in and out through their noses so they can feed and breathe without breaking the latch."
3. "Everything about babies is small. It truly is amazing how everything works so well."
4. "You are right. I will report the baby's small nasal openings to the primary healthcare provider right away."

30. The nursery charge nurse is assessing a 1-day-old female neonate on morning rounds. Which of the following findings should be reported to the primary healthcare provider as soon as possible? **Select all that apply.**

1. A spot of blood in the diaper.
2. Grunting during expiration.
3. Deep red coloring on one side of the body with normal skin coloring on the other side.
4. Flaring of the nares during inspiration.

31. A mother calls the nurse to her room because "My baby's eyes are bleeding." The nurse notes bright red hemorrhages in the sclerae of both of the baby's eyes. Which of the following actions by the nurse is appropriate at this time?

1. Notify the primary healthcare provider immediately and report the finding.
2. Notify the social worker about the probable maternal abuse.
3. Reassure the mother that the trauma resulted from pressure changes at birth and that the hemorrhages will slowly disappear.
4. Obtain an ophthalmoscope from the nursery to evaluate the red reflex and condition of the retina in each eye.

32. Which of the following full-term babies requires immediate nursing intervention?

1. Baby with seesaw breathing.
2. Baby with irregular breathing and 10-second apnea spells.
3. Baby with coordinated thoracic and abdominal breathing.
4. Baby with respiratory rate of 52.

33. Which of the following drawings is consistent with a baby who was in the frank breech position in utero?

1.
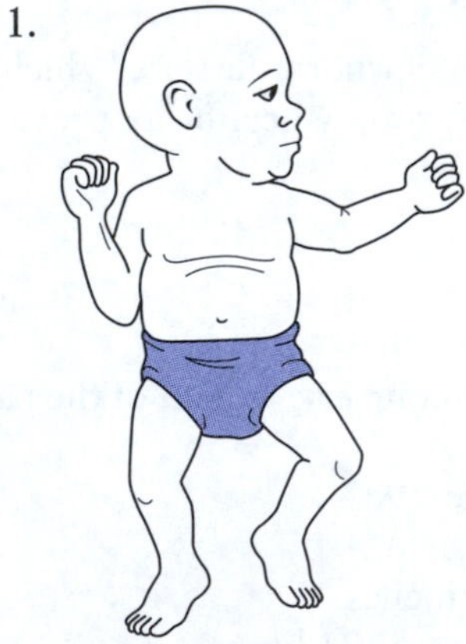

2.
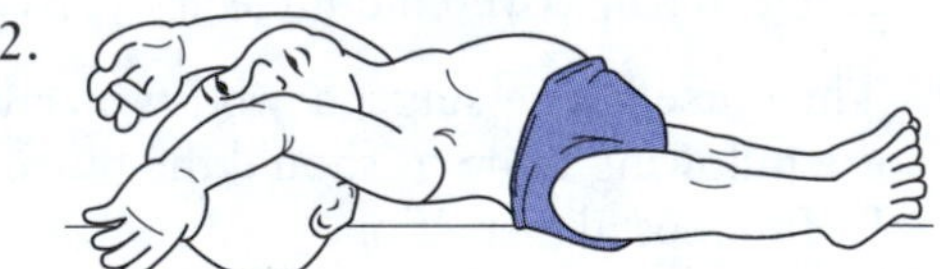

3.
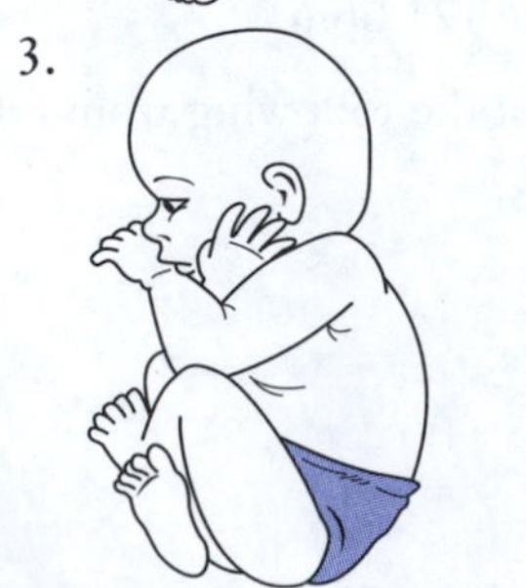

4.
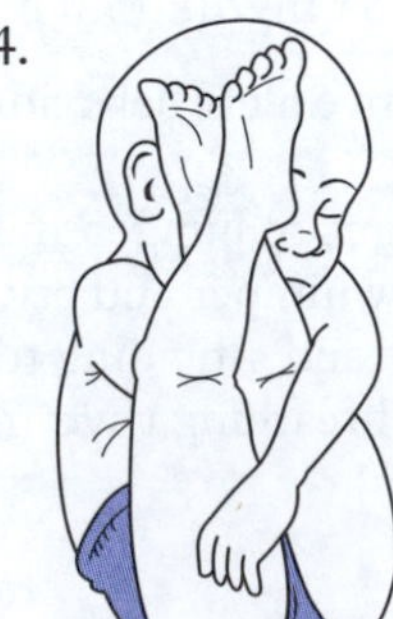

34. The following four babies are in the newborn nursery. Which of these babies should be seen by the primary healthcare provider?
1. 1-day-old, HR 100 bpm, in deep sleep.
2. 2-day-old, T 97.7° F (36.5° C), slightly jaundiced.
3. 3-day-old, breastfeeding every 4 hours, jittery.
4. 4-day-old, crying, papular rash on an erythematous base.

35. In which of the following situations would it be appropriate for the nurse to suggest that a new father place his baby in the "en face" position to promote neonatal bonding?
1. The baby is asleep with little to no eye movement, regular breathing.
2. The baby is asleep with rapid eye movement, irregular breathing.
3. The baby is awake, looking intently at an object, irregular breathing.
4. The baby is awake, placing hands in the mouth, irregular breathing.

36. Four newborns were admitted into the newborn nursery 1 hour ago. Which of the babies should the nurse ask the primary healthcare provider to evaluate?
1. The neonate with a temperature of 98.9° F (37.2° C) and weight of 6 lbs 6 oz (3,000 grams).
2. The neonate with white spots on the bridge of the nose.
3. The neonate with raised white specks on the gums.
4. The neonate with irregular respirations of 72 and heart rate of 166 bpm.

37. The nurse is about to elicit the Moro reflex. Which of the following responses should the nurse expect to see?
1. When the cheek of the baby is touched, the newborn turns toward the side that is touched.
2. When the lateral aspect of the sole of the baby's foot is stroked, the toes extend and fan outward.
3. When the baby is suddenly lowered or startled, the neonate's arms straighten outward and the knees flex.
4. When the newborn is supine and the head is turned to one side, the arm on that same side extends.

38. To check for the presence of Epstein pearls, the nurse should assess which part of the neonate's body?
1. Feet.
2. Hands.
3. Back.
4. Mouth.

39. The nurse is assessing a neonate in the newborn nursery. Which of the following findings in a newborn should be reported to the primary healthcare provider?
1. The eyes cross and uncross when they are open.
2. The ears are positioned in alignment with the inner and outer canthus of the eyes.
3. Axillae and femoral folds of the baby are covered with a white cheesy substance.
4. The nostrils flare whenever the baby inhales.

40. A newborn at 40 weeks' gestation is in the first period of reactivity. Which of the following actions should the nurse take at this time?
1. Encourage the parents to bond with their baby.
2. Notify the primary healthcare provider of the finding.
3. Perform the gestational age assessment.
4. Place the baby under the overhead warmer.

41. The nurse notes that a newborn who is 5 minutes old exhibits the following characteristics: heart rate 108 bpm, respiratory rate 29 respirations per minute with lusty cry, pink body with bluish hands and feet, some flexion. What does the nurse determine the baby's Apgar score to be?
    1. 6.
    2. 7.
    3. 8.
    4. 9.

THE APGAR SCORE

Assessment	0 points	1 point	2 points
Color	Central cyanosis	Acrocyanosis	All pink
Heart rate	No heart rate	1–99 bpm	Equal to or greater than 100 bpm
Respiratory rate	No respirations	Slow and irregular	Good lusty cry
Reflex irritability	No response	Grimace	Good lusty cry
Tone	Flaccid	Some flexion	Marked flexion or active movement

42. The mother notes that her baby has a "bulge" on the back of one side of the head. She calls the nurse into the room to ask what the bulge is. The nurse notes that the bulge covers the right parietal bone but does not cross the suture lines. The nurse explains to the mother that the bulge results from which of the following?
    1. Molding of the baby's skull so that the baby could fit through her pelvis.
    2. Swelling of the tissues of the baby's head from the pressure of her pushing.
    3. The position that the baby took in her pelvis during the last trimester of her pregnancy.
    4. Small blood vessels that broke under the baby's scalp during birth.

43. A nurse is providing discharge teaching to the parents of a newborn. Which of the following should be included when teaching the parents how to care for the baby's umbilical cord?
    1. Cleanse it with hydrogen peroxide if it starts to smell.
    2. Remove it with sterile tweezers at one week of age.
    3. Call the doctor if greenish drainage appears.
    4. Cover it with sterile dressings until it falls off.

44. A mother asks the nurse which powder she should purchase to use on the baby's skin. What should the nurse's response be?
    1. "Any powder made especially for babies should be fine."
    2. "It is recommended that powder not be put on babies."
    3. "There is no real difference except that many babies are allergic to cornstarch so it should not be used."
    4. "As long as you put it only on the buttocks area, you can use any brand of baby powder that you like."

45. The nurse is teaching the parents of a 1-day-old baby how to give a sponge bath. Which of the following actions should be included?
    1. Clean the eyes from outer canthus to inner canthus.
    2. Cleanse the ear canals with a cotton swab.
    3. Assemble all supplies before beginning the bath.
    4. Check the temperature of the bath water with the fingertips.

46. The nurse is teaching the parents of a female baby how to change the baby's diapers. Which of the following should be included in the teaching?
1. Always wipe the perineum from front to back.
2. Remove any vernix caseosa from the labial folds.
3. Put powder on the buttocks every time the baby stools.
4. Weigh every diaper to assess hydration status.

47. The nurse has provided anticipatory guidance to a couple who has just delivered a baby. Which of the following is an appropriate goal for the care of their new baby?
1. The baby will have a bath with soap every morning.
2. During a supervised play period, the baby will be placed on the tummy every day.
3. The baby will be given a pacifier after each feeding.
4. For the first month of life, the baby will sleep on his or her side in a crib next to the parents.

48. A nurse is advising a mother of a neonate being discharged from the hospital regarding car seat safety. Which of the following should be included in the teaching plan? **Select all that apply.**
1. Place the baby's car seat in the front passenger seat of the car.
2. Position the car seat rear facing until the baby reaches 2 years of age.
3. Attach the car seat to the car at two latch points at the base of the car seat.
4. Check that the installed car seat moves no more than 1 inch side to side or front to back.
5. Make sure that there is at least a 3-inch space between the straps of the seat and the baby's body.

49. A nurse is providing anticipatory guidance to a couple regarding the baby's immunization schedule. Which of the following statements by the parents shows that the teaching by the nurse was successful? **Select all that apply.**
1. The first hepatitis B injection is given by 1 month of age.
2. The first polio injection will be given at 2 months of age.
3. The measles, mumps, and rubella (MMR) immunization should be administered before the first birthday.
4. Three diphtheria, tetanus, and acellular pertussis (DTaP) shots will be given during the first year of life.
5. The varicella immunization will be administered after the baby turns 1 year of age.

50. A nurse is advising the parents of a newborn regarding when they should call their pediatrician. Which of the following responses show that the teaching was effective? **Select all that apply.**
1. If the baby repeatedly refuses to feed.
2. If the baby's breathing is irregular.
3. If the baby has no tears when he cries.
4. If the baby is repeatedly difficult to awaken.
5. If the baby's temperature is above 100.4° F (38° C).

51. A nurse is providing anticipatory guidance to a couple before they take home their newborn. Which of the following should be included? **Select all that apply.**
1. If their baby is sleeping soundly, they should not awaken the baby for a feeding.
2. If their baby is exposed to the sun, they should put sunscreen on the baby.
3. They should purchase liquid acetaminophen to be used when ordered by the primary healthcare provider.
4. They should notify their primary healthcare provider when the umbilical cord falls off.
5. When strapping their baby into a car seat, they should position the top of the chest clip at the level of the baby's belly button.

52. A baby with mucousy secretions is being left with the parents for the first time after delivery. Which of the following should the nurse teach the parents regarding use of the bulb syringe?
   1. Suction the nostrils before suctioning the mouth.
   2. Make sure to suction the back of the throat.
   3. Insert the bulb syringe before compressing the bulb.
   4. Dispose of the drainage in a tissue or a cloth.

53. Please put an "X" on the site where the nurse should perform a heel stick on the neonate.

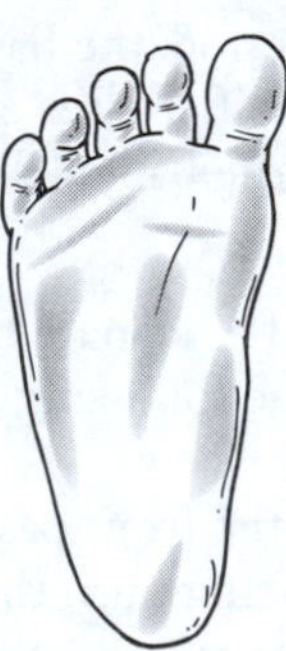

54. A nurse must give phytonadione 0.5 mg IM to a newly born baby. Which of the following needles should the nurse choose for the injection?
   1. 5/8 inch, 18 gauge.
   2. 5/8 inch, 25 gauge.
   3. 1 inch, 18 gauge.
   4. 1 inch, 25 gauge.

55. A nurse is practicing the procedures for conducting cardiopulmonary resuscitation (CPR) in the neonate. Which site should the nurse use to assess the pulse of a baby?
   1. Carotid.
   2. Radial.
   3. Brachial.
   4. Pedal.

56. A baby has just been admitted into the newborn nursery. Before taking the newborn's vital signs, the nurse should warm his or her hands and the stethoscope to prevent heat loss resulting from which of the following?
   1. Evaporation.
   2. Conduction.
   3. Radiation.
   4. Convection.

57. The nurse is developing a teaching plan for parents who are taking home their 2-day-old breastfeeding baby. Which of the following should the nurse include in the plan?
   1. Wash hands well before picking up the baby.
   2. Refrain from having visitors for the first month.
   3. Wear a mask to prevent transmission of a cold.
   4. Sterilize the breast pump supplies after every use.

58. It is time for a baby who is in the drowsy behavioral state to breastfeed. Which of the following techniques could the mother use to arouse the baby? **Select all that apply.**
   1. Swaddle or tightly bundle the baby.
   2. Hand express milk onto the baby's lips.
   3. Talk with the baby while making eye contact.
   4. Remove the baby's shirt and/or change the baby's diaper.
   5. Play pat-a-cake with the baby.

59. A bottle feeding mother is providing a return demonstration of how to burp the baby. Which of the following would indicate that the teaching was successful? **Select all that apply.**
   1. The woman gently strokes and pats her baby's back.
   2. The woman positions the baby in a sitting position on her lap.
   3. The woman waits to burp the baby until the baby's feeding is complete.
   4. The woman states that a small amount of regurgitated formula is acceptable.
   5. The woman remarks that the baby does not need to burp after trying for 1 full minute.

60. A breastfeeding baby is born with a tight frenulum. Which of the following is an important assessment for the nurse to make?
   1. Integrity of the baby's uvula.
   2. Presence of maternal nipple damage.
   3. Presence of neonatal tongue injury.
   4. The baby's breathing pattern.

61. A mother is told that she should bottle feed her child for medical reasons. Which of the following maternal disease states are consistent with the recommendation? **Select all that apply.**
   1. Untreated, active tuberculosis (TB).
   2. Hepatitis B surface antigen positive.
   3. Human immunodeficiency virus positive.
   4. Chorioamnionitis.
   5. Mastitis.

62. A nurse has brought a 2-hour-old baby to its mother from the nursery. The nurse is going to assist the mother with the first breastfeeding experience. Which of the following actions should the nurse perform first?
   1. Compare mother's and baby's identification bracelets.
   2. Help the mother into a comfortable position.
   3. Teach the mother about a proper breast latch.
   4. Tickle the baby's lips with the mother's nipple.

63. A nurse determines that which of the following is an appropriate short-term goal for a full-term, breastfeeding newborn?
   1. The baby will regain birth weight by 4 weeks of age.
   2. The baby will sleep through the night by 4 weeks of age.
   3. The baby will stool every 2 to 3 hours by 1 week of age.
   4. The baby will urinate 6 to 10 times per day by 1 week of age.

64. A mother is attempting to latch her newborn baby to the breast. Which of the following actions by the mother require follow up and more education by the nurse to the mother? **Select all that apply.**
   1. The mother places the baby on his or her back in the mother's lap and leans down, toward the baby.
   2. The mother holds the baby at the level of her breasts in a tummy-to-tummy position.
   3. The mother waits until the baby opens its mouth wide before attempting a latch.
   4. The mother points the baby's nose to her nipple.
   5. The mother waits until the baby's tongue is pointed toward the roof of its mouth before attempting a latch.

65. The nurse is evaluating the effectiveness of an intervention when assisting a woman whose baby has been latched to just the nipple rather than to the nipple and the areola. Which response would indicate that further intervention is needed?
   1. The client states that the pain has decreased.
   2. The nurse hears the baby swallow after each suck.
   3. The baby's jaws move up and down once every second.
   4. The baby's cheeks move in and out with each suck.

66. The parents and their full-term, breastfed newborn were discharged from the hospital. Which behavior 2 days later indicates a positive response by the parents to the nurse's discharge teaching? **Select all that apply.**
1. The parents count their baby's diapers.
2. The parents measure the baby's intake.
3. The parents give one bottle of formula every day.
4. The parents take the baby to see the primary healthcare provider.
5. The parents time the baby's feedings.

67. The nurse does not hear the baby swallow when suckling even though the baby appears to be latched properly to the breast. Which of the following situations may be the reason for this observation?
1. The mother reports a pain level of 4 on a 5-point scale.
2. The baby has been suckling for over 10 minutes.
3. The mother uses the cross-cradle hold while feeding.
4. The baby lies with the chin touching the under part of the breast.

68. The nurse is concerned that a bottle-fed baby may become obese because of which activity by the mother?
1. She encourages the baby to finish the bottle at each feed.
2. She feeds the baby every 3 to 4 hours.
3. She feeds the baby a soy-based formula.
4. She burps the baby every 1/ 2 to 1 ounce.

69. A 2-day-old, exclusively breastfed baby is to be discharged home. Under what conditions should the nurse teach the parents to call the primary healthcare provider?
1. If the baby feeds 8 to 12 times each day.
2. If the baby urinates 6 to 10 times each day.
3. If the baby has stools that are watery and bright yellow.
4. If the baby has eyes and skin that are tinged yellow.

70. A newborn weighed 7 lbs 2 oz (3,278 grams) at birth. On day 2 of life, the baby weighed 6 lbs 7 oz (3,042 grams). What percentage of weight loss did the baby experience? **Calculate to the nearest hundredth.**

_____ %

71. A mother is preparing to breastfeed her baby. Which of the following actions would encourage the baby to open its mouth wide for feeding?
1. Holding the baby in the "en face" position.
2. Pushing down on the baby's lower jaw.
3. Tickling the baby's lips with the nipple.
4. Giving the baby a trial bottle of formula.

72. A breastfeeding mother mentions to the nurse that she has heard that babies sleep better at night if they are given a small amount of rice cereal in the evening. Which of the following comments by the nurse is appropriate?
1. "That is correct. The rice cereal takes longer for them to digest so they sleep better and longer."
2. "It is recommended that babies receive only breast milk for the first 4 to 6 months of their lives."
3. "It is too early for rice cereal, but I would recommend giving the baby a bottle of formula at night."
4. "A better recommendation is to give apple sauce at 3 months of age and apple juice 1 month later."

73. On admission to the maternity unit, it is learned that a mother has smoked two packs of cigarettes per day and expects to continue to smoke after discharge. The mother also states that she expects to breastfeed her baby. The nurse's response should be based on which of the following?
1. Breastfeeding is contraindicated if the mother smokes cigarettes.
2. Breastfeeding is protective for the baby and should be encouraged.
3. A two-pack-a-day smoker should be reported to child protective services for child abuse.
4. A mother who admits to smoking cigarettes may also be abusing illicit substances.

74. A breastfeeding mother who is 2 weeks postpartum is informed by her primary healthcare provider that her 4-year-old has chickenpox (varicella). The mother calls the nursery nurse because she is concerned about having the baby in contact with the sick sibling. The mother had chickenpox as a child. Which of the following responses by the nurse is appropriate?
1. "The baby received passive immunity through the placenta, plus the breast milk will also be protective."
2. "The baby should stay with relatives until the ill sibling recovers from the episode of chickenpox."
3. "Chickenpox is transmitted by contact route so careful hand washing should prevent transmission."
4. "Because chickenpox is a spirochetal illness, both the child and baby should receive the appropriate medications."

75. A client is preparing to breastfeed her newborn son in the cross-cradle position. Which of the following actions should the woman make?
1. Place a pillow in her lap.
2. Position the head of the baby in her elbow.
3. Put the baby on his back.
4. Move the breast toward the mouth of the baby.

76. A mother who gave birth 5 minutes ago states that she would like to breastfeed. The baby's Apgar score is 9/9. Which of the following actions should the nurse perform first?
1. Assist the woman to breastfeed.
2. Dress the baby in a shirt and diaper.
3. Administer the ophthalmic prophylaxis.
4. Take the baby's rectal temperature.

77. A 4-day-old breastfeeding neonate whose birth weight was 5 lbs 9 oz (2,678 grams) has lost 100 grams since the cesarean birth. Which of the following actions should the nurse take?
1. Nothing because this is an acceptable weight loss.
2. Advise the mother to supplement feedings with formula.
3. Notify the primary healthcare provider of the excessive weight loss.
4. Give the baby dextrose water between breast feedings.

78. A breastfeeding client at 2 days postpartum is complaining of pain during feedings. Which of the following may be causing the pain?
1. The neonate's frenulum is attached to the tip of the tongue.
2. The baby's tongue forms a trough around the breast during the feedings.
3. The newborn's feeds last for 30 minutes every 2 hours.
4. The baby is latched to the nipple and to about 1 inch of the mother's areola.

79. A newly delivered mother states, "I have not had any alcohol since I decided to become pregnant. I have decided not to breastfeed because I would really like to go out and have a good time for a change." Which of the following is the best response by the nurse?
   1. "I understand that being good for so many months can become very frustrating."
   2. "Even if you bottle feed the baby, you will have to refrain from drinking alcohol for at least the next six weeks to protect your own health."
   3. "Alcohol can be consumed at any time while you are breastfeeding."
   4. "You may drink alcohol while breastfeeding, although it is best to wait until the alcohol has been metabolized before you feed again."

80. A primary healthcare provider writes in a breastfeeding mother's chart, "Ampicillin 500 mg q 6 h po. Baby should be bottle-fed until medication is discontinued." What should be the nurse's next action?
   1. Follow the order as written.
   2. Call the provider and question the order.
   3. Follow the antibiotic order but ignore the order to bottle feed the baby.
   4. Refer to a text to see whether the antibiotic is safe while breastfeeding.

81. Four pregnant women advise the nurse that they wish to breastfeed their babies. Which of the mothers should be advised to bottle feed her child?
   1. The woman with a neoplasm requiring chemotherapy.
   2. The woman with cholecystitis requiring surgery.
   3. The woman with a concussion.
   4. The woman with thrombosis.

82. A woman states that she is going to bottle feed her baby because, "I hate milk and I know that to make good breast milk I will have to drink milk." The nurse's response about producing high-quality breast milk should be based on which of the following?
   1. The mother must drink at least three glasses of milk per day to absorb sufficient quantities of calcium.
   2. The mother should consume at least one glass of milk per day but should also consume other dairy products such as cheese.
   3. The mother can consume a variety of good calcium sources such as broccoli and fish with bones as well as dairy products.
   4. The mother must monitor her protein intake more than her calcium intake because the baby needs the protein for growth.

83. A client asks whether or not there are any foods that she must avoid eating while breastfeeding. Which of the following responses by the nurse is appropriate?
   1. "No, there are no foods that are strictly contraindicated while breastfeeding."
   2. "Yes, the same foods that were dangerous to eat during pregnancy should be avoided."
   3. "Yes, foods like onions, cauliflower, broccoli, and cabbage make babies very colicky."
   4. "Yes, spices from hot and spicy foods get into the milk and can bother your baby."

84. A woman who has just delivered has decided to bottle feed her full-term baby. Which of the following should be included in the patient teaching?
   1. The baby's stools will appear bright yellow and will usually be loose.
   2. The bottle nipples should be enlarged to ease the baby's suckling.
   3. It is best to heat the baby's bottle in the microwave before feeding.
   4. It is important to hold the bottle so as to keep the nipple filled with formula.

85. Please choose the picture of the breastfeeding baby that shows correct position and latch on.

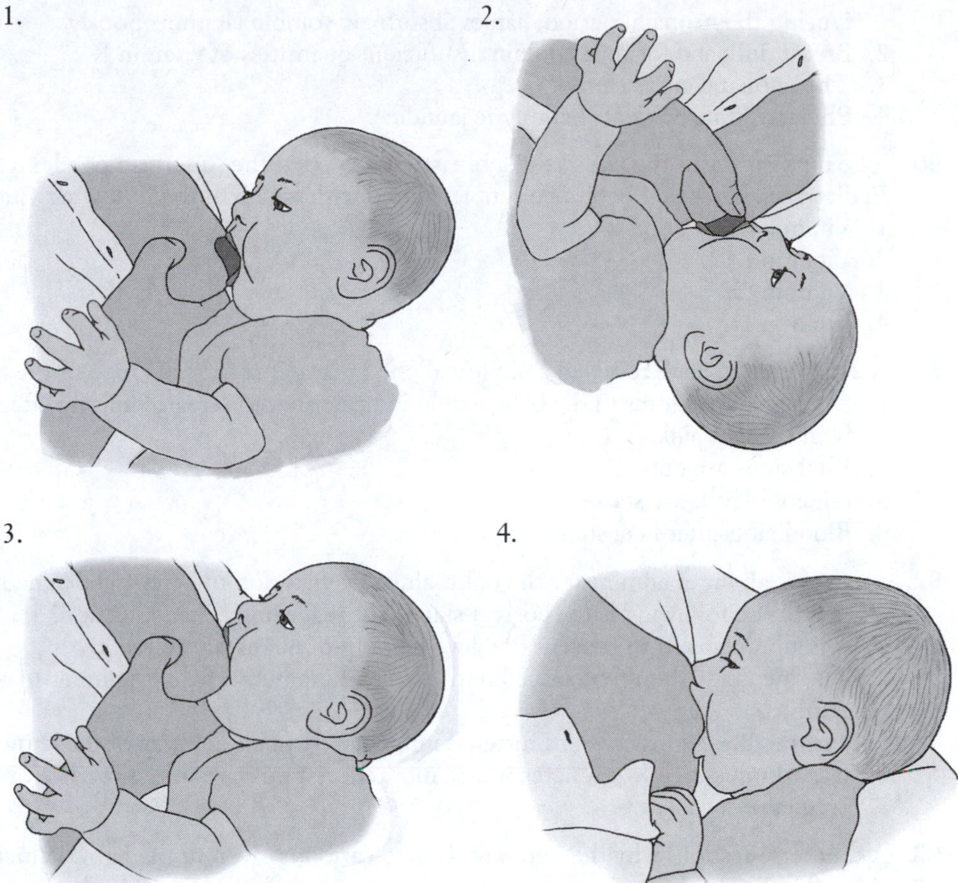

86. A full-term neonate, Apgars 9/9, has just been admitted to the nursery after a planned cesarean delivery, fetal position left mentum anterior (LMA), under epidural anesthesia. Which of the following physiological findings would the nurse expect to see?
1. Soft pulmonary rales.
2. Absent bowel sounds.
3. Depressed Moro reflex.
4. Positive Ortolani sign.

87. A full-term neonate has brown adipose fat tissue (BAT) stores that were deposited during the latter part of the third trimester. What does the nurse understand is the function of BAT stores?
1. To promote melanin production in the neonatal period.
2. To provide heat production when the baby is hypothermic.
3. To protect the bony structures of the body from injury.
4. To provide calories for neonatal growth between feedings.

88. A neonate has an elevated bilirubin and is slightly jaundiced on day 3 of life. What is the probable reason for these changes?
1. Hemolysis of neonatal red blood cells by the maternal antibodies.
2. Physiological destruction of fetal red blood cells during the extrauterine period.
3. Pathological liver function resulting from hypoxemia during the birthing process.
4. Delayed meconium excretion resulting in the production of direct bilirubin.

89. The primary healthcare provider writes the following order for a term newborn: phytonadione 1 mg IM. Which of the following responses provides a rationale for this order?
1. During the neonatal period, babies absorb fat-soluble vitamins poorly.
2. Breast milk and formula contain insufficient quantities of vitamin K.
3. The neonatal gut is sterile.
4. Phytonadione prevents hemolytic jaundice.

90. The nurse informs the parents of a breastfed baby that the American Academy of Pediatrics advises that babies be supplemented with which of the following vitamins?
1. Vitamin A.
2. Vitamin B12.
3. Vitamin C.
4. Vitamin D.

91. A 2-day-old neonate received a phytonadione injection at birth. Which of the following signs/symptoms in the baby would indicate that the treatment was effective?
1. Skin color is pink.
2. Vital signs are normal.
3. Glucose levels are stable.
4. Blood clots after heel sticks.

92. A nurse is about to administer the ophthalmic preparation to a newly born neonate. Which of the following is the correct statement regarding the medication?
1. It is administered to prevent the development of neonatal cataracts.
2. The medicine should be placed in the lower conjunctiva from the inner to outer canthus.
3. The medicine must be administered immediately upon delivery of the baby.
4. It is administered to neonates whose mothers test positive for gonorrhea during pregnancy.

93. A mother questions why the ophthalmic medication is given to the baby. Which of the following responses by the nurse would be appropriate to make at this time?
1. "I am required by law to give the medicine."
2. "The medicine helps to prevent eye infections."
3. "The medicine promotes neonatal health."
4. "All babies receive the medicine at delivery."

94. A certified nursing assistant (CNA) is working with a registered nurse (RN) in the neonatal nursery. Which of the following actions should the RN perform rather than delegating it to the CNA?
1. Bathe and weigh a 1-hour-old baby.
2. Take the apical heart rate and respirations of a 4-hour-old baby.
3. Obtain a stool sample from a 1-day-old baby.
4. Provide discharge teaching to the mother of a 4-day-old baby.

95. Four babies with the following conditions are in the well-baby nursery. The baby with which of the conditions is at high risk for physiologic jaundice?
1. Cephalohematoma.
2. Caput succedaneum.
3. Harlequin coloring.
4. Mongolian spotting.

96. A full-term baby's bilirubin level is 12 mg/dL (205.2 μmol/L) on day 3. Which of the following neonatal behaviors would the nurse expect to see?
1. Excessive crying.
2. Increased appetite.
3. Lethargy.
4. Hyperreflexia.

97. A 2-day-old baby's blood values are: Blood type, O– (negative). Direct Coombs, negative. Hematocrit, 50%. Bilirubin, 1.5 mg/dL (25.6 μmol/L). The mother's blood type is A+ (positive). What should the nurse do at this time?
1. Do nothing because the results are within normal limits.
2. Assess the baby for opisthotonic posturing.
3. Administer RhoGAM to the mother per doctor's order.
4. Call the doctor for an order to place the baby under bili-lights.

98. A 4-day-old baby born via cesarean section is slightly jaundiced. The laboratory reports a bilirubin assessment of 6 mg/dL (102.6 μmol/L). Which of the following would the nurse expect the primary healthcare provider to order for the baby at this time?
1. To be placed under phototherapy.
2. To be discharged home with the parents.
3. To be prepared for a replacement transfusion.
4. To be fed glucose water between routine feeds.

99. A nurse is assessing the bonding of the father with his newborn baby. Which of the following actions by the father would be of concern to the nurse?
1. He holds the baby in the "en face" position.
2. He calls the baby by a full name rather than a nickname.
3. He tells the mother to pick up the crying baby.
4. He falls asleep in the chair with the baby on his chest.

100. The nurse is conducting a state-mandated evaluation of a neonate's hearing. Infants are assessed for deficits because hearing-impaired babies are at high risk for which of the following?
1. Delayed speech development.
2. Otitis externa.
3. Poor parental bonding.
4. Choanal atresia.

101. A baby has just been circumcised. If bleeding occurs, which of the following actions should be taken first?
1. Put the baby's diapers on as tightly as possible.
2. Apply light pressure to the area with sterile gauze.
3. Call the physician who performed the surgery.
4. Assess the baby's heart rate and oxygen saturation.

102. A nurse reads that the neonatal mortality rate in the United States for a given year was 5. The nurse interprets that information as:
1. Five babies less than 28 days old per 1,000 live births died.
2. Five babies less than 1 year old per 1,000 live births died.
3. Five babies less than 28 days old per 100,000 births died.
4. Five babies less than 1 year old per 100,000 births died.

103. A mother tells the nurse that because of family history she is afraid her baby son will develop colic. Which of the following colic management strategies should the parents be taught? **Select all that apply.**
1. Small, frequent feedings.
2. Prone sleep positioning.
3. Tightly swaddling the baby.
4. Rocking the baby while holding him face down on the forearm.
5. Maintaining a home environment that is cigarette smoke-free.

104. When providing discharge teaching to parents, a nurse emphasizes actions to prevent plagiocephaly and to promote gross motor development in their full-term newborn. Which of the following actions should the nurse advise the parents to take?
1. Breastfeed the baby frequently.
2. Make sure the baby receives vaccinations at recommended intervals.
3. Change the diapers regularly.
4. Minimize supine positioning during supervised play periods.

105. A mother and her 2-day-old baby are preparing for discharge. Which of the following situations would require the baby's discharge to be cancelled?
1. The parents own a car seat that only faces the rear of the car.
2. The baby's bilirubin is 19 mg/dL (324.9 μmol/L).
3. The baby's blood glucose is 65 mg/dL (3.6 mmol/L).
4. There is a large bluish spot on the left buttock of the baby.

106. A mother confides to a nurse that she has no crib at home for her baby. The mother asks the nurse which of the following places would be best for the baby to sleep. Of the following choices, which location should the nurse suggest?
1. In bed with his 5-year-old brother.
2. In a waterbed with his mother and father.
3. In a large empty dresser drawer.
4. In the living room on a pull-out sofa.

107. It has just been discovered that a newborn is missing from the maternity unit. The nursing staff should be watchful for which of the following individuals?
1. A middle-aged male.
2. An underweight female.
3. Pro-life advocate.
4. Visitor of the same race.

108. Which of the following behaviors should nurses know are characteristic of infant abductors? **Select all that apply.**
1. Act on the spur of the moment.
2. Create a diversion on the unit.
3. Ask questions about the routine of the unit.
4. Choose rooms near stairwells.
5. Wear over-sized clothing.

109. The nurse is providing anticipatory guidance to a formula feeding mother who is concerned about how much formula she should offer her newborn infant at each feeding. The nurse would know that teaching was effective when the mother makes which of the following statements?
1. "I should expect my baby to drink about 3 ounces of formula every 3 hours or so."
2. "At the end of each pediatric appointment, the provider will tell me how much formula to feed my baby."
3. "By the time we go home from the hospital, I should expect him to drink at least 4 ounces per feeding."
4. "I should give my baby enough formula to make him sleep for 4 hours between feedings."

110. After advising the parents of a 1-day-old baby that the baby must have a "heart defect test," the mother states, "Why? My baby is healthy. The primary healthcare provider told me so." Which of the following responses by the nurse is appropriate?
1. "I must have misread the name on the chart. It must be another baby who has to have the test."
2. "We do this test on all of the babies before discharge, and I'm sure your baby's heart is healthy."
3. "This is a screening test done on all babies. It is performed to find any possible heart problems before babies are discharged."
4. "Your baby just had some minor symptoms that need to be checked. The test won't hurt the baby."

111. When administering the neonatal screening for critical congenital heart defects (CCHD) on a baby in the well baby nursery, the nurse should perform which of the following actions? **Select all that apply.**
1. Obtain parental consent before performing the screen.
2. Take the baby's electrocardiogram.
3. Wait until the baby is at least 24 hours old.
4. Record the baby's heart rate fluctuations for 1 full minute.
5. Report pulse oximetry readings of 96% on the hand and 92% on the foot.

ANSWERS AND RATIONALES

The correct answer number and rationale for why it is the correct answer are given in **boldface blue type.** Rationales for why the other possible answer options are incorrect also are given, but they are not in boldface type.

1. **Answers 1 and 2 are correct.**
   1. **If the baby does not take in enough breastmilk, the bilirubin may not be adequately eliminated from the baby's body.**
   2. **Although physiologic jaundice that occurs after the first 24 hours of life can be normal, it must be monitored.**
   3. Two wet diapers a day is normal for the first 2 days of life.
   4. Baby's vital signs are within normal limits.
   5. It is standard practice to cover a gomco clamp circumcision with a small square of gauze slathered with petroleum jelly to prevent the gauze from sticking to the penis. There is nothing in the stem to indicate that petroleum jelly was not used.

TEST-TAKING HINT: Newborn physiologic jaundice is most often a benign condition. Physiologic jaundice occurs in 60% of newborns after 24 hours of birth and may persist for up to 2 weeks (AAP, 2004). If jaundice occurs before 24 hours of age, or rises beyond a certain level, it could lead to pathologic jaundice, a much more serious condition that can lead to kernicterus. As such, jaundice is monitored very closely in the newborn.

2. **Answers 1, 4, 5, and 6 are correct.**
   1. **The collection of blood within the cephalohematoma can contribute to jaundice.**
   2. At 6 lbs (2,721 grams) the baby is not small for gestational age.
   3. The circumcision has nothing to do with breastfeeding issues or jaundice, the two issues of concern.
   4. **The mother is a primipara, so her milk may not come in for 3 to 5 days.**
   5. **The end product of normal RBC hemolysis is bilirubin.**
   6. **The mother is holding the baby's head in her hand while breastfeeding. She could be causing pain by pressing on the cephalohematoma. This could be why the baby is crying and refusing to breastfeed.**

TEST-TAKING HINT: The two primary issues of concern are breastfeeding issues and newborn jaundice. The baby's cephalohematoma can contribute to higher levels of jaundice as the blood within the hematoma is broken down. Because the mother is a primipara, her milk will not likely come in fully for another day or two, so the baby's level of jaundice, weight loss, intake, and output must be monitored closely until everything is stable. A different breastfeeding position should be used to prevent pressure on the cephalohematoma and promote newborn comfort for successful infant feeding.

3. **Answers 1a and 2d are correct.**

   1 a. **The nurse's plan for care will be guided by the newborn's level of jaundice. The number of stools, effective latch, and baby's weight loss will inform the next steps related to the level of jaundice. Of the four choices on the list, jaundice is the risk of highest concern because it can rise quickly with devastating results if interventions are not made in a timely manner. When the number of choices is limited, the test taker should select the answer that relates to the condition of highest, life-threatening risk.**

   1 b. The baby has had a meconium stool. It is important that the baby have frequent stools in order to remove the bilirubin from the intestines, but this is not the primary assessment at this time until we know what the jaundice level is.

   1 c. Latch assessment is not primary at this point even though the baby must latch efficiently in order to stimulate milk production and to transfer colostrum from the breast. Even after the baby achieves a successful latch, however, the healthcare providers cannot make a decision on whether or not supplementation with formula is necessary until they know the level of jaundice and follow its progression.

   1 d. The baby's weight is an important and routine assessment, but it is not primary at this point. Assessing the jaundice level and risk factors for rising levels is the first step.

   2 a. Jaundice is the primary assessment as indicated above.

   2 b. The baby is stooling. There is nothing in the stem of the question to indicate this is a concern that needs further assessment.

2 c. Newborn latch is necessary for maternal breastmilk production, but this is not one of the top two priorities for assessment at this time.

2 d. All babies lose some weight initially. The percentage of weight loss and the level of jaundice inform the next steps of whether or not formula supplementation is indicated. Significant weight loss can be a sign of dehydration, which predisposes the infant to severe hyperbilirubinemia (Huang et al., 2012). The best way to decrease bilirubin levels it to help remove it through adequate feedings, leading to increased bowel movements that excrete the bilirubin. The normal percentage of newborn weight loss in the first few days of life is up to 10% (Paul et al., 2016). This percentage does not present a health hazard for the newborn, and the weight is expected to begin to rise by day 7.

TEST-TAKING HINT: Both of the correct answers for this question relate to assessments for the hazardous risk of physiologic jaundice that may require urgent interventions. The key to answering this question is in noticing that it asks for "assessments,"

4. Answers 2 and 3 are correct.

1. The baby's weight loss is within a normal range and there is nothing in the stem of the question to suggest he needs phototherapy.
2. **Breastfeeding success will benefit the mother's self-confidence and reduce her anxiety. It will also assist in adequate milk production for the baby which will, in turn, lead to more frequent stools, weight gain, and reduction of jaundice.**
3. **It is standard practice in most hospitals to check all babies' jaundice levels with a non-invasive transcutaneous bilirubin (TcB) measurement tool. This electronic device gives a reading that indicates whether or not the baby's jaundice is in a range between low risk, low intermediate risk, high intermediate risk, and high risk. The risk factor is interpreted by the baby's age in hours (AAP, 2004).**
4. There is nothing in the stem of the question to suggest the newborn's blood glucose should be checked.

TEST-TAKING HINT: Phototherapy would require a provider's order and would be based on the TcB test results among other things. It is one of the last steps in treatment of jaundice. In this case study, the nurse is taking the first steps to identify, "What can I do?" Both answers refer to those initial steps.

5.
1. A TcB of 10 at 48 hours is in the low intermediate risk zone, within normal, and does not require a phone call to the primary healthcare provider.
2. There is nothing to indicate this baby needs phototherapy.
3. There is nothing to indicate this baby needs a CBC.
4. **Assisting with successful breastfeeding to hydrate the baby and promote the production of feces is the most important action for the nurse to take next.**

TEST-TAKING HINT: This baby's weight loss, transcutaneous bilirubin measurement, and output are all within normal. The baby does have three clinically significant risk factors for hyperbilirubinemia: (1) exclusive breastfeeding; (2) jaundice before discharge; and (3) cephalohematoma. However, none of these factors by itself is a predictor of significant hyperbilirubinemia. If the parents are provided with written and verbal information that includes (1) an explanation of jaundice, (2) the need to monitor the baby for further jaundice, (3) what to report to the primary healthcare provider, and (4) a pre-scheduled follow-up visit with the provider in 3 to 4 days, the nurse can have confidence that this family has what they need to monitor the baby's condition.

All newborn bilirubin levels, whether obtained by TcB or by a blood test, are interpreted according to the infant's age in hours, using the Bhutani nomogram (see following graph). To calculate the neonate's bilirubin risk zone, the nurse finds the neonate's age in hours on the line at the bottom. Following that line up to where it intersects with the neonate's bilirubin results in mg/dL in the vertical list on the left or in standard international units (μmol/L) on the right, the nurse can determine the neonate's risk zone.

For more information on physiologic jaundice, see the appendix. For a history of phototherapy and the physiology of how it works, see https://nursing.ceconnection.com/ovidfiles/00149525-201110001-00003.pdf.

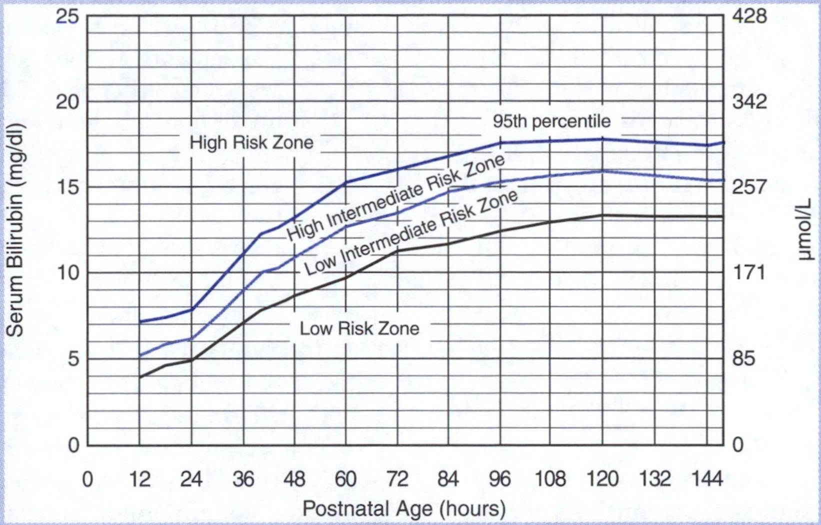

6. Answers 1, 2, and 3 are correct.

1. **Passage of stool eliminates bilirubin and prevents reabsorption of bilirubin.**
2. **A drop of milk in the baby's mouth indicates mother's milk is present and will likely increase.**
3. **A TcB measurement in the low intermediate risk is expected with this baby's risk factors.**
4. It is important to warn mothers not to fall asleep with the baby in their arms, if possible. Breastfeeding releases prolactin from the mother's pituitary gland. This often makes her feel sleepy and relaxed. Because this might happen, the baby and the mother's arms should be supported appropriately during a feeding in order to prevent the baby from sliding to the floor or getting trapped between the bed coverings and pillows.

TEST-TAKING HINT: The nurse must be aware of normal findings and the anticipated trends, or progression of those findings in order to support clients appropriately. Teaching the client about behaviors to avoid, such as falling asleep with the baby in her arms, is also appropriate.

7. Answers 1, 2, 3, and 5 are correct.

1. **Congenital hypothyroidism is a malfunction of or complete absence of the thyroid gland that is present from birth. In the U.S., it is screened for in all 50 states.**
2. **Sickle cell disease is an autosomal recessive disease resulting in abnormally shaped red blood cells. In the U.S., it is screened for in all 50 states.**
3. **Galactosemia is an incurable autosomal recessive disease characterized by the absence of the enzyme required to metabolize galactose. In the U.S., it is screened for in all 50 states.**
4. Cerebral palsy (CP) is a disorder characterized by motor dysfunction resulting from a nonprogressive injury to brain tissue. The injury may occur during pregnancy, labor, delivery, or shortly after delivery. Physical examination is required to diagnose CP. Blood screening is not an appropriate means of diagnosis.
5. **Cystic fibrosis is an autosomal recessive illness characterized by the presence of thick mucus in many organ systems, most notably the respiratory tract. In the U.S., it is screened for in all 50 states.**

TEST-TAKING HINT: It is important to realize that neonatal screening is state- and country-specific. In the U.S., each state determines which diseases will be screened for. In March 2015, the Advisory Committee on Heritable Disorders in Newborns and Children recommended that all newborns be screened for 35 core disorders and 26 secondary disorders. Most states screen for 29 of the 35 core conditions. Individual states make those decisions based on several factors including (1) the laws of the state; (2) the financial costs of screening; (3) the frequency of the disorder in the state; (4) the availability of treatments and follow-up for each condition; and (5) the funding sources for the newborn screening program (for specific state information see babysfirsttest.org).

8. 1. Meconium is a sterile stool. The newborn will not produce gastrointestinal bacteria until a few days after delivery.

2. Amniotic fluid is a reservoir for viral diseases like HIV and hepatitis B. If the woman is infected with those viruses, the amniotic fluid will be infectious.

3. Fetal urine is not highly alkaline.

4. Although babies are at high risk for infection, there is no need for nurses to wear gloves routinely when caring for the babies. Immediately after delivery the nurse is protecting himself or herself from the baby, not the other way around.

TEST-TAKING HINT: By wearing gloves, the nurse is practicing standard precautions per the Centers for Disease Control and Prevention (CDC) to protect himself or herself from viruses that may be present in the amniotic fluid and on the neonate's body. This question illustrates how important it is for the test taker to read each possible answer very carefully. For example, the test taker may be tempted to choose choice 1 but the fact that the option states that meconium contains "enteric bacteria" makes that answer incorrect.

9. 1. When newborns are wet they can become hypothermic from heat loss resulting from evaporation. They may then develop cold stress.

2. The first Apgar score is not done until 60 seconds after delivery. The wet blankets should have been removed from the baby well before that time.

3. Eye prophylaxis can be delayed until after the parents have begun bonding with their baby.

4. Although the baby's central nervous system must be carefully assessed, reflex assessment should be postponed until after the baby is dried and is breathing on his or her own.

TEST-TAKING HINT: This is a prioritizing question. Every one of the actions will be performed after the birth of the baby. The nurse must know which action is performed first. Because hypothermia can compromise a neonate's transition to extrauterine life, it is essential to dry the baby immediately to minimize heat loss through evaporation. It is important for the test-taker to review cold stress in the newborn.

10. 1. Hypothermia in the neonate is defined as a temperature below 97.7° F (36.5° C). Cold stress may develop if the baby's temperature is below that level.

2. A healthy neonate does not need supplemental feedings. And if supplements are needed, they should be either formula or breast milk, not glucose water.

3. There is no indication in the stem that glucose assessments are needed for this baby.

4. Babies should be breastfed every 2 to 3 hours. Feedings every 4 hours are not frequent enough.

TEST-TAKING HINT: It is important for the test taker to remember that a baby weighing 6 lbs 3 oz (2,900 grams) is an average-sized baby. (Normal weight range is 5 lbs 5 oz to 8 lbs 8 oz or 2,500 to 4,000 grams). Blood glucose levels are generally recommended for macrosomic babies, which includes those weighing 8 lbs 8 oz to 9 lbs 9 oz (4,000 to 4,500 grams) or more. Because no other information is included in the stem, the test taker must assume that the baby is healthy. The answers, therefore, should be evaluated in terms of the healthy newborn. Hypoglycemia can result when a baby develops cold stress because babies must metabolize food to create heat. When they use up their food stores, they become hypoglycemic (Patel, 2020).

11. Answers 2, 3, and 5 are correct.

1. All of the babies' senses are well developed at birth.

2. Babies respond to all forms of taste. They prefer sweet things.

3. Babies' sense of touch is considered to be the most well-developed sense.

4. Babies see quite well at 8 to 12 inches. They prefer to look at the human face.

5. Babies hear quite well once the amniotic fluid is absorbed from the ear canal. All newborns' hearing is tested prior to discharge from the newborn nursery. If a baby is found to have a hearing impairment, the baby should receive early intervention.

TEST-TAKING HINT: Many parents believe that babies are incapable of receptive communication. On the contrary, they are amazingly able to give and receive communication. All five senses are intact and function well, though some, such as vision, operate at an immature level.

12. 1. Petechiae can be present as a result of an infectious disease, for example, meningococcemia. In this situation, however, there is no indication that an infection is present.

2. When neonates speed through the birth canal during rapid deliveries, the presenting parts become bruised. The bruising often takes the form of petechial hemorrhages.
3. Erythema toxicum, the newborn rash, is characterized by papules or pustules on an erythematous base.
4. There is nothing in the scenario to suggest that child abuse has occurred.

TEST-TAKING HINT: Although this question is about the neonate, the key to answering the question is knowledge of the normal length of a vaginal labor and delivery. The average length of labor for a multiparous client is about 8 to 10 hours; a primiparous client may be in labor for more than 20 hours. The 3-hour labor noted in the stem of the question is significantly shorter than the average labor. The neonate, therefore, has progressed rapidly through the birth canal and, as a result, the face is bruised.

13. 1. The baby has lost less than 4% of its birth weight. Babies often lose between 5% and 10% of their birth weight. A loss greater than 10% is considered pathologic.
2. The weight loss is within normal limits.
3. Supplementation is not needed at this time.
4. There is no indication in the stem that the baby is at high risk for hypoglycemia.

TEST-TAKING HINT: Most neonates lose weight after birth. The weight loss is not considered pathologic unless it exceeds 10%. Only then must the baby's weight loss be reported to the newborn's healthcare provider. Supplementary feedings with formula might be necessary at that time.

14. 1. Meconium should pass within 24 hours of delivery.
2. This baby's glucose level is within normal limits.
3. Normal neonatal breathing is irregular at 30 to 60 breaths per minute. This baby is tachypneic.
4. A milky discharge—sometimes referred to as witch's milk or neonatal galactorrhea—is normal. It results from the drop in maternal hormones in the neonatal system following delivery.

TEST-TAKING HINT: Clinical judgment is guided by the question, "What is normal?" Unless the nurse understands the characteristics of a normal newborn, it may be impossible to recognize subtle changes that require further assessment or treatment.

15. 0.25 mL
Standard ratio and proportion formula:

$$\frac{\text{Known volume : known dosage}}{\text{desired volume : desired dosage}} =$$

$$2 : 1 \text{ mL} = 0.5 : x$$

The means are multiplied together and extremes are multiplied together.

$$2x = 0.5$$
$$x = 0.25 \text{ mL}$$

Dimensional analysis method for calculating the volume of medication to be administered:

Known volume	Desired dosage	= Desired volume
Known dosage		

1 mL	0.5 mg	= 0.25 mL
2 mg		

TEST-TAKING HINT: This is an alternate-form question. Test takers will be required to do mathematical calculations using the calculator within the test, and input their answers. Test takers must be familiar with med math calculations and with simple clinical calculations. Note that the units—in this case, mL—are included in the question and that the question indicates how many decimal places to calculate the answer to.

16. Answers 1, 2, 3, and 5 are correct.
1. With the baby placed flat on its back, the practitioner grasps the baby's thighs using thumbs and index fingers.
2. When assessing for Ortolani sign, the baby's thighs are abducted. When performing the Barlow test, the baby's thighs are adducted.
3. With the baby's hips and knees at 90-degree angles, the hips are abducted. With DDH, the trochanter dislocates from the acetabulum. The provider would feel the dislocation while palpating the trochanter.
4. When performing both the Ortolani and Barlow tests, the baby is placed flat on its back. When assessing for symmetry of leg lengths and tissue folds, the baby is placed in both the supine and prone positions.
5. Legs are extended to assess for equal leg lengths and for equal thigh and gluteal folds.

TEST-TAKING HINT: This test is not generally performed by a nurse. To assess for developmental dysplasia of the hip, the Ortolani and the Barlow tests are performed by the provider. The order of

the steps of the Ortolani procedure is (1) the baby is placed on its back; (2) the provider grasps the baby's thighs with a thumb on the inner aspect and forefingers over the trochanter; (3) with the knees flexed at 90-degree angles, the hips are abducted; and (4) the provider palpates the trochanter to assess for hip laxity. The Barlow test is performed by (1) adducting the baby's legs; (2) gently pushing the legs posteriorly; and (3) feeling to note any slippage of the trochanter out of the acetabulum. Galeazzi sign, to assess for uneven knee heights, can also be performed.

17.
1. There is no evidence in the stem that would warrant placing the child in an isolette.
2. Cyanotic hands and feet are not signs of hypoxia in the neonate.
3. **The baby's extremities are cyanotic as a result of the baby's immature circulatory system. Swaddling or placing the baby skin-to-skin on a parent's chest will help to warm the baby's hands and feet.**
4. There is no evidence in the stem that would warrant monitoring with the pulse oximeter.

TEST-TAKING HINT: The nurse must be familiar with the differences between normal findings of the newborn and those of an older child or adult. Acrocyanosis—bluish/cyanotic hands and feet—is normal in the very young neonate resulting from his or her immature circulation to the extremities (Dosanjh, 2018). It is a benign finding that may persist for 24 to 48 hours.

18.
1. There is no evidence that circumcision status affects a boy's self-image.
2. No official statements have been published regarding the rationality of performing circumcisions.
3. The CDC has made no policy statement on circumcision.
4. **The AAP, although acknowledging that there are some advantages to circumcision, states that there is not enough evidence to suggest that all baby boys be circumcised.**

TEST-TAKING HINT: In this question, authorities were cited—namely, the Centers for Disease Control and Prevention (CDC) and the American Academy of Pediatrics (AAP). The nurse should be familiar with authorities in the fields of maternity, including the CDC, AAP, American College of Obstetricians and Gynecologists (ACOG), and the Association of Women's Health, Obstetric, and Neonatal Nursing (AWHONN). It is helpful to cite authorities when responding to parents' questions about emotionally charged issues such as circumcision. In the end, however, it is the parents' decision and nurses must not attempt to force their personal beliefs on the parents.

19.
1. Circumcision is a surgical procedure that requires a sterile field and sterile technique. The nurse is performing safe practice in this situation.
2. **The nurse is being a patient advocate because the baby is unable to ask for pain medication. The AAP has made a policy statement that pain medications be used during all circumcision procedures.**
3. If a baby feeds immediately before the circumcision, he may aspirate his feeds. This is safe practice.
4. Making sure the baby is not hemorrhaging at the incision site is also an example of safe nursing practice.

TEST-TAKING HINT: This question requires differentiating between safe practice and client advocacy. Nurses perform a variety of roles. Being a safe practitioner is an essential role of the nurse. Just as important and quite different, however, is the role of client advocate. Answers 1, 3, and 4 are examples of safe practice. Only question 2 demonstrates client advocacy, defined loosely as providing support for the rights of a clients who are unable to speak for or support themselves.

20. Answers 4 and 5 are correct.
1. Although assessed in other pain scales, the heart rate is not part of the NIPS.
2. Blood pressure is not assessed in any infant pain scale.
3. Temperature is not assessed in any infant pain scale.
4. **Facial expression is one variable that is evaluated as part of the NIPS.**
5. **Breathing pattern is one variable that is evaluated as part of the NIPS.**

TEST-TAKING HINT: The nurse should be familiar with the pain-rating scales and use them clinically because neonates cannot communicate their pain to the nurse. The scoring variables that are evaluated when assessing neonatal pain using the NIPS are facial expression, crying, breathing patterns, movement of arms and legs, and state of arousal. Other tools for assessing pain in the neonate are the Pain Assessment Tool (PAT), the Neonatal Post-op Pain Scale (CRIES), and the Premature Infant Pain Profile (PIPP).

21.
1. Hydrogen peroxide is not used when cleansing the circumcised penis.
2. Antifungals are not indicated in this situation.

3. **Squeezing water over the penis cleanses the area without irritating the site and causing the site to bleed.**
4. Dry dressings are not applied to the circumcised penis. It is, however, usually recommended to liberally apply petroleum jelly to the site before diapering. The petroleum jelly may be applied directly to the penis via a sterile dressing or via a petroleum jelly–impregnated gauze.

TEST-TAKING HINT: This question requires the test taker to read all answers carefully to avoid misinterpreting them. In this case, question 3 refers to squeezing water over the glans. It is followed by question 4 which asks about a dry dressing. The test taker must not assume this refers to a dry, replacement dressing that includes petroleum jelly, unless petroleum jelly is mentioned in the stem or in the answer. The circumcised penis has undergone a surgical procedure, but to apply a dry dressing is potentially injurious. If the dressing adheres to the newly circumcised penis, the incision could bleed. The test taker should be aware that with routine cleaning, as cited previously, circumcisions usually heal quickly and rarely become infected.

22. **The "X" should be placed on the baby in the supine position (on its back, "as though looking at the sun") on the vastus lateralis on either the left or right thigh—that is, the anterior-lateral portion of the middle third of the thigh from the trochanter to the patella. This is the only safe site for intramuscular injections in infants.**

TEST-TAKING HINT: This is another alternate-form question. The test taker must place the "X" on the appropriate picture—the baby in the supine position—and be careful to place the "X" at the precise location where the injection can safely be given. If the "X" extends past the area of safety, the question will be marked as incorrect.

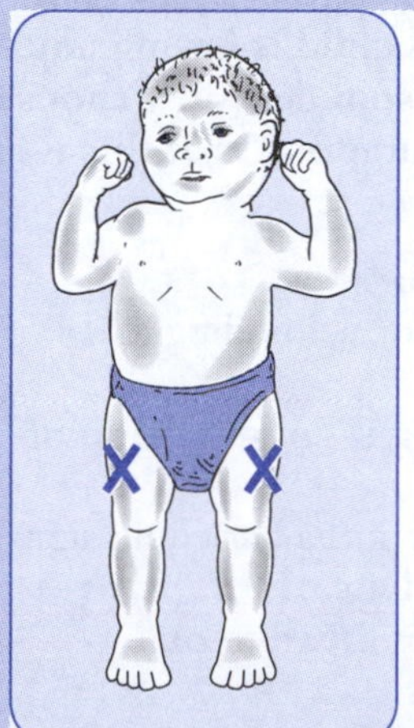

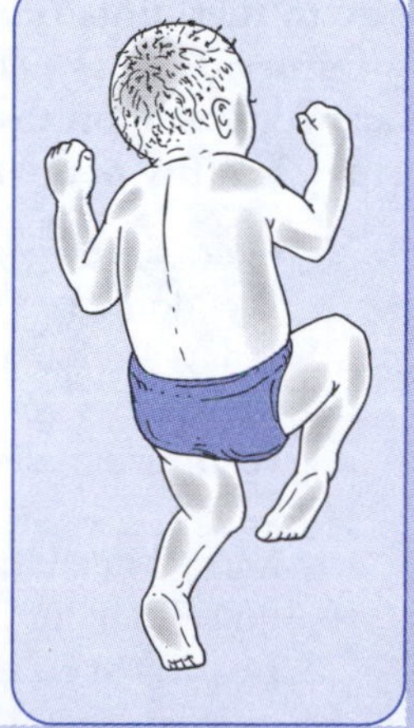

23. **The "X" should be placed on the posterior fontanelle or the triangle-shaped area on the occiput of the baby's head.**

TEST-TAKING HINT: It is important not only to know the shape and size of the fontanelles but also to know the ages when the fontanelles usually close. The nurse will need to know this to provide anticipatory guidance to the parents as well as to be able to assess the child for normal growth and development.

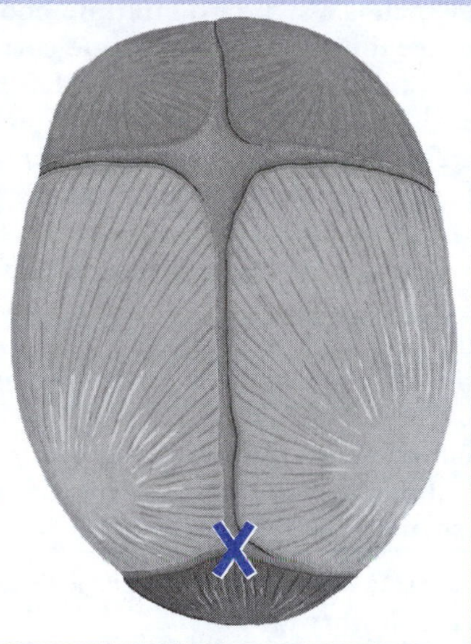

24.
1. A three-vessel cord is a normal finding.
2. The anterior fontanelle is diamond-shaped.
3. **Undescended testes—cryptorchidism—is an unexpected finding. It is one sign of prematurity.**
4. Although multiple café au lait spots are seen in some neurological anomalies, the presence of one area of pigmentation is a normal finding.

TEST-TAKING HINT: It is important for the nurse to be able to discriminate between normal and abnormal findings. In addition, it is important to be able to discern when the amount or degree of a finding is abnormal, as in the presence of multiple café au lait spots.

25. **Answers 1, 2, and 3 are correct.**
1. **The patches are called Mongolian spots and they are commonly seen in babies of color. They will fade and disappear with time.**
2. **The whitish discharge has been called witch's milk in the past and is currently referred to as *neonatal milk*, or *neonatal galactorrhea*. It is excreted as a result of the drop in maternal hormones in the baby's system. The discharge is temporary.**
3. **The bloody discharge is called pseudo-menses and occurs as a result of the drop in maternal hormones in the baby's system. The discharge is temporary.**

4. The demarcated area is a port wine stain, or capillary angioma. It is a permanent birthmark.
5. The dimple may be a pilonidal cyst or a small defect into the spinal cord (spina bifida). An ultrasound should be done to determine whether or not a pathological condition is present.

TEST-TAKING HINT: A multiple-response type of question is often a more difficult type of question to answer than is a standard multiple-choice item because there is not simply one correct response to the question. The test taker must look at each answer option to see whether or not it accurately answers the stem of the question. A useful approach is to read each answer on its own, as a true or false answer to the question, "What is normal?" If the response is "true," it is one of the answers; if it is "false," it doesn't apply. In this question, purple-colored patches are considered normal in an African American neonate. The other findings, a whitish discharge from the breasts, and a bloody vaginal discharge, are normal findings in all female newborns, regardless of ethnicity.

26. **1. Intercostal retractions are a sign of respiratory distress.**
2. Caput succedaneum is a normal finding in a neonate.
3. Epstein pearls are often seen in the mouths of neonates.
4. Harlequin sign, although odd-appearing, is a normal finding in a neonate.

TEST-TAKING HINT: Each of the normal findings is seen in newborns, although not seen later in life. The nurse must be familiar with these age-specific normal findings. It is also important to remember that, based on the hierarchy of needs, respiratory problems often take precedence.

27. 1. Respiratory rate between 30 and 60 and oxygen saturation above 95% are normal findings.
2. Although the Apgar score of 9 is excellent, the baby's weight—10 lbs 2 ounces (4,660 grams)—is well above the average of 5 lbs 5 ounces to 8 lbs 8 ounces (2,500 to 4,000 grams). Babies who are large for gestational age (LGA) are at high risk for hypoglycemia.
3. This is within normal newborn vital signs, which are: temperature 97.7° F (36.5° C) to 99° F (37.2° C) and length 18 to 22 inches.
4. Blood glucose 40 to 60 mg/dL (2.2 to 3.3 mmol/L) and heart rate 110 bpm to 160 bpm are normal findings.

TEST-TAKING HINT: This is a prioritizing question requiring very subtle discriminatory ability. The nurse must know normal values and conditions as well as the consequences that may occur if findings outside of normal are noted.

28. **1. Showing signs of hunger and frustration describes the active alert or active awake state.**
2. Starting to whimper and cry describes the crying behavioral state.
3. A baby who is wide awake and attending to the mother's face is in the quiet alert state; sometimes called wide-awake state.
4. Sleeping and breathing regularly describe deep or quiet sleep.

TEST-TAKING HINT: It is essential that the test taker be able to discern the differences between the various behaviors of the neonate to teach clients about the inherent behavioral expressions of their babies. Babies are in a transition period during the active alert period. Caregivers often can meet the needs of the baby in the active alert state to preclude the need for the baby to resort to crying.

29. 1. This is actually a true statement. Babies do rarely open their mouths to breathe. However, it is not the best response that the nurse could provide.
2. This statement provides the mother with the knowledge that babies are obligate nose breathers so that they are able to suck, swallow, and breathe while feeding.
3. Again, this statement is inherently true, but it is a meaningless platitude that will not satisfy the mother's need for information.
4. This response is inappropriate. Healthy newborns have small nares but aerate effectively as obligate nose breathers.

TEST-TAKING HINT: Some test takers might be tempted to respond to this question by choosing answer 4. It is important, however, to respond to the question as it is posed. There is nothing in the stem that hints that this child is having any respiratory distress. The responder must choose an answer based on the assumption that this is a normal, healthy neonate.

30. **Answers 2 and 5 are correct.**
1. Pseudomenses is a normal finding in a 1-day-old female.
2. Expiratory grunting is an indication of respiratory distress.
3. This is a description of the harlequin sign, a normal neonatal finding.
4. Nasal flaring is an indication of respiratory distress.

TEST-TAKING HINT: Pseudo-menses is seen in many 1-day-old female neonates. Expiratory grunting and nasal flaring, however, are not normal. Respiratory difficulties always need to be assessed fully. The transient harlequin sign (unilateral erythema) is usually a normal finding. It is much different than the "harlequin fetus" which is a rare and serious skin condition (Tang et al., 2010).

31. 1. This is not an emergent problem needing physician intervention.
2. There is nothing in the stem that implies that the child has been abused.
3. Subconjunctival hemorrhages are a normal finding and are not pathological. They will disappear over time. Explaining this to the mother is the appropriate action.
4. There is nothing in the stem that implies that there has been any intraocular damage. It is not within the nurse's scope of practice to diagnose the condition of the retina.

TEST-TAKING HINT: The key to answering this mother's concern is knowing what is normal and what is abnormal in a neonate. Hemorrhages in the sclerae are considered normal, resulting from pressure changes at birth. Although the mother is frantic, the nurse's assessment shows that this is a normal finding. The nurse, therefore, provides the mother with the accurate information.

32. **1. Seesaw breathing is an indication of respiratory distress.**
2. This is the normal breathing pattern of a neonate.
3. When babies breathe, their abdomens and thoraces rise and fall in synchrony.
4. The normal respiratory rate is 30 to 60 respirations per minute.

TEST-TAKING HINT: The nurse must be knowledgeable of the normal variations of neonatal respirations. Apnea spells of 10 seconds or less are normal, but apnea spells longer than 20 seconds should be reported to the primary healthcare provider. Normally, when a baby breathes, the abdomen and chest rise and fall in synchrony. When they rise and fall arrhythmically, as in seesaw breathing, it is an indication that the baby is in respiratory difficulty.

33. 1. This is an image of a baby in the tonic neck position.
2. This is an image of a baby in the opisthotonic posture.
3. This is an image of a baby in the classic fetal position.
4. This is an image of a baby in the frank breech posture.

TEST-TAKING HINT: Babies often assume a posture after delivery that reflects the posture they were in while in utero. Babies in the frank breech position in utero are bent at the waist with both legs adjacent to the head. That same posture is seen in the baby after delivery.

34. 1. Slight drop in heart rate is normal when babies are in deep sleep.
2. Slight jaundice is within normal limits on the second day of life. Pathologic jaundice appears within the first 24 hours of life, whereas physiologic jaundice appears after 24 hours of life. Temperature is within normal limits of 97.7° F (36.5° C) to 99° F (37.2° C).
3. Babies who breastfeed fewer than eight times a day are not receiving adequate nutrition. Jitters are indicative of hypoglycemia.
4. The rash is a normal newborn rash—erythema toxicum. Crying, without other signs and symptoms, is a normal response by babies.

TEST-TAKING HINT: A baby can be at risk of hypoglycemia whether it is newly born or several days old, if it isn't feeding often enough, or if the milk supply is limited. A 3-day-old baby breastfeeding every 4 hours, rather than every 2 to 3 hours, is not consuming enough nutrients. As a result, the baby is jittery, which could be a sign of low serum glucose. Infants of mothers with diabetes may develop hypoglycemia for up to 10 days of age (AAP, 2011).

35. 1. This baby is asleep. Placing the baby en face will not promote neonatal bonding.
2. This baby is asleep. Placing the baby en face will not promote neonatal bonding.
3. This baby is in the quiet alert behavioral state. Placing the baby en face will foster bonding between the father and baby.
4. This baby is showing hunger cues. The baby likely needs to be fed at this time.

TEST-TAKING HINT: The test taker could make an educated guess regarding this question even if the term "en face" were unfamiliar. The expression means "face to face," which is clearly implied by the term. Because bonding between parent and child is so important, whenever a baby exhibits the quiet alert behavior, the nurse should encourage the interaction. Although the father may bond with a sleeping baby who is in the en face position, the baby is unable to interact or bond with its parent.

36. 1. The normal temperature of a neonate is 97.7° F (36.5° C) to 99° F (37.2° C) and the weight of a term neonate is between 5 lbs 5 oz to 8 lbs 8 oz (2,500 to 4,000 grams).
2. Milia—white spots on the bridge of the nose—are exposed sebaceous glands. They are normal.
3. Epstein pearls—raised white specks on the gums or on the hard palate—are normal findings in the neonate.
4. The normal resting respiratory rate of a neonate is 30 to 60 breaths per minute and the normal resting heart rate of a neonate is 110 to 160 bpm.

TEST-TAKING HINT: Only one of these groups of findings is not normal. The nurse new to obstetrics should focus first on, "what is normal?" By having normal parameters for newborn vital signs, weights, and physical findings ingrained in one's mind for immediate access, newborn assessments can be quickly and efficiently sorted into those of concern and those outside of normal that need a provider's notification or assessment.

37. 1. This is a description of the rooting reflex.
2. This is a description of the Babinski reflex.
3. This is a description of the Moro reflex. When the baby is suddenly lowered or startled, the neonate's arms straighten outward and the knees flex.
4. This is a description of the tonic neck reflex.

TEST-TAKING HINT: The nurse must be familiar not only with the reason for eliciting reflexes but also with the correct technique for eliciting the actions.

38. 1. Epstein pearls are not found on the feet.
2. Epstein pearls are not found on the hands.
3. Epstein pearls are not found on the back.
4. Epstein pearls—small white specks (keratin-containing cysts)—are located on the palate and gums.

TEST-TAKING HINT: This question is not a trick question. Some test takers, when asked a fairly direct question, believe that the question is a trick and choose an alternate response to try to outfox the examiner. The test taker should remember that the NCLEX test will include some straightforward questions such as this one. Take each question at face value and don't try to read into the question or to out-psych the test.

39. 1. Pseudostrabismus—eyes cross and uncross when they are open—is normal in the neonate because of poor tone of the muscles of the eye.
2. Ears positioned in alignment with the inner and outer canthus of the eyes is the normal position. In Down's syndrome, ears are low set.
3. Vernix caseosa covers and protects the skin of the fetus. Depending on the gestational age of the baby, there is often some left on the skin at birth.
4. Nasal flaring is a symptom of respiratory distress.

TEST-TAKING HINT: To answer this question, the test taker should first consider each statement as a true or false statement that answers the question, "What is normal?" After identifying the normal findings described here, the test taker will be left with one response that is not normal. That is nasal flaring, a symptom of respiratory distress. This is the symptom that must be reported to the primary healthcare provider.

40. 1. Babies are awake and alert for approximately 30 minutes to 1 hour immediately after birth. This is the perfect time for the parents to begin to bond with their babies.
2. There is no reason to notify the primary healthcare provider.
3. This is a full-term baby. There is no need to perform a gestational age assessment.
4. Warmth can be maintained, preferably by placing the baby skin to skin with the mother or, if required, by swaddling the baby in one or more blankets.

TEST-TAKING HINT: After the first period of reactivity, babies enter a phase of inactivity when they sleep. They may be in the sleep phase for a number of hours. It is important, therefore, for parental bonding to be initiated during the reactivity phase and, if the mother plans to breastfeed, to have the baby go to breast at this time as well.

41. 1. The baby's Apgar is not 6.
2. The baby's Apgar is not 7.
3. The baby's Apgar is 8.
4. The baby's Apgar is not 9.

TEST-TAKING HINT: Apgar scoring is usually a nursing responsibility. To determine the correct response, the nurse must know the Apgar scoring scale given below and add the points together: 2 for heart rate, 2 for respiratory rate, 1 for color, 2 for reflex irritability, 1 for flexion. The total score for this baby is 8. Apgar "normals" are NOT the same as clinical normals. For example, the normal heart rate of a neonate is defined as 110 to 160 bpm. The baby will receive the maximum 2 points for heart rate, however, with a heart rate of greater than or equal to 100 bpm. In most hospitals or birth centers, the Apgar is posted for easy reference and the parameters need not be memorized for recall, although they do become second nature in time.

THE APGAR SCORE

Assessment	0 points	1 point	2 points
Color	Central cyanosis	Acrocyanosis	All pink
Heart rate	No heart rate	1–99 bpm	Equal to or greater than 100 bpm
Respiratory rate	No respirations	Slow and irregular	Good lusty cry
Reflex irritability	No response	Grimace	Good lusty cry
Tone	Flaccid	Some flexion	Marked flexion or active movement

42. 1. Molding is characterized by the overlapping of the cranial bones. It is rarely one sided and would feel like a ridge rather than a bulge.
2. Swelling of the tissues of the baby's head occurs over the entire cranium and is called caput succedaneum.
3. Positioning usually results in molding.
4. **Cephalohematomas are subcutaneous swellings of accumulated blood from the trauma of delivery. The bulges may be one-sided or bilateral and the swellings do not cross suture lines.**

TEST-TAKING HINT: The key to the correct response is the fact that the bulge has not crossed the suture lines. Because the fluid collection is between the periosteum and the skull, the boundaries of a cephalohematoma are defined by the underlying bone and a cephalohematoma does not cross the suture lines. Although each of the answer options is a common finding in neonates, only one is consistent with the assessments made by the nurse. The nurse can explain that the bleeding is gradual and may not be evident at the birth. It often develops during the hours or days following birth. Mothers also benefit from knowing that because the collection of blood is sitting on top of the skull and not under it, there is no pressure placed on the brain. It will resolve on its own but may take a few weeks.

43. 1. There is controversy in the literature regarding what should be used to clean the umbilical cord, but hydrogen peroxide is not one of the recommended agents. Previously, the cord was wiped with an alcohol swab at each diaper change, but more current literature indicates that nothing should be applied to the umbilical cord and that it should be allowed to air dry.
2. The cord should fall off on its own. This usually happens 7 to 10 days after birth.
3. **The green drainage may be a sign of infection. The cord should become dried and shriveled.**
4. There is no need to cover the umbilicus.

TEST-TAKING HINT: Using the strategy of the right answer being the one most at risk of causing serious illness or death, the answer that refers to a sign of infection is definitely the only correct answer.

44. 1. It is recommended that powders, even if advertised for the purpose, not be used on babies.
2. **This is true. It is recommended that powders, even if advertised for the purpose, not be used on babies in order to avoid the babies inhaling the powder, regardless of how careful the mother may be during the diaper change.**
3. There is no evidence that most babies are allergic to cornstarch.
4. It is irrelevant where the powder is being used; it is recommended that powders, even if advertised for the purpose, not be used on babies.

TEST-TAKING HINT: Sometimes answer options include qualifiers. For example, in this question, choice 4 includes the qualifier "As long as you put it only on the buttocks area." Test takers should be wary of qualifiers. They are often used to draw one to an incorrect response.

45. 1. To prevent infection, the eyes should be cleaned from inner canthus to outer canthus.
2. To prevent injury, parents should be advised never to put anything smaller than their fingertips into the baby's nose or ears.
3. **If items must be obtained while the bath is being given, the baby should be removed from the water and kept warm while being carried by the parent to obtain the needed supplies.**
4. The safest way to check the temperature of the water is with a thermometer or, if none is available, with the elbow or forearm.

TEST-TAKING HINT: When removed from water, a baby may become hypothermic from evaporation resulting from exposure to the air when wet. As such, the room should be warm and without

drafts, and the baby should be dried as soon as possible after being removed from the water, if an immersion bath has been done. Safety issues are especially important when providing parent education. The nurse must be familiar with actions that promote safety as well as those that put the neonate at risk.

46. **1. The perineum of female babies should always be cleansed from front to back to prevent bacteria from the rectum from entering the bladder and causing infection.**
2. Vernix may be in the labial folds at delivery. It is a natural lanolin that will be absorbed over time. Actively removing the vernix can actually irritate the baby's tissues.
3. Powder is not recommended for use on babies, especially in the diaper area. When mixed with urine, powders can produce an irritating paste.
4. Until the mother's milk is established and the baby's weight is stable, the number of a baby's diapers used in each 24-hour period should be counted to assess for hydration, but weighing the diapers of full-term babies is rarely needed.

TEST-TAKING HINT: It is important for nurses to provide needed education to parents for the care of their new baby. Diapering, although often seen as a skill that everyone should know, must be taught. And it is especially important to advise parents that introducing bacteria from the rectum can cause urinary tract infections in their female babies because of the relatively short urethra in females.

47. 1. Babies do not need to have a full bath each day. Daily soap baths can dry the newborn's skin.
2. Tummy time, while awake and while supervised, helps to prevent plagiocephaly and to promote growth and development.
3. There is no recommendation that babies be given a pacifier after every feeding. In fact, some experts believe that pacifier use interferes with the success of breastfeeding.
4. It is strongly recommended that babies always be placed on their backs for sleep.

TEST-TAKING HINT: The test taker must not be confused by recommendations that appear contradictory such as giving baby tummy time but putting it to sleep on its back. The recommendation for "supervised" tummy time is one that includes safety measures and is the right answer. It is also the only correct answer, based on current expert recommendations.

48. Answers 2, 3, and 4 are correct.
1. Because air bag deployment can seriously injure young children, it is recommended that no child under 13 years of age be seated in the front seat of a car.
2. The baby should be facing the rear in the back seat of the car until he or she is 2 years of age, or meets specified weight requirements.
3. Since 2002, infant car seats have been designed with two attachment points at the base of the car seat. The car seat should be attached to the seat of the car using both attachment points.
4. After being installed, if a car seat moves more than 1 inch back and forth or side to side, it is not installed properly.
5. The straps of a car seat should fit snugly, allowing only two fingers to be inserted between them and the baby.

TEST-TAKING HINT: Nurses should be aware that recommendations and guidelines often change over time. In 2018, the American Academy of Pediatrics (AAP) released updated recommendations on infant and child seat restraint systems. The new recommendations encourage rear facing for as long as possible, until a child reaches the highest weight or height allowed by the manufacturer (Durbin et al, 2018).

49. Answers 1, 2, 4, and 5 are correct.
1. The first of three injections of the hepatitis B vaccine is often given in the newborn nursery, but, if not, it is recommended that it be given by 1 month of age.
2. It is recommended that the first of three injections of the Salk polio vaccine be given at the 2-month health maintenance checkup.
3. Because the baby has received passive immunity from the mother, the MMR is not given until the second year of life.
4. Three DTaP (diphtheria, tetanus, and pertussis) injections are given during the first year of life and boosters are given as the child grows. Note that babies receive DTaP injections and mothers receive Tdap injections. The capital letters "D" and "P" for the newborn, refer to higher levels of diphtheria and pertussis antigen concentrations for babies than for adults. Mothers and other adults receive a booster for protection from the same diseases, which is a different formulation referred to as Tdap (tetanus, diphtheria, and pertussis).

5. **Because the baby has received passive immunity from the mother, the varicella vaccine is not given until during the second year of life.**

TEST-TAKING HINT: Many recommendations are age-specific (AAP, 2016). The CDC changes immunization recommendations when new research emerges. The nurse should periodically review reliable sites like www.cdc.gov (Centers for Disease Control and Prevention) and www.aap.org (American Academy of Pediatrics) to check recommendations.

50. **Answers 1, 4, and 5 are correct.**
    1. **Babies do not starve themselves intentionally. If a baby refuses to eat, it may mean that the baby is seriously ill. For example, babies with cardiac defects often refuse to eat.**
    2. Newborns normally breathe irregularly. Apnea spells of 10 seconds or less are normal.
    3. Newborns do not tear when they cry. If a baby does tear, he or she may have a blocked lacrimal duct.
    4. **Although babies who are in the deep sleep state are difficult to arouse, the deep sleep state lasts no more than an hour. If the baby continues to be nonarousable, the pediatrician should be notified.**
    5. **A temperature above 100.4° F (38° C) is a febrile state for a newborn and the pediatrician should be notified. Many pediatricians advise parents to report a temperature above 99° F (37.2° C).**

TEST-TAKING HINT: The test taker must judge each answer option independently of the others when completing a multiple-response item. These items require more comprehensive knowledge because there is not simply one best response but rather, many correct answers.

51. **Answers 2 and 3 are correct.**
    1. Some newborn babies do not respond to their own hunger cues. It is especially important to note that breastfed babies must feed at least eight times in a 24-hour period to grow and for the mother to produce a sufficient milk supply. Parents should awaken a newborn if they do not awaken for a feeding when anticipated.
    2. **Babies should always be shielded from direct sunlight, preferably under an umbrella or other cover. If they must be in direct sunlight, sunscreen should be applied to all exposed areas, including the scalp.**
    3. **Liquid acetaminophen should be available in the home, but it should not be administered until the parent speaks to the primary healthcare provider.**
    4. There is no need to notify the doctor when the cord falls off.
    5. The top of the car seat chest clip should be positioned at the level of the baby's armpits.

TEST-TAKING HINT: A nurse who gives parents anticipatory guidance is providing the couple with knowledge that they will need for the future. Anticipatory guidance can prevent crises from occurring. Here, the nurse is providing accurate information so that the parents will be prepared to ensure that their child feeds often enough and is given medication only when it is needed. In addition, positioning the chest clip in the correct location would prevent abdominal injuries should the baby be in an automobile accident.

52. 1. The mouth should be suctioned before the nose.
    2. If the back of the throat is suctioned, it will stimulate the gag reflex.
    3. The bulb should be compressed before it is inserted into the baby's mouth.
    4. **The drainage should be evaluated by the nurse. The drainage, therefore, should be disposed of in a tissue or cloth.**

TEST-TAKING HINT: To remember whether the nose or the mouth should be suctioned first, remember "m" comes before "n"—the mouth should be suctioned before the nose. This order is recommended to prevent the baby from aspirating oral secretions when startled during the more uncomfortable nasal suction.

53. **The "X" should be placed on one of the lateral aspects of the heel, the safe sites for heel sticks. If other sites are used, the baby's nerves, arteries, or fat pad may be damaged.**

TEST-TAKING HINT: When responding to "X marks the spot" questions, it is essential that the "X" be placed as accurately as possible. Trying to guess by placing the "X" between sites will result in an incorrect response.

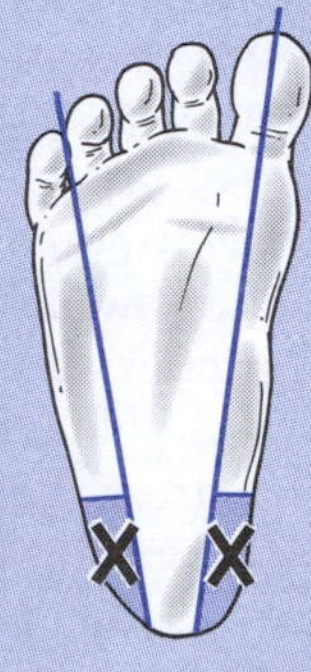

54. 1. An 18-gauge needle is too thick to be used.
    2. A 5/8-inch, 25-gauge needle is an appropriate needle for a neonatal IM injection.
    3. A 1-inch needle is too long and the gauge is too thick.
    4. Although the gauge is appropriate, a 1-inch needle is too long.

TEST-TAKING HINT: The larger the gauge of a needle, the narrower the needle width and vice versa. The 25-gauge needle, therefore, is narrow, whereas the 18-gauge needle is thick.

55. 1. The recommended site for assessing the pulse of a neonate is the brachial pulse. The carotid pulse is used to assess the pulse of an adult as well as that of a child over 1 year of age.
    2. The radial pulse is never recommended for use during CPR.
    3. The recommended site for assessing the pulse of a neonate undergoing CPR is the brachial pulse.
    4. The pedal pulse is never recommended for use during CPR.

TEST-TAKING HINT: Neonates and infants have very short necks. It is very difficult to access the carotid pulse in them. The brachial pulse is easily accessible and is a relatively strong pulse.

56. 1. Heat loss resulting from evaporation occurs when the baby is wet and exposed to the air.
    2. Heat loss resulting from conduction occurs when the baby comes in contact with cold objects (hands or stethoscope).
    3. Heat loss resulting from radiation occurs when the baby is exposed to cool objects that the baby is not in direct contact with.
    4. Heat loss resulting from convection occurs when the baby is exposed to the movement of cooled air—for example, air-conditioning currents.

TEST-TAKING HINT: Heat loss can lead to cold stress in the neonate. All four causes of heat loss must be understood and actions must be taken to prevent the baby from situations that would foster heat loss from any of the causes.

57. **1. Although this baby is being breastfed, the baby is still susceptible to illness. The best way to prevent transmission of pathogens is to wash hands carefully before touching the baby.**
    2. Visitors, too, should wash hands before touching the baby, but it is unnecessary to isolate the baby from them.
    3. The best way to prevent the transmission of a cold is to wash hands. Also, this baby is receiving protective antibodies through the breast milk. Masks are not necessary.
    4. All washable pieces of the equipment should be washed thoroughly after each use and sanitized daily, but not after each use. Sanitizing may be done by boiling the equipment in water or by using steam bags especially made for this purpose.

TEST-TAKING HINT: The test taker should choose responses that dictate behavior very carefully. For example, the statement, "Refrain from having visitors for the first month" is not the best response because there are very few instances when social interaction is prohibited. Certainly, the mother is free to tighten restrictions on visitors and to use a mask if she wishes to, but current literature does not suggest that this is necessary. It is important to remember that the most important action that can be taken to prevent communicable disease transmission is washing one's hands. This question and the answers do not reflect the societal practices during the coronavirus pandemic. Certainly, at that time, visitors were restricted. The test taker must understand that infection control practices may be different during unique circumstances, but must answer the questions about infection control in general, unless the stem of the question specifically states a pandemic is present.

58. Answers 2, 3, 4, and 5 are correct.
    1. Babies who are in the drowsy behavioral state and who are tightly swaddled often fall asleep rather than become aroused.
    2. The smell and/or the taste of the milk will often arouse a drowsy baby.
    3. Drowsy babies will open their eyes when spoken to or when placed in the "en face" position.
    4. Performing manipulations like diapering will arouse a drowsy baby.
    5. Performing manipulations like playing pat-a-cake will often arouse a drowsy baby.

TEST-TAKING HINT: It is important to distinguish a drowsy baby from a baby in the quiet alert or active alert state. For example, a baby who is in the active alert state may actually benefit from being swaddled because he or she is upset and needs to be calmed. Conversely, a baby in a drowsy state may need to be stimulated by manipulating or playing with the baby or by expressing milk onto the baby's lips.

59. Answers 1, 2, and 4 are correct.
    1. Stroking and patting the baby's back are very effective ways of burping.

2. **Babies can be burped in many different positions, including over the shoulder, lying flat across the lap, and in a sitting position. When placing the baby in the sitting position, the mother should carefully support the baby's chin. Positioning the baby face down on the lap can be very effective, and some mothers feel more secure using this position because the baby is unlikely to be dropped from this position.**
3. In the first few weeks of life, it is important to burp babies frequently throughout feedings. Bottle-fed babies often take in a great deal of air. Babies who burp only at the end of the feed often burp up large quantities of formula. Further teaching is needed.
4. **A small amount of "spit up" is within normal limits. Breastfed babies also may spit up curdled milk. This is normal.**
5. It may take quite a few minutes of patting before the baby burps effectively. If the baby does not burp well, they may regurgitate large quantities of the feeding.

TEST-TAKING HINT: It is important to distinguish between babies who are bottle-fed and those who are breastfed. Breastfed babies usually ingest much less air than do bottle-fed babies. Breastfed babies should be burped at least once in the middle of their feeds, generally before transfer to the second breast, whereas bottle-fed babies should be burped every 1/2 to 1 ounce because they take in more air during feedings.

60. 1. The uvula and frenulum are distinctly different structures in the mouth.
2. **Babies who are tongue-tied—that is, have a tight frenulum—have difficulty extending their tongues while breastfeeding. The mothers' nipples often become damaged as a result.**
3. A tight frenulum does not result in injury to the baby's tongue.
4. There is no relationship between breathing ability and being tongue-tied.

TEST-TAKING HINT: The baby's tongue must perform many actions in order to breastfeed successfully. One of the first actions the tongue must make is to extend past the gum line. A tight frenulum precludes the baby from being able to fully extend their tongue. As a result, the baby may "chew" on the mother's nipple with the gums, causing nipple soreness and injury.

61. Answers 1 and 3 are correct.
1. **A mother with active, untreated TB should be separated from her baby until the mother has been on antibiotic therapy for about 2 weeks. She can, however, pump her breast milk and have it fed to the baby through an alternate feeding method.**
2. Being hepatitis B surface antigen positive (HBsAg+) is not a contraindication to breastfeeding.
3. **Mothers who are HIV positive are advised not to breastfeed because there is an increased risk of transmission of the virus to the infant, even when both the mother and the infant are being treated for the virus.**
4. Acute bacterial infections, such as chorioamnionitis, are not contraindications to breastfeeding unless the medication given to the mother is contraindicated. There are, however, very few antibiotics that are incompatible with breastfeeding.
5. It is recommended that a mother with mastitis continue to breastfeed. She must keep draining her breasts of milk to prevent the development of a breast abscess. Again, only antibiotics compatible with breastfeeding should be administered.

TEST-TAKING HINT: There are very few instances when breastfeeding is contraindicated. When there is a restriction, it is generally because the disease is transmitted through breast milk, or because the mother's medications can be toxic to the baby.

62. 1. **The first action the nurse should always perform is to make sure that the correct baby is being given to the correct mother by comparing identification bracelet numbers.**
2. Helping the mother get comfortable is an important action but it is not the first action.
3. Teaching the mother about proper breast latching is an important action but it is not the first action.
4. Tickling the baby's lips with the mother's nipple is an important action but it is not the first action.

TEST-TAKING HINT: When establishing priorities, it is essential that the most important action be taken first. Even though the question discusses breastfeeding, the feeding method is irrelevant to the scenario. The most important action is to check the identity of the mother and baby to make sure that the correct baby has been taken to the correct mother.

63. 1. Breastfed babies usually regain their birth weights by about day 10.
2. Rarely do babies sleep through the night by 4 weeks of age.

3. By 1 week of age, breastfed babies should have three to four bright yellow stools in every 24-hour period, although some babies do stool more frequently.
4. **By 1 week of age, breastfed babies should be urinating at least six times in every 24-hour period.**

TEST-TAKING HINT: The test taker must avoid answering questions based on their personal experience. For example, although the test-taker's baby may have slept through the night at 4 weeks of age, this should not be an expectation given to clients. Even bottle-fed babies usually awaken for feeds during the night for several weeks or months after the birth.

64. Answers 1, 4, and 5 require follow up by the nurse.

1. **This requires follow up. The mother will be very uncomfortable if she must lean forward during the entire feeding, which could take up to half an hour. She might either give up breastfeeding altogether, or shorten the feedings.**
2. This is the ideal position, tummy-to-tummy at the level of the mother's breast. Because the neonate's mouth muscles are relatively weak, it is important for the baby to be placed at the level of the breast. If the baby is placed lower, they are likely to "slip to the tip" of the nipple and cause nipple abrasions. In addition, babies must face the breast for effective feeding because they cannot swallow when their heads are turned.
3. This process does not require follow up. To achieve an effective latch of both the nipple and the areolar tissue, the baby must have a wide-open mouth.
4. **This requires follow up. A baby whose nose is pointed toward the mother's nipple is not in good alignment. Babies latch best when they are positioned at the breast, in preparation to opening their mouths, with their *chins* pointed toward their mothers' nipples.**
5. **This requires follow up. The baby's tongue must be below and surrounding the nipple to achieve effective suckling. This is not possible if the baby's tongue is pointed toward the roof of its mouth, leaving the space under the tongue for the nipple.**

TEST-TAKING HINT: The NCLEX does not ask negative questions, such as "what should not be done?" However, some questions are phrased as in this question, by asking, "What requires follow-up?" To answer the question, the test-taker must first identify which answers reflect the standard of care, or best practice. Answers that do not meet the standard or recommendations require follow up.

65.
1. This is good news. Unless the nipples have been damaged extensively, once babies are latched correctly, pain usually subsides.
2. This is a good sign. Audible swallowing is an excellent indicator of breastfeeding success.
3. Slow, rhythmic jaw movement is an indicator of breastfeeding success.
4. **Babies whose cheeks move in and out during feeds are attempting to use negative pressure to extract the milk from the breasts. This action is not an indicator of breastfeeding success.**

TEST-TAKING HINT: This question refers to the last phase of the nursing process—evaluation. When doing a breastfeeding evaluation, the nurse should apply the principles of successful breastfeeding—audible swallowing, rhythmic jaw extrusion, and pain-free feeding.

66. Answers 1 and 4 are correct.

1. **Until the mother's breastmilk is successfully established and the baby is showing signs of weight gain, the parents should count the number of wet and soiled diapers the baby has throughout every day to determine that the baby is consuming sufficient quantities of breast milk.**
2. There is no physical way to measure breastfeeding intake unless the baby is weighed immediately before and immediately after feeds. This action is not routinely recommended.
3. To promote milk production, it is recommended that babies breastfeed at each feeding until at least 1 month of age.
4. **The baby should be seen by the primary healthcare provider within a few days of discharge and at regular intervals.**
5. Breastfeedings should not be timed. Some babies are rapid eaters, whereas others eat more slowly. The baby should decide when they have finished a feeding.

TEST-TAKING HINT: All babies should be seen by the primary healthcare provider at 3 to 5 days of age to assess for the presence of jaundice, dehydration, or other complications. Because most babies are discharged on day 2 of life, they need to be taken to the primary healthcare provider within 3 days of discharge.

67. **1. When the mother is anxious, overly fatigued, and/or in pain, the secretion of oxytocin is inhibited, and this, in turn, inhibits the milk ejection reflex and insufficient milk may be consumed.**
2. If a baby is suckling effectively at the breast, the baby will swallow breast milk even after 10 minutes.
3. The cross-cradle hold is one of the recommended breastfeeding positions.
4. Ideally, the baby's chin should touch the underside of the mother's breast.

TEST-TAKING HINT: The breast is never empty of milk. Even if the baby has suckled for a long period of time, the baby will still be able to extract milk from the breast. The role of oxytocin in breastfeeding is of primary importance and should be fully understood.

68. **1. It has been shown that bottle-fed babies are at higher risk for obesity than breastfed babies. One of the reasons is the insistence by some mothers that the baby finish the formula in a bottle even if the baby initially rejects it. The increased calorie intake leads to increased weight gain.**
2. Bottle-fed babies usually feed every 3 to 4 hours.
3. All formulas for full-term babies supply the same number of calories per ounce.
4. It is recommended that bottle-fed babies burp every 1/2 to 1 ounce when they are very young.

TEST-TAKING HINT: The feeding patterns of bottle-fed and breastfed babies are different. Bottle feeding mothers should be strongly encouraged to allow their babies to determine how much formula they wish to consume at each feeding.

69. 1. It is expected that the baby will feed 8 to 12 times a day.
2. It is expected that the baby will void a minimum of 6 to 10 times a day.
3. Breastfed babies' stools are watery and yellow in color.
4. **If the baby has yellow sclerae, the baby is exhibiting signs of jaundice and the primary healthcare provider should be contacted.**

TEST-TAKING HINT: When nurses discharge patients with their newborns the nurses must provide anticipatory guidance regarding hyperbilirubinemia. Jaundice is the characteristic skin color of a baby with elevated bilirubin. The parents must be taught to notify their primary healthcare provider if the baby is jaundiced because high levels of bilirubin are neurotoxic.

70. **7.19%**

To determine how many grams the baby has lost, subtract the new weight from the birth weight:

$$\begin{array}{r} 3{,}278 \\ -3{,}042 \\ \hline 236 \end{array}$$ grams of weight loss

Then, to determine the percentage of weight loss, divide the difference by the original weight and multiply by 100%:

$$\frac{236}{3{,}278} = 0.0719$$

$$0.0719 \times 100 = 7.19\%$$

TEST-TAKING HINT: To calculate percentage of weight loss, which is needed in a variety of clinical settings as well as in the neonatal nursery, the nurse must subtract the new weight from the old weight, divide the difference by the old weight, and then multiply the result by 100%.

71. 1. The "en face" position is an ideal position for interacting with a baby who is in the quiet alert behavioral state but not to encourage a baby to open wide for feeding.
2. Although sometimes needed, it is not routinely recommended that mothers push down on their baby's lower jaw to encourage the baby to open his or her mouth for feeding. Sometimes this action has the opposite effect.
3. **Tickling the baby's lips with the nipple is the recommended method of encouraging a baby to open his or her mouth for feeding.**
4. Bottles should not be used to entice babies to breastfeed. Expressing breast milk onto the baby's lips may encourage the baby to open wide.

TEST-TAKING HINT: The "en face" position is not the best preamble to breastfeeding.

72. 1. Babies digest cereal poorly before the age of 4 to 6 months.
2. **This is the correct response.**
3. It is recommended that babies receive breast milk at all feedings. When formula feeds are substituted, breastfeeding success is often compromised.
4. Apple juice is added to the diet when recommended by the primary healthcare provider, usually after cereals have been introduced.

TEST-TAKING HINT: Common beliefs must be separated from scientific fact. Although many grandmothers strongly encourage the addition of solids early in a baby's diet, it is important for the nurse to provide the parents with up-to-date information followed by a rationale. It is recommended that solid foods not be introduced into a baby's diet until the baby is 4 months, to preferably, 6 months of age. The rationale for this recommendation relates to allowing the baby to benefit from maternal breastmilk as long as possible. The benefits include reducing the risk of obesity, diabetes, respiratory and ear infections, improving the baby's immune system through maternal antibodies in the breast milk, reducing allergies, and so forth (AAP, 2012). Some studies have shown no difference in newborn sleep patterns related to solid foods.

73. 1. Although it is recommended that the mother stop smoking, breastfeeding is not contraindicated when the mother smokes.
2. This is true. The baby received nicotine from the mother's blood during the pregnancy. Breastfeeding can prevent the newborn from suffering nicotine withdrawal. However, the mother should be advised to avoid smoking while holding the baby and while breastfeeding.
3. Maternal smoking does not warrant a report to child protective services.
4. This statement is not true. There is no evidence to show that women who smoke at the time they deliver have a high incidence of illicit drug use.

TEST-TAKING HINT: Nurses must not make assumptions about client behavior. Even though smoking is discouraged because of the serious health risks associated with the addiction, it is a legal act. It is best for the nurse to promote behaviors that will mitigate the negative impact of smoking. Breastfeeding the baby is one of those behaviors, as is encouraging the mother to refrain from smoking inside the house and, even more importantly, when in direct contact with the baby. Because the benefits of breastmilk are higher than the risk of small amounts of nicotine the baby receives through the milk and because these small amounts of nicotine may reduce the discomfort of nicotine withdrawal for the baby, the AAP does not discourage breastfeeding by mothers who smoke (AAP, 2013).

74. 1. This statement is accurate. The baby has already been exposed to the chickenpox, including during the prodromal period. The baby received passive antibodies through the placenta and is now receiving antibodies via the breast milk.
2. The baby has already been exposed and has received antibodies through the placenta and breastmilk. Therefore, there is no need to remove the baby from the home.
3. Chickenpox is highly contagious via droplet and contact routes. Good handwashing can reduce transmission, but cannot prevent it.
4. Chickenpox is not a spirochetal illness; it is transmitted via the herpes zoster virus.

TEST-TAKING HINT: One of the important clues to answering this question is the age of the baby. Antibodies passed by passive immunity are usually evident in the neonatal system for at least 3 months. Because this baby is only 2 weeks old, the antibodies should protect the baby. Plus, because the baby is breastfeeding, the baby is receiving added protection.

75. 1. This is true. The baby must be at the level of the breast to feed effectively.
2. In the cross-cradle position, the baby's head is in the mother's hand. This position is different from the more familiar cradle position. It requires a pillow or breastfeeding support for the baby. The mother uses one hand to bring the baby's head to her breast, and the other hand to compress the breast to fit the shape of the baby's mouth.
3. The baby should be positioned facing the mother—"tummy-to-tummy."
4. The baby should be brought to the mother rather than the mother moving her body to the baby.

TEST-TAKING HINT: Even if the nurse is unfamiliar with the cross-cradle position, making sure that the baby is at the level of the breast is one of the important principles for successfully breastfeeding a neonate. "Tummy-to-tummy" positioning and having the baby brought to the mother rather than vice versa are also important.

76. 1. Breastfeeding should be instituted as soon as possible to promote milk production, stability of the baby's glucose levels, and meconium excretion, as well as to stabilize the baby's temperature through skin-to-skin contact.
2. Although the baby will eventually need to be dressed in a shirt and diaper, skin-to-skin contact—baby's naked chest against mother's naked body—facilitates successful breastfeeding and newborn temperature regulation.

3. Ophthalmic prophylaxis should be delayed until after the first feeding. The drops/ointment can impact bonding by impairing the baby's vision.
4. Skin-to-skin contact with the mother during breastfeeding effectively stabilizes neonatal temperatures.

TEST-TAKING HINT: Unless the health of the baby is compromised, one of the first actions that should be made after delivery is placing the baby skin-to-skin at the breast, with a warm blanket covering both mother and baby. The baby's temperature will normalize, and the baby will receive needed nourishment from the colostrum.

77. 1. This baby has lost only 3.7% of its birth weight—100/2,678 × 100% = 3.7%. The accepted weight loss is 5% to 10% and this is not even there yet.
2. There is no need to supplement this baby's feeds.
3. The weight loss is not excessive.
4. Dextrose water is not recommended for babies.

TEST-TAKING HINT: To answer this question, the test taker can either estimate the maximum accepted weight loss for this baby or calculate the exact weight loss for this baby. The calculation is shown in the answer above. The best way to "estimate" the accepted weight loss is to multiply the birth weight by 0.1 to calculate a 10% weight loss (2,678 × 0.1 = 267.8 g) and then to divide 267.8 by 2 (267.8 ÷ 2 = 133.9 g) to calculate the 5% weight loss. A 100-gram loss is below both figures.

78. 1. Babies with short frenulums—tongue-tied babies—are unable to extend their tongues enough to form a trough and achieve a sufficient grasp. Painful and damaged nipples often result.
2. The baby's tongue should be troughed to feed effectively.
3. This is, on average, the feeding pattern of breastfed babies.
4. Babies should latch to both the nipple and areola.

TEST-TAKING HINT: If the term "frenulum" is not familiar to the test taker, the nurse who understands normal breastfeeding behaviors can figure out that the first answer is the best option. Anything attached to the tip of the baby's tongue can cause problems with breastfeeding because the baby cannot position the tongue properly.

79. 1. This response acknowledges the client's feelings but it does not provide her with the information she needs regarding alcohol consumption and breastfeeding.
2. Alcohol is not restricted during the postpartum period.
3. Alcohol is found in the breast milk in exactly the same concentration as in the mother's blood. Because of this, the woman should breastfeed immediately *before* consuming a drink and then wait 1 to 2 hours to metabolize the drink before feeding again. If she decides to have more than one drink, she can pump and dump her milk for a feeding or two.
4. Alcohol consumption is not incompatible with breastfeeding, but the woman should try to avoid breastfeeding within 1 to 2 hours after drinking. This will avoid transfer of the alcohol and metabolites to the baby.

TEST-TAKING HINT: In relation to alcohol consumption, the transfer of possibly harmful substances to the baby through breastfeeding is different from the transfer of harmful substances before birth, through the placenta. The difference is that the newborn is at the breast intermittently, not continually.

While in utero, the placenta was consistently transferring substances from the mother to the baby so there was no way to reduce the risk during the pregnancy. With breastfeeding, the alcohol can be consumed after the feeding so it is metabolized in time before the next breastfeeding. In this way, the baby receives very little alcohol and metabolites. The mother can be educated to consume alcohol in moderation and with some minor restrictions and guidelines. It is best, however, to avoid all alcohol when breastfeeding.

80. 1. Most medications are safely consumed by the breastfeeding mother. To blindly follow this order is poor practice.
2. Ultimately, this probably will be the nurse's action but they must have a rationale for questioning the order.
3. It is unacceptable to completely ignore an order even though the nurse may disagree with the order.
4. Once the reference has been consulted, the nurse will have factual information to relay to the physician—specifically that ampicillin is compatible with breastfeeding. A call to the doctor would then be appropriate.

TEST-TAKING HINT: Nurses are not only responsible for instituting the orders made

by physicians and other primary healthcare providers; they also have independent practice for which they are accountable. In this scenario, the nurse is accountable to the client. Because the medication is compatible with breastfeeding, but the physician was apparently unaware of that fact, it is the nurse's responsibility to convey that information to the doctor and to advocate for the client. The National Institutes of Health (NIH) has created a Web site—LactMed—where the potential danger of medications during lactation can be checked. There also is a free app that nurses can download to their mobile phones (NIH, n.d.-a).

81. 1. **Breastfeeding is contraindicated when a woman is receiving chemotherapy.**
    2. Neither the medical problem—in this case, cholecystitis—nor the planned surgery precludes breastfeeding. The mother may have to "pump and dump" a few feedings depending on the short-term medications that she will receive, but, ultimately, she will still be able to breastfeed.
    3. Breastfeeding is not contraindicated with a diagnosis of a concussion. Again, the mother may have to "pump and dump" a few feedings if she must take any incompatible short-term medications, but, ultimately, she will still be able to breastfeed.
    4. Breastfeeding is not contraindicated with a diagnosis of thrombosis. Again, the mother may have to "pump and dump" a few feedings if she must take any incompatible short-term medications, but, ultimately, she will still be able to breastfeed.

TEST-TAKING HINT: By and large, mothers who wish to breastfeed should be enthusiastically encouraged to do so. It is the responsibility of the nurse to make sure that any medications that the woman is taking are compatible with breastfeeding. A reliable source should be consulted, such as LactMed (NIH, n.d.-a) or Hale and Rowe (2014). In addition, it is the nurse's responsibility to advocate for breastfeeding mothers who must undergo surgery or who are diagnosed with acute illnesses that are compatible with breastfeeding.

82. 1. The woman does not have to consume three glasses of milk per day.
    2. It is unnecessary for the mother to consume any dairy products.
    3. **Dairy foods provide protein and other nutrients, including the important mineral calcium. The calcium can, however, be obtained from a number of other foods, such as broccoli and fish with bones.**
    4. Protein can be obtained from many other foods, including meat, poultry, rice, legumes, and eggs.

TEST-TAKING HINT: Breast milk is synthesized in the glandular tissue of the mother from the raw materials in the mother's bloodstream. There is, therefore, no need for the mother to consume milk as long as she receives the needed nutrients in another manner. Calcium-rich, non-dairy food items as well as calcium supplements, if needed, can provide the needed mineral.

83. 1. **There are no foods that are absolutely contraindicated during lactation. Some babies may react to certain foods, but this must be determined on a case-by-case basis.**
    2. Food restrictions such as sushi are lifted once the baby is born.
    3. Some babies may be bothered by gas-producing foods, but this is not universal.
    4. Some babies may be bothered by hot and spicy foods, but this is not universal.

TEST-TAKING HINT: There is a popular belief that mothers who breastfeed must restrict their eating habits. This is not true. In fact, it is important for the test taker to realize that breastfed babies often are less fussy eaters because the flavor of breast milk changes depending on the mother's diet. Mothers should be encouraged to have a varied diet, and only if their baby appears to react to a certain food should it be eliminated from the diet.

84. 1. Stools in breastfed babies are bright yellow and loose. In bottle-fed babies, they are brownish and pasty.
    2. To prevent aspiration, bottle nipples should not be enlarged.
    3. Microwaving can overheat the formula, causing burns.
    4. **To minimize the ingestion of large quantities of air, the bottle should be held so that the nipple is always filled with formula.**

TEST-TAKING HINT: It is important for the nurse to teach parents never to place formula in the microwave for warming. This is a safety issue. The microwave does not change the composition of the formula, but it can overheat the fat globules in the formula, resulting in severe burns in the baby's mouth.

85. 1. This baby's mouth is pursed. The baby seems to be chewing on the nipple and may cause nipple damage.
2. This baby's head is lower than its body. Swallowing will be required to go uphill, which may lead to choking.
3. This baby's mouth is also pursed, and is not spread around the nipple. This can also cause nipple damage.
4. This baby is latched well.

TEST-TAKING HINT: It is important for the test-taker to not only be able to choose a correct answer from a word description but also to be able to assess a mother–infant dyad and determine whether or not the breastfeeding positioning is ideal. In the picture below, the baby's mouth is open wide, covering the breast as well as the nipple, and the baby's lips are flanged.

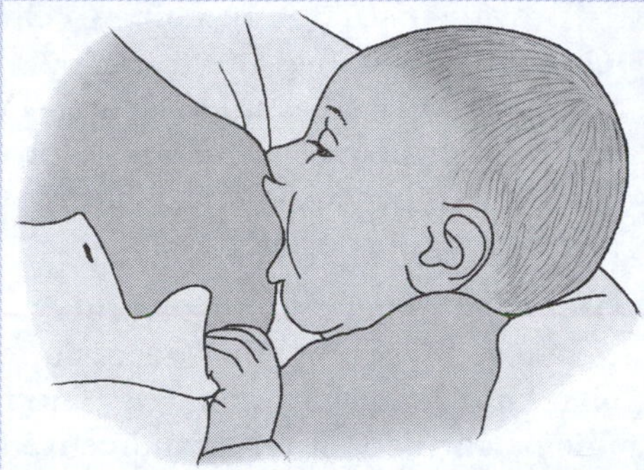

86. **1. Soft rales are expected because babies born via cesarean section do not have the advantage of having the amniotic fluid squeezed from the pulmonary system as occurs during a vaginal birth.**
2. The bowel sounds should be normal.
3. The Moro reflex should be normal.
4. Babies in the LMA position are not at high risk for developmental dysplasia of the hip. Breech babies are at high risk for DDH.

TEST-TAKING HINT: Cesarean section (C/S) babies often respond differently in the immediate postdelivery period than babies born vaginally. Remembering that one of the triggers for neonatal respirations is the mechanical compression of the thorax, which results in the forced expulsion of amniotic fluid from the baby's lungs, is important here. Because C/S babies do not traverse the birth canal, they do not have the benefit of that compression.

87. 1. Melanin production is not related to the presence of BAT.
2. Babies do not shiver. Rather, to produce heat, they utilize chemical thermogenesis, also called non-shivering thermogenesis. BAT is metabolized during hypothermic episodes to maintain body temperature. Unfortunately, this can lead to metabolic acidosis if prolonged.
3. BAT is unrelated to injury prevention.
4. Sufficient calories for growth are provided from breast milk or formula.

TEST-TAKING HINT: Neonates have immature thermoregulatory systems. To compensate for their inability to shiver to produce heat, full-term babies have BAT stores that were laid down during the latter part of the third trimester. Preterm babies, however, do not have sufficient BAT stores.

88. 1. This is a description of pathologic jaundice resulting from maternal–fetal blood incompatibilities.
2. With lung oxygenation, the neonate no longer needs large numbers of red blood cells. As a result, excess red blood cells are destroyed. Jaundice often results on days 2 to 4.
3. There is nothing in the scenario to suggest that this was a traumatic delivery.
4. There is nothing in the scenario to suggest that meconium excretion was delayed.

TEST-TAKING HINT: One of the important clues in this question is the age of the baby. The timing of jaundice is very important. Physiologic jaundice, seen in a large number of neonates, is observed after the first 24 hours. Pathologic jaundice, a much more serious problem, is seen during the first 24 hours. For more information on jaundice, see the appendix.

89. 1. Healthy babies are able to absorb fat-soluble vitamins.
2. Vitamin K is synthesized in the gut in the presence of normal flora.
3. It takes about 1 week for the baby to be able to synthesize vitamin K. The gut, at birth, is sterile.
4. Vitamin K has no function in relation to the development of pathologic jaundice.

TEST-TAKING HINT: It is important for the test taker to review how vitamin K is synthesized by the intestinal flora. Because the neonate is deficient in intestinal flora until 1 week of age, the baby is unable to manufacture vitamin K until that time. Phytonadione is important, especially for babies who will be circumcised, because it is needed to activate coagulation factors synthesized in the liver.

90. 1. Breast milk contains sufficient quantities of vitamin A.
2. Breast milk contains sufficient quantities of vitamin B12.

3. Breast milk contains sufficient quantities of vitamin C.
4. **Many babies are vitamin D deficient because of the recommendation that they be kept out of direct sunlight to protect their skin from sunburn. For this reason, supplementation with vitamin D is recommended.**

TEST-TAKING HINT: Breast milk is sufficient in vitamins and minerals for the healthy full-term baby. The AAP recommends that babies be supplemented with 400 international units of vitamin D per day (Casey et al., 2010).

91. 1. The therapeutic action of vitamin K is not related to skin color.
2. The therapeutic action of vitamin K is not related to vital signs.
3. The therapeutic action of vitamin K is not related to glucose levels.
4. **Vitamin K is needed for adequate blood clotting.**

TEST-TAKING HINT: It is essential that the nurse be familiar with the actions, normal dosages, recommended routes, and so on, of all standard medications administered to the neonate.

92. 1. The ophthalmic preparation is administered to prevent ophthalmia neonatorum, which is caused by gonorrhea and/or chlamydial infections. It is not given to prevent cataracts.
2. **This is the correct method of instillation of the ophthalmic prophylaxis.**
3. The medication can be delayed until the baby has had its first feeding and has begun the bonding process.
4. Ophthalmic prophylaxis is given to all neonates at birth whether or not their mothers are positive for gonorrhea.

TEST-TAKING HINT: The eye prophylaxis clouds the vision of the neonate. Even though it is state law in all 50 of the United States that the medication be given, it is best to delay the instillation of the medication for an hour or so after birth so that eye contact and parent–infant bonding can occur during the immediate post-uterine period.

93. 1. Although this is a true statement, it does not provide a rationale for the medication administration.
2. **This response gives the mother a brief scientific rationale for the medication administration.**
3. This response is too vague.
4. Although this is a true statement, it does not provide a rationale for the medication administration.

TEST-TAKING HINT: When asked a direct question by a client, it is important for the nurse to give as complete a response as possible. Trite responses like "All babies receive the medication at birth" do not provide information to the client. It is the right of all clients to receive accurate and complete information about their own treatments and, because the neonate is a dependent, the parents have the right to receive accurate and complete information about their baby's treatments or to refuse treatments.

94. 1. With training, unlicensed personnel are able to take newborn vital signs.
2. With training, unlicensed personnel are able to take newborn vital signs.
3. With training, unlicensed personnel are able to obtain stool specimens.
4. **It is the registered nurse's responsibility to provide discharge teaching to clients. Only the RN knows the scientific rationales as well as the teaching–learning principles necessary to provide accurate information and answer questions appropriately.**

TEST-TAKING HINT: There are important differences between actions that necessitate professional knowledge and skill and actions that may be performed either by unlicensed personnel or by licensed practical nurses. Patient teaching is a task that the registered nurse cannot delegate.

95. 1. **Red blood cells in the cephalohematoma will have to be broken down and excreted. The by-product of the destruction—bilirubin—increases the baby's risk for jaundice.**
2. A caput is merely a collection of edematous fluid. There is no relation between the presence of a caput and jaundice.
3. Harlequin coloration is related to the dilation of blood vessels on one side of the baby's body. There is no relation between the presence of harlequin coloring and jaundice.
4. Mongolian spots are hyperpigmented areas primarily seen on the buttocks. There is no relation between the presence of mongolian spots and jaundice.

TEST-TAKING HINT: During the early newborn period, whenever a situation exists that results in the breakdown of red blood cells, the baby is at high risk for hyperbilirubinemia and resulting jaundice. In this case, the baby is at high risk from a cephalohematoma, a collection of blood

between the skull and the periosteal membrane. In addition, the neonate is at high risk for hyperbilirubinemia because of the immaturity of the newborn liver.

96. 1. Excessive crying is not a symptom of hyperbilirubinemia.
2. Babies often feed poorly when their bilirubin levels are elevated.
3. **Lethargy is one of the most common early symptoms of hyperbilirubinemia.**
4. Hyperreflexia is seen with prolonged periods of markedly elevated serum bilirubin.

TEST-TAKING HINT: The nurse should be familiar with the normal bilirubin values of the healthy full-term baby as well as those values that may result in kernicterus—a disease characterized by an infiltration of bilirubin into neural tissue. When bilirubin levels rise, babies will exhibit some neurological depression, such as lethargy and poor feeding. When levels are markedly elevated, permanent brain damage can result.

97. 1. **When bilirubin levels elevate to toxic levels, babies can develop kernicterus.**
2. Erythroblastosis fetalis is a syndrome resulting from the antigen–antibody reaction related to maternal–fetal blood incompatibility.
3. This bilirubin level is above the level most primary healthcare providers consider acceptable for discharge.
4. Phototherapy is ordered when hyperbilirubinemia is present or when the development of hemolytic jaundice is very likely.

TEST-TAKING HINT: This question asks the test-taker to identify a client care goal for a newborn with physiologic jaundice. The client care goal reflects the nurse's desired patient care outcome. The development of kernicterus is a potential pathological outcome resulting from hyperbilirubinemia. The client care goal, therefore, is that the neonate not develop kernicterus.

98. 1. **These findings are all within normal limits.**
2. There is no indication that this child has developed any signs of kernicterus, which is associated with opisthotonic posturing.
3. The mother is Rh-positive. Only mothers who are Rh-negative and who deliver babies who are Rh-positive receive RhoGAM.
4. The bilirubin level is very low. There is no indication that phototherapy is needed.

TEST-TAKING HINT: Blood incompatibilities are seen when the mother is Rh-negative (Rh-) and the baby is Rh-positive or when the mother is type O and the baby is either type A or type B. When the baby is either Rh- or type O, there is actually a reduced risk that pathologic jaundice will result. For more information on ABO incompatibility see the appendix.

99. 1. With the baby in the en face position, the father is holding the baby "face to face" so that he is looking directly into the baby's eyes.
2. Parents who call their babies by name, whether full or nickname, are exhibiting one sign of positive bonding.
3. **A father who expects his partner to quiet a crying baby may not be accepting or may be fearful of accepting the parenting role.**
4. Although this may not be the safest position for a baby to be sleeping in, the father is showing a sign of positive bonding.

TEST-TAKING HINT: This question should be read carefully. The question is not asking about safe sleep practices—although the nurse should discuss safe sleep practices with this father. Rather, the question is asking about evidence of poor bonding.

100. 1. **Babies learn to speak by imitating the speech of others in their environment. If they are hearing impaired, there is a likelihood of delayed speech development.**
2. Otitis externa is an inflammation of the ear canal outside of the eardrum. It is often called "swimmer's ear."
3. Parents bond well with babies who are deaf. As a matter of fact, parents are often unaware that their babies have hearing deficits.
4. Choanal atresia is a congenital condition when the nasal passages are blocked. Babies who have choanal atresia often choke during feedings because they are not able to breathe through their noses.

TEST-TAKING HINT: It is important that the test-taker not be lured to an answer simply because the question includes an unfamiliar technical term, such as otitis externa or choanal atresia.

101. 1. Putting the baby's diapers on tightly will put pressure on the area and help to stop the bleeding, but it is not the first or best response.
2. **Putting direct pressure on the site is the best way to stop the bleeding.**
3. The nurse must first apply pressure and then notify the physician.
4. Only after performing first aid should the nurse assess the vital signs.

TEST-TAKING HINT: This is a prioritizing question. The nurse's first action must be to provide immediate first aid to best stop the bleeding. Then the nurse must obtain assistance and assess the baby's vital signs to see if they have deviated.

102. **1. The neonatal period is defined as the first 28 days of life. The neonatal mortality rate is defined as neonatal deaths per 1,000 live births. Therefore, five babies less than 28 days old per 1,000 live births died.**

2. The neonatal period is defined as the first 28 days of life, whereas the infancy period is defined as the period between birth and 1 year of life.
3. The neonatal mortality rate is defined as neonatal deaths per 1,000 live births, not per 100,000 live births.
4. The neonatal period is defined as the first 28 days of life, the infancy period is defined as the period between birth and 1 year of life, and the neonatal mortality rate is defined as neonatal deaths per 1,000 live births, not per 100,000 live births.

TEST-TAKING HINT: The term "neonatal" refers to the first 28 days of life. Therefore, answer options 2 and 4 can be eliminated. A neonatal death rate of 5 means that five babies less than 28 days old per 1,000 live births died. The ability to interpret statistical data enables the nurse to compare and contrast healthcare outcomes from state to state and country to country.

103. **Answers 1, 3, 4, and 5 are correct.**

1. **Small, frequent feedings reduce the symptoms of colic in some babies.**
2. The prone sleep position is not recommended for babies under 1 year of age.
3. **Some babies' symptoms have decreased when they were tightly swaddled.**
4. **This is called the colic hold. The position does help to soothe some colicky neonates.**
5. **Babies who live in an environment where adults smoke have a higher incidence of colic than babies who live in a smoke-free environment.**

TEST-TAKING HINT: It is essential to read each possible answer option carefully. Even though it has been shown that colicky babies sometimes find relief when they are placed prone on a hot water bottle, it is not recommended that the babies be left in that position for sleep. It is recommended that healthy babies, whether colicky or not, be placed in the prone position only while awake and while supervised.

104. 1. Breastfeeding does not prevent the development of plagiocephaly nor does it promote gross motor development.

2. Vaccinations do not prevent the development of plagiocephaly nor do they promote gross motor development.
3. Changing the baby's diapers will not prevent the development of plagiocephaly nor will it promote gross motor development.
4. **As a result of sleeping on their backs, and spending long periods of time in this supine position, the backs of babies' heads may be flattened (plagiocephaly). When the baby is awake and under adult supervision, however, it can be in the prone position safely. Being placed in the prone position while awake helps to prevent plagiocephaly and allows babies to practice gross motor skills like rolling over.**

TEST-TAKING HINT: Even if the exact definition of plagiocephaly is unknown, the test taker can surmise that the word is related to the skull because the term "cephalic" or "cephaly" pertains to the head. Neither breastfeeding, nor vaccinations, nor diaper changing is related to head development.

105. 1. The neonate should be placed in a rear-facing car seat.

2. **A bilirubin of 19 mg/dL (324.9 µmol/L) is above the expected level. Therapeutic intervention is needed.**
3. A blood glucose level of 65 mg/dL (3.6 mmol/L) is within normal levels for a neonate.
4. Mongolian spots are normal variations seen on the neonatal skin.

TEST-TAKING HINT: The bilirubin level of 19 mg/dL (324.0 µmol/L) is well above normal, and because bilirubin levels peak on day 3 to 5, it is likely that the level will rise even higher. Because it is likely that a therapeutic intervention, such as phototherapy, will be ordered for this baby, the baby should not be discharged, and the primary healthcare provider should be notified of the bilirubin level.

106. 1. Sleeping with a sibling has been shown to put babies at high risk for SIDS.

2. Sleeping in an adult bed has been shown to put babies at high risk for SIDS.
3. **A large empty drawer has a firm bottom so that the baby is unlikely to re-breathe his or her own carbon dioxide and the sides of the drawer will prevent the baby from falling out of "bed."**
4. Pull-out sofas have been shown to put babies at high risk for SIDS.

TEST-TAKING HINT: Creative strategies are sometimes required to meet the needs of clients with limited assets. When compared with the other three responses, the empty drawer provides the baby with the safest possible environment. The nurse should also refer this mother and baby to a social worker for assistance.

107. 1. Males are rarely newborn abductors.
2. Females who abduct neonates are often overweight. They rarely appear underweight.
3. Pro-life advocates have not been shown to be high risk for neonatal abduction.
4. Abductors usually choose newborns of their same race.

TEST-TAKING HINT: An abductor of a newborn is usually a female who is unable to have a child of her own. Because she wishes to have her own child, she targets babies who are similar in appearance to her.

108. Answers 2, 3, 4, and 5 are correct.
1. Abductors usually plan their strategies carefully before taking the baby.
2. A common diversion is pulling the fire alarm to distract the staff.
3. Those who are inquisitive about where babies are at different times of the day may be planning an abduction.
4. Rooms near stairwells provide the abductor with a quick and easy get-away.
5. The abductor is able to hide a baby under oversized clothing or in large bags.

TEST-TAKING HINT: The nurse should be familiar with the many characteristics of the typical neonatal abductor. In addition to those cited above, individuals who are emotionally immature, suffer from low self-esteem, and have a history of manipulative behavior may attempt infant abduction.

109. 1. Newborn infants typically consume 2 to 3 ounces of formula every 3 to 4 hours during the first month of life.
2. The nurse should provide the mother with guidance regarding the typical amounts babies consume during the early neonatal period.
3. Most infants will consume 4 ounces or more per feeding at about 1 month of age.
4. Formula fed babies typically sleep between 3 and 4 hours after each feeding. The mother should not expect the baby always to sleep 4 hours at a stretch.

TEST-TAKING HINT: Although it is important to inform parents about the quantity of formula they should expect their baby to consume, it is just as important to advise them that their baby will likely consume slightly different amounts at each feeding. They should follow their baby's lead in order not to underfeed or overfeed their child.

110. 1. This statement is incorrect. The critical congenital heart defect (CCHD) screen is performed on all neonates.
2. It is correct to advise the parent that the screening test is performed on all neonates, but it is ill-advised to inform the client that the baby has no defects. That may not be true.
3. This statement is true. The test is administered to all neonates prior to discharge.
4. This statement is incorrect. The test is not performed following the appearance of symptoms. It is a screening test performed on all neonates.

TEST-TAKING HINT: Almost 2% of all babies are born with a congenital heart defect. They can be life threatening, requiring early intervention. Unfortunately, many of the defects are undetected during prenatal ultrasounds. In addition, many babies with defects exhibit no apparent symptoms in the early neonatal period. They only become ill after discharge from the hospital. The CCHD screen is performed to identify those babies who may have an undiagnosed congenital heart defect (AAP, n.d.).

111. Answers 3 and 5 are correct.
1. Parental consent is not needed for the CCHD screen.
2. Pulse oximetry is assessed during a CCHD screen; an electrocardiogram is not performed.
3. This statement is correct. To prevent false-negative results, the test is performed after the baby is at least 24 hours old.
4. During the CCHD screen, heart rate fluctuations are not assessed or recorded.
5. This statement is correct. A positive screen is defined as a difference of 3 percentage points between the pulse oximetry reading on the neonate's right hand and the reading on the right foot.

TEST-TAKING HINT: The CCHD screen is mandated to be performed on all neonates who are at least 24 hours old in order to identify those babies with undiagnosed cyanotic cardiac defects (AAP, n.d.).

7 Normal Postpartum

The postpartum period begins immediately after the delivery of the placenta and lasts until the uterus has returned to its fully involuted state, about 6 weeks later. The first hour after delivery is often referred to as the fourth stage of labor, and might seem more appropriate in the labor and delivery chapter. However, questions about the fourth stage of labor have been included in this chapter because the assessments and concerns of that hour relate more directly to the postpartum period as breastfeeding is established, fundal checks begin, and the client adjusts to being a mother of one or more children. If this is her first child, she might be referred to as a *nullipara during labor, and a primipara after the baby is born*; if it is her second child or more, she is a *multipara*. Each of these parities brings its own unique risks and concerns.

The postpartum nurse must be vigilant in monitoring the mother's physiological adjustment to the nonpregnant state, whether the client delivered vaginally or via cesarean section. Sharing benchmarks and information about these physiological changes with the client can assist her in making the needed adjustments to this new stage of life.

Equally important to the physiological adjustments are the emotional adjustments to parenthood. The responsibilities of mothering are challenging and unique to each client. They are different than the physiological and hormonal readjustments of the body to the nonpregnant state, which are fairly predictable. Educational goals for the client must include self-care needs and baby care (see Chapter 6, Normal Newborn). A gentle word of warning to the mother about the often unexpected but normal burden of fatigue and emotional stress she may feel is warranted. The postpartum nurse is a resource and coach who plays an important part in the success of each newly created or expanded family unit.

KEYWORDS

The following words include English vocabulary, nursing/medical terminology, concepts, principles, or information relevant to content specifically addressed in the chapter or associated with topics presented in it. English dictionaries, your nursing textbooks, and medical dictionaries such as *Taber's Cyclopedic Medical Dictionary* are resources that can be used to expand your knowledge and understanding of these words and related information.

Cesarean section
Complementary therapy
Diaphoresis
Discharge teaching
Docusate sodium
Engorgement
Epidural anesthesia
Episiotomy
Forceps delivery
Fourth stage of labor
Fundal assessment
Homans sign
Kegel exercises
Laceration (1°, 2°, 3°, and 4°)
"Letting go" phase
Lochia (rubra, serosa, alba)
Methylergonovine
Multipara
Narcotic analgesia
Nonimmune
Nullipara
Patient-controlled analgesia (PCA)
Postnatal post-traumatic stress disorder
Postpartum
Postpartum blues
Postpartum depression

Postpartum exercises
Postpartum psychosis
Primipara
Puerperium
Puerperal fever
Quantitative blood loss
REEDA scale
Rubella vaccine
Sitz bath
Spinal anesthesia
Spontaneous vaginal delivery
"Taking hold" phase
"Taking in" phase
Vacuum extraction

QUESTIONS

CASE STUDY: *The first six questions below are part of an evolving case study. All six questions follow the Next Generation NCLEX® question format of six steps:*

1. Recognize cues—What matters most?
2. Analyze cues—What could it mean?
3. Prioritize hypotheses—Where do I start?
4. Generate solutions—What can I do?
5. Take action—What will I do?
6. Evaluate outcomes—Did it help?

(National Council of State Boards of Nursing [NCSBN], 2020). For more information on the Next Generation NCLEX (NGN) question formats, see NGN quarterly newsletters at https://www.ncsbn.org.
NCLEX questions assume the nurse has a provider's order for listed interventions, unless noted otherwise.

A 26-year-old G3 P3003 in the immediate postpartum phase who delivered approximately 1 hour ago calls the nurse into her room. The nurse has learned in report that the client's prenatal course was uncomplicated. She was induced at 41 weeks' gestation. She has a history of asthma. Her prenatal Hct was 32%. She was in labor for over 20 hours, had an epidural, and pushed for 3 hours. Eventually, she had an instrumented delivery with forceps over a 3rd degree episiotomy for a nonreassuring fetal heart rate. The baby was in the occiput posterior position. The baby weighed 9 lbs 14 oz (4,110 grams). After delivery, the placenta delivered spontaneously, and the episiotomy was repaired. Quantitative blood loss at the time of delivery was 490 mL. The client's lochia has been moderate and her fundus has been massaged to firm two times in the past hour.

The client's epidural catheter has been removed. She has not voided. She states that after sitting up and taking a few bites of a sandwich and a few sips of orange juice, she felt light-headed and lowered the head of the bed. She appears pale and is lying flat in bed, breathing slowly with her eyes closed. An intravenous infusion of 20 units oxytocin in 1,000 mL lactated ringer's solution is running at 50 mL/hour by pump.

1. **Recognize cues. What matters most?** Which of the following assessments requires **immediate** follow-up? **Select all that apply.**
   1. Light-headedness.
   2. Voiding.
   3. Fundal tone.
   4. Respirations.

2. **Analyze cues. What could it mean?** Based on a review of the client's medical history, obstetrical history, and reported symptoms, which of the following potential issues is the client at risk for developing? **Select all that apply.**
   1. Hyponatremia.
   2. Hematoma.
   3. Uterine atony.
   4. Vaginal wall laceration.
3. **Prioritize hypotheses. Where do I start?**

   Note: This is a two-part question. In the NCLEX exam, the test taker will have two drop-down boxes of four options each, from which to select an answer.

   The client is at highest risk for developing:
   1. Seizure.
   2. Dysrhythmia.
   3. Hemorrhage.
   4. Hypoxia.

   As evidenced by the client's:
   a. Fundal assessments.
   b. Respirations.
   c. Lethargy.
   d. Multiparity.
4. **Generate solutions. What can I do?** The nurse has determined that the client is at highest risk of uterine atony. Which of the following interventions is appropriate? **Select all that apply.**

Possible Nursing Intervention	(a) Indicated	(b) Nonessential	(c) Contraindicated
1. Fundal massage			
2. Encourage breastfeeding			
3. Increase oxytocin rate			
4. Ambulate to bathroom to void			
5. Catheterize client			
6. Initiate oxygen by mask			
7. Encourage the client to finish her meal			
8. Calculate intake and output			

5. **Take action. What will I do?** The nurse has completed fundal massage, and turned up the oxytocin rate to 125 mL/hour. The client voided 400 mL on the bedpan. Because there is little improvement in fundal tone, and because of the risk of the oxytocin receptors being full and unresponsive to the oxytocin, the nurse has administered the next medication on the order sheet, 0.2 mg methylergonovine IM. The nurse has paged the provider to call back stat and reviews the other uterotonic medication options on the provider's orders. Which medication is contraindicated for this client?
   1. Methylergonovine 0.2 mg IM q 2–4 hrs prn, up to 5 doses.
   2. Prostaglandin F2 Alpha, 250 mcg IM, repeat q 15–90 minutes prn, maximum 8 doses.
   3. Prostaglandin E2 suppositories 20 mg per rectum q 2 hrs prn.
   4. Misoprostol 1,000 mcg per rectum x1, prn.

6. **Evaluate outcomes. Did it help?** The obstetrical provider completed a bedside assessment an hour ago. On examination, she found no evidence of hematoma or vaginal wall laceration. The provider manually removed some clots from the lower uterine segment and returned to her office. The nurse administered misoprostol 1,000 mcg per rectum 30 minutes ago. The nurse is performing a follow-up assessment. Which signs would indicate declining and/or worsening status? **Select all that apply.**
   1. Reduced blood pressure.
   2. Reduced heart rate.
   3. Clammy skin.
   4. Confusion

7. A breastfeeding mother is preparing for discharge at 3 days postpartum. She is not immune to rubella and has signed a consent form to receive the rubella vaccine at discharge. Which of the following must the nurse include in the client's discharge teaching regarding the vaccine?
   1. The client should not become pregnant for at least 4 weeks.
   2. The client should pump and dump her breast milk for 1 week.
   3. Surgical masks must be worn by the mother when she holds the baby.
   4. Antibodies transported through the breast milk will protect the baby.

8. A client who delivered 3 days ago questions why she is to receive the rubella vaccine before leaving the hospital. Which of the following rationales should guide the nurse's response?
   1. The client's obstetric status is optimal for receiving the vaccine.
   2. The client's immune system is highly responsive during the postpartum period.
   3. The client's baby will be at high risk for acquiring rubella if the client does not receive the vaccine.
   4. The client's insurance company will pay for the shot if it is given during the immediate postpartum period.

9. A client with an obstetrical history of G2 P1102, who delivered her baby 8 hours ago, now has a temperature of 100.2° F (37.8° C). Which of the following is the appropriate nursing intervention at this time?
   1. Notify the doctor to get an order for acetaminophen.
   2. Request an infectious disease consult from the doctor.
   3. Provide the client with cool compresses.
   4. Encourage intake of water and other fluids.

10. To prevent infection, the nurse teaches postpartum clients to perform which of the following tasks?
    1. Apply antibiotic ointment to the perineum daily.
    2. Change the peripad at each voiding.
    3. Void at least every two hours.
    4. Spray the perineum with povidone-iodine after toileting.

11. A postpartum client who is breastfeeding is being assessed. She delivered 3 days ago. Her breasts are firm and warm to the touch. When asked when she last fed the baby her reply is, "I fed the baby last evening. I let the nurses feed him in the nursery last night. I needed to rest." Which of the following actions should the nurse take at this time?
    1. Explain the benefits of exclusive breastfeeding.
    2. Have the client massage her breasts hourly.
    3. Obtain an order to culture her expressed breast milk.
    4. Take the temperature and pulse rate of the client.

12. A breastfeeding client has been counseled on how to prevent engorgement. Which of the following actions by the mother shows that the teaching was effective?
    1. She pumps her breasts after each feeding.
    2. She feeds her baby every 2 to 3 hours.
    3. She feeds her baby 10 minutes on each side.
    4. She supplements each feeding with formula.
13. A breastfeeding client at 2 days postpartum states, "I am sick of being fat. When can I go on a diet?" Which of the following responses is appropriate?
    1. "It is fine for you to start dieting right now as long as you drink plenty of milk."
    2. "Your breast milk will be low in vitamins if you start to diet while breastfeeding."
    3. "You must eat at least 3,000 calories per day in order to produce enough milk for your baby."
    4. "Many mothers lose weight when they breastfeed because the baby consumes about 600 calories a day."
14. A client with an obstetrical history of G2 P2002 who had a spontaneous vaginal delivery 6 hours ago is assessed. The nurse notes that the fundus is firm at the umbilicus, there is heavy lochia rubra, and perineal sutures are intact. Which of the following actions should the nurse take at this time?
    1. Do nothing. This is a normal finding.
    2. Massage the client's fundus.
    3. Accompany the client to the bathroom to void.
    4. Notify the client's primary healthcare provider.
15. A client informs the nurse that she intends to bottle feed her baby. Which of the following actions should the nurse encourage the client to perform? **Select all that apply.**
    1. Increase her fluid intake for a few days.
    2. Massage her breasts every 4 hours.
    3. Apply heat packs to her axillae.
    4. Wear a supportive bra 24 hours a day.
    5. Stand with her back toward the shower water.
16. The nurse in the obstetric clinic received a telephone call from a bottle-feeding mother whose baby is 3 days old. The mother states that her breasts are firm, red, and warm to the touch. Which of the following is the best action for the nurse to advise the client to perform?
    1. Intermittently apply ice packs to her axillae and breasts.
    2. Apply lanolin to her breasts and nipples every 3 hours.
    3. Express milk from the breasts every 3 hours.
    4. Ask the primary healthcare provider to order a milk suppressant.
17. A multigravid, postpartum client reports severe abdominal cramping whenever she nurses her baby. Which of the following responses by the nurse is appropriate?
    1. Suggest that the client bottle feed for a few days.
    2. Instruct the client on how to massage her fundus.
    3. Instruct the client to feed using an alternate position.
    4. Discuss the action of breastfeeding hormones.
18. The nurse is caring for a breastfeeding mother who asks for advice on foods that will provide both vitamin A and iron. Which of the following should the nurse recommend?
    1. ½ cup raw celery dipped in 1 ounce cream cheese.
    2. 8 ounces yogurt mixed with 1 medium banana.
    3. 12 ounces strawberry milk shake.
    4. 1½ cups raw broccoli.

19. A breastfeeding mother states that she has sore nipples. In response to the complaint, the nurse assists with latching the baby and recommends that the mother do which of the following?
1. Use a nipple shield at each breastfeeding.
2. Cleanse the nipples with soap 3 times a day.
3. Rotate the baby's positions at each feed.
4. Bottle feed for 2 days and then resume breastfeeding.

20. Which of the following statements is true about breastfeeding mothers as compared to bottle-feeding mothers?
1. Breastfeeding mothers usually complete uterine involution completely by 3 weeks postpartum.
2. Breastfeeding mothers have decreased incidence of diabetes mellitus later in life.
3. Breastfeeding mothers show higher levels of bone density after menopause.
4. Breastfeeding mothers are prone to fewer bouts of infection immediately postpartum.

21. A breastfeeding woman who delivered 6 weeks ago calls the advice nurse at the obstetrician's office. She states, "I am very embarrassed but I need help. Last night I had an orgasm when my husband and I were making love. You should have seen the milk. We were both soaking wet. What is wrong with me?" The nurse should base the response to the client on which of the following?
1. The client is exhibiting signs of pathological galactorrhea.
2. The same hormone stimulates orgasms and the milk ejection reflex.
3. The client should have a serum galactosemia assessment done.
4. The baby is stimulating the client to produce too much milk.

22. A client who is 3 days postpartum asks the nurse, "When may my husband and I begin having sexual relations again?" The nurse should encourage the couple to wait until after which of the following has occurred?
1. The client has had her 6-week postpartum checkup.
2. The episiotomy has healed and the lochia has stopped.
3. The lochia has turned to pink and the vagina is no longer tender.
4. The client has had her first postpartum menstrual period.

23. A breastfeeding client at 7 weeks postpartum, complains to an obstetrician's triage nurse that when she and her husband had intercourse for the first time after the delivery, "I couldn't stand it. It was so painful. The doctor must have done something terrible to my vagina." Which of the following responses by the nurse is appropriate?
1. "After a delivery the vagina is always very tender. It should feel better the next time you have intercourse."
2. "Does your baby have thrush? If so, you should be assessed for a yeast infection in your vagina."
3. "Women who breastfeed often have vaginal dryness. A vaginal lubricant may remedy your discomfort."
4. "Sometimes the stitches of episiotomies heal too tight. Why don't you come in to be checked?"

24. The nurse monitors postpartum clients carefully because which of the following physiological changes occurs during the early postpartum period?
1. Decreased urinary output.
2. Increased blood pressure.
3. Decreased blood volume.
4. Increased estrogen level.

25. A client who gave birth 24 hours ago is complaining of profuse diaphoresis. She has no other complaints. Which of the following actions by the nurse is appropriate?
   1. Take the client's temperature.
   2. Advise the client to decrease her fluid intake.
   3. Reassure the client that this is normal.
   4. Notify the neonate's pediatrician.

26. Which of the following laboratory values would the nurse expect to see in a normal postpartum client?
   1. Hematocrit, 39%.
   2. White blood cell count, 16,000 cells/mm^3.
   3. Red blood cell count, 5 million cells/mm^3.
   4. Hemoglobin, 15 grams/dL.

27. A nurse reports that a client has moderate lochia. Which of the following pads would be consistent with her evaluation? (Please mark the appropriate pad with an "X.")

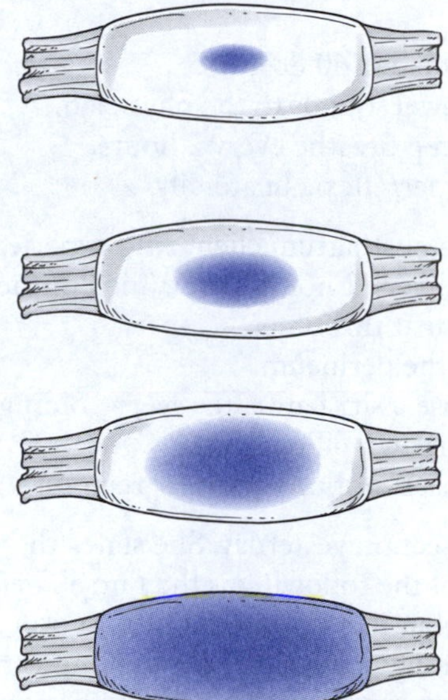

28. The nurse is discussing the importance of doing Kegel exercises during the postpartum period. Which of the following should be included in the teaching plan?
   1. She should repeatedly contract and relax her rectal and thigh muscles.
   2. She should practice by stopping the urine flow midstream every time she voids.
   3. She should get on her hands and knees whenever performing the exercises.
   4. She should be advised that her Kegel exercises should be performed during all bowel movements.

29. The nurse is evaluating the uterine involution of a client who is 3 days postpartum. Which of the following findings would the nurse evaluate as normal?
   1. Fundus 1 cm above the umbilicus, lochia rosa.
   2. Fundus 2 cm above the umbilicus, lochia alba.
   3. Fundus 3 cm below the umbilicus, lochia rubra.
   4. Fundus 4 cm below the umbilicus, lochia serosa.

30. During a home visit, the nurse assesses a client 2 weeks after delivery. Which of the following signs/symptoms should the nurse expect to see?
   1. Diaphoresis.
   2. Lochia alba.
   3. Cracked nipples.
   4. Hypertension.

31. The day after delivery, a client whose fundus is firm at 1 cm below the umbilicus and who has moderate lochia tells the nurse that something must be wrong: "All I do is go to the bathroom." Which of the following is an appropriate nursing response?
   1. Catheterize the client per doctor's orders.
   2. Measure the client's next voiding.
   3. Inform the client that polyuria is normal.
   4. Check the specific gravity of the next voiding.

32. A breastfeeding client with an obstetrical history of G10 P6408, delivered 10 minutes ago. Which of the following assessments is most important for the nurse to perform at this time?
   1. Pulse.
   2. Fundus.
   3. Bladder.
   4. Breast.

33. The nurse is caring for a client who had a cesarean section under spinal anesthesia less than 2 hours ago. Which of the following nursing actions is appropriate at this time?
   1. Elevate the head of the bed 60 degrees.
   2. Report absence of bowel sounds to the physician.
   3. Have her turn and deep breathe every 2 hours.
   4. Assess for patellar hyperreflexia bilaterally.

34. The nurse is caring for a postpartum client who experienced a second-degree perineal laceration at delivery 2 hours ago. Which of the following interventions should the nurse perform at this time?
   1. Apply an ice pack to the perineum.
   2. Advise the client to use a sitz bath after every voiding.
   3. Advise the client to sit on a pillow.
   4. Teach the client to insert nothing into her rectum.

35. A client had a cesarean section yesterday. She states that she needs to cough but that she is afraid to. Which of the following is the nurse's best response?
   1. "I know that it hurts but it is very important for you to cough."
   2. "Let me check your lung fields to see if coughing is really necessary."
   3. "If you take a few deep breaths in, that should be as good as coughing."
   4. "If you support your incision with a pillow, coughing should hurt less."

36. A client is receiving patient-controlled analgesia (PCA) post–cesarean section. Which of the following must be included in the client teaching?
   1. The client should monitor how often she presses the button.
   2. The client should report any feelings of nausea or itching to the nurse.
   3. The family should press the button whenever they feel the client is in pain.
   4. The family should inform the nurse if the client becomes sleepy.

37. The nurse is caring for a client who had an emergency cesarean section a day ago, with her husband in attendance. The baby's Apgar scores were 9/9. The client and her husband had attended childbirth education classes and had anticipated having a water birth with family present. The client states, "I guess I didn't have a very natural childbirth." Which of the following comments by the nurse is appropriate?
   1. "Sometimes babies just don't deliver the way we expect them to."
   2. "With all of your preparations, it must have been disappointing for you to have had a cesarean."
   3. "I know you had to have surgery, but you are very lucky that your baby was born healthy."
   4. "At least your husband was able to be with you when the baby was born."

38. A client is to receive morphine 4 mg q 3–4 hr subcutaneously for pain. The morphine is available on the unit in premeasured syringes of 10 mg/1 mL. When the nurse administers the medication, how many milliliters (mL) of morphine will be wasted? **Calculate to the nearest tenth.**

____ mL

39. The obstetrician has ordered a client's patient-controlled analgesia (PCA) to be discontinued. The client had a cesarean section the day before. Which of the following actions by the nurse is appropriate?
1. Discard the remaining medication in the presence of another nurse.
2. Recommend waiting until her pain level is zero to discontinue the medicine.
3. Discontinue the medication only after the analgesia is completely absorbed.
4. Return the unused portion of medication to the narcotics cabinet.

40. A client is receiving an epidural infusion of a narcotic for pain relief after a cesarean section. Which of the following assessments would the nurse report to the anesthesia provider?
1. Respiratory rate 8 per minute.
2. Complaint of thirst.
3. Urinary output of 250 mL/hr.
4. Numbness of feet and ankles.

41. A client who had a cesarean section 2 days ago complains to the nurse that she has yet to have a bowel movement since the surgery. Which of the following responses by the nurse would be appropriate at this time?
1. "That is very concerning. I will request that your physician order an enema for you."
2. "Two days is not that bad. Some clients go four days or longer without a movement."
3. "You have been taking antibiotics through your intravenous line. That is probably why you are constipated."
4. "Food and exercise often help to combat constipation. Take a stroll around the unit, drink lots of fluid, and order something on the menu that sounds good."

42. A post–cesarean section, breastfeeding client whose subjective pain level is 2/5 requests her prn narcotic analgesics every 3 hours. She states, "I have decided to make sure that I feel as little pain from this experience as possible." Which of the following should the nurse conclude in relation to this client's behavior?
1. The client needs a stronger narcotic order.
2. The client is at high risk for severe constipation.
3. The client's breast milk volume may drop while taking the medicine.
4. The client's newborn may become addicted to the medication.

43. A nurse is assessing a client who had her baby by cesarean section. Which of the following should the nurse report to the surgeon?
1. Fundus at the umbilicus.
2. Nodular breasts.
3. Pulse rate 60 bpm.
4. Pad saturation every 30 minutes.

44. The nurse is assessing the midline episiotomy on a postpartum client. Which of the following findings should the nurse expect to see?
1. Moderate serosanguinous drainage.
2. Well-approximated edges.
3. Ecchymotic area distal to the episiotomy.
4. An area of redness adjacent to the incision.

45. A client with an obstetrical history now of G1 P1001 had an epidural and has just delivered a daughter over a mediolateral episiotomy. The physician used low forceps. The baby's Apgar scores were 9/9. While recovering, the client states, "I'm a failure. I couldn't stand the pain and couldn't even push my baby out by myself!" Which of the following is the best response for the nurse to make?
   1. "You'll feel better later after you have had a chance to rest and to eat."
   2. "Don't say that. There are many women who would be ecstatic to have that baby."
   3. "I am sure that you will have another baby. I bet that it will be a natural delivery."
   4. "To have things work out differently than you had planned is disappointing."

46. The nurse is developing a standard care plan for postpartum clients who have had midline episiotomies. Which of the following interventions should be included in the plan?
   1. Assist with stitch removal on the third postpartum day.
   2. Administer analgesics every 4 hours per doctor's orders.
   3. Teach the client to contract her buttocks before sitting.
   4. Irrigate the incision twice daily with antibiotic solution.

47. A primiparous client who had a spontaneous vaginal delivery 1 hour ago without an epidural states that she needs to urinate. Which of the following actions by the nurse is appropriate at this time?
   1. Provide the client with a bedpan.
   2. Advise the client that the feeling is likely related to the trauma of delivery.
   3. Remind the client that she had a catheter in place from the delivery.
   4. Assist the client to the bathroom.

48. A nurse is assessing the fundus of a client during the immediate postpartum period. Which of the following actions indicates that the nurse is performing the skill correctly?
   1. The nurse measures the fundal height using a paper centimeter tape.
   2. The nurse stabilizes the base of the uterus with the nondominant hand.
   3. The nurse palpates the fundus with the tips of the fingers.
   4. The nurse precedes the assessment with a sterile vaginal exam.

49. A client who delivered 24 hours ago states, "I think I have a urinary tract infection. I have to go to the bathroom all the time." Which of the following actions should the nurse take?
   1. Assure the client that frequent urination is normal after delivery.
   2. Obtain an order for a urine culture.
   3. Assess the urine for cloudiness.
   4. Ask the client if she is prone to urinary tract infections.

50. The nurse is assessing the laboratory report on a G1 P1001 client who delivered 2 days ago. The client had a normal postpartum assessment this morning. Which of the following results should the nurse report to the primary healthcare provider?
   1. White blood cells, 12,500 cells/mm^3.
   2. Red blood cells, 4,500,000 cells/mm^3.
   3. Hematocrit, 26%.
   4. Hemoglobin, 11 g/dL.

51. A client who delivered vaginally 1½ weeks ago and is bottle feeding her baby, calls the obstetric office to state that she has saturated two pads in the past 1 hour. Which of the following responses by the nurse is appropriate?
   1. "You must be doing too much. Lie down for a few hours and call back if the bleeding has not subsided."
   2. "You are probably getting your period back. You will bleed like that for a day or two and then it will lighten up."
   3. "It is not unusual to bleed heavily every once in a while after a baby is born. It should subside shortly."
   4. "It is important for you to be examined by the doctor today. Let me check to see when you can come in."

52. A client, 2 days postpartum from a spontaneous vaginal delivery, asks the nurse about postpartum exercises. Which of the following responses by the nurse is appropriate?
1. "You must wait to begin to perform exercises until after your 6-week postpartum checkup."
2. "You may begin Kegel exercises today, but do not do any other exercises until the doctor tells you that it is safe."
3. "By next week you will be able to return to the exercise schedule you had before you were pregnant."
4. "You can do some Kegel exercises today and then slowly increase your toning exercises over the next few weeks."

53. The nurse is examining a client at 2 days postpartum. Her fundus is 2 cm below the umbilicus. Bright red lochia saturates about 4 inches of a pad in 1 hour. What should the nurse document in the nursing record?
1. Abnormal involution, lochia rubra heavy.
2. Abnormal involution, lochia serosa scant.
3. Normal involution, lochia rubra moderate.
4. Normal involution, lochia serosa heavy.

54. The nurse palpates a distended bladder on a client who delivered vaginally 2 hours earlier. The client refuses to go to the bathroom. "I really don't need to go." Which of the following responses by the nurse is appropriate?
1. "Okay. I must be palpating your uterus."
2. "I understand but it's important to try to empty your bladder."
3. "You still must be numb from the local anesthesia."
4. "That is a problem. I will have to catheterize you."

55. A client with an obstetrical history of G1 P0101 is assessed on postpartum day 1. The nurse notes that the client's lochia rubra is moderate and her fundus is boggy, 2 cm above the umbilicus and deviated to the right. Which of the following actions should the nurse take first?
1. Notify the client's primary healthcare provider.
2. Massage the client's fundus.
3. Escort the client to the bathroom to urinate.
4. Check the quantity of lochia on the peripad.

56. The nurse has admitted a client to the postpartum unit and has taught her about pericare. Which of the following indicates that the client understands the procedure? **Select all that apply.**
1. The client performs the procedure twice a day.
2. The client washes her hands before and after the procedure.
3. The client sits in warm tap water for 10 minutes three times a day.
4. The client sprays her perineum from front to back.
5. The client mixes warm tap water with hydrogen peroxide.

57. The nurse informs a postpartum client that which of the following is the reason that ibuprofen is especially effective for afterbirth pains?
1. Ibuprofen is taken every 2 hours.
2. Ibuprofen has an anti-prostaglandin effect.
3. Ibuprofen is given via the parenteral route.
4. Ibuprofen can be administered in high doses.

58. A client had a 6 lb 6 oz (3,000 grams) baby via normal spontaneous vaginal delivery 12 hours ago. Place an "X" on the location where the nurse would expect to palpate her fundus.

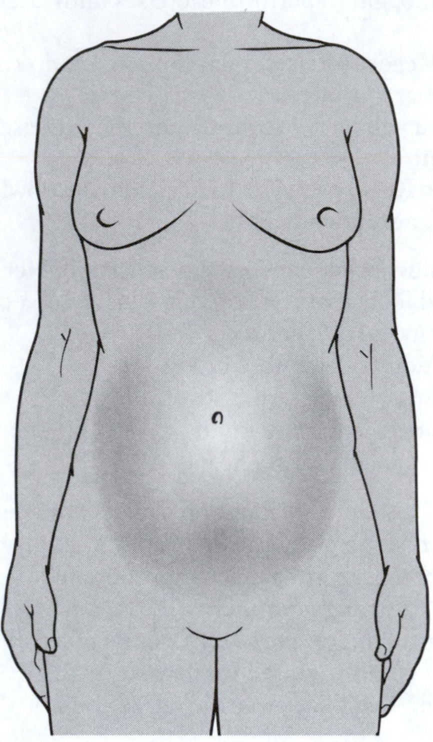

59. A physician has ordered an iron supplement for a postpartum client. The nurse strongly suggests that the client take the medicine with which of the following drinks?
1. Skim milk.
2. Ginger ale.
3. Orange juice.
4. Chamomile tea.

60. On admission to the labor and delivery unit, a client's hemoglobin (Hgb) was assessed at 11 g/dL and her hematocrit (Hct) at 33%. Which of the following values would the nurse expect to see 2 days after a normal spontaneous vaginal delivery?
1. Hgb 12.5 g/dL; Hct 37%.
2. Hgb 11 g/dL; Hct 33%.
3. Hgb 10.5 g/dL; Hct 31%.
4. Hgb 9 g/dL; Hct 27%.

61. During a postpartum assessment, it is noted that a client with an obstetrical history of G1 P1001 who delivered vaginally over an intact perineum has a cluster of hemorrhoids. Which of the following would be appropriate for the nurse to include in the client's health teaching? **Select all that apply.**
1. The client should use a sitz bath daily as a relief measure.
2. The client should digitally replace external hemorrhoids into her rectum.
3. The client should breastfeed frequently to stimulate oxytocin to reduce the size of the hemorrhoids.
4. The client should be advised that the hemorrhoids will increase in size and quantity with subsequent pregnancies.
5. The client should apply topical anesthetic as a relief measure.

62. Which of the following is the priority nursing action during the immediate postpartum period?
1. Palpate fundus.
2. Check pain level.
3. Perform pericare.
4. Assess breasts.

63. Immediately after delivery, a client is shaking uncontrollably. Which of the following nursing actions is most appropriate?
1. Provide the client with warm blankets.
2. Put the client in the Trendelenburg position.
3. Notify the primary healthcare provider.
4. Increase the intravenous infusion.

64. Which of the following nursing interventions would be appropriate for the nurse to perform to prevent thrombophlebitis?
1. Encourage early ambulation.
2. Promote oral fluid intake.
3. Massage the legs of the client twice daily.
4. Provide the client with high-fiber foods.

65. The nurse is developing a plan of care for the postpartum client during the "taking in" phase. Which of the following should the nurse include in the plan?
1. Teach baby-care skills such as diapering.
2. Discuss the labor and birth with the mother.
3. Discuss contraceptive choices with the mother.
4. Teach breastfeeding skills such as pumping.

66. The nurse is developing a plan of care for the postpartum client during the "taking hold" phase. Which of the following should the nurse include in the plan?
1. Provide the client with a nutritious meal.
2. Encourage the client to take a nap.
3. Assist the client with activities of daily living.
4. Assure the client that she is meeting the needs of her baby very well.

67. The nurse takes a newborn to a primiparous mother for a feeding. The mother holds the baby "en face," strokes his cheek, and states that this is the first newborn she has ever held. Which of the following nursing assessments is most appropriate?
1. Positive bonding and client needs little teaching.
2. Positive bonding but teaching related to newborn care is needed.
3. Poor bonding and referral to a child abuse agency is essential.
4. Poor bonding but there is potential for positive mothering.

68. A primipara at 2 hours postpartum requests that the nurse diaper her baby after a feeding because "I am so tired right now. I just want to have something to eat and take a nap." Based on this information, the nurse concludes that the client is exhibiting signs of which of the following?
1. Social deprivation.
2. Child neglect.
3. Normal postpartum behavior.
4. Postpartum depression.

69. A nurse is counseling a client about postpartum blues. Which of the following should be included in the discussion?
1. The father may become sad and weepy.
2. Postpartum blues last about a week or two.
3. Medications are available to relieve the symptoms.
4. Very few women experience postpartum blues.

70. An Asian client's temperature 10 hours after delivery is 100.2° F (37.8° C) but, when encouraged to drink ice water, she refuses. Which of the following nursing actions is most appropriate?
1. Ask the client what she would like instead.
2. Notify the client's healthcare provider.
3. Reassess the temperature in one-half hour.
4. Remind the client that drinking is very important.

71. A medication order reads: Methylergonovine 0.2 mg PO q 6 h × 4 doses. For which of the following clients should the nurse question the dose before administering the medication? **Select all that apply.**
1. Client with heavy flow.
2. Client with a blood pressure (BP) of 140/90.
3. Client with type 1 diabetes.
4. Client with Raynaud's disease.

72. Which of the following complementary therapies can a nurse suggest to a multiparous client who is complaining of severe afterbirth pains?
1. Lie prone with a small pillow cushioning her abdomen.
2. Contract her abdominal muscles for a count of ten.
3. Slowly ambulate in the hallways.
4. Drink iced tea with lemon or lime.

73. The nurse should warn a client who is about to receive methylergonovine of which of the following side effects?
1. Headache.
2. Nausea.
3. Cramping.
4. Fatigue.

74. The third stage of labor has just ended for a client who has decided to bottle feed her baby. Which of the following maternal hormones will increase sharply at this time?
1. Estrogen.
2. Prolactin.
3. Human placental lactogen.
4. Human chorionic gonadotropin.

75. The nurse hears the following information on a newly delivered client during shift report: 21 years old, married, G1 P1001, 8 hours post-spontaneous vaginal delivery over an intact perineum; vitals 110/70, 98.6° F (37° C), pulse 82, respiratory rate 18; fundus firm at umbilicus; moderate lochia rubra; ambulated 4 times to the bathroom to void; breastfeeding every 2 hours. Which of the following conditions should the nurse anticipate in planning care for this client?
1. Fluid volume deficit r/t excess blood loss.
2. Impaired skin integrity r/t vaginal delivery.
3. Impaired urinary elimination r/t excess output.
4. Knowledge deficit r/t lack of parenting experience.

76. A client who delivered an 8 lb 6 oz (3,900 grams) baby vaginally over a right mediolateral episiotomy states, "How am I supposed to have a bowel movement? The stitches are right there!" Which of the following is the best response by the nurse?
1. "I will call the doctor to order a stool softener for you."
2. "Your stitches are actually far away from your rectal area."
3. "If you eat high-fiber foods and drink fluids you should have no problems."
4. "If you use your topical anesthetic on your stitches you will feel much less pain."

77. After a client's placenta is delivered, the obstetrician states, "Please add 20 units of oxytocin to the lactated ringer's and increase the drip rate to 250 mL/hr." The client has 750 mL in her IV and the macro IV tubing delivers fluid at the rate of 10 gtt/mL. To what drip rate should the nurse set the infusion?

____ gtt/min

78. A client has just been transferred to the postpartum unit from labor and delivery. Which of the following nursing care goals is of highest priority?
1. The client will breastfeed her baby every 2 hours.
2. The client will consume a normal diet.
3. The client will have a moderate lochial flow.
4. The client will ambulate to the bathroom every 2 hours.

79. A client has just been transferred to the postpartum unit from labor and delivery. Which of the following tasks should the registered nurse delegate to the certified nursing assistant (CNA)?
1. Assess client's fundal height.
2. Teach client how to massage her fundus.
3. Take the client's vital signs.
4. Document quantity of lochia in the chart.

80. A client who is now G2 P1102, is 30 minutes postpartum from a low forceps vaginal delivery over a right midline episiotomy. Her physician has just finished repairing the incision. The client's legs are in stirrups and she is breastfeeding her baby. Which of the following actions should the nurse perform?
1. Assess her feet and ankles for pitting edema.
2. Advise the client to stop feeding her baby while her blood pressure is assessed.
3. Lower both of her legs at the same time.
4. Measure the length of the episiotomy and document the findings in the chart.

81. A maternity nurse knows that obstetric clients are most at high risk for cardiovascular compromise during the one hour immediately following a delivery because of which of the following?
1. Weight of the uterine body is significantly reduced.
2. Excess blood volume from pregnancy is circulating in the client's peripheral circulation.
3. Cervix is fully dilated and the lochia flows freely.
4. Maternal blood pressure drops precipitously once the baby's head emerges.

82. The nurse must initiate discharge teaching regarding the need for an infant car seat for the day of discharge. Which of the following responses indicates that the nurse acted appropriately? The nurse discussed the need with the client:
1. After admission to the labor room.
2. In the client room after the delivery.
3. When the client put the baby to the breast for the first time.
4. The day before the client and baby are to leave the hospital.

83. The nurse is preparing to place a peripad on the perineum of a client who delivered her baby 10 minutes earlier. The client states, "I don't use those. I always use tampons." Which of the following actions by the nurse is appropriate at this time?
1. Remove the peripad and insert a tampon into the client's vagina.
2. Advise the client that for the first two days she will be bleeding too heavily for a tampon.
3. Remind the client that a tampon would hurt until the soreness from the delivery resolves.
4. State that it is unsafe to place anything into the vagina until involution is complete.

84. A client has been transferred to the post-anesthesia care unit following a cesarean delivery. The client had spinal anesthesia for the surgery. Which of the following interventions should the nurse perform at this time?
1. Assess the level of the anesthesia.
2. Encourage the client to urinate in a bedpan.
3. Provide the client with the diet of her choice.
4. Check the incision for signs of infection.

85. The surgeon has removed the surgical cesarean section dressing from a client the day after surgery. Which of the following actions by the nurse is appropriate?
1. Irrigate the incision twice daily.
2. Monitor the incision using the REEDA scale.
3. Apply steri strips to the incision line.
4. Palpate the incision and assess for pain.

86. A nurse is performing a postpartum assessment on a client who delivered vaginally. Which of the following actions will the nurse perform? **Select all that apply.**
1. Palpate the breasts.
2. Auscultate the carotid.
3. Check vaginal discharge.
4. Assess the extremities.
5. Inspect the perineum.

87. During a postpartum assessment, the nurse assesses the calves of a client's legs. The nurse is checking for which of the following signs/symptoms? **Select all that apply.**
1. Pain.
2. Warmth.
3. Discharge.
4. Ecchymosis.
5. Redness.

88. A nurse is performing a postpartum assessment on a client whose baby was delivered by cesarean section. Which of the following actions will the nurse perform? **Select all that apply.**
1. Auscultate the abdomen.
2. Palpate the fundus.
3. Assess the nipple skin integrity.
4. Assess the central venous pressure.
5. Auscultate the lung fields.

89. A postpartum nurse is caring for a client who received epidural anesthesia during her labor and delivery. The nurse should advise the client that she may experience which of the following side effects of the medication during the postpartum period?
1. Backache.
2. Light-headedness.
3. Hypertension.
4. Footdrop.

90. A nurse is caring for a postpartum client who has stated that her plans include adoption for her newborn son. The client asks the nurse to help her breastfeed her baby. Which of the following responses by the nurse is appropriate?
1. "Are you sure you want to try breastfeeding? You won't be able to do it once you give your baby away."
2. "Let's place your baby on a lap pillow and have your baby face you. Then wait for the baby to open his mouth before moving the baby toward your breast."
3. "If you stimulate your breasts to produce milk by having the baby breastfeed, you may become engorged when your baby leaves you."
4. "You should be forewarned that breastfeeding is such an intimate experience that if you start feeding your baby that way, you won't want to give him up."

91. A mother who delivered her first baby vaginally an hour ago, is transferred to the postpartum unit. She pushed for 45 minutes and the placenta was delivered 10 minutes after the birth. The baby weighed 6 lbs 2 oz (2,800 grams). The client is receiving intravenous fluids with 20 units oxytocin added to 1,000 mL of lactated ringer's solution. The student nurse receiving report questions why the oxytocin was added to the IV bag. Which of the following responses by the transferring nurse is most likely?
1. "The medication was added 10 minutes ago to prevent excess bleeding during her transfer."
2. "The medication was added immediately after the baby's birth to promote placental delivery."
3. "The medication was added after the placenta was delivered because of its rapid separation."
4. "The medication was added while she was pushing to speed up the baby's birth."

CASE STUDY: *The next three questions are part of a case study. This is based on a bowtie, or stand-alone question format that nursing graduates may see in the NGN NCLEX© exam (NCSBN, 2021). On the computerized test, the test taker will drag the appropriate answer into the appropriate box. Note that the first answer applies to the center box, with answers to question 2 in the boxes on the left, and answers to question 3 in the boxes on the right. For the purposes of this book, the test taker can select the correct answers as in any multiple-choice question. The bowtie diagram is given to provide familiarity with the format.*

A community health nurse is making a home visit to a postpartum client who delivered her baby 6 days ago. The client's obstetrical history is G1 P1001. The client has reported having breastfeeding issues and is considering feeding her baby a bottle instead of breastfeeding because of nipple pain. The client reports "I feel like I have the flu, and I'm trying to breastfeed every time she cries, which is all the time, but she won't latch on. It really hurts, so I've given her a bottle the last two feedings. I don't want to make her sick." The baby's weight is 3 ounces less than her birth weight. She appears well fed and is not jaundiced. The client reports the baby is having more than 4 wet diapers a day, and loose, yellow stools.

92. Select a complication for which the client is at increased risk.
1. Postpartum psychosis.
2. Mastitis.
3. Candidiasis.
4. Breast abscess.

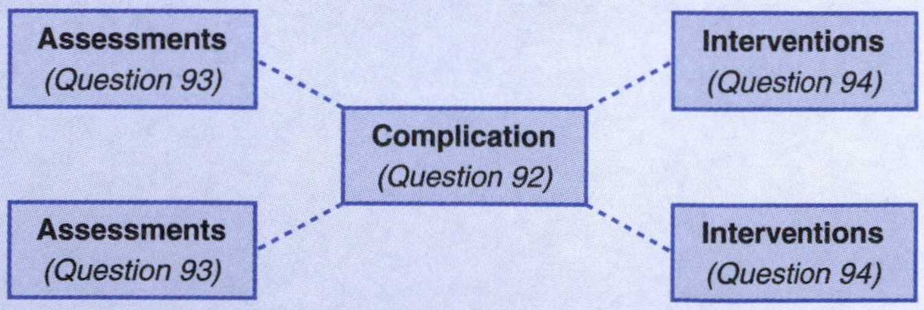

93. Which of the following assessments are important for the nurse to make to identify the complication? **Select two.**
1. Breast letdown reflex.
2. Breast firmness and tenderness.
3. Breast erythema and warmth.
4. Breast milk quantity removed at each feeding.

94. The client's vital signs are T 100° F (37.7° C), P 76, R 18, BP 128/72. The nurse notes a wedge-shaped area of erythema approximately 4 cm in diameter on the outer aspect of the client's right breast, near the areola. There is no nipple injury. **Specify two immediate interventions** the nurse should perform as a way to reduce the risks of the identified complication.

1. Assist with breastfeeding.
2. Obtain breastmilk cultures.
3. Reduce fluid intake for 24 hours.
4. Apply warm compresses to breast.

ANSWERS AND RATIONALES

The correct answer number and rationale for why it is the correct answer are given in **boldface blue type.** Rationales for why the other possible answer options are incorrect also are given, but they are not in boldface type.

1. **Answers 1, 2, and 3 are correct.**
   1. **Although she is understandably tired after the difficult labor and delivery, light-headedness and lethargy are not expected.**
   2. **A full bladder can contribute to fundal atony and bleeding.**
   3. **Fundal tone has been unstable.**
   4. She is breathing slowly, but there is nothing in the question stem to indicate her respirations are slower than normal.

TEST-TAKING HINT: At this point, the nurse is noticing in general, the client's pertinent symptoms that need more attention. What is relevant, and what is irrelevant? Light-headedness can be a normal finding, but should not be dismissed, especially in light of the blood loss of nearly 500 mL at delivery. The client's reported history of fundal massage two times in the past hour should be further investigated. She has not voided in the past hour, and her bladder fullness and position should be assessed. Her respiratory rate is not said to be abnormally slow and is irrelevant.

2. **Answers 2, 3, and 4 are correct.**
   1. A prolonged oxytocin induction can contribute to hyponatremia (also called water intoxication) as a result of oxytocin's antidiuretic properties, but the client's symptoms do not suggest that this is the problem.
   2. **The forceps delivery puts her at risk of hematoma. Hematoma can cause unseen hypovolemia. Her symptoms of light-headedness are consistent with this.**
   3. **Her long induction of 20 hours and fetal weight above 4,000 grams put her at risk for uterine atony and hemorrhage. Her symptoms are consistent with this.**
   4. **The forceps delivery and fetal weight put her at risk of vaginal wall laceration and bleeding. Her symptoms are consistent with this.**

TEST-TAKING HINT: This is the step in which the test taker interprets the information provided in the case study by considering if the client's symptoms are consistent with each potential condition. This helps to narrow down the focus of nursing interventions in the next step of prioritizing hypotheses. Consider multiple possibilities at this point. Although hyponatremia, also called "water intoxication" is a possible side effect of oxytocin, it is more commonly seen at high rates of oxytocin infusion. The client's symptoms do not suggest that is an issue.

3. **Answers 3 and a are correct.**
   1. There is nothing to suggest the client might have a seizure.
   2. There is nothing to suggest the client might have a dysrhythmia.
   3. **The client is at highest risk for developing a hemorrhage.**
   4. There is nothing to suggest the client will develop hypoxia, even though she's breathing slowly.

   a. **The obstetrical recovery documentation indicates that within the first hour after delivery, the fundus required massage two times.**
   b. The client is breathing "slowly," but she is not apneic.
   c. Lethargy could indicate the client is hypovolemic. But the question asks the test taker to identify in the second section (a–d answers) the client condition that could be causing the identified risk in the first part of the question (answers 1–4). Lethargy does not *cause* hypovolemia.
   d. Although multiparity can contribute to hemorrhage, other factors such as induction, fetal size, and forceps use are more direct and focused contributors.

TEST-TAKING HINT: In prioritizing the hypothesis, the nurse ranks them in order of priority. What is most likely; what is most urgent? In answering these questions, the nurse must determine "why" a particular hypothesis is prioritized. In this situation, the fundus is "most likely" atonic again, as evidenced by the previous need for massage two times. Although the nurse palpates the fundus every 15 minutes during the first hour to confirm it is well contracted, an atonic fundus that requires focused massage till firm, is worrisome. In the NCLEX exam, this format will contain two dropdown lists. Note that the first part (answers 1–4) asks the nurse to identify broadly the highest risk to the client. The second part (answers a–d) identifies the reason "why" that is of highest risk.

4. Answers 1 (a), 2 (a), 3 (a), 4 (c), 5 (c), 6 (b), 7 (c), and 8 (a) are correct.

Possible Nursing Intervention	(a) Indicated	(b) Nonessential	(c) Contraindicated
1. Fundal massage	X		
2. Encourage breastfeeding	X		
3. Increase oxytocin rate	X		
4. Ambulate to bathroom to void			X
5. Catheterize client			X
6. Initiate oxygen by mask		X	
7. Encourage the client to finish her meal			X
8. Calculate intake and output	X		

1a. Fundal massage is likely indicated, especially in light of being necessary two times previously.

2a. Breastfeeding is indicated once the nurse has completed fundal massage. Breastfeeding stimulates the release of intrinsic oxytocin, which can assist with uterine contraction.

3a. Increased oxytocin rate is indicated. At a rate of 50 mL/hour, the IV oxytocin solution is not running rapidly enough to support an atonic uterus. The nurse must either increase the rate of the oxytocin infusion or request an order to add oxytocin to the infusion to make it more concentrated.

4c. Bladder emptying is indicated to promote uterine contractility, but ambulating to the bathroom is contraindicated because of the risk of fainting. Until the client's condition is stable, she should not ambulate to the bathroom to void. Having bled 490 mL during childbirth, the additional bleeding in the last hour has no doubt moved her physiologically into a postpartum hemorrhage calculation. She is at risk of passing out if she stands up. A bedpan would be the best thing to try. If she refuses that, a bedside commode can be suggested.

5c. Catheterization is contraindicated at this time as a first step to bladder emptying, as it can introduce infection.

6b. Oxygen is nonessential. She is not having breathing difficulties.

7c. This is contraindicated. The client is not likely light-headed because of hypoglycemia. Until she is stable, she should remain NPO in case surgical intervention becomes necessary.

8a. An up-to-date tally of intake and output should be calculated to inform the nurse and the provider of any additional treatments that may be indicated. Sometimes generating solutions includes obtaining more information, as in this case.

TEST-TAKING HINT: When generating solutions, the nurse must identify goals for the client. In this case, managing the client's bleeding is the primary goal. A second goal is to avoid a fall, should the client try to walk to the bathroom in her light-headed condition. The table does not include all the possible nursing interventions the nurse could employ, such as vital sign assessments. It is designed to evaluate less obvious clinical judgments. The nurse must be aware that surgical intervention is a possibility. As such, the client should not eat or drink any more. Until the client's uterus remains firm, the risk of needing a perineal examination and laceration or hematoma repair under anesthesia, or a dilation and curettage, is high. For that reason, it is best if the client keeps her stomach as empty as possible. There is nothing in this question to indicate this client received an oxytocin bolus or injection after the birth, and the current IV rate is at 50 mL/hour, which is not rapid enough to stimulate uterine contractility. The Association of Women's Health, Obstetric, and Neonatal Nurses (AWHONN) recommends that the use of guidelines prepared by the California Maternal Quality Care Collaborative (CMQCC) be implemented to reduce maternal morbidity and mortality (AWHONN, 2021). These guidelines include the recommendation for oxytocin: 10 to 40 units per 500 to 1000 mL IV fluid at ≥500 mL/hour, titrated to response

(CMQCC, 2015, p. 1). Because her induction was so long, it's possible the oxytocin receptors in her uterus are full and are not responding to the oxytocin. It's possible she will need an additional uterotonic such as methylergonovine to stimulate uterine contractility.

5. **Answer 2 is correct.**
   1. Another dose of methylergonovine is not contraindicated, but the use of a third uterotonic is a better choice. The American College of Obstetricians and Gynecologists (ACOG) recommends that with postpartum hemorrhage, multiple agents should be used, and in the presence of ongoing hemorrhage, they should follow in rapid succession (ACOG, 2017d). As such, if this client is bleeding in spite of the oxytocin IV solution and methergine, a third uterotonic should be administered as fundal massage continues (ACOG, 2017d).
   2. **Prostaglandin F2 Alpha is contraindicated for clients with asthma, as it can cause bronchospasm.**
   3. There is no contraindication for prostaglandin E2.
   4. There is no contraindication for misoprostol.

TEST-TAKING HINT: The nurse must be aware of specific differences in medications that may be used for more than one condition, that sound alike, or that have similar ingredients. Three of these medications contain prostaglandins, as indicated in their generic names (prostaglandin F2 Alpha and prostaglandin E2). Misoprostol includes prostaglandins, as well. Two of these medications—prostaglandin E2 suppositories (PGE2) and misoprostol—may also be used for labor induction intravaginally. Misoprostol may alternatively be administered orally. When used for labor induction, both medications are used in lower doses than when used for hemorrhage. As such, the nurse cannot simply take an order for "prostaglandins" without asking for the specifics of type, dose, and route of administration. The nurse must also be aware of the client's risk factors for the medication, such as asthma in this case.

6. **Answers 1, 3, and 4 are correct.**
   1. **A dropping blood pressure can indicate hypovolemic shock.**
   2. A reduced heartrate would indicate that the client was stable.
   3. **Clammy skin is another sign of hypovolemic shock.**
   4. **Confusion is a sign of hypovolemic shock.**

TEST-TAKING HINT: Risk factors that are present on admission, such as multigravid status, fetus that is large for gestational age, polyhydramnios, twin pregnancy, and other factors should be noted. As labor progresses, additional factors should also be noted and shared in report, in order to provide for timely responses if necessary. This client seemed to have no risk factors on admission. However, by the time she delivered, several risk factors were present for the astute nurse to be alert for: long, induced labor; 3-hour second stage in a multipara; occiput posterior fetal position requiring use of forceps; 490 mL quantitative blood loss, which is very close to the definition of postpartum hemorrhage. Quantitative blood loss is the practice of weighing all pads and using a delivery drape with a calibrated cone for measuring blood loss after the birth of the baby. This practice is much more accurate than subjectively estimating blood loss. If the client has had heavy flow over the past 30 minutes to an hour, she has no doubt lost much more than 500 mL of blood. All pads should be weighed, if they weren't previously, to determine the total quantitative blood loss that has occurred in order to guide further treatment. In this client's case, since she is showing additional signs of postpartum hemorrhage, it is likely she will need to go to the operating room for a more thorough evaluation and possible dilation and curettage. That likelihood begins another series of clinical judgments and prioritizing of decisions for this client.

7. 1. **This statement is correct. The rubella vaccine contains a live attenuated virus. Severe birth defects can develop if the woman becomes pregnant within 4 weeks of receiving the injection.**
   2. This is unnecessary. There is no risk to the baby whether the mother is bottle feeding or breastfeeding.
   3. This statement is incorrect. There is no risk to the baby.
   4. This statement is incorrect.

TEST-TAKING HINT: If rubella is contracted during pregnancy, the fetus is at very high risk for injury. Whenever pregnant clients are found to be non-immune to rubella—defined as a titer of 1:8 or lower—they are advised to receive the vaccine during the early postpartum period and are counseled regarding the teratogenic properties of the vaccine. Pregnancy should be prevented for at least 3 months after the injection. A titer of 1:10 is generally the measurement used to indicate a person is rubella immune and does not need

the injection. A reading between 1:8 and 1:10 is considered equivocal, or uncertain to predict immunity. Vaccination is encouraged for these clients.

8. 1. **This statement is correct. Because the vaccine is teratogenic, the best time to administer it is when the client is not pregnant. Having just delivered her baby, there is no question that she is not currently pregnant.**
2. This statement is incorrect. The immune systems of women during their pregnancies and immediately postpartum are slightly depressed.
3. This statement is incorrect. The baby will be susceptible to rubella whether or not the woman receives the vaccine.
4. In general, insurance companies will pay for vaccinations whenever they are needed.

TEST-TAKING HINT: A woman's obstetric status immediately after delivery is optimal for receiving the medication, precisely because she is not pregnant and is very unlikely to become pregnant soon.

9. 1. A temperature of 100.2° F (37.8° C) is not a febrile temperature. It is unlikely that this client needs acetaminophen.
2. A temperature of 100.2° F (s7.8° C) is not a febrile temperature. It is unlikely that this client is infected.
3. A temperature of 100.2° F (37.9° C) is not a febrile temperature. It is unlikely that this client needs cool compresses.
4. **It is likely that this client is dehydrated. She should be advised to drink fluids.**

TEST-TAKING HINT: In the early postpartum period up to 24 hours after delivery, the most common reason for clients to have slight temperature elevations is dehydration. During labor, clients work very hard, often utilizing breathing techniques as a form of pain control. As a result, the clients lose fluids through insensible loss via the respiratory system and sweating.

10. 1. It is unnecessary to apply antibiotic ointment to the perineum after delivery.
2. **Clients should be advised to change their pads at each voiding.**
3. The clients should void about every 2 hours, but this action is not an infection control measure.
4. It is unnecessary to spray the perineum with a povidone-iodine solution. Plain water, however, should be sprayed on the perineum.

TEST-TAKING HINT: Postpartum clients should be advised to perform three actions to prevent infections: (1) change their peripads at each toileting because blood is an excellent medium for bacterial growth; (2) spray the perineum from front to back with clear water to cleanse the area; and (3) wipe the perineum from front to back after toileting to prevent pulling the rectal flora forward and contaminating the urethra or perineum. This is especially important if the client had lacerations or an episiotomy and has stitches in the area.

11. 1. **Clients should be strongly encouraged to exclusively breastfeed their babies to prevent engorgement and to maintain milk supply.**
2. Massaging of the breast will stimulate more milk production. That is not the best action to take.
3. It is unnecessary to culture the breast. This client is engorged; she does not have an infection.
4. It is unnecessary to assess this client's temperature and pulse rate. This client is engorged; she is not infected.

TEST-TAKING HINT: The lactating breast produces milk continuously, whether or not it is being stimulated. When a feeding is skipped, milk is still produced for the baby. When the baby is not fed, breast congestion or engorgement results. Not only is engorgement uncomfortable, it also gives the body the message to stop producing milk, resulting in an insufficient milk supply. In addition, engorgement makes it difficult for the baby to latch onto the breast to empty it, creating a vicious circle that often leads to a woman giving up breastfeeding.

12. 1. Clients are not recommended to pump their breasts after feedings unless there is a specific reason to do so.
2. **This statement is true. The best way to prevent engorgement is to feed the baby on demand, or at least every 2 to 3 hours.**
3. Clients should not restrict babies' feeding times. Babies feed at different rates. Babies themselves, therefore, should regulate the amount of time they need to complete their feeds.
4. Clients are not recommended to supplement with formula unless there is a specific reason to do so.

TEST-TAKING HINT: This question is similar to the preceding question except that this question tests the nurse's ability to evaluate a client's response rather than to perform a nursing action.

13. 1. It is not recommended that breastfeeding mothers go on weight-reduction diets. In addition, it is not necessary for mothers to drink milk to make breast milk.
2. When a breastfeeding woman has a poor diet, the quality of her breast milk changes very little. In fact, if a mother consumes a poor diet, it is her own body that will suffer.
3. Mothers do not need to eat 3,000 calories a day while breastfeeding.
4. **Many mothers who consume approximately the same number of calories while breastfeeding as they did when they were pregnant do lose weight while breastfeeding.**

TEST-TAKING HINT: Mothers should be advised to eat a well-balanced diet and drink sufficient quantities of fluids while breastfeeding. There is no absolute number of calories that the mother should consume, but if she does go on a restrictive diet, it is likely that her milk supply may dwindle. Babies do take in about 600 calories a day at the breast, meaning mothers lose or burn approximately 600 calories a day. This includes calories required to make the milk and calories excreted in the milk for the baby to burn. Therefore, mothers can be advised that breastfeeding may result in at least some weight loss.

14. 1. Heavy lochia is not a normal finding. Moderate lochia, which is similar in quantity to a heavy menstrual period, is a normal finding.
2. The client's fundus is firm. There is no need to massage the fundus.
3. The fundus is at the umbilicus and it is firm. It is unlikely that her bladder is full.
4. **Because of the heavy lochia, the nurse should notify the client's healthcare provider.**

TEST-TAKING HINT: The nurse must do some detective work when observing unexpected signs/symptoms. This client is bleeding more heavily than the nurse would expect. When the nurse assesses the two most likely sources of the bleeding—the fundus and the perineal sutures—normal findings are noted. The next most likely source of the bleeding—a laceration in the birth canal—is unobservable to the nurse because performing a postpartum internal examination is not a nursing function. The nurse, therefore, must notify the primary healthcare provider of the problem.

15. **Answers 4 and 5 are correct.**
1. It is unnecessary for a bottle-feeding mother to increase her fluid intake.
2. It is inadvisable for a bottle-feeding mother to massage her breasts.
3. It is inadvisable for a bottle-feeding mother to apply heat to her breasts.
4. **The mother should be advised to wear a supportive bra 24 hours a day for a week or so.**
5. **The mother should be advised to stand with her back toward the warm shower water.**

TEST-TAKING HINT: The postpartum body naturally prepares to breastfeed a baby. To suppress the milk production, the mother should refrain from stimulating her breasts. Both massage and heat stimulate the breasts to produce milk. Mothers, therefore, should be encouraged to refrain from touching their breasts and to direct the warm water toward their backs rather than toward their breasts when showering. A supportive bra will help to minimize any engorgement that the client may experience.

16. 1. **The client should apply ice packs to her axillae and breasts.**
2. Engorgement will not be relieved by applying lanolin to the breasts. And the act of applying the lanolin may actually stimulate milk production.
3. If the client expresses milk from her breasts, she will stimulate the breasts to produce more milk.
4. The Food and Drug Administration (FDA) recommends that milk suppressants not be administered because of the serious side effects of the medications.

TEST-TAKING HINT: Breast milk is produced in the glandular tissue of the breast. An adequate blood supply to the area is required for milk production. When cold is applied to the breast, the blood vessels constrict, decreasing the blood supply to the area. This is a relatively easy, nonhazardous action that helps to suppress breast milk production. The use of medications to suppress lactation is no longer recommended. The approval for bromocriptine, specifically, has been withdrawn in the United States and is discouraged in other countries because of increased risk of maternal health hazards such as stroke, seizures, cardiovascular disorders, death, and possibly psychosis (NIH, n.d.-a). Because engorgement resolves on its own within 7 to 10 days after the birth, the risks of medication that can cause lifelong health disorders or

death very clearly outweigh the benefits of such medication.

17. 1. It is inappropriate to advise a breastfeeding mother to switch to the bottle unless there is a specific medical reason for her to do so.
2. Massaging the fundus will not relieve the client's discomfort.
3. An alternate position will not relieve the client's discomfort.
4. **The nurse should discuss the action of oxytocin in particular.**

TEST-TAKING HINT: Oxytocin, the hormone of labor, also stimulates the uterus to contract in the postpartum period to reduce blood loss at the placental site. Oxytocin is the same hormone that regulates the milk ejection reflex. Therefore, whenever a mother breastfeeds, oxytocin stimulates her uterus to contract. In essence, breastfeeding benefits the mother naturally by contracting the uterus and preventing excessive bleeding. Taking a prescribed anti-inflammatory medication such as ibuprofen at least 30 minutes before breastfeeding can be of help for those with severe discomfort.

18. 1. Celery is especially high in vitamin K, but it contains very little iron or vitamin A. Cream cheese is very high in fat.
2. Yogurt is high in calcium but is not high in either iron or vitamin A. Bananas are high in vitamin B6, potassium, and vitamin C, but they are not high in either iron or vitamin A.
3. Strawberries are very high in vitamin C, but they are not high in either iron or vitamin A.
4. **Broccoli is very high in vitamin A and also contains iron.**

TEST-TAKING HINT: Breastfeeding clients should be advised to consume a well-balanced diet high in vitamins and minerals. As a result, nurses must be prepared to suggest foods that meet those needs.

19. 1. Nipple shields should be used sparingly. Other interventions should be tried first.
2. Soap will deplete the breast of its natural lanolin. It is recommended that women wash their breasts with only warm water during the breastfeeding period.
3. **Rotating positions at feedings is one action that can help to minimize the severity of sore nipples.**
4. It is inappropriate to recommend that the client switch to formula at this time.

TEST-TAKING HINT: If a mother rotates positions at each breastfeeding, the baby is likely to put pressure on varying points on the nipple. A good, deep latch, however, is the most important way to prevent nipple soreness and cracking. The mother could also apply lanolin to her breasts after each feeding.

20. 1. Although breastfeeding does have a protective effect on postpartum blood loss, involution can take up to 6 weeks in breastfeeding women as well as in bottle-feeding women.
2. **There is evidence to show that women who breastfeed their babies are less likely to develop type 2 diabetes later in life.**
3. Women who breastfeed have not been shown to have higher levels of bone density later in life.
4. Breastfed babies are less likely to develop infections than are bottle-fed babies. The mothers, however, have not been shown to have the same protection.

TEST-TAKING HINT: Breastfeeding has many beneficial properties for both mothers and babies. It is the responsibility of the nurse to provide women with the knowledge they need to make fact-based decisions about how they will feed their babies. Breastfeeding support, especially in the early days and weeks postpartum can increase breastfeeding duration and exclusivity (van Dellen et al., 2019).

21. 1. The client is not exhibiting symptoms of galactorrhea, which occurs when a woman produces breast milk even though she has not delivered a baby.
2. **This is true. Oxytocin stimulates sexual orgasm and is also the hormone that stimulates the milk ejection reflex.**
3. This is incorrect. Galactosemia is a genetic disease. Babies who have the disease are unable to digest galactose, the predominant sugar in breast milk.
4. Excessive milk production is an unlikely explanation of the problem.

TEST-TAKING HINT: It is important for the nurse in the obstetrician's office to inform breastfeeding clients of this potential situation. Because clients are strongly encouraged to refrain from having intercourse until they are 6 weeks postpartum, the postpartum nurse may not include this information in the client's discharge instructions. When the client is seen for her postpartum check, however, the information should be included.

22. **1. This response is correct. The couple is encouraged to wait until after involution is complete.**
2. Although some clients do begin having intercourse once the episiotomy is healed and lochia stops, it is recommended that clients wait the full 6 weeks.
3. The couple is encouraged to wait until after involution is complete, not to base the decision on lochial color or vaginal tenderness.
4. The couple is encouraged to wait until after involution is complete, not to base the decision on resumption of menses. A breastfeeding woman may not have another period for several months after the birth.

TEST-TAKING HINT: Like many other time frames that are recommended in medicine, the 6-week postpartum recovery period is based more on tradition than evidence. Before modern medicine, 1 in 10 women died from postpartum infections called "puerperal fever." To avoid the risk of this often life-threatening condition, physicians recommended "pelvic rest" for the first 6 weeks after childbirth. After 6 weeks, it was highly likely that the uterus was completely involuted, meaning uterine blood vessel access to the maternal blood system was completely closed down, and possible vaginal wall tears were healed. Sexual intercourse or insertion of tampons into the vagina are not as likely to cause infection after that time. Some healthcare providers refer to the 40 *weeks* of gestation, and compare that to the 42 *days* (approximately 6 weeks) of healing that follow.

23. 1. This response is inappropriate. It is likely that as long as the client breastfeeds she will experience vaginal dryness.
2. This is an inappropriate response. It is unlikely that a proliferation of *Candida* is the problem.
3. This response is correct. The client should be encouraged to use a lubricating jelly or oil.
4. It is unlikely that the problem is related to the episiotomy repair.

TEST-TAKING HINT: When women breastfeed, their estrogen levels remain low. As a result, they often complain of vaginal dryness and dyspareunia. The client should be advised to try an over-the-counter lubricant. If that is not helpful, the client may be prescribed an estrogen-based vaginal cream by her primary healthcare provider.

24. 1. The urinary output increases during the early postpartum period.
2. The blood pressure should remain stable during the postpartum period.
3. The blood volume does drop precipitously during the early postpartum period.
4. The estrogen levels drop during the early postpartum period.

TEST-TAKING HINT: The combination of reduced blood volume and decreased systemic vascular resistance of pregnancy can lead to postural hypotension during the postpartum period. Major arteries reduce their vascular resistance by 35% to 40% during pregnancy and become stretchy. In pregnancy, this decreased resistance accommodates the increased blood volume of almost 50% and prevents hypertension during pregnancy as a result. It is similar to using a larger hose to dispense larger volumes of water in order to reduce the pressure within the hose. It is normal for a woman to lose up to 500 mL of blood after a vaginal delivery. In addition, within a few hours after delivery, a shift of fluid from the extravascular to intravascular space occurs. At the same time, marked diuresis and diaphoresis occurs, in response to hormonal changes post delivery. This is why postpartum clients must be monitored very carefully for hypotension and increased bleeding during the early postpartum period due to decreased vascular tone.

25. 1. It is unlikely that the client is febrile.
2. The client should maintain an adequate fluid intake.
3. Diaphoresis is normal during the postpartum period.
4. There is no need to report the diaphoresis to the baby's pediatrician.

TEST-TAKING HINT: Because the client's blood volume is returning to its nonpregnant level, the client loses fluids via both the kidneys and through insensible loss by sweating. As a result, postpartum women often awaken from sleep with their nightwear saturated with perspiration.

26. 1. The hematocrit is often low in postpartum clients.
2. The nurse would expect to see an elevated white cell count.
3. The red blood cell count is often low in postpartum clients.
4. The hemoglobin is often low in postpartum clients.

TEST-TAKING HINT: Familiarity with normal laboratory values will help the test taker to

deduce the answer to this question by comparing the values. Three of the values—hematocrit, hemoglobin, and red blood cell count—relate to the oxygen-carrying properties of the blood, and all of these values are lower than normal during the postpartum phase. Only one answer, white blood cell count, is elevated. The white blood cell count elevates late in the third trimester and stays elevated during labor and the early postpartum period to protect the mother from infection during the delivery and puerperium.

27. **The pad with the moderate amount of lochia flow would be marked with an "X."**

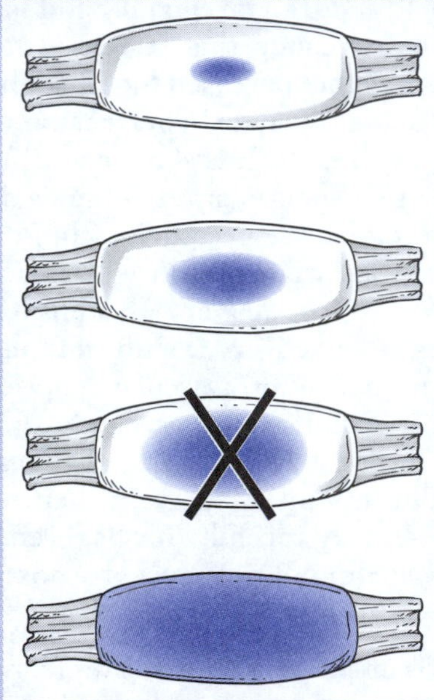

TEST-TAKING HINT: Determining the amount of lochial flow does include some subjectivity. The best guidelines to follow for a 1-hour time frame are up to 1 inch of lochia on the peripad—a scant amount; less than 4 inches on the pad— light amount; 4 to 6 inches on the pad—moderate amount; and saturated pad—heavy amount.

28. 1. To perform Kegel exercises, the client should be advised to contract and relax the muscles that stop the urine flow.
    2. **This is a correct statement. Stopping the urine mid-flow during voiding is the essence of Kegel exercises.**
    3. Kegel exercises can be performed in any position.
    4. Kegels can be performed at any time of day and in any position but, to determine which muscles are contracted during Kegels, the client should be taught to stop her urine flow midstream.

TEST-TAKING HINT: Kegel exercises are sometimes called clench and release exercises. They can help to strengthen the pelvic floor, which can ultimately assist in reducing urinary incontinence, if this is an issue after childbirth. Clients should be advised to perform them periodically throughout the day. They can be performed in any position and in any location.

29. 1. The fundus should have descended below the umbilicus and there is no such lochia as "lochia rosa."
    2. The fundus should have descended below the umbilicus and the lochia usually does not turn to alba until about 10 days postpartum.
    3. **The fundus is usually 3 cm below the umbilicus on day 3 and the lochia continues to be red, or rubra until day 4.**
    4. The fundus is usually 3 cm below the umbilicus on day 3 and the lochia usually has turned to serosa by day 4.

TEST-TAKING HINT: The fundus of the uterus is usually 1 cm, or 1 fingerbreadth below the umbilicus at 24 hours after the birth. It continues to descend about 1 cm per day. Although each client's postpartum course is slightly different, on day 3 postpartum, the nurse would expect the fundus of most clients to be 3 cm, or 3 fingerbreadths below the umbilicus and the lochia to still be dark red, rubra.

30. 1. Diaphoresis has usually subsided by this time.
    2. **The nurse would expect that the client would have lochia alba.**
    3. The nurse would not expect the client's nipples to be cracked.
    4. The nurse would not expect the client to be hypertensive.

TEST-TAKING HINT: The normal progression of lochial change is as follows: lochia rubra, days 1 to 3; lochia serosa, days 3 to 10; and lochia alba, days 10 until discharge stops. There is some variation in the exact timing of the lochial changes, but it is important for the client to know that the lochia should not revert backward. In other words, if a client whose lochia is alba begins to have bright red discharge, she should notify her primary healthcare provider.

31. 1. It is unlikely that this client needs to be catheterized.
    2. It is unnecessary to measure this client's output.
    3. **This response is correct. Polyuria is normal.**
    4. It is unnecessary to do a specific gravity on the client's output.

TEST-TAKING HINT: This client's physical assessment is normal. If the client's bladder were

distended, the client's fundus would be elevated in the abdomen and deviated to the right, and the client would have excess blood loss. It is unnecessary, therefore, to either catheterize the client or to measure her output. Diuresis occurs in response to the normal shift of fluid from the tissues to the blood (from extravascular to intravascular space) after childbirth. The average amount is 6 to 8 liters of total body water. This occurs as a result of hormonal changes that promote urinary sodium excretion. For the first 2 weeks after childbirth, it is not uncommon to have a urinary output of 3,000 mL/day, depending on the amount of fluid the woman retained during pregnancy (Chauhan & Tadi, 2020).

32. 1. An assessment of the client's pulse rate is important, but it is not the most important assessment.
    2. **An assessment of the client's fundus is the most important assessment to perform on this client.**
    3. An assessment of the client's bladder is important, but it is not the most important assessment.
    4. An assessment of the client's breasts is important, but it is not the most important assessment.

TEST-TAKING HINT: This client's gravidity and parity indicate that she is a grand multipara. She has been pregnant 10 times, carrying 6 babies to term and 4 babies preterm. Because her uterus has been stretched so many times, she is at high risk for uterine atony during the postpartum period. The nurse must, therefore, monitor the postpartum contraction of her uterus very carefully. Breastfeeding can assist in stimulating the uterus to contract, and as a result, this client would likely benefit from taking an anti-inflammatory medication regularly in the immediate postpartum period to reduce the pain from uterine contractions.

33. 1. This response is incorrect. Clients who have had spinal anesthesia are at high risk for spinal headaches when they are elevated soon after surgery.
    2. It is unnecessary to report absent bowel sounds to the client's physician immediately after surgery.
    3. **The client should turn, cough, and deep breathe every 2 hours.**
    4. There is no indication in the scenario that this client needs patellar reflex assessments every 2 hours.

TEST-TAKING HINT: It is recommended that clients who have had spinals be elevated only slightly during the early postoperative period. Sixty degrees is too much. Spinal anesthesia is administered directly into the spinal column. As a result, spinal fluid is able to escape through the puncture wound. When there is a drop in the amount of spinal fluid, clients often develop severe headaches. To maintain pulmonary health, however, it is essential that clients perform respiratory exercises frequently during the postoperative period. In addition, changing positions every 2 hours can prevent pressure damage to the skin.

34. 1. **It is appropriate to apply an ice pack to the area.**
    2. The sitz bath is an appropriate intervention beginning on the second postpartum day, not 2 hours after delivery. Sitz baths are usually performed 2 to 3 times a day for up to 20 minutes at a time.
    3. It is not necessary for the client to sit on a pillow.
    4. It is unnecessary for the client to be advised to put nothing in her rectum. Second-degree lacerations do not reach the rectum.

TEST-TAKING HINT: A second-degree laceration affects the skin, vaginal mucosa, and underlying muscles. It does not affect the rectum or rectal sphincter. Because of the injury, the area often swells, causing pain. Ice packs help to reduce the inflammatory response of swelling and numb the area.

35. 1. This response is accurate, but the nurse is exhibiting a lack of caring.
    2. This response is inappropriate. Even if the lung fields are clear, the client should perform respiratory exercises.
    3. This response is inappropriate. Simply breathing deeply may not be as effective as coughing.
    4. **This is the appropriate response. The nurse is providing the client with a means of reducing the discomfort of postsurgical coughing.**

TEST-TAKING HINT: Clients with abdominal incisions experience significant postoperative pain. Because their abdominal muscles have been incised, the pain is increased when the clients breathe in and cough. Bracing the abdominal muscles with a pillow or a blanket helps to reduce the discomfort.

36. 1. This is unnecessary. PCA pumps monitor the number of attempts clients make.
    2. **This information is correct. Clients often experience nausea and/or itching when PCA narcotics are administered.**

3. This is a false statement. Family members should not press the button for the client.
4. This information is untrue. It is unnecessary for family members to inform the nurse. It is not unusual for clients to fall asleep when receiving PCA.

TEST-TAKING HINT: It is important for the nurse to teach a client's family members that they must not control the PCA pump. Even though the pump is programmed with a minimum time between medication attempts, there is a possibility that the client could receive an overdose of medication if someone else controls the administrations. If a client is able to push the button herself, she is, by definition, awake and alert.

37. 1. This comment is inappropriate. It does not acknowledge the client's likely disappointment about having to have a cesarean section.
2. This comment conveys sensitivity and understanding to the client.
3. This comment may be true, but it does not acknowledge the client's likely disappointment about having to have a cesarean section.
4. This comment may be true, but it does not acknowledge the client's likely disappointment about having to have a cesarean section.

TEST-TAKING HINT: Clients who must have cesarean sections when they had developed birth plans for vaginal deliveries are often very disappointed. They may express regret and/or anger over the experience. The nurse must realize that such clients are not angry with the nurse but rather at the situation. It is essential for the nurse to accept the clients' feelings with understanding and caring. However, if the client has not expressed disappointment, it would not be appropriate for the nurse to assume or to suggest that emotion.

38. 0.6 mL.

The standard ratio and proportion formula for calculating the volume of medication to be wasted is:

$$\frac{\text{Known dosage}}{\text{Known volume}} = \frac{\text{Desired dosage}}{\text{Desired volume}}$$

$$\frac{10 \text{ mg}}{1 \text{ mL}} = \frac{6 \text{ mg}}{x\text{ml}}$$

$$10x = 6$$

$$x = 0.6 \text{ mL}$$

The dimensional analysis method for calculating the volume of medication to be wasted is:

Known volume	Desired dosage	= Desired volume
Known dosage		

1 mL	6 mg	= 0.6 mL
10 mg		

***The desired over have* or *formula* method is to divide the amount desired by the amount you have. It works very well in this situation since there are 10 mg of morphine in 1 mL: 4 mg (the desired dose) divided by 10 mg/1 mL (the dose you have) = 0.4 mL per dose. The nurse would waste 0.6 mL.**

TEST-TAKING HINT: Since the medication on hand is 10 mg and the nurse is to give 4 mg, the nurse must waste 6 mg. The nurse, therefore, must determine the volume that is equivalent to 6 mg.

39. 1. This answer is correct. Because the medication in a PCA pump is a controlled substance, the medication must be wasted in the presence of another nurse.
2. This answer is inappropriate. A pain level of 0 is unrealistic after abdominal surgery. The nurse, however, should request that the doctor order one of the many oral analgesics to control the client's discomfort.
3. This answer is inappropriate. Unless the nurse has a rationale to question the order, they should discontinue the medication as soon as the order has been received.
4. This answer is inappropriate. Once the intravenous solution bag or cartridge has been punctured and used for one client, the bag cannot be reused.

TEST-TAKING HINT: There are a number of considerations that the nurse must make when giving medications, especially when administering controlled substances. The nurse is legally bound to account for the administration of, or the disposal of narcotic medications. If any narcotic is wasted, a second nurse must cosign the disposal. The nurse must also anticipate the client's upcoming needs for oral pain medications and consider administering that at the same time the PCA is discontinued to assure ongoing pain control.

40. 1. This action is appropriate. This client's respiratory rate of 8 is below normal and should be reported to the anesthesia provider.

2. A complaint of thirst is within normal. There is no need to notify the anesthesia provider.
3. This urinary output is normal for a postpartum client. There is no need to notify the anesthesia provider.
4. Clients who have received epidurals will have numbness of their feet and ankles until the medication has metabolized. There is no need to notify the anesthesia provider.

TEST-TAKING HINT: One of the serious complications of narcotic administration is respiratory depression. This client's respiratory rate is well below expected. The nurse should continue to monitor the client carefully and notify the anesthesia provider of the complication.

41. 1. It is not unusual for post–cesarean section clients to have had no bowel movements. The client should be advised to drink fluids and to ambulate to stimulate peristalsis.
2. This response is inappropriate. This client is obviously very concerned about her bowel pattern.
3. This response is inaccurate. Clients who have received antibiotics often complain of diarrhea as a result of the change in their intestinal flora. Narcotic analgesics, however, are constipating medications.
4. Consuming fluids and fiber and exercising, can help clients to reestablish normal bowel function. If the provider has ordered "diet as tolerated," the nurse should recommend that the client order regular food from the menu.

TEST-TAKING HINT: This client is 2 days into the postoperative period, following a cesarean section. Many providers write postoperative orders that allow for the client to "advance diet as tolerated." In the past, clients who had abdominal surgery were not allowed to advance to soft or solid foods until they passed flatus. More recently, however, the literature highly recommends that a postoperative client be offered solid foods within 2 hours after surgery. This was found to enhance an earlier return to normal bowel function, increase client satisfaction, and to reduce postoperative nausea and length of stay (Macones et al., 2019).

42. 1. The client's subjective pain level is 2/5. It is unlikely that she needs stronger medication.
2. This statement is correct. One of the common side effects of narcotics is constipation.
3. This statement is incorrect. As long as the client feeds her baby frequently, the use of narcotics should not affect her milk production.
4. This statement is incorrect. This client's narcotic use is short term. Postoperative narcotic medications are considered safe for the breastfeeding baby. If the mother were a chronic narcotic user, the baby's response would be a concern.

TEST-TAKING HINT: Because clients who take narcotics are at high risk for constipation, the nurse should inform clients of the potential and advise them to take necessary precautions. For example, the clients should be advised to drink fluids, eat high-fiber foods, and ambulate regularly. In addition, the client should be advised of the potential for unintended narcotic dependency.

43. 1. This fundal height is within normal limits. The uterus of a client who had a cesarean section will often involute at a slightly slower pace than that of clients who have had vaginal deliveries.
2. This finding is normal. Pregnant clients and clients in the early postpartum period have nodular breasts in preparation for lactation.
3. This pulse rate is normal. Once the placenta is delivered, the reservoir for the large blood volume is gone. Clients often develop bradycardia as a result.
4. This blood loss is excessive, especially for a postoperative cesarean section client. The surgeon should be notified.

TEST-TAKING HINT: Because the placenta is manually removed and the uterine cavity is often manually wiped with sterile lap sponges during cesarean deliveries, it is common for postoperative clients to have a scanty lochial flow. This client is having a heavy loss. After the fundal assessment is complete, the observations should be reported to the surgeon.

44. 1. The nurse would not expect to see any drainage.
2. The nurse would expect to see well-approximated edges.
3. The nurse would not expect to see ecchymosis.
4. The nurse would not expect to see redness.

TEST-TAKING HINT: The best tool to use when assessing any incision is the REEDA scale. The nurse assesses for: R—redness, E—edema, E—ecchymosis, D—drainage, and A—poor approximation. If there is evidence of any of the findings, they should be documented, monitored, and reported.

45. 1. Even though this response may be true, the client's feelings are being ignored by the nurse.
2. This response is inappropriate. Even though the baby is well, the client feels disappointed with her performance.
3. Even though this response may be true, the client's feelings are being ignored by the nurse.
4. This response shows that the nurse has an understanding of the client's feelings.

TEST-TAKING HINT: When clients express their feelings, nurses must provide acceptance and implicit approval to encourage the clients to continue to express those feelings. Comments like "Don't say that. There are many women who would be ecstatic to have that baby" close down conversation and communicate disapproval. This sounds like it was a difficult delivery. The nurse must also consider that this client may be at risk of an emerging condition that has only recently been recognized: Postnatal Post-Traumatic Stress Disorder. Although there is a paucity of research on this topic, early research has indicated it can be triggered by the experience of a difficult birth, or one in which the birth plan was not met and the woman felt out of control and at mortal risk (Rodríguez-Almagro et al., 2019).

46. 1. Episiotomy sutures are not removed.
2. Clients who have had episiotomies may or may not require pain medication. The medicine should be offered throughout the day because it is usually ordered prn.
3. This statement is correct. When clients contract their buttocks before sitting, they usually feel less pain than when they sit directly on the suture line.
4. It is not recommended to irrigate episiotomy incisions.

TEST-TAKING HINT: Clients who have had episiotomies often avoid sitting normally. In addition to encouraging them to take medications as needed, nurses should encourage clients to contract their buttocks before sitting, and to sit normally rather than trying to favor one buttock over the other. Mediolateral incisions, which are incisions that are cut at approximately a 45-degree angle from the perineum, tend to be more painful than midline incisions (those cut posteriorly from the vagina toward the rectum). Median, or midline episiotomies are more commonly performed in the United States, while mediolateral episiotomies are more common in other parts of the world. An ACOG Practice Bulletin published in 2006 and reaffirmed in 2016 (ACOG, 2016a) determined that median episiotomy is associated with higher rates of injury to the anal sphincter and rectum than mediolateral episiotomy. They recommended restricted use of episiotomy in clinical practice (level A recommendation). In 2007, the United Kingdom published similar guidelines advocating against routine episiotomy, and recommending the use of mediolateral episiotomy when indicated (National Collaborating Centre for Women's and Children's Health, 2007).

47. 1. The client should ambulate. There is nothing in the scenario indicating that the client must use a bedpan.
2. It is likely that the client needs to urinate.
3. Indwelling catheters are rarely inserted for clients without epidurals during labor who have vaginal deliveries. There is nothing in the stem to indicate she had a catheter during labor.
4. This is the appropriate action by the nurse. The client should be accompanied to the bathroom.

TEST-TAKING HINT: Because pregnancy increases a client's clotting factors, postpartum clients are at high risk for thrombus formation. As such, ambulation should be encouraged. Clients who can ambulate safely to the bathroom should be encouraged to do so to prevent pooling of blood in the dependent blood vessels. Clients should be *accompanied* to the bathroom during the early postpartum period, however, because they may be light-headed from the stress and work of labor and delivery and from the fluid shifts as a result of giving birth.

48. 1. Fundal height is measured using a centimeter tape during pregnancy, not in the postpartum period.
2. The nurse should stabilize the base of the uterus with the nondominant hand.
3. The fundus should be palpated using the flat surface of the fingers.
4. No vaginal examination should be performed by the nurse.

TEST-TAKING HINT: If the base of the uterus is not stabilized during the assessment, there is a possibility that the uterus may invert or prolapse. While stabilizing the base, the nurse should gently assess for the fundus by palpating the abdomen firmly with the flat part of the fingers until the fundus is felt. The motion is one of moving the fingers and palm of the hand down, vertically toward the bed, then down horizontally toward the pubic bone to palpate the uterus.

49. 1. **This response is correct. Reassuring the client is appropriate.**
2. It is unlikely that the client has a urinary tract infection.
3. The urine will be blood tinged from the lochia.
4. This question is unnecessary. It is unlikely that the client has a urinary tract infection.

TEST-TAKING HINT: There is nothing in this question to indicate the client is at risk of a urinary tract infection. Frequent urination is normal after a delivery. The urine of a postpartum client will be blood tinged. This does not mean that the client has red blood cells in her bladder, but rather that the lochia from the vagina has contaminated the sample. Unless a catheterized sample is obtained, it is virtually impossible to obtain an uncontaminated urine sample in the postpartum period.

50. 1. The white blood cell count is within normal limits for a postpartum client.
2. The red blood cell count is within normal limits for a postpartum client.
3. **The client's hematocrit is well below normal. This value should be reported to the client's primary healthcare provider.**
4. The hemoglobin is within normal limits for a postpartum client.

TEST-TAKING HINT: The hematocrit of a postpartum client is likely to be below the "normal" of 35% to 45%, but a hematocrit of 30% or lower is considered abnormal and should be reported to the client's healthcare provider. It is likely that the client will be prescribed iron supplements.

51. 1. This response is not appropriate. This client is bleeding heavily and she is not breastfeeding.
2. It is unlikely that this client is menstruating since she is only 1½ weeks postpartum.
3. This response is not appropriate. The client should not bleed heavily, especially so long after delivery.
4. **This response is appropriate. The client should be examined to assess her uterine involution.**

TEST-TAKING HINT: One important piece of information in this question is the fact that the client is bottle feeding her baby. If she were breastfeeding, she could be encouraged to put the baby to breast and see if the bleeding subsided. Since oxytocin is released when babies suckle at the breast, this is a noninvasive method of promoting uterine contraction.

52. 1. This response is not accurate. Clients can begin to perform some exercises during the postpartum period.
2. The client can begin Kegel exercises, and little by little she can add other muscle-toning exercises during the postpartum period.
3. It is inappropriate to make this statement to a client. Her pre-pregnancy exercise schedule may be beyond her physical abilities at this time.
4. **This statement is correct. The client should begin with Kegel exercises shortly after delivery, move to abdominal tightening exercises in the next couple of days, and then slowly progress to stomach crunches, and so on.**

TEST-TAKING HINT: It is important for the postpartum client to begin muscle toning early in the postpartum period. However, she should not do any weight lifting or high-impact or stressful aerobic exercising until after her 6-week postpartum checkup.

53. 1. The involution is normal, at approximately 1 cm per postpartum day.
2. The involution is normal and the lochia is rubra.
3. **This response is correct. The involution is normal and the lochia is rubra.**
4. The lochia is not heavy, it is moderate rubra.

TEST-TAKING HINT: The first step in answering this question is to consider whether or not the involution is normal or abnormal. That will eliminate 2 of the question options. In this case, the client is experiencing normal involution of 2 cm at 2 days postpartum. The nurse would expect the fundus to descend below the umbilicus approximately 1 cm per postpartum day. In other words, at 1 day postpartum, the fundus is usually felt 1 cm below the umbilicus; 2 days postpartum, it is usually felt 2 cm below the umbilicus, and so on.

Lochia rubra is bright red, lochia serosa is pinkish to brownish, and lochia alba is whitish. It is common to have lochia rubra for the first 3 days after childbirth.

54. 1. This is an incorrect statement.
2. **This statement is accurate. Mothers often do not feel bladder pressure after delivery.**
3. Local anesthesia does not affect a client's ability to feel bladder distention.
4. This statement is inappropriate. The nurse should escort the client to the bathroom to urinate.

TEST-TAKING HINT: During pregnancy, the bladder loses its muscle tone because of the pressure exerted on it by the gravid uterus. As a result, after delivery, mothers are often unaware that their bladders have become distended unless they stand up and the weight of the bladder puts pressure on the urethra. This simple explanation can often be helpful to a client who might otherwise resist.

55. 1. Notifying the client's primary healthcare provider may be appropriate eventually, but it is not the first action that should be taken.
2. Massaging the client's fundus is the first action that the nurse should take.
3. Escorting the client to the bathroom may be needed, but it is not the first action that should be taken.
4. Assessing the client's lochial flow is needed, but it is not the first action that should be taken.

TEST-TAKING HINT: When a postpartum client's bladder is distended, the uterus becomes displaced and boggy because it cannot contract as it should. Deviation of the bladder to the right indicates a full bladder. The client should be escorted to the bathroom to void. However, before escorting the client to urinate, the nurse should assess the flow of lochia and gently massage the uterus to remove any large clots that might fall to the floor when the client stands up, causing a slippery surface on the floor.

56. Answers 2 and 4 are correct.
1. The client should perform pericare at each toileting and whenever she changes her peripad.
2. This statement is correct. The client should wash her hands before and after performing pericare.
3. When a client sits in a warm water bath, she is taking a sitz bath.
4. This statement is accurate. The client sprays the water from front to back.
5. Hydrogen peroxide is not added to a perineal irrigation bottle (peri bottle).

TEST-TAKING HINT: A postpartum client is taught to spray warm tap water on the perineum from front to back, after each toileting and whenever she changes her peripads. She should also be taught to wash her hands before and after the procedure.

57. 1. Ibuprofen is usually administered every 4 to 6 hours, depending on the dose.
2. This statement is correct. Ibuprofen has an anti-prostaglandin effect.
3. Ibuprofen is administered orally.
4. Administration of a high dose is not the reason ibuprofen is especially effective for postpartum cramping.

TEST-TAKING HINT: Natural prostaglandins are produced as part of the inflammatory response. They cause pain and inflammation. When ibuprofen is administered, the client benefits from both the pain-reducing action of the medication as well as its anti-inflammation properties. Ibuprofen can be thought of as an aid in neutralizing the painful acidic effects of physiologic prostaglandins.

58. An "X" should be placed on the line drawing at the level of the umbilicus.

TEST-TAKING HINT: By 12 hours after delivery, the fundus is usually felt at the level of the umbilicus. Every postpartum day thereafter, the fundus will descend about 1 cm, often documented as "one finger breadth" below the umbilicus.

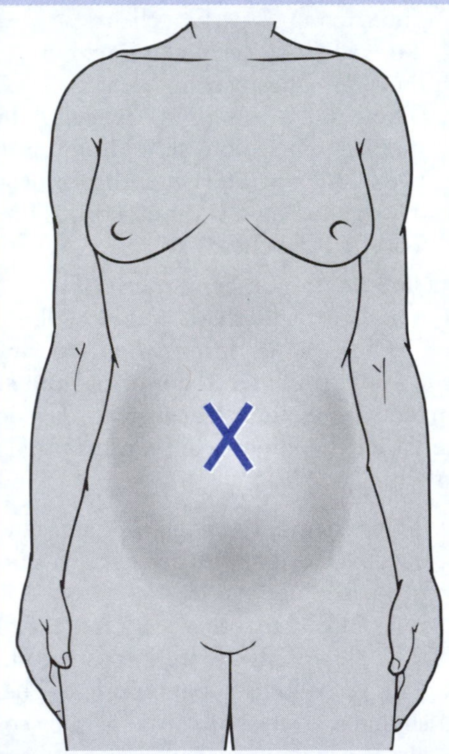

59. 1. Milk inhibits the absorption of iron. Milk and iron should not be consumed at the same time.
2. There is no recommendation that iron be taken with ginger ale.
3. The nurse would recommend that the iron be taken with orange juice because ascorbic acid, which is in orange juice, promotes the absorption of iron into the body.
4. There is no recommendation that iron be taken with chamomile tea.

TEST-TAKING HINT: **Since ascorbic acid promotes the absorption of iron into the body, it is appropriate for the nurse to recommend that the client take her iron supplement with a food source high in ascorbic acid, such as orange juice.**

60. 1. The nurse would not expect the values to rise. These results may indicate that the client is dehydrated or third spacing fluids (i.e., fluid is shifting into her interstitial spaces).
2. The nurse would not expect the values to remain the same. On average, clients lose about 500 mL of blood during spontaneous vaginal deliveries.
3. The nurse would expect these values—a slight decrease in both hemoglobin and hematocrit values.
4. The nurse would not expect the values to drop to these levels.

TEST-TAKING HINT: **The test taker must begin with the understanding that these two blood values drop slightly after delivery. Each potential response must then answer the question, "Is this a slight drop?" Answer 1 is eliminated because it indicates a higher result. Answer 2 is eliminated because it indicates an unchanged result. That leaves answers 3 and 4. Answer 3 indicates a slight drop, and answer 4 indicates a severe drop, which is abnormal. Therefore, answer 3 is the correct answer. Because clients lose blood during their deliveries, the nurse would expect to see approximately a 2% drop in the hematocrit and about a 0.5 gm/dL drop in the hemoglobin. If the hematocrit drops below 30%, the nurse should notify the primary healthcare provider.**

61. Answers 1, 2, and 5 are correct.
1. Sitz baths do have a soothing effect for clients with hemorrhoids.
2. Clients often feel some relief when external hemorrhoids are reinserted into the rectum.
3. Oxytocin will have no effect on the hemorrhoids.
4. It is impossible to tell whether or not the hemorrhoids will change with subsequent pregnancies.
5. Topical anesthetics can provide relief from the discomfort of hemorrhoids.

TEST-TAKING HINT: **Hemorrhoids are varicose veins of the rectum. They develop as a result of the weight of the gravid uterus on the client's dependent blood vessels. In addition to the actions noted previously, the client should be advised to eat high-fiber foods and drink fluids to prevent constipation, since straining with stools can lead to hemorrhoids.**

62. 1. Fundal assessment is the priority nursing action.
2. Pain level assessment is important, but it is not the priority nursing action.
3. Performing pericare is important, but it is not the priority nursing action.
4. Breast assessment is important, but it is not the priority nursing action.

TEST-TAKING HINT: **Hemorrhage is one of the primary causes of morbidity and mortality in postpartum women. It is essential, therefore, that nurses repeatedly assess a client's postpartum uterine tone. When the uterus is well contracted, a woman is unlikely to bleed heavily after delivery.**

63. 1. The appropriate action is to provide the client with warm blankets.
2. Postpartum shaking is very common. It is unnecessary to place the client in the Trendelenburg position.
3. Postpartum shaking is very common. It is unnecessary to notify the client's primary healthcare provider.
4. Postpartum shaking is very common. It is unnecessary to increase the client's intravenous fluid rate.

TEST-TAKING HINT: **Postpartum shaking is thought to be caused by nervous responses and/or vasomotor changes. The shaking is very common and, unless accompanied by a fever, is of no physiological concern. The best action by the nurse is supportive care—providing the client with a warm blanket and reassuring her that the response is within normal limits.**

64. 1. Early ambulation does help to prevent thrombophlebitis.
2. Oral fluid intake does not directly prevent thrombophlebitis.
3. Massaging of the legs is not helpful and in some situations can actually be harmful. If there is a clot in one of a client's lower extremity blood vessels, it can be dislodged when the leg is vigorously massaged.
4. High-fiber foods will prevent constipation, not thrombophlebitis.

TEST-TAKING HINT: **Postpartum clients are at high risk for thrombophlebitis because of an increase in the quantity of circulating clotting factors. To prevent clot formation, clients should ambulate as soon as possible after delivery. If they must be on bedrest because of complications, the nurse should contact the physician for an order for anti-embolic stockings and/or anti-embolic pressure boots and have the client perform active range-of-motion exercises.**

65. 1. Clients in the taking in phase are not receptive to teaching.

2. During the taking in phase, clients need to internalize their labor experiences. Discussing the labor process is appropriate for this postpartum phase.

3. Clients in the taking in phase do not focus on future issues or needs.

4. Clients in the taking in phase are not receptive to teaching.

TEST-TAKING HINT: The "taking in" postpartum phase is the first phase that clients pass through after they deliver their baby. During this time they are especially "me oriented." They wish and need to be cared for. This is a time when they should be given a chance to freshen up if desired, and/or be allowed to rest. They take in nourishment and take in the experience that they have just been through. They may want to review the experience with the nurse and seek validation that they did well. Primigravid and cesarean section clients often proceed more slowly through this phase than other clients.

66. 1. Nourishment is a need of the client in the taking in phase.

2. Rest is a need of the client in the taking in phase.

3. Assistance with self-care is a need of the client in the taking in phase.

4. Clients in the taking hold phase need assurance that they are learning the skills they will need to care for their new baby.

TEST-TAKING HINT: During the "taking hold" phase, clients regain their independence. They care for their own bodies and are very receptive to learning about child care as well as self-care. Primigravida clients are especially open to learning about caring for their baby during this phase and are especially vulnerable if they feel incompetent when performing baby-care tasks.

67. 1. Although the client is showing signs of positive bonding, she definitely needs a great deal of teaching.

2. This response is correct. The client is showing signs of positive bonding—"en face" positioning and stroking of the baby's cheeks. Because she is a primipara, she can benefit from information on child care.

3. This action is absolutely inappropriate at this time. There are no signs of poor bonding or of abuse.

4. There are no signs of poor bonding.

TEST-TAKING HINT: This client has never held a newborn before. The nurse, therefore, should be prepared to provide the client with information on newborn care. Two signs of positive bonding are holding a baby in the "en face position"—so that the mother is looking directly into the baby's eyes—and stroking the baby's cheeks.

68. 1. The client is not exhibiting signs of social isolation.

2. The client is not exhibiting signs of child neglect.

3. The client is exhibiting normal postpartum behavior.

4. The client is not exhibiting signs of postpartum depression.

TEST-TAKING HINT: This client is exhibiting signs of the postpartum "taking in" phase. She is a primigravida who delivered only 2 hours earlier. Her comments are well within those expected of a client at this point during her postpartum period.

69. 1. Although there is evidence that some fathers experience postpartum depression during the months following a birth, fathers have not been shown to experience postpartum blues.

2. This information is correct. The blues usually resolve within 2 weeks of delivery, in contrast to postpartum depression that can linger much longer and which may require medication and/or talk therapy.

3. Medications are usually not administered to relieve postpartum blues. Medications can be prescribed for clients who experience postpartum depression or postpartum psychosis.

4. This information is incorrect. The majority of women will experience postpartum blues during the first week or two postpartum.

TEST-TAKING HINT: There are three psychological changes that mothers may experience after the birth: postpartum blues, postpartum depression, and postpartum psychosis. Postpartum blues is a normal phenomenon experienced by the majority of women and is related to fatigue, hormonal shifts, and the enormous responsibility of becoming a mother. Postpartum depression and postpartum psychosis are pathological conditions that only some women experience.

70. 1. This action is appropriate. Although many Asian people believe in the hot-cold theory of disease and will often not drink cold fluids or eat cold foods during the postpartum period, the nurse must not assume this is the case.

2. The primary healthcare provider does not need to be informed.

3. There is no need to re-take the temperature. It is unlikely that the temperature will change significantly in 30 minutes.
4. This information is correct and the client may agree. She simply does not want ice water. The nurse must take into consideration the client's beliefs and traditions.

TEST-TAKING HINT: The knowledge that consuming fluids is important is not in conflict with this client's traditions. There is no reason the client must consume cold fluids. The nurse should first seek to understand the client's hesitation and then provide the client with warm fluids if she prefers.

71. **Answers 2 and 4 are correct.**
1. Methylergonovine is appropriate for a client with a heavy flow, who could be at risk of hemorrhaging. Of course, the nurse must also confirm that the client has no factors that would contraindicate the medication, such as pre-eclampsia.
2. **The order should be questioned for this client. A systolic blood pressure of 140 or higher, or a diastolic pressure of 90 or higher, or both, meet criteria for hypertension. Methylergonovine should not be given to clients with hypertension.**
3. Methylergonovine is not contraindicated for clients with diabetes.
4. **The order should be questioned for this client. Methylergonovine is not appropriate for a client with Raynaud's disease.**

TEST-TAKING HINT: Methylergonovine is an oxytoxic agent that works directly on the myofibrils of the uterus to maintain uterine contraction and prevent hemorrhage. The smooth muscle of the vascular tree is also affected. The blood pressure may elevate, therefore, to dangerous levels. The medication should be held if the blood pressure is 130/90 or higher and the client's primary healthcare provider should be notified if appropriate. Because Raynaud's syndrome is a vascular disease that causes intermittent blood flow to the extremities, methylergonovine should not be administered to clients with this condition, as it can aggravate the condition.

72. 1. **Lying prone on a pillow helps to relieve some women's afterbirth pains.**
2. Contracting the abdominal muscles has not been shown to alleviate afterbirth pains.
3. Ambulation has not been shown to alleviate afterbirth pains.
4. Drinking iced tea has not been shown to alleviate afterbirth pains.

TEST-TAKING HINT: Afterbirth pains can be quite uncomfortable, especially for multiparous women. The nurse should suggest that the clients take prn medications—ibuprofen is especially helpful—and try complementary therapies like lying on a small pillow on her abdomen or placing a hot water bottle on the abdomen.

73. 1. The client should not develop a headache from methylergonovine.
2. The client should not become nauseated from methylergonovine.
3. **Cramping is an expected outcome of the administration of methylergonovine.**
4. The client should not become fatigued from methylergonovine.

TEST-TAKING HINT: Methylergonovine is administered to postpartum clients to stimulate their uterus to contract. As a consequence, clients frequently complain of cramping after taking the medication. The nurse can administer the prn pain medication to the client at the same time the methylergonovine is administered to help to mitigate the client's discomfort.

74. 1. Estrogen drops precipitously after the placenta is delivered.
2. **Prolactin will elevate sharply in the client's bloodstream.**
3. Human placental lactogen drops precipitously after the placenta is delivered.
4. Human chorionic gonadotropin is produced by the fertilized ovum.

TEST-TAKING HINT: At the end of the third stage of labor, following delivery of the placenta, the hormones of pregnancy once produced by the placenta—progesterone and estrogen—drop precipitously. Prolactin is no longer inhibited and, therefore, rises. The woman's body prepares to provide milk for the baby, whether or not the woman plans to breastfeed. The hormone prolactin, referred to by some as *pro lactation*, begins to stimulate milk production once the placenta is delivered.

75. 1. This client's lochia flow and vital signs are normal. She is exhibiting no signs of fluid volume deficit.
2. This client has had no episiotomy or perineal laceration. She is exhibiting no signs of impaired skin integrity.
3. This client is voiding as expected—approximately every 2 hours. She is exhibiting no signs of impaired urinary elimination.
4. **This client is a primigravida. The nurse would anticipate that she is in need of teaching regarding newborn care as well as self-care.**

TEST-TAKING HINT: This is a difficult analysis level question. The test taker must determine, based on the facts given, which conditions to anticipate. This question, however, should be approached the same way that all other questions are approached: (1) determine what is being asked; (2) develop possible answers to the question BEFORE reading the given responses; (3) read the responses and answer them individually as true or false questions; and (4) choose the one response that is true.

76. 1. Offering to request a stool softener is not the best response because the answer implies that the stitches are near the rectum. The stitches are not near the rectal area.
    2. **This is the best response. A right mediolateral episiotomy is angled away from the perineum and rectum.**
    3. Recommending high fiber foods and liquids is not the best response because the answer implies that the stitches are near the rectum. The stitches are not near the rectal area.
    4. Recommending the use of anesthetic spray on the stitches is not the best response because the answer implies that the stitches are near the rectum. The stitches are not near the rectal area.

TEST-TAKING HINT: Women often are fearful of having a bowel movement when they have had an episiotomy or a laceration. Unless they have a third- or fourth-degree laceration, they should be assured that the stitches are a distance away from the rectal area, especially if they had a mediolateral episiotomy, which avoids the rectal area.

77. **42 gtt/min**

The standard formula to calculate an intravenous drip rate is:

$$\frac{\text{Volume} \times \text{Drop factor}}{\text{Time in minutes}} = \text{Drip rate (gtt/min)}$$

$$\frac{250 \text{ mL} \times 10 \text{ gtt/mL}}{60 \text{ min}} = \frac{2,500}{60} = 42 \text{ gtt/min}$$

The dimensional analysis method formula is:

$$\frac{\text{Volume ordered}}{\text{Time for infusion}} \bigg| \frac{\text{Drops}}{\text{per mL}} \bigg| \frac{\text{Time conversion}}{\text{in minutes (if needed)}} \bigg| \frac{\text{Volume conversion}}{\text{(if needed)}} = \text{Infusion rate (gtt/min)}$$

$$\frac{250 \text{ mL}}{60 \text{ min}} \bigg| \frac{10 \text{ gtt}}{} = \frac{2,500}{60} = 42 \text{ gtt/min}$$

TEST-TAKING HINT: There are three things to remember when calculating the answer to this question: (1) the quantity of fluid left in the IV is irrelevant because the physician has ordered the rate per hour; (2) the dosage of the medication is irrelevant because the volume of the fluid is not related to the medication dosage; and (3) time is always converted to minutes when a drip rate is calculated. (When a pump is being calibrated, on the other hand, the drip rate is generally programmed in mL/hr.)

78. 1. Although breastfeeding the newborn every 2 hours is an important goal, it is not the most important.
    2. Although consuming a normal diet is an important goal, it is not the most important.
    3. **Moderate (not heavy) lochial flow is the most important goal during the immediate postdelivery period.**
    4. Although ambulating to the bathroom every 2 hours is an important goal, it is not the most important.

TEST-TAKING HINT: When establishing priorities, the test taker should consider the client's most important physiological functions—that is, the C-A-B—circulation, airway, and breathing. If the client were to bleed heavily, her circulation would be compromised. None of the other goals is directly related to the C-A-Bs. Another consideration should be which of the answers relates to the lowest, most basic level of Maslow's hierarchy of needs—survival. The prevention of maternal hemorrhage is the one possible answer related to that need.

79. 1. It is not appropriate for the nurse to delegate fundal height assessments to the CNA. Physical assessment is a skill that requires professional nursing judgment.
2. It is not appropriate for the nurse to delegate client teaching to the CNA. Teaching is a skill that requires professional nursing knowledge.
3. It is appropriate for the nurse to delegate taking the client's vital signs to the CNA. Once the vital signs are checked, the CNA can report the results to the nurse for their interpretation.
4. It is not appropriate for the nurse to delegate documentation of lochial amount to the CNA. The chart is a legal document. Assessing the lochial amount is the responsibility of the nurse and nurses should document their own findings.

TEST-TAKING HINT: Delegation is an important skill. Nurses are unable to meet all the needs of all of their clients. They must ask other healthcare workers, for example, licensed practical nurses and certified nursing assistants (CNAs), to meet some of the clients' needs. It is essential, however, that the nurse delegate appropriately. Some state boards of nursing define "delegation" as tasks assigned in a community healthcare environment, and use the term "assign" in the acute care setting, rather than the term "delegate." In the end, the process of delegating means handing over a task to a healthcare worker who is not a Registered Nurse. Assessment, teaching, and documentation of nursing care are tasks that should not be delegated to nursing assistants. The nurse is responsible for confirming that the healthcare worker taking on the assigned or delegated tasks has had the proper training and is competent to do the task/s.

80. 1. There is nothing in the scenario that indicates that the client's feet and ankles need to be assessed.
2. This is unnecessary. The blood pressure can be assessed while a client is breastfeeding.
3. This action is very important. If the legs are removed from the stirrups one at a time, the client is at high risk for back and hip injuries.
4. It is unnecessary to measure the episiotomy. The provider will document the necessary information about the episiotomy that was performed.

TEST-TAKING HINT: Stirrups are not generally used during normal spontaneous deliveries; however, when forceps or vacuum extractors are used, physicians often request that the client's legs be placed in stirrups for stability. The nurse should raise the client's legs simultaneously when placing her legs in stirrups and lower her legs simultaneously when the delivery is complete, to prevent injury. The nurse should also position the legs with care. Pressure on the popliteal space can lead to thrombus formation.

81. 1. Although the uterine weight does drop precipitously when the baby is born, this is not the primary reason for the client's cardiovascular compromise.
2. This response is true. Once the placenta is delivered and the uterus contracts, the uterine circulatory reservoir for the mother's large blood volume is gone. Her peripheral circulation receives a 300 to 500 mL auto-transfusion of blood that once circulated throughout the uterus.
3. This response is not accurate. The cervix begins to contract shortly after delivery and the lochial flow is not related to the cardiovascular compromise that affects all postpartum clients.
4. This is a false statement. Maternal blood pressure does not drop precipitously when the baby's head emerges.

TEST-TAKING HINT: It is essential that the nurse closely monitor the vital signs of a newly delivered client. Because of the surge in blood volume from the uterus, the client is at high risk for cardiovascular compromise.

82. **1. Discharge teaching should be initiated at the time of admission. This nurse is correct in initiating the process in the labor room.**
2. Discharge teaching should be initiated at the time of admission, not right after the delivery.
3. Discharge teaching should be initiated at the time of admission, not when the baby begins breastfeeding for the first time.
4. Discharge teaching should be initiated at the time of admission; it should not wait until the day of discharge. There is too much information for the client to absorb all at once.

TEST-TAKING HINT: Discharge teaching should begin upon entry to the hospital. If nurses wait until the time of discharge, clients are expected to process a large amount of information during a very stressful time. Even when initiated early in the hospital stay, the nurse will likely need to repeat the instructions many times before the client is fully prepared to leave the hospital.

83. 1. Nothing must be placed in the vagina by the nurse, the client, or her partner before involution is complete.
2. This response is inappropriate. The amount of discharge does not determine the type of pad that can be used.
3. This response is inappropriate. The client's pain does not determine the type of pad that can be used.
4. **This response is correct. It is unsafe to place anything in the vagina before involution is complete.**

TEST-TAKING HINT: This question examines whether or not the test taker is aware of changes in care that are determined by the situation. Because the cervix is not fully closed and the uterine body is at high risk for infection, it is unsafe to insert anything into the vagina until involution is complete.

84. 1. **This answer is correct. The nurse should assess the level of anesthesia every 15 minutes while in the post-anesthesia care unit.**
2. This answer is inappropriate. The client had an indwelling catheter inserted for the surgery. And even if the catheter were removed immediately after the operation, she is paralyzed from the spinal anesthesia and unable to void.
3. This answer is inappropriate. The client has had major surgery. She will be consuming clear fluids, at the most, immediately after the cesarean section.
4. This answer is inappropriate. Immediately after surgery, the incision is covered by a dressing. Plus, it is too early for an infection to have appeared.

TEST-TAKING HINT: The key to answering this question is the fact that the client has just moved from the operating room. The nurse in the post-anesthesia care unit (PACU) is concerned with monitoring for immediate postoperative and postpartum complications and the client's recovery from the anesthesia.

85. 1. Cesarean section incisions do not routinely need to be irrigated.
2. **This is appropriate. The nurse should assess for all signs on the REEDA scale.**
3. The incision is held together with sutures or staples. It is unnecessary to apply steri strips at this time.
4. It is inappropriate for the nurse to palpate the suture line.

TEST-TAKING HINT: Once the dressing has been removed, the nurse on each shift should monitor the incision line for all signs on the REEDA scale—redness, edema, ecchymosis, discharge, and approximation.

86. **Answers 1, 3, 4, and 5 are correct.**
1. **The nurse should palpate the breasts to assess for fullness and/or engorgement.**
2. The postpartum assessment does not include carotid auscultation.
3. **The nurse should check the client's vaginal discharge.**
4. **The nurse should assess the client's extremities.**
5. **The nurse should inspect the client's perineum.**

TEST-TAKING HINT: If a nurse benefits from using acronyms, the acronym BUBBLE HE may help to remember the items in the postpartum assessment.. The letters stand for: B—breasts; U—uterus; B—bladder; B—bowels and rectum (for hemorrhoids and to inquire about most recent bowel movement); L—lochia; E—episiotomy (and perineum); H—hormones (for emotions); and E—extremities. It is important to note that Homan's sign is no longer recommended. Rather, careful inspection of the calves without dorsiflexing the foot for signs of DVT should be performed.

87. **Answers 1, 2, and 5 are correct.**
1. **The nurse would assess for pain.**
2. **The nurse would assess for warmth.**
3. The nurse would not be assessing for discharge.
4. The nurse would not be assessing for ecchymosis.
5. **The nurse would assess for redness.**

TEST-TAKING HINT: Postpartum clients are at high risk for deep vein thrombosis (DVT). At each postpartum assessment the nurse assesses the calves for signs of the complication, that is, those seen in any inflammatory response: pain, warmth, redness, and edema. If those signs/symptoms are noted, the nurse should notify the primary healthcare provider and discuss diagnostic tests to be performed, such as a Doppler series.

88. **Answers 1, 2, 3, and 5 are correct.**
1. **The nurse should auscultate the abdomen for presence of bowel sounds.**
2. **The nurse should palpate the firmness of the fundus.**
3. **The nurse should assess the nipple skin integrity, especially if the client is breastfeeding.**

4. The central venous pressure is not assessed.
5. **The nurse should auscultate the lung fields.**

TEST-TAKING HINT: Cesarean clients are surgical clients as well as postpartum clients. They should be monitored for complications associated with major abdominal surgery such as paralytic ileus and pneumonia. They should also be monitored for complications associated with labor, delivery, and the postpartum phases, such as boggy uterus and cracked nipples. Some nurses are reticent to palpate the fundus because of the pain it causes, but if the fundus does not contract effectively, the client is at high risk for hemorrhage—a very serious postpartum complication.

89. 1. **Many clients who have received epidurals during labor complain of a backache during the postpartum period.**
2. Light-headedness is rarely a complaint of post-epidural clients in the postpartum phase
3. Hypertension is not a complication seen in post-epidural clients.
4. Footdrop is very rarely a complication of epidural anesthesia.

TEST-TAKING HINT: Although a serious complication or a long-lasting side effect of epidural anesthesia is rare, clients who received epidurals during their labor and delivery frequently complain of backache. The clients should be counseled that the backaches usually resolve in a few weeks and that heat and over-the-counter analgesics are often effective in relieving the discomfort.

90. 1. Even though this statement is accurate, it is an inappropriate nursing response.
2. **The nurse should accurately respond to the client's request. This is her body and her baby.**
3. Even though this statement may be true, it is an inappropriate nursing response.
4. Even though this statement may be true, it is an inappropriate nursing response.

TEST-TAKING HINT: After much thought, some pregnant women decide that the best decision for themselves and their baby is to place the baby for adoption. While in the hospital, however, the woman is the baby's mother and may care for the baby herself. This may include breastfeeding, if she wishes. In some instances, women then decide to keep the baby rather than surrendering the baby to adoptive parents. This is still the client's decision, not the nurse's. The nurse must avoid making decisions for the client.

91. 1. Client transfer from labor and delivery to postpartum does not stimulate excess bleeding. It is unlikely that this is the rationale for the medication administration.
2. **It is likely that the medication was added during the third stage of labor to promote placental delivery and prevent postpartum hemorrhage.**
3. The placental separation was not rapid. Placental delivery usually occurs between 5 minutes and 30 minutes after the birth. A 10-minute timeframe is within normal parameters.
4. Twenty units of oxytocin is an unsafe dosage to be administered before the fetus is born and goes against all standards of obstetrical care.

TEST-TAKING HINT: Postpartum hemorrhage (PPH) is a leading cause of maternal death. One effective means of preventing PPH is active management of the third stage of labor. In other words, oxytocin is administered after the birth of the baby to promote uterine contraction and placental delivery. The oxytocin is usually added to the client's IV infusion and the infusion is continued until the fluid is fully absorbed.

92. 1. There is no indication the client is at risk of postpartum psychosis.
2. **The client is at risk of mastitis because she is engorged and has missed some feedings.**
3. There is no indication the client is at risk of candidiasis, or thrush.
4. Although the client may develop a breast abscess if this condition is not treated, there is no indication at this time that she is developing a breast abscess.

TEST-TAKING HINT: Inflammation of the breast, or mastitis, may or may not indicate a client has a breast infection. It occurs on a trajectory of breast engorgement to non-infective mastitis then infective mastitis, then breast abscess (Amir et al., 2014). Mastitis may occur in response to a number of factors that include a plugged duct, missed feedings, overproduction of milk, and/or poor attachment of the baby to the breast, resulting in inadequate emptying of the breasts (Amir & The Academy of Breastfeeding Medicine Protocol Committee, 2014). It is not uncommon for the client to have flu-like symptoms, but a fever is not always present. In this question, although a breast abscess is possible in the future, the most pressing, current likelihood of risk is non-infective mastitis.

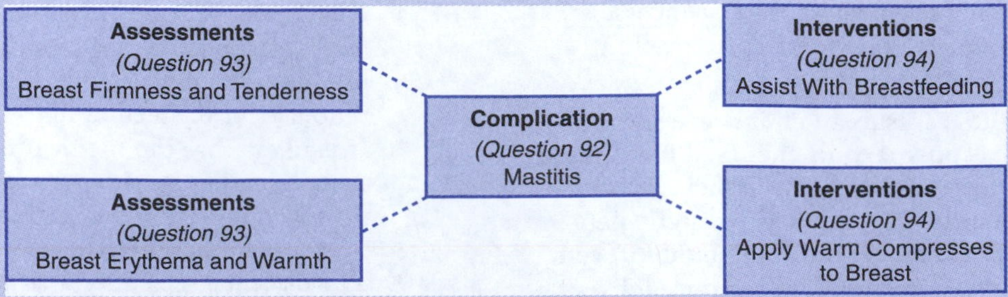

93. Answers 2 and 3 are correct.

1. The breast letdown reflex is not an assessment for mastitis.
2. **Breast firmness and tenderness can suggest engorgement, the first step toward mastitis.**
3. **Breast erythema and warmth are not normal findings in lactation and suggest mastitis.**
4. The amount of milk removed from the breast by the baby at each feeding would be important if the baby seemed undernourished or was not gaining weight. There is nothing in the stem to indicate concerns with the baby's nutrition.

TEST-TAKING HINT: Having recognized and analyzed cues, the nurse has identified mastitis as a priority hypothesis. The nurse's assessments focus on characteristics of the breast that support that hypothesis. In addition, a complete assessment will include vital signs, although a fever is not always present with non-infective mastitis.

94. Answers 1 and 4 are correct.

1. **It is important to assess the baby's latch and positioning at the breast in order to foster breastfeeding success and avoid a worsening mastitis, nipple injury, and/or breast abscess.**
2. Breastmilk cultures are not a first step in mastitis treatment. They are done, however, in certain situations such as no response to antibiotics after 48 hours, hospital-acquired mastitis, and/or recurrent mastitis (Amir & The Academy of Breastfeeding Medicine Protocol Committee, 2014).
3. Increased hydration—not a reduction in fluids—is recommended for mastitis treatment.
4. **Warm compresses to the breast can be soothing, can promote healing by bringing blood to the area, and can promote the breast let-down reflex, which aids in effective milk removal. After the feeding is over, the client may apply ice packs to the breasts and take analgesics as ordered by her primary healthcare provider, to reduce the discomfort. However, warm packs are more helpful than ice during the time that infant feeding is planned. Alternatively, the client may be encouraged to stand in a warm shower with her back to the water before the next feeding, and manually express some of the milk to soften the breasts and enhance the baby's breast attachment.**

TEST-TAKING HINT: In this case study, the nurse completed five steps of the NCSBN clinical judgment model in a condensed way: (1) recognize cues, (2) analyze cues, (3) prioritize hypotheses, (4) generate solutions, and (5) take action. The final step of evaluating outcomes may not be completed until a few days later, when the nurse returns for a follow-up visit. The test taker must keep these steps in mind, including the last one, (6) evaluate outcomes, when answering test questions and when caring for clients.

8 High-Risk Antepartum

Although pregnancy is considered to be a healthy state, there are several complications that may occur during the antepartum period, some of which result from preexisting conditions and some of which develop during the pregnancy. Any of these can affect the mother and/or the developing fetus. Questions in this chapter cover a number of topics that include spontaneous abortion (miscarriage), gestational diabetes, infectious diseases, pregnancy with multiple fetuses, and third trimester bleeding. To answer these questions, the nurse must be familiar not only with the pathophysiology of the conditions but also with the potential impact of the complications on the current pregnancy, future pregnancies, and lifelong health. In addition, because a healthy pregnancy is the expectation, any complication, no matter how small, can negatively impact the client's emotional state and dash her dreams about the joy she anticipated experiencing while pregnant. Instead of joy, the client and her family experience fear and anxiety. Accurate and up-to-date information is necessary as the nurse and other healthcare providers guide and support clients through a complicated pregnancy to what can still be a joyous birth.

KEYWORDS

The following words include English vocabulary, nursing/medical terminology, concepts, principles, or information relevant to content specifically addressed in the chapter or associated with topics presented in it. English dictionaries, your nursing textbooks, and medical dictionaries such as *Taber's Cyclopedic Medical Dictionary* are resources that can be used to expand your knowledge and understanding of these words and related information.

ABO incompatibility
Absent end diastolic flow (related to UA Doppler studies)
Adolescent pregnancy
Amniocentesis
Biophysical profile
Caudal agenesis
Cervical cerclage
Cervical insufficiency
Clonus
Complementary therapy
Coombs test
Diabetic ketoacidosis (DKA)
Euglycemic diabetic ketoacidosis (EDKA)
Dilation and curettage (D&C)
Dizygotic twins
Eclampsia
Ectopic pregnancy
Erythroblastosis fetalis
Fern test
Fetal kick count
Gestational diabetes mellitus (GDM)
Gestational trophoblastic disease
Glucose tolerance test (GTT)
Glycosylated hemoglobin (HbA1c)
HELLP syndrome (hemolysis, elevated liver enzymes, low platelet count)
Hemoglobin A1c (HbA1c)
Human placental lactogen (hPL)
Hydatidiform mole
Hydramnios (polyhydramnios)
Hyperemesis gravidarum
Hypertensive illnesses of pregnancy
Incompetent cervix
Lecithin/sphingomyelin ratio (L/S ratio)
Listeriosis
Monozygotic twins
Nonstress test (NST)
Oligohydramnios
Oral glucose tolerance test (OGTT)
Placenta previa
Placental abruption

Pre-eclampsia with and without severe features
Preterm labor
Preterm premature rupture of the membranes (PPROM)
Pseudocyesis
Reflex assessment
Reverse end diastolic flow (related to UA Doppler studies)
Rh incompatibility
Rho(d) immune globulin human
Rubella
Shake test (foam test)
Sickle cell disease
Spina bifida
Spontaneous abortion
SSRI (selective serotonin reuptake inhibitor)
Teratogen
Third-trimester bleed
Toxemia
Toxoplasmosis
Umbilical artery (UA) Doppler study
Vaginal birth after cesarean section (VBAC)

QUESTIONS

CASE STUDY: *The first six questions below are part of an evolving case study. All six questions follow the Next Generation NCLEX© question format of six steps:*

1. Recognize cues—What matters most?
2. Analyze cues—What could it mean?
3. Prioritize hypotheses—Where do I start?
4. Generate solutions—What can I do?
5. Take action—What will I do?
6. Evaluate outcomes—Did it help?

(National Council of State Boards of Nursing [NCSBN], 2020). For more information on the Next Generation NCLEX (NGN) question formats, see NGN quarterly newsletters at https://ncsbn.org.
NCLEX questions assume the nurse has a provider's order for listed interventions, unless noted otherwise.

1700: A 25-year-old woman at 35 weeks' gestation is brought to the labor and delivery unit by her husband. She is lethargic and complains of low abdominal pain. Her husband states she started vomiting the previous day and hasn't eaten anything since then. This is her first pregnancy. Her medical history includes type 1 diabetes mellitus (T1DM) for 2 years. Until the pain started, her insulin regimen was to administer an intermediate-acting insulin twice a day, and a short-acting insulin at each meal. Her husband states she has not been checking her blood sugar regularly because of the vomiting, and he's not sure she's been taking insulin since she has not been eating. He checked her blood sugar 30 minutes ago, before bringing her in and it was 320 mg/dL (17.8 mmol/L). The client's vital signs are T 98.6° F (37° C), P 110, R 24, BP 106/ 70. Her electronic medical record indicates a weight of 180 lb at her last office visit 7 days ago.

1. **Recognize cues. What matters most?** What additional information requires immediate follow-up? **Select all that apply.**
   1. Fundal height.
   2. Fetal heart rate.
   3. Capillary blood glucose (CBG).
   4. Urinalysis.
   5. Height and weight

2. **Analyze cues. What could it mean?** The client's provider does not use standing orders for diabetic clients. The nurse prepares to call the physician. Which of the following orders can the nurse anticipate receiving? **Select all that apply.**
   1. Intravenous fluid hydration.
   2. Serum blood glucose.
   3. Insulin IV bolus.
   4. Continuous insulin drip per pump.
   5. Orange juice, ¼ cup.
   6. Arterial blood gas analysis.

1730: The fetal monitor shows the fetal heart rate (FHR) at 120 bpm with minimal variability and no decelerations. In addition, the client is having irregular contractions every 5 to 7 minutes, lasting 30 to 45 seconds. They are mild on palpation.

The nurse has received orders from the physician. The following lab samples are sent to the appropriate departments and processed: (1) a urine sample for a urinalysis, culture, and sensitivity; (2) blood for arterial blood gases; and (3) blood for CBC and electrolytes. The client's urinalysis and culture are pending. Arterial blood gases are pH of 7.036, HCO3 of 2.6 mmol/L and PCO2 of 9.5 mm Hg. Serum blood glucose is 350 mg/dL (19.4 mmol/L). Potassium is 3.2 mmol/l. The provider indicates the client has diabetic ketoacidosis (DKA)

3. **Prioritize hypotheses. Where do I start?**

   Note: This is a two-part question. In the NCLEX exam, the test taker will have two drop-down boxes of four options each, from which to select an answer.

   The nurse is planning care for this client. The nurse should *first* address the client's:
   1. Blood glucose findings.
   2. Fetal heart rate pattern.
   3. Contraction pattern.
   4. Dehydration.

   Followed by the client's:
   a. Blood glucose findings.
   b. Fetal heart rate pattern.
   c. Contraction pattern.
   d. Dehydration.

4. **Generate solutions. What can I do?** Select words from the choices below to fill in each blank found in the following sentences:

   The best outcomes for the client would be to (1) _____ and (2) ________. To achieve optimal outcomes, the nurse should (3) _______ and (4) _______.
   a. Rehydrate.
   b. Accelerate fetal lung maturity.
   c. Insert urinary catheter.
   d. Achieve normoglycemia.
   e. Administer IV fluids.
   f. Achieve term delivery.
   g. Administer insulin.

5. **Take action. What will I do?** The nurse is initiating treatment for this client. Select two interventions that must be completed first. **Select two.**
   1. Insert indwelling catheter.
   2. Administer intravenous insulin therapy.
   3. Administer intravenous fluid therapy.
   4. Administer subcutaneous insulin therapy.
   5. Administer bicarbonate.
   6. Assess capillary blood glucose.
   7. Administer steroids for fetal lung maturity.

6. Evaluate outcomes. Did it help?

2130: The client has been hydrated with an IV infusion of normal saline. She has also received an insulin IV bolus per piggyback pump, and the nurse is setting the pump for a continuous insulin infusion. What outcomes are reasonable to anticipate over the next few hours as a result of these nursing interventions? **Select all that apply.**

1. FHR in normal range with moderate variability.
2. FHR with tachycardia and minimal variability.
3. Oxytocin induction.
4. Cesarean section.
5. Normoglycemia.

7. A client at 32 weeks' gestation with a severe headache and ankle swelling is admitted to the hospital with pre-eclampsia. Her vital signs are as follows: T 98.6° F (37° C), pulse rate 100, RR 20, BP 160/112. The blood pressure was repeated in 15 minutes and was 140/70. The nurse is preparing to call the primary healthcare provider. Which of the anticipated provider's orders can the nurse consider to be indicated, nonessential, or contraindicated?

Potential Order	Indicated (a)	Nonessential (b)	Contraindicated (c)
1. Magnesium sulfate 4 gm bolus over 20 minutes, followed by maintenance infusion of 2 gm/hour IV per pump.			
2. Insert indwelling catheter and send urine specimen to lab.			
3. Continuous fetal monitoring.			
4. Corticosteroids.			
5. Begin oxytocin induction.			
6. Begin 24-hour urine collection for protein.			
7. Antihypertensive medication.			

8. A nurse is counseling a pre-eclamptic client about her diet. Which should the nurse encourage the woman to do?

1. Restrict sodium intake.
2. Increase intake of fluids.
3. Eat a well-balanced diet.
4. Avoid simple sugars.

9. The nurse is evaluating the effectiveness of bedrest for a client with pre-eclampsia without severe features. Which of the following signs/symptoms would the nurse determine is a finding that suggests pre-eclampsia with severe features?

1. Platelet count 95,000/mcL.
2. 2+ proteinuria.
3. Increase in plasma protein.
4. Serum creatinine greater than 1.3 mg/dL.

10. A client at 32-weeks' gestation was last seen in the prenatal clinic 4 weeks ago, at 28 weeks' gestation. Which of the following changes should the nurse bring to the attention of the certified nurse midwife?

1. Weight change from 128 pounds to 138 pounds.
2. Pulse rate change from 88 bpm to 92 bpm.
3. Blood pressure change from 120/80 to 118/78.
4. Respiratory rate change from 16 to 20.

11. A client at 24 weeks' gestation is being seen in the prenatal clinic. She states, "I have had a terrible headache for the past 2 days." Which of the following is the most appropriate action for the nurse to perform next?
   1. Inquire whether or not the client has allergies.
   2. Take the woman's blood pressure.
   3. Assess the woman's fundal height.
   4. Ask the woman about stressors at work.

12. A nurse remarks to a client who has come to the clinic at 38 weeks' gestation, "It looks like your face and hands are swollen." The client responds, "Yes, you're right. Why do you ask?" The nurse's response is based on the fact that the changes may be caused by which of the following?
   1. Altered glomerular filtration.
   2. Cardiac failure.
   3. Hepatic insufficiency.
   4. Altered splenic circulation.

13. A client has pre-eclampsia with severe features. The nurse would expect the primary healthcare provider to order tests to assess the fetus for which of the following?
   1. Severe anemia.
   2. Hypoprothrombinemia.
   3. Craniosynostosis.
   4. Intrauterine growth restriction.

14. A gravid client with 4+ proteinuria and 4+ reflexes is admitted to the hospital. The nurse must closely monitor the woman for which of the following?
   1. Grand mal seizure.
   2. High platelet count.
   3. Explosive diarrhea.
   4. Jaundice.

15. A client is admitted to the hospital with a diagnosis of pre-eclampsia with severe features. The nurse is assessing for clonus. Which of the following actions should the nurse perform?
   1. Strike the woman's patellar tendon.
   2. Palpate the woman's ankle.
   3. Dorsiflex the woman's foot.
   4. Position the woman's feet flat on the floor.

16. The nurse is grading a woman's reflexes. Which of the following grades would indicate reflexes that are slightly brisker than normal?
   1. +1.
   2. +2.
   3. +3.
   4. +4.

17. A woman at 26 weeks' gestation is diagnosed with pre-eclampsia with severe features and HELLP syndrome. The nurse will assess for which of the following signs/symptoms?
   1. Low serum creatinine.
   2. High serum protein.
   3. Bloody stools.
   4. Epigastric pain.

18. A woman at 29 weeks' gestation with a diagnosis of pre-eclampsia with severe features is noted to have a blood pressure of 170/112, 4+ proteinuria, and a weight gain of 10 pounds over the past 2 days. Which of the following signs/symptoms would the nurse also expect to see?
   1. Fundal height of 32 cm.
   2. Oliguria.
   3. Patellar reflexes of +2.
   4. Nystagmus.

19. A client diagnosed with pre-eclampsia without severe features has been advised to stop working and be on light activities and bedrest at home. She asks why this is necessary. Which of the following is the best response for the nurse to give the client?
    1. "Bedrest will help you to conserve energy for your labor."
    2. "Bedrest will help to relieve your nausea and anorexia."
    3. "Reclining will increase the amount of oxygen that your baby gets."
    4. "The position change will prevent the placenta from separating."

20. In anticipation of a complication that may develop in the second half of pregnancy, the nurse teaches a client at 18 weeks' gestation to call the office if she experiences which of the following?
    1. Headache and decreased output.
    2. Puffy feet.
    3. Hemorrhoids and vaginal discharge.
    4. Backache.

21. Which of the following clients is at highest risk for developing a hypertensive illness of pregnancy?
    1. G1 P0000, age 41 with history of diabetes mellitus.
    2. G2 P0101, age 34 with history of rheumatic fever.
    3. G3 P1102, age 27 with history of scoliosis.
    4. G3 P1011, age 20 with history of celiac disease.

22. The nurse has assessed four primigravid clients in the prenatal clinic. Which of the women would the nurse refer to the nurse midwife for further assessment?
    1. 10 weeks' gestation, complains of fatigue with nausea and vomiting.
    2. 26 weeks' gestation, complains of ankle edema and chloasma.
    3. 32 weeks' gestation, complains of epigastric pain and facial edema.
    4. 38 weeks' gestation, complains of bleeding gums and urinary frequency.

23. A client's previous clinic assessment at 32 weeks was: BP 90/60; TPR 98.6° F (37° C), P 92, R 20; weight 145 lb; and urine negative for protein. Which of the following findings at the 34-week appointment should the nurse highlight for the certified nurse midwife?
    1. BP 110/70; TPR 99.2° F (37° C), P 88, R 20.
    2. Weight 155 lb; urine protein +2.
    3. Urine protein trace; BP 88/56.
    4. Weight 147 lb; TPR 99° F (37° C), P 76, R 18.

24. A nurse is caring for a 25-year-old client who has just had a spontaneous first trimester abortion. Which of the following comments by the nurse is appropriate?
    1. "You can try again very soon."
    2. "It is probably better this way."
    3. "At least you weren't very far along."
    4. "I'm here to talk if you would like."

25. The blood work of a client hospitalized on the antepartum unit of the hospital is as follows: hematocrit 30% and hemoglobin 10 gm/dL. In light of the laboratory data, which of the following meal choices should the nurse recommend to this client?
    1. Chicken livers, sliced tomatoes, and dried apricots.
    2. Cheese sandwich, tossed salad, and rice pudding.
    3. Veggie burger, cucumber salad, and wedge of cantaloupe.
    4. Bagel with cream cheese, pear, and hearts of lettuce.

26. A gravid woman has just been admitted to the emergency department subsequent to a head-on automobile accident. Her body appears to be uninjured. The nurse carefully monitors the woman for which of the following possible complications of pregnancy? **Select all that apply.**
   1. Placenta previa.
   2. Transverse fetal lie.
   3. Placental abruption.
   4. Pre-eclampsia with severe features.
   5. Preterm labor.

27. A 25-year-old client is admitted with the following history: 12 weeks pregnant, vaginal bleeding, no fetal heartbeat seen on ultrasound. The nurse would expect the doctor to write an order to prepare the client for which of the following?
   1. Cervical cerclage.
   2. Amniocentesis.
   3. Nonstress testing.
   4. Dilation and curettage.

28. Which of the following long-term goals is appropriate for a client at 10 weeks' gestation who is diagnosed with gestational trophoblastic disease (hydatidiform mole)?
   1. Client will be cancer-free 1 year from diagnosis.
   2. Client will deliver her baby at full term without complications.
   3. Client will be pain-free 3 months after diagnosis.
   4. Client will have normal hemoglobin and hematocrit at delivery.

29. Which of the following findings should the nurse expect when assessing a client at 8 weeks' gestation with gestational trophoblastic disease (hydatidiform mole)?
   1. Protracted pain.
   2. Variable fetal heart decelerations.
   3. Dark-brown vaginal bleeding.
   4. Suicidal ideations.

30. Which of the following findings would the nurse expect to see when assessing a first-trimester gravida client suspected of having gestational trophoblastic disease (hydatidiform mole) that the nurse would not expect to see when assessing a first-trimester gravida with a normal pregnancy? **Select all that apply.**
   1. Hematocrit 39%.
   2. Grape-like clusters passed from the vagina.
   3. Markedly elevated blood pressure.
   4. White blood cell count 8,000/mcL.
   5. Hypertrophied breast tissue.

31. Which finding should the nurse expect when assessing a client with placenta previa?
   1. Severe occipital headache.
   2. History of thyroid cancer.
   3. Previous premature delivery.
   4. Painless vaginal bleeding.

32. A nurse is caring for four prenatal clients in the clinic. Which of the clients is at high risk for placenta previa? **Select all that apply.**
   1. Jogger with low body mass index.
   2. Primigravida who smokes 1 pack of cigarettes per day.
   3. Infertility client who is carrying in-vitro triplets.
   4. Registered nurse who works 12-hour shifts.
   5. Police officer on foot patrol.

33. A woman has been diagnosed with a ruptured ectopic pregnancy. Which of the following signs/symptoms is characteristic of this diagnosis?
   1. Dark-brown rectal bleeding.
   2. Severe nausea and vomiting.
   3. Sharp unilateral pain.
   4. Marked hyperthermia.

34. A pregnant client with an obstetrical history of G2 P1001, telephones the gynecology office complaining of left-sided pain. Which of the following questions by the triage nurse would help to determine whether the one-sided pain is due to an ectopic pregnancy?
1. "When did you have your pregnancy test done?"
2. "When was the first day of your last menstrual period?"
3. "Did you have any complications with your first pregnancy?"
4. "How old were you when you first got your period?"

35. A woman, 8 weeks pregnant, is admitted to the obstetrical unit with a diagnosis of threatened abortion. Which of the following tests would help to determine whether the woman is carrying a viable or a nonviable pregnancy?
1. Luteinizing hormone level.
2. Endometrial biopsy.
3. Hysterosalpingogram.
4. Serum progesterone level.

36. A woman with a diagnosis of ectopic pregnancy is to receive medical intervention rather than a surgical interruption. Which of the following intramuscular medications would the nurse expect to administer?
1. Dexamethasone.
2. Methotrexate.
3. Menotropin.
4. Progesterone.

37. A woman who has been diagnosed with an ectopic pregnancy is to receive methotrexate 50 mg/m^2 IM. The woman weighs 136 lb and is 5 ft 4 in. tall. What is the maximum safe dose in mg of methotrexate that this woman can receive? **(If rounding is needed, please round to the nearest tenth.)**

______ mg

38. A woman is to receive methotrexate IM for an ectopic pregnancy. The drug reference states that the recommended safe dose of the medicine is 50 mg/m^2. She weighs 52 kg and is 148 cm tall. What is the maximum safe dose in mg of methotrexate that this woman can receive? **(If rounding is needed, please round to the nearest tenth.)**

______ mg

39. A woman is to receive methotrexate IM for an ectopic pregnancy. The nurse should teach the woman about which of the following common side effects of the therapy? **Select all that apply.**
1. Nausea and vomiting.
2. Abdominal pain.
3. Fatigue.
4. Light-headedness.
5. Breast tenderness.

40. The nurse is caring for a client who was just admitted to the hospital to rule out ectopic pregnancy. Which of the following orders is the most important for the nurse to perform?
1. Take the client's temperature.
2. Document the time of the client's last meal.
3. Obtain urine for urinalysis and culture.
4. Assess for complaint of dizziness or weakness.

41. A client is admitted with a diagnosis of third-trimester bleeding. It is a priority for the nurse to assess for a change in which of the following vital signs?
1. Temperature.
2. Pulse.
3. Respirations.
4. Blood pressure.

42. A client with an obstetrical history of G6 P5005, has been admitted to the hospital at 24 weeks' gestation with placenta previa. Which of the following is an appropriate long-term goal for this client?
1. The client will state an understanding of need for complete bedrest.
2. The client will have a reactive nonstress test (NST) on day 2 of hospitalization.
3. The client will be symptom-free until at least 37 weeks' gestation.
4. The client will have normal vital signs on admission.

43. Which of the following statements is appropriate for the nurse to say to a client with a complete placenta previa?
1. "During the first phase of labor you will do slow chest breathing."
2. "You should ambulate in the halls at least two times each day."
3. "The doctor will deliver you once you reach 25 weeks' gestation."
4. "It is important that you inform me if you become constipated."

44. A client at 12 weeks' gestation presents in the emergency department with abdominal cramps and scant, dark-red bleeding. For which of the following signs/symptoms should the nurse assess this client? **Select all that apply.**
1. Tachycardia.
2. Referred shoulder pain.
3. Headache.
4. Fetal heart dysrhythmias.
5. Hypertension.

45. A client is on total bedrest at 32 weeks' gestation with placenta previa. The physician expects her to be hospitalized on bedrest until her cesarean section, which is scheduled for 38 weeks' gestation. To prevent complications while in the hospital, the nurse should do which of the following? **Select all that apply.**
1. Perform passive range-of-motion exercises.
2. Restrict the fluid intake of the client.
3. Decorate the room with pictures of family.
4. Encourage the client to eat a high-fiber diet.
5. Teach the client deep-breathing exercises.

46. A client is pregnant with monochorionic twins. For which of the following complications should this pregnancy be monitored?
1. Oligohydramnios.
2. Placenta previa.
3. Cephalopelvic disproportion.
4. Twin-to-twin transfusion.

47. On ultrasound, it is noted that the pregnancy of a hospitalized woman who is carrying monochorionic twins is complicated by twin-to-twin transfusion. The nurse should carefully monitor this client for which of the following?
1. Rapid fundal growth.
2. Vaginal bleeding.
3. Projectile vomiting.
4. Congestive heart failure.

48. A nurse is performing assessments on four clients at 22 weeks' gestation. The nurse reports to the obstetrician that which of the clients may be carrying twins?
1. The client whose progesterone levels are elevated.
2. The client with a weight gain of 13 pounds.
3. The client whose fundal height measurement is 26 cm.
4. The client whose alpha-fetoprotein level is one-half normal.

49. Which of the following pregnant clients is most high risk for preterm premature rupture of the membranes (PPROM)? **Select all that apply.**
1. 31 weeks' gestation with prolapsed mitral valve (PMV).
2. 32 weeks' gestation with urinary tract infection (UTI).
3. 33 weeks' gestation with twins post–in vitro fertilization (IVF).
4. 34 weeks' gestation with gestational diabetes (GDM).
5. 35 weeks' gestation with deep vein thrombosis (DVT).

50. A grand multipara with an obstetrical history of G8 P3406 is being seen at 14 weeks' gestation in the prenatal clinic. During the nurse's prenatal teaching session, the nurse will emphasize that the woman should notify the obstetric office immediately if she notes which of the following?
1. Change in fetal movement.
2. Signs and symptoms of labor.
3. Swelling of feet and ankles.
4. Appearance of spider veins.

51. A woman at 12 weeks' gestation with an obstetrical history of G4 P0210 has been admitted to the labor and delivery suite for a cerclage procedure. Which of the following long-term outcomes is average for this client?
1. The client will gain less than 25 pounds during the pregnancy.
2. The client will deliver after 38 weeks' gestation.
3. The client will have a normal blood glucose throughout the pregnancy.
4. The client will deliver a baby who is average for gestational age.

52. A woman with an obstetrical history of G5 P0311 is in the post-anesthesia care unit (PACU) after a cervical cerclage procedure. During the immediate post-procedure period, what should the nurse carefully monitor this client for?
1. Hyperthermia.
2. Hypotension.
3. Uterine contractions.
4. Fetal heart dysrhythmias.

53. A multigravida at 30 weeks' gestation with an obstetrical history of G3 P1011 is admitted to the labor suite. She is contracting every 5 minutes, with a contraction duration of 40 seconds. Which of the comments by the client would be most informative regarding the etiology of the client's present condition?
1. "For the past day I have felt burning when I urinate."
2. "I have a daughter who is 2 years old."
3. "I jogged 1½ miles this morning."
4. "My miscarriage happened a year ago today."

54. A client who works as a waitress and is 35 weeks pregnant telephones the labor suite after getting home from work and states, "I am feeling tightening in my groin about every 5 to 6 minutes." Which of the following comments by the nurse is appropriate at this time?
1. "Please lie down and drink about four full glasses of water or juice."
2. "You are having false labor pains so you need not worry about them."
3. "It is essential that you get to the hospital immediately."
4. "That is very normal for someone who is on her feet all day."

55. A client with type 1 diabetes mellitus (T1DM) has developed polyhydramnios. She is 34 weeks pregnant. The client should be taught to report which of the following?
    1. Uterine contractions.
    2. Reduced urinary output.
    3. Marked fatigue.
    4. Puerperal rash.

56. A pregnant client with diabetes has been diagnosed with polyhydramnios. Which of the following would explain this finding?
    1. Excessive fetal urination.
    2. Recurring hypoglycemic episodes.
    3. Fetal sacral agenesis.
    4. Placental vascular damage.

57. A client with type 1 diabetes mellitus (T1DM) is being seen for preconception counseling. The nurse should emphasize that during the first trimester the woman may experience which of the following?
    1. Needing less insulin than normal
    2. More frequent hyperglycemic episodes.
    3. Polyhydramnios.
    4. A need to be hospitalized for fetal testing.

58. The results of a 75-gram oral glucose tolerance test (OGTT) for a client at 25 weeks' gestation are:

    - Fasting—100 mg/dL (5.5 mmol/L)
    - One hour—200 mg/dL (11.1 mmol/L)
    - Two-hour—160 mg/dL (8.9 mmol/L).

    Which of the following information is appropriate for the nurse to give the client at this time?
    1. Inform the client that the glucose results are normal.
    2. Inform the client that an additional 3-hour 100-gram oral glucose test is necessary for follow-up.
    3. Inform the client that the primary healthcare provider will likely order an oral hypoglycemic agent.
    4. Inform the client that the primary healthcare provider will likely order a referral to a registered dietitian.

59. The nurse is educating a client who has been diagnosed with gestational diabetes how to perform home blood glucose testing. Which of the following information should be included in the teaching session?
    1. When pricking the fingertip, always prick the center of the fingertip.
    2. One-hour postprandial glucose values should be 146 mg/dL (8 mmol/L) or lower.
    3. Blood glucose testing should be performed 2 times per day—before breakfast and before bedtime.
    4. All blood glucose results should be kept in a log for evaluation by the nurse and primary healthcare provider.

60. In analyzing the need for health teaching in a client with an obstetrical history of G5 P4004 who has been diagnosed with gestational diabetes, the nurse should ask which of the following questions?
    1. "How old were you at your first pregnancy?"
    2. "Do you exercise regularly?"
    3. "Is your partner diabetic?"
    4. "Do you work outside of the home?"

61. A client at 36 weeks' gestation with type 1 diabetes mellitus (T1DM) has just had a biophysical profile (BPP). Which of the following results should be reported to the obstetrician?
 1. One fetal heart acceleration in 20 minutes.
 2. Three episodes of fetal rhythmic breathing in 30 minutes.
 3. Two episodes of fetal extension and flexion of 1 arm.
 4. One amniotic fluid pocket measuring 3 cm.

62. A client at 27 weeks' gestation has been diagnosed with gestational diabetes. Which of the following therapies will most likely be ordered for this client?
 1. Oral hypoglycemic agents.
 2. Diet control with exercise.
 3. Regular insulin injections.
 4. Inhaled insulin.

63. A client has just done a fetal kick count assessment. She noted 6 movements during the past hour. If taught correctly, what should her next action be?
 1. Nothing, because further action is not warranted.
 2. Call the primary healthcare provider to discuss next steps.
 3. Redo the test during the next half hour.
 4. Drink a glass of orange juice and redo the test.

64. A nurse who is caring for a pregnant client with type 1 diabetes mellitus (T1DM) should carefully monitor the client for which of the following? **Select all that apply.**
 1. Urinary tract infection.
 2. Multiple gestation.
 3. Metabolic acidosis.
 4. Pathologic hypotension.
 5. Hypolipidemia.

65. A client with gestational diabetes who requires insulin therapy to control her blood glucose levels telephones the hospital's obstetrical unit, complaining of dizziness and a racing pulse. Which of the following actions should the nurse take at this time?
 1. Have the client proceed to the office to see her primary healthcare provider.
 2. Advise the client to drink a glass of juice and then call back.
 3. Instruct the client to inject herself with regular insulin.
 4. Tell the client to telephone her primary healthcare provider immediately.

66. A client with diabetes is to receive 5 units regular and 15 units NPH insulin at 0800. To administer the medication appropriately, what is the best approach?
 1. Draw 5 units regular in one syringe and 15 units NPH in a second syringe and inject in different locations.
 2. Draw 5 units regular first and 15 units NPH second into the same syringe and inject.
 3. Draw 15 units NPH first and 5 units regular second into the same syringe and inject.
 4. Mix 5 units regular and 15 units NPH in a vial before drawing the full 20 units into a syringe and inject.

67. The nurse is caring for a client with type 1 diabetes mellitus (T1DM) who wishes to become pregnant. The nurse notes that the client's glycohemoglobin, or glycosylated hemoglobin (Hgb A1c), result was 7% today and the fasting blood glucose result was 100 mg/dL (5.5 mmol/L). Which of the following interpretations by the nurse is correct in relation to these data?
 1. The client has been hyperglycemic for the past 3 months and is within target levels today.
 2. The client has been normoglycemic for the past 3 months and is within target today.
 3. The client has been normoglycemic for the past 3 months and is within target today.
 4. The client has been within target for the past 3 months and is hyperglycemic today.

68. A client with insulin-dependent diabetes will require higher doses of insulin as which of the following pregnancy hormones increases in her body?
   1. Estrogen.
   2. Progesterone.
   3. Human chorionic gonadotropin.
   4. Human placental lactogen.

69. A client has just been diagnosed with gestational diabetes. She cries, "Oh no! I will never be able to give myself shots!" Which of the following responses by the nurse is appropriate at this time?
   1. "I am sure you can learn for your baby."
   2. "I will work with you until you feel comfortable giving yourself the insulin."
   3. "We will be giving you pills for the diabetes."
   4. "If you follow your diet and exercise you will probably need no insulin."

70. A client with insulin-dependent diabetes and an obstetrical history of G3 P0200, is being seen at 38 weeks' gestation, in the labor and delivery suite. The client states she has had nausea and vomiting for the past 24 hours and thinks she has a bladder infection. The nurse knows that which of the following maternal blood values presents the highest risk to her unborn baby?
   1. Glucose 150 mg/dL (8.3 mmol/L).
   2. pH 7.25.
   3. PCO2 34 mm Hg.
   4. Hemoglobin A1c 6%.

71. A 30-year-old client with an obstetrical history of G3 P1201, states she is planning to become pregnant again. She reports that 8 years ago she gave birth to a premature baby boy who died shortly after delivery from an infection secondary to spina bifida. Which of the following interventions is most important for this client?
   1. Grief counseling.
   2. Nutrition counseling.
   3. Infection control counseling.
   4. Genetic counseling.

72. A client at 42 weeks' gestation has just had a 20-minute nonstress test (NST). Which of the following results would the nurse interpret as a reactive test?
   1. Moderate fetal heart rate (FHR) baseline variability.
   2. Maternal heart rate accelerations to 140 bpm lasting at least 20 seconds.
   3. Two fetal heart rate accelerations of 15 bpm lasting at least 15 seconds.
   4. Absence of maternal premature ventricular contractions.

73. A client with an obstetrical history of G1 P0000, is at 40 5/7 weeks' gestation. Her Bishop score is 4. Which of the following complementary therapies might be recommended? **Select all that apply.**
   1. Sexual intercourse.
   2. Aromatherapy.
   3. Breast stimulation.
   4. Ingestion of castor oil.
   5. Aerobic exercise.

74. A client at 24 weeks' gestation has been diagnosed with severe choledocholithiasis and is scheduled for a cholecystectomy under general anesthesia. In addition to routine surgical and postsurgical care, the nurses should pay special attention to which of the following? **Select all that apply.**
    1. The circulating nurse should place the woman supine and slightly tilted to the left during the surgical procedure.
    2. An obstetrical nurse should assess the fetal heart rate regularly following the surgery.
    3. The post-anesthesia care nurse should monitor the client's lochia and the firmness of her fundus.
    4. The post-anesthesia care nurse should monitor the woman carefully for nausea and vomiting.
    5. The circulating nurse should place anti-embolic stockings on the woman's legs preoperatively.

75. A pregnant woman has sickle cell anemia. Which of the following situations could precipitate a vaso-occlusive crisis in this woman?
    1. Hypoxia.
    2. Alkalosis.
    3. Fluid overload.
    4. Hyperglycemia.

76. A pregnant woman with sickle cell anemia is admitted in vaso-occlusive crisis. Which of the following is the priority intervention that the nurse must perform?
    1. Administer narcotic analgesics.
    2. Apply heat to swollen joints.
    3. Place on strict bedrest.
    4. Infuse intravenous solution.

77. A pregnant woman with obesity is being seen in the prenatal clinic. The nurse will monitor this client carefully throughout her pregnancy because she is at high risk for which of the following complications of pregnancy? **Select all that apply.**
    1. Placenta previa.
    2. Gestational diabetes.
    3. Deep vein thrombosis.
    4. Pre-eclampsia.
    5. Chromosomal defects.

78. A client with obesity is being seen by the nurse during her prenatal visit. Which of the following comments by the nurse is appropriate at this time?
    1. "We will want you to gain the same amount of weight we would encourage any pregnant woman to gain."
    2. "To have a healthy baby we suggest that you go on a weight-reduction diet right away."
    3. "To prevent birth defects we suggest that you gain weight during the first trimester and then maintain your weight for the rest of the pregnancy."
    4. "Weight gain is expected throughout your pregnancy, but the guidelines are lower for women in your weight category."

79. The physician has ordered a nonstress test (NST) to be done on a client at 41 weeks' gestation. During the test, the nurse observed three periods of fetal heart accelerations that were 15 beats per minute above the baseline and that lasted 15 seconds each. No contractions were observed. Based on these results, what should the nurse do next?
    1. Report positive results to the medical doctor and send the client home if ordered.
    2. Perform a nipple stimulation test to assess the fetal heart in response to contractions.
    3. Prepare the client for induction with intravenous oxytocin.
    4. Place the client on her side with oxygen via face mask.

80. A 39-year-old client at 18 weeks' gestation has had an amniocentesis. Before discharge, the nurse teaches the woman to call her doctor if she experiences which of the following conditions? **Select all that apply.**
1. Fever or chills.
2. Lack of fetal movement.
3. Abdominal pain.
4. Rash or pruritus.
5. Vaginal bleeding or fluid.

81. The fetus of a client at 38 weeks' gestation has been diagnosed with intrauterine growth restriction (IUGR). The nurse would expect that which of the following diagnostic assessments would be appropriate for the primary healthcare provider to order at this time? **Select all that apply.**
1. Biophysical profile (BPP).
2. Nonstress test (NST).
3. Umbilical artery (UA) Doppler assessment.
4. Chorionic villus sampling (CVS).
5. Human chorionic gonadotropin test (HCG)

82. A biophysical profile (BPP) has been performed on a full-term client who has pre-eclampsia with severe features. Which of the following interpretations should the nurse make regarding the BPP results of 4?
1. Fetal well-being is compromised.
2. Client's blood pressure is returning to normal.
3. Client is at high risk for seizure.
4. Fetus's amniotic sac is about to rupture.

83. A lecithin/sphingomyelin (L/S) ratio has been ordered by a pregnant woman's obstetrician. Which of the following data will the nurse learn from this test?
1. Coagulability of maternal blood.
2. Maturation of the fetal lungs.
3. Potential for fetal development of erythroblastosis fetalis.
4. Potential for maternal development of gestational diabetes.

84. The laboratory reported the L/S ratio results from an amniocentesis as 1:1. How should the nurse interpret the result?
1. The baby is premature.
2. The mother is at high risk for hemorrhage.
3. The infant has kernicterus.
4. The mother is at high risk for eclampsia.

85. A client is being taught fetal kick counting. Which of the following should be included in the client teaching?
1. The client should choose a time when their baby is least active.
2. The client should lie on their side
3. The client should report fetal kick counts of greater than 10 in an hour.
4. The client should refrain from eating immediately before counting.

86. An ultrasound is being done on an Rh-negative woman. Which of the following pregnancy findings would indicate that the baby has developed erythroblastosis fetalis?
1. Caudal agenesis.
2. Cardiomegaly.
3. Oligohydramnios.
4. Hyperemia.

87. A woman is to receive Rh_o(D) immune globulin at 28 weeks' gestation. Which of the following actions must the nurse perform before giving the injection?
1. Validate that the baby is Rh-negative.
2. Assess that the direct Coombs test is positive.
3. Verify the identity of the woman.
4. Reconstitute the globulin with sterile water.

88. A nurse is about to inject Rho(D) immune globulin into an Rh-negative (Rh–) mother. Which of the following is the preferred site for the injection?
1. Deltoid.
2. Dorsogluteal.
3. Vastus lateralis.
4. Ventrogluteal.

89. A client is recovering at the gynecologist's office following a late first-trimester spontaneous abortion. At this time, it is essential for the nurse to check which of the following?
1. Maternal varicella titer.
2. Past obstetric history.
3. Maternal blood type.
4. Cervical patency.

90. At 28 weeks' gestation, an Rh-negative (Rh–) woman receives Rho(D) immune globulin. What is the expected outcome of administering the medication?
1. The baby's Rh status changes to Rh-negative (Rh–)
2. The mother produces no Rh antibodies.
3. The baby produces no Rh antibodies.
4. The mother's Rh status changes to Rh-positive (Rh+).

91. It is discovered that a client at 24 weeks' gestation is leaking amniotic fluid. Before the client is sent home on bedrest, the nurse teaches her which of the following?
1. Perform a nitrazine test every morning upon awakening.
2. Immediately report any breast tenderness to the primary healthcare provider.
3. Abstain from engaging in intercourse for the rest of the pregnancy.
4. Carefully weigh all of her saturated peripads.

92. A client at 32 weeks' gestation states that she thinks she is leaking amniotic fluid. Which of the following tests could be performed to determine whether the membranes had ruptured?
1. Fern test.
2. Biophysical profile.
3. Amniocentesis.
4. Kernig assessment.

93. A nurse is interviewing a prenatal client. Which of the following factors in the client's history should the nurse highlight for the primary healthcare provider?
1. That she is eighteen years old.
2. That she owns a cat and a dog.
3. That she eats peanut butter daily.
4. That she works as a surgeon.

94. A pregnant client is being seen in the prenatal clinic with diarrhea, fever, stiff neck, and headache. Upon inquiry, the nurse learns that the woman drinks unpasteurized milk and eats soft cheese daily. For which of the following bacterial infections should this woman be assessed?
1. *Staphylococcus aureus.*
2. *Streptococcus albicans.*
3. *Pseudomonas aeruginosa.*
4. *Listeria monocytogenes.*

95. A pregnant client has been diagnosed with listeriosis. She eats rare meat and raw smoked seafood. Which of the following signs/symptoms would this woman exhibit?
1. Fever and muscle aches.
2. Rash and thrombocytopenia.
3. Petechiae and anemia.
4. Amnionitis and epistaxis.

96. A client who is 24 weeks pregnant has been diagnosed with syphilis. She asks the nurse how the infection will affect the baby. The nurse's response should be based on which of the following?
1. She is at high risk for premature rupture of the membranes.
2. The baby will be born with congenital syphilis.
3. Penicillin therapy will reduce the risk to the fetus.
4. The fetus will likely be born with a cardiac defect.

97. Prenatal teaching for a pregnant woman should include instructions to do which of the following?
1. Refrain from touching her pet bird.
2. Wear gloves when gardening.
3. Cook pork until medium well done.
4. Avoid sleeping with the dog.

98. A child has been diagnosed with rubella. What must the pediatric nurse teach the child's parents to do?
1. Notify any exposed pregnant friends.
2. Give oral penicillin every 6 hours for 10 full days.
3. Observe the child for signs of respiratory distress.
4. Administer diphenhydramine every 4 hours as needed.

99. A client at 37 weeks' gestation has been advised that she is positive for group B streptococcus (GBS). Which of the following comments by the nurse is appropriate at this time?
1. "The doctor will prescribe intravenous antibiotics for you. A visiting nurse will administer them to you in your home."
2. "You are at very high risk for an intrauterine infection. It is important for you to check your temperature every day."
3. "The bacteria are living in your vagina. They will not hurt you, but we will give you medicine in labor to protect your baby from getting sick."
4. "The bacteria cause scarlet fever. If you notice that your tongue becomes very red and that you feel feverish you should call the doctor immediately."

100. Nurses working in obstetric clinics know that, in general, teen pregnancies are high risk because of which of the following?
1. High probability of chromosomal anomalies.
2. High oral intake of manganese and zinc.
3. High numbers of post-term deliveries.
4. High incidence of late prenatal care.

101. A 14-year-old client is seeking obstetric care. Which of the following vital signs must be monitored very carefully during this woman's pregnancy?
1. Heart rate.
2. Respiratory rate.
3. Blood pressure.
4. Temperature.

102. A 16-year-old client is being seen for her first prenatal visit. Which of the following comments by the young woman is highest priority for the nurse to respond to?
1. "My favorite lunch is a burger with fries."
2. "I've been dating my new boyfriend for 2 weeks."
3. "On weekends we go out and drink a few beers."
4. "I dropped out of school about 3 months ago."

103. A 14-year-old client is seeking obstetrical care. Which of the following is an appropriate goal for the nurse to encourage this client to accomplish? The client will:
1. Bring her partner to all prenatal visits.
2. Terminate the pregnancy.
3. Continue her education.
4. Undergo prenatal single gene analysis.

104. A nurse works in a clinic with a high adolescent pregnancy population. The nurse provides teaching to the young women to prevent which of the following high-risk complications of pregnancy?
1. Preterm birth.
2. Gestational diabetes.
3. Macrosomic babies.
4. Polycythemia.

105. Which of the following would be the best approach to take with an unmarried 14-year-old girl who tells the nurse that she is undecided whether or not to maintain an unplanned pregnancy?
1. "You should consider an abortion since you are so young."
2. "It is a difficult decision. What have you thought about so far?"
3. "Studies show that babies living with teen mothers often become teen parents."
4. "Why don't you keep the pregnancy? You could always opt for adoption later."

106. A 15-year-old client is being seen for her first prenatal visit. Because of this client's special nutritional needs, the nurse evaluates the client's intake of:
1. Protein and magnesium.
2. Calcium and iron.
3. Carbohydrates and zinc.
4. Pyroxidine and thiamine.

107. A client with a history of congestive heart disease is 36 weeks pregnant. Which of the following findings should the nurse report to the primary healthcare provider?
1. Presence of striae gravidarum.
2. Dyspnea on exertion.
3. 4-pound weight gain in a month.
4. Patellar reflexes +2.

108. During a prenatal examination, the nurse notes scarring on and around the woman's genitalia. Which of the following questions is most important for the nurse to ask in relation to this observation?
1. "Have you ever had vaginal or clitoral surgery?"
2. "Have you worn any piercings in your genital area?"
3. "Have you had a tattoo removed from your genital area?"
4. "Have you ever been forced to have sex?"

109. A woman enters the prenatal clinic accompanied by her partner. When she is asked by the nurse about her reason for seeking care, the woman looks down as her male partner states, "She says she thinks she's pregnant. She constantly complains of feeling tired. And her vomiting is disgusting!" Which of the following is the priority action for the nurse to perform?
1. Ask the woman what times of the day her fatigue seems to be most severe.
2. Recommend to the couple that they have a pregnancy test done as soon as possible.
3. Continue the interview of the woman in private.
4. Offer suggestions on ways to decrease the vomiting.

110. The nurse is providing health teaching to a group of women of childbearing age. One woman who states that she smokes, asks about smoking's impact on the pregnancy. The nurse responds that which of the following fetal complications can develop if the mother smokes? **Select all that apply.**
1. Genetic changes in the fetal reproductive system.
2. Extensive central nervous system damage.
3. Fetal dependence on nicotine.
4. Fetal intrauterine growth restriction.

111. A pregnant client mentions to the clinic nurse that she and her husband enjoy working together on projects around the house and says, "I always wear protective gloves when I work." The nurse should advise the woman that even when she wears gloves, which of the following projects could be high risk to the baby's health?
1. Replacing a light fixture in the nursery.
2. Sanding the paint from an antique crib.
3. Planting tulip bulbs in the side garden.
4. Shoveling snow from the driveway.

112. A pregnant client who is 25 years old is diagnosed with gallstones. She asks her nurse, "Aren't I too young to get gallstones?" The nurse bases her response on which of the following?
1. Progesterone slows emptying of the gallbladder, making gravid women at high risk for the disease.
2. Gallbladder disease has a strong genetic component, so the woman should be advised to see a genetic counselor.
3. Older women are no more prone to gallstones than are younger women.
4. Gallbladder disease is related to a high dietary intake of carbohydrates.

113. A client has been diagnosed with pseudocyesis. Which of the following signs/symptoms would the nurse expect to see?
1. 4+ pedal edema.
2. No fetal heartbeat.
3. Hematocrit above 40%.
4. Denial of quickening.

114. The nurse should be aware that which of the following clients is at highest risk for pseudocyesis?
1. The client with lymphatic cancer.
2. The client with celiac disease.
3. The client with multiple miscarriages.
4. The client with grand multiparity.

115. The nurse is caring for a multigravid client at 32 weeks with an obstetrical history of G8 P7007. She has been diagnosed with placenta previa. Which of the following interventions would the nurse expect to see on the provider's orders? **Select all that apply.**
1. Daily contraction stress tests.
2. Blood type and cross match.
3. Bedrest with passive range-of-motion exercises.
4. Daily serum electrolyte assessments.
5. Weekly biophysical profiles.

116. A client has been admitted with a diagnosis of hyperemesis gravidarum. Which of the following laboratory blood values would be consistent with this diagnosis?
1. PO2 90, PCO2 35, HCO3 19 mEq/L, pH 7.3.
2. PO2 100, PCO2 30, HCO3 21 mEq/L, pH 7.5.
3. PO2 60, PCO2 50, HCO3 28 mEq/L, pH 7.3.
4. PO2 90, PCO2 45, HCO3 30 mEq/L, pH 7.5.

117. A client has been admitted with a diagnosis of hyperemesis gravidarum. Which of the following orders written by the primary healthcare provider is highest priority for the nurse to complete?
1. Obtain complete blood count.
2. Start infusion with multivitamins.
3. Check admission weight.
4. Obtain urine for urinalysis.

118. An ultrasound has identified that a client's pregnancy is complicated by oligohydramnios. The nurse would expect that an ultrasound may show that the baby has which of the following structural defects?
1. Multicystic dysplastic kidneys.
2. Coarctation of the aorta.
3. Hydrocephalus.
4. Hepatic cirrhosis.

119. An ultrasound has identified that a client's pregnancy is complicated by polyhydramnios. The nurse would expect that an ultrasound may show that the baby has which of the following structural defects?
1. Pulmonic stenosis.
2. Tracheoesophageal fistula.
3. Ventriculoseptal defect.
4. Developmental hip dysplasia.

120. A client at 8 weeks gestation has been diagnosed with a bicornuate uterus. Which of the following signs should the nurse teach the client to carefully monitor for?
1. Hyperthermia.
2. Palpitations.
3. Cramping.
4. Oliguria.

121. The nurse suspects that a client is third-spacing fluid. Which of the following signs will provide the nurse with the best evidence of this fact?
1. Client's blood pressure.
2. Client's appearance.
3. Client's weight.
4. Client's pulse rate.

122. A client is being stabilized in the labor suite following a diagnosis of eclampsia. The fetal heart rate tracing shows moderate variability with intermittent late decelerations. Which of the following actions by the nurse is appropriate at this time?
1. Tape a tongue blade to the head of the bed.
2. Pad the side rails and head of the bed.
3. Provide the client with needed stimulation.
4. Provide the client with grief counseling.

123. A client is seen at 8 weeks' gestation for her first prenatal visit. During her last gynecological visit, the client's blood pressure was 100/60. Her blood pressure is now 150/90. For which of the following pregnancy-related illnesses should this client be assessed?
1. Hyperemesis gravidarum.
2. Hydatidiform mole.
3. Pre-eclampsia.
4. Gestational diabetes.

124. A client at 36 weeks' gestation is having cultures taken to determine whether she is colonized with group B strep. Which of the following sites is being cultured? **Select all that apply.**
1. Throat.
2. Nipple.
3. Vagina.
4. Rectum.
5. Nostrils.

125. A client with a BMI of 31.2, is seen for her first prenatal visit at 7 weeks' gestation. The nurse requests an order from the primary healthcare provider for which of the following tests?
1. Electroencephalogram.
2. Oral glucose tolerance test.
3. Biophysical profile.
4. Lecithin/sphingomyelin ratio.

CASE STUDY: *The next six questions are part of an evolving case study. All six questions follow the Next Generation NCLEX© question format of six steps:*

1. Recognize cues—What matters most?
2. Analyze cues—What could it mean?
3. Prioritize hypotheses—Where do I start?
4. Generate solutions—What can I do?
5. Take action—What will I do?
6. Evaluate outcomes—Did it help?

(National Council of State Boards of Nursing [NCSBN], 2020). For more information on the Next Generation NCLEX (NGN) question formats, see NGN quarterly newsletters at https://www.ncsbn.org.
NCLEX questions assume the nurse has a provider's order for listed interventions, unless noted otherwise.

0900: A client with an obstetrical history of G5 P3104 has been on the antepartum unit for 5 days with bleeding from a placenta previa. She has had two cesarean sections, followed by two successful VBACs (vaginal birth after cesarean). She is currently at 33 5/7 weeks' gestation. Vital signs are T 98.6° F (37° C), P 80, R 20, BP 120/68. She is no longer bleeding, but the nurses have documented intermittent dark, spotty blood on her pads. She is allowed to be up and about in her room.

The fetal monitor strip that was completed two hours ago showed FHR 150 bpm with moderate variability and irregular, mild contractions. These findings were reported to the primary healthcare provider and the decision was made to consider magnesium sulfate administration to reduce the contraction frequency, if necessary. The client is standing by the window in her room. She has called the nurse to her room and states, "All this sitting around has given me a backache. Can I have a heating pad or acetaminophen?" She rates her back pain as 5/10 on the pain scale.

126. Recognize cues. What matters most? The nurse should recognize that:
1. Preterm labor is associated with placenta previa.
2. Intermittent backache can indicate she is in early labor.
3. A heating pad is contraindicated with placenta previa.
4. Intermittent backache is a sign of placental abruption.
5. A vaginal exam is indicated to confirm early labor.

127. Analyze cues. What could it mean? What can the nurse anticipate might happen next? **Select all that apply.**
1. The contractions will become stronger.
2. She will resume bleeding.
3. Intrauterine fetal death.
4. A cesarean section will be necessary.

128. Prioritize hypotheses. Where do I start? The nurse prepares to notify the provider of the client's current status. Which orders are likely to be anticipated or nonessential?

Potential Order	(a) Anticipated	(b) Nonessential
1. IV antibiotics.		
2. Administer acetaminophen.		
3. Preparation for surgery.		
4. Administer magnesium sulfate.		
5. Corticosteroids.		
6. Continuous fetal monitoring.		

129. Generate solutions. What can I do? What would be the goal(s) of care at this time? **Select all that apply.**

1. Reduce anxiety.
2. Determine labor status.
3. Prevent hemorrhage.
4. Maintain fetal well-being.

130. Take action. What will I do? Which three provider's orders should the nurse complete right away? **Select three.**

1. Acetaminophen 325 mg, two tabs PO q 6 hrs, prn.
2. Betamethasone 12 mg IM q 24 hours x 2 doses.
3. Magnesium sulfate 4 g loading dose IV over 20 minutes followed by maintenance dose of 2 g IV per hour.
4. Place electronic fetal monitor.
5. Assess client's vital signs.
6. Heating pad to back prn.

131. Evaluate outcomes. Did it help?

1030: The nurse has administered betamethasone, has completed the magnesium sulfate bolus, and has placed the electronic fetal monitor. In addition, she administered acetaminophen and the heating pad for the client's backache. The client is resting in bed with her eyes closed. The client's vital signs are T 98.6° F (37° C), P 88, R 20, BP 120/68. The nurse's assessments are shown below. For each assessment finding, indicate whether the client's condition has improved, demonstrates no change, or has declined or worsened.

Assessment Findings	(a) Improved	(b) No change	(c) Declined
1. Fetal heart rate 150 bpm with moderate variability.		X	
2. Contractions every 10 minutes, lasting 30–45 seconds.			X
3. Contractions are mild on palpation.		X	
4. The client reports dark blood on her pad.		X	
5. Back pain 3/10.	X		

132. The antepartum nurse has just received shift report on four pregnant clients at 0700. Which of the clients should the nurse assess first?
a. G5 P2202, 32 weeks, placenta previa, today's hemoglobin 11.6 g/dL.
b. G2 P0101, 39 weeks, type 2 diabetes mellitus (T2DM), fasting blood glucose 85 mg/dL (4.7 mmol/L).
c. G1 P0000, 32 weeks, partial placental abruption, fetal heart rate (FHR) 120 bpm 15 minutes ago.
d. G2 P1001, 28 weeks, Rh-negative (Rh–). 1 day post cerclage placement.

133. Which of the following signs or symptoms would the nurse expect to see in a client with a placental abruption?
a. Sinusoidal fetal heart rate.
b. Pain-free vaginal bleeding.
c. Fetal heart accelerations.
d. Hyperthermia with leukocytosis.

134. A nurse is caring for four antepartum clients. Which of the clients will the nurse carefully monitor for signs of placental abruption?
a. G2 P0010, 27 weeks' gestation, polyhydramnios.
b. G3 P1101, 36 weeks' gestation, flu.
c. G4 P2101, 32 weeks' gestation, cancer survivor.
d. G5 P1211, 24 weeks' gestation, cocaine use.

135. An antepartum nurse is caring for a client at 38 weeks' gestation, who has been diagnosed with symptomatic placenta previa. Which of the following orders by the primary healthcare provider should the nurse question?
a. Begin oxytocin drip rate at 0.5 milliunits/min.
b. Assess fetal heart rate every 10 minutes.
c. Weigh all vaginal pads.
d. Assess hematocrit and hemoglobin.

136. The doctor writes the following order for a client at 31 weeks' gestation with symptomatic placenta previa: Weigh all vaginal pads and estimate blood loss. The nurse weighs one of the client's saturated pads at 24 grams and a dry pad at 4 grams. How many milliliters (mL) of blood can the nurse estimate the client has bled? **Calculate to the nearest whole number.**

__________ mL

137. A client at 29 weeks' gestation is admitted to the antepartum unit with vaginal bleeding. To differentiate between placenta previa and abruptio placentae, the nurse should assess which of the following?
a. Leopold's maneuver results.
b. Quantity of vaginal bleeding.
c. Presence of abdominal pain.
d. Maternal blood pressure.

138. A client with a complete placenta previa is on the antepartum clinical unit in preparation for delivery. Which of the following should the nurse include in a teaching session for this client?
a. Coughing and deep breathing.
b. Phases of the first stage of labor.
c. Lamaze labor techniques.
d. Leboyer hydro-birthing.

ANSWERS AND RATIONALES

The correct answer number and rationale for why it is the correct answer are given in **boldface blue type**. Rationales for why the other possible answer options are incorrect also are given, but they are not in boldface type.

1. Answers 2, 3, and 4 are correct.

1. Although fundal height is an important assessment, it is not urgent.
2. **A maternal blood sugar of 320 mg/dL (17.8 mmol/L) and the maternal vital signs put the fetus at risk of hypoxia. As such, fetal status must be assessed urgently by continuous external fetal monitoring (EFM).**
3. **Although the client's husband reports a recent CBG, the nurse should retest with the hospital's CBG monitor to establish a baseline and to get a current reading.**
4. **Low abdominal pain suggests both preterm labor and a urinary tract infection (UTI).**
5. Although the client's height and weight are important assessments, they are not urgently needed.

TEST-TAKING HINT: Of the assessments listed, the test taker is asked to identify assessments that require *immediate* follow-up. This is not intended to be a complete list, just an assessment of the test taker's ability to prioritize items within the list. Blood glucose is a priority in diabetic conditions. In pregnant women, both the fetus and abdominal pain are also priorities. A urinalysis will help to define a possible cause of the abdominal pain.

The mother has been vomiting. Maternal dehydration leads to decreased uteroplacental blood flow, causing impaired oxygen delivery to the fetus. This complicates the fetal demand for oxygen, which is increased by fetal hyperglycemia and hyperinsulinemia and an increased metabolism.

2. Answers 1, 2, 3, 4, and 6 are correct

1. **Correcting dehydration is the most important treatment this client needs initially. Aggressive hydration is done before administering an insulin bolus or insulin drip. IV fluids decrease stress hormones, which contribute to acidemia. In addition, IV fluids perfuse the cells, and dilute the blood, which effectively reduces the hyperglycemia and increases the response to insulin therapy when it is started (Sibai & Viteri, 2014).**
2. **An initial capillary blood glucose may be obtained on admission and may be used for titrating insulin during care, but a serum blood glucose is more accurate for a client in this type of emergency situation and should be drawn to establish a baseline (Mohan et al., 2017).**
3. **The nurse can anticipate orders to administer an insulin bolus after hemodilution has been achieved.**
4. **Following the insulin bolus, a low dose, continuous insulin drip is started per pump for maintenance until the client's blood sugars are stable enough to return to subcutaneous insulin injections.**
5. This client does not need any more glucose. Orange juice is contraindicated.
6. **A person with type 1 diabetes mellitus (T1DM) is at risk for diabetic ketoacidosis if insulin is not administered regularly. An arterial blood gas analysis will confirm the level of metabolic acidosis and can guide further decisions for treatment.**

TEST-TAKING HINT: The nurse should always consider the CAB of client stabilization—Circulation, Airway, Breathing. This client's circulation and ability of the blood to deliver oxygen to the cells is at risk because of the high blood sugar. The tissues that are oxygenated by the tiny capillaries will be impaired if blood cannot flow through those vessels easily as a result of the viscosity of the blood. The syrupy blood must be diluted with IV solutions in order to improve circulation and bring adequate oxygen to the cells. There is nothing in this question to suggest the client has a problem with her airway or breathing.

3. Answers 4 and (a) are correct.

1. The client's hyperglycemia needs treatment, but the dehydration should be addressed first.
2. The client's dehydration should be addressed first. The fetal heart rate pattern bears watching because of the minimal variability. What is reassuring, however, is that the rate is within normal limits and there are no decelerations. Minimal variability could indicate a fetal sleep cycle. It is very likely that restoring the mother to normoglycemia will also improve the

fetal variability as placental oxygenation improves.

3. The client's dehydration should be addressed first. The contraction pattern may also improve with a reduction in contractions as the mother is hydrated and normoglycemia is restored.
4. **The client's dehydration should be addressed first.**

The assessments above should be followed by (a) below.

a. **The client's hyperglycemia is addressed after the client is hydrated. After rehydration, insulin will be administered per a pump for precise regulation in order to bring glucose into the cells and reduce the body's production of ketone bodies, which will reduce the level of acidemia. None of these changes happens quickly, and both the client and the fetus will remain at high risk until homeostasis is achieved.**
b Maternal hydration comes first even though the fetal heart rate pattern is important. The FHR will likely improve as the mother's status improves.
c. The client's dehydration should be addressed first, as it will likely reduce the contractions.
d. The client's dehydration should be addressed first, before insulin is administered.

TEST-TAKING HINT: All of the interventions are important for this client. However, the test taker must demonstrate the ability to prioritize care. With appropriate critical thinking that links interventions to broad outcomes (such as improvements in fetal heart rate and reduction in contractions as a result of restoring hydration and normoglycemia), the test taker demonstrates more complex clinical judgment than in a knowledge-based question.

This client has diabetic ketoacidosis (DKA) and metabolic acidosis. DKA is always accompanied by dehydration as a result of hyperglycemia. The blood is like syrup, and pulls fluid from the extracellular fluid by osmosis, in an effort to thin out the concentration. Some of the sugar overflows into the urine, taking salt and potassium with it. All of this takes a toll on cellular function. Without insulin, the cells cannot take in glucose. With acidosis, the drop in the pH causes oxygen to bind to hemoglobin. This results in limited oxygen release to the cells, and anaerobic metabolism begins, in which fatty acids are burned for energy, releasing more acids and further decreasing the pH of the blood. Burning fatty acids is a bit like burning wet firewood. In the same way that burning wet firewood releases acrid smoke, burning fatty acids releases toxic ketone bodies—acetone, acetoacetate, and beta-hydroxybutyrate. The rising levels of ketone bodies in the blood contribute to further acidemia, leading to vomiting, which contributes to further fluid loss and dehydration. This vicious cycle can lead to death if not reversed early enough.

4. **Answers 1 (a or d), 2 (d or a), 3 (e or g), and 4 (g or e) are correct.**
The best outcomes for the client would be to **1(a) rehydrate** and **2(d) achieve normoglycemia.** To achieve optimal outcomes, the nurse should **3(e) administer IV fluids** and **4(g) administer insulin.**

TEST-TAKING HINT: The nurse will have several goals of treatment for this client and must focus on the two most important goals. These include correction of dehydration, in order to supply adequate oxygen to body systems, followed by insulin administration to facilitate transfer of blood glucose into cells. In addition, monitoring of electrolytes, ketones, and blood sugar will be ongoing. Correction of dehydration is the first step in treating DKA and is key to maternal and fetal stabilization and treatment. Cells respond better to insulin once they are hydrated (Mohan et al., 2017). As such, insulin administration to achieve normoglycemia is the second primary goal, which follows hydration.

The test taker should indicate that both hydration and a return to normoglycemia are the best outcomes for this client in this specific situation. Note that although both *a* and *d* are correct, and neither is specific to answer 1 or 2, it is best to answer in the most logical order or prioritization of goals. That is, 1(a) and 2(d).

This question requires the test taker to remain focused on the current client condition and nursing interventions, not on pregnancy as a whole. To that end, the answer "accelerate fetal lung maturity" (b) is not applicable. In addition, "achieve term delivery" (f) is not the best answer because it is too broad. Acceleration of fetal lung maturity with corticosteroids is recommended for pregnancies between 24 0/7 weeks' and 33 6/7 weeks' gestation if the client is at risk of delivering within 7 days (American College of Obstetricians and Gynecologists [ACOG], 2017c). This client is at 35 weeks' gestation so the medication is not recommended. In addition, if the fetal response to maternal normoglycemia is positive, the fetus will not need to be delivered prematurely.

To achieve optimal outcomes, the nurse must administer IV fluids and insulin. A urinary catheter may be ordered to measure hourly urine output to assist in following the improvement in rehydration, but insertion of the catheter is not an outcome, it is a specific action. Insertion of the catheter will not change the client's condition in the way that IV fluids and administration of insulin can do, even though it is an important action.

When caring for an actual diabetic client with this condition, it is obvious that client education is indicated to assist this client with self-care. A review of diabetes principles can be included in small, memorable bits during treatment, once the client is stabilized. Since she was diagnosed with type 1 diabetes mellitus (T1DM) just 2 years ago, and this is her first pregnancy, she will need information about the differences between diabetes before pregnancy, during pregnancy, during the postpartum phase while breastfeeding, and ongoing.

5. **Answers 1 and 3 are correct.**
   1. **An indwelling catheter is inserted to assess hydration and hourly output (Mohan et al., 2017).**
   2. The client must be hydrated before she is given insulin, and initially, the insulin will likely be per intravenous bolus by pump, over 20 minutes.
   3. **Intravenous fluid therapy is the first step in treatment for DKA.**
   4. Subcutaneous insulin therapy is implemented once the client is stabilized, not initially.
   5. The use of bicarbonate is not recommended, and may actually be harmful to both the mother and the fetus (Mohan et al., 2017).
   6. It is not necessary to assess the capillary blood glucose. Treatment has been determined by the recent serum blood glucose.
   7. Steroids for fetal lung maturity are not indicated because this client is beyond 33 6/7 weeks' gestation; in addition, steroids would increase both her blood sugar levels and the baby's.

TEST-TAKING HINT: This question asks the test taker to identify specific nursing actions. Unlike the previous question which asked for outcome planning, this one is more focused on actions. To recap, this client has type 1 diabetes mellitus (T1DM), meaning her pancreas does not secrete insulin and it must be administered by injection or intravenously by pump. This regimen went awry because she stopped taking her insulin, and began vomiting. See the steps in development of this condition in the appendix, under Diabetic Ketoacidosis. The test taker is asked to prioritize treatment to give evidence of focusing on priorities. The nurse is completing the first nursing actions toward the identified outcomes in the previous question. Intravenous fluids are being administered, and an indwelling catheter is inserted to monitor output.

6. **Answers 1 and 5 are correct.**
   1. **It is reasonable to anticipate an FHR in the normal range with moderate variability within 4 to 8 hours after correction of maternal DKA (Mohan et al., 2017, p. 59).**
   2. The FHR is currently 120 bpm. Maternal temperature is not elevated. As such, it is not reasonable to anticipate fetal tachycardia, or for minimal variability to continue once the maternal DKA has been corrected.
   3. Oxytocin induction is not indicated and it is not an outcome of nursing interventions; it is a medical intervention.
   4. There is nothing in the case study to indicate a cesarean section is indicated. Even if it were, it is not an outcome of nursing interventions, it is a medical intervention.
   5. **It is reasonable to anticipate normoglycemia within 8 hours of treatment with insulin (Mohan et al., 2017).**

TEST-TAKING HINT: The nurse must be aware of anticipated improvements in the client's condition and the estimated time frames, so the goalposts can be shared with the client as a means of encouragement as she recovers.

7. **Answers 1(a), 2(b), 3(a), 4(a), 5(c), 6(a) and 7(a) are correct.**
   - **1(a) Magnesium sulfate is indicated for this client to prevent seizures.**
   - **2(b) The client doesn't need an indwelling catheter at this point.**
   - **3(a) The fetus must be monitored continuously.**
   - **4(a) Steroids are indicated to enhance fetal lung maturity in case a premature delivery becomes necessary.**
   - **5(c) At this point, there is nothing in the client's presentation to require an oxytocin induction.**
   - **6(a) A 24-hour urine collection for protein assessment can guide the patient's plan of care, that may include an indwelling catheter and complete bedrest, steroids, and an oxytocin induction. However, at this point there is nothing to indicate those interventions are necessary.**
   - **7(a) Antihypertensive medication is indicated to prevent a stroke.**

Potential Order	(a) Indicated	(b) Nonessential	(c) Contraindicated
1. Magnesium sulfate 4 gm bolus over 20 minutes, followed by maintenance infusion of 2 gm/hour IV per pump.	X		
2. Insert indwelling catheter and send urine specimen to lab.		X	
3. Continuous fetal monitoring.	X		
4. Corticosteroids.	X		
5. Begin oxytocin induction.			X
6. Begin 24-hour urine collection for protein.	X		
7. Antihypertensive medication.	X		

TEST-TAKING HINT: Pre-eclampsia is a very serious, multiorgan disease process of pregnancy that carries a genetic component (Williams & Pipkin, 2011). The primary characteristic is new onset hypertension after 20 weeks' gestation. In addition, the client may demonstrate proteinuria, thrombocytopenia, renal insufficiency, impaired liver function, pulmonary edema, or cerebral or visual symptoms. This client's blood pressure of 160/112 indicates pre-eclampsia with severe features (ACOG, 2020c). Antihypertensive medication is indicated. Both maternal and fetal well-being must be considered at the same time. The use of magnesium sulfate to prevent maternal seizures (not hypertension) will benefit the fetus by avoiding a maternal seizure, which would create a tetanic contraction and a hypoxic event for the fetus. Antihypertensives will prevent constriction of maternal blood vessels, thus providing adequate oxygenation for the fetus. Finally, corticosteroids will promote fetal lung development in advance of a preterm delivery, which will likely be necessary. Progressive deterioration of both mother and fetus is to be expected in pre-eclampsia with severe features. The goal is "expectant management" to maintain the pregnancy until at least 34 weeks, if possible (ACOG, 2020c).

8. 1. Sodium restriction is not recommended.
   2. There is no need to increase fluid intake.
   3. It is important for the client to eat a well-balanced diet.
   4. Although not the most nutritious of foods, there is no need to restrict the intake of simple sugars.

TEST-TAKING HINT: Clients with pre-eclampsia are losing albumin through their urine. They should eat a well-balanced diet with sufficient protein to replace the lost protein. Even though pre-eclamptic clients are hypertensive, it is not recommended that they restrict salt—they should have a normal salt intake—because during pregnancy the kidney is salt sparing. When salt is restricted, the kidneys become stressed.

9. Answers 1, 2, and 4 are correct.
   1. A platelet count of less than 100,000 per microliter is a sign of pre-eclampsia with severe features. A normal platelet level in pregnancy is 150,000 per microliter.
   2. This client is losing protein. A reading of greater than 1+ indicates worsening kidney insufficiency.
   3. An increase in serum protein is a positive sign.
   4. Serum creatinine greater than 1.1 mg/dL indicates worsening renal insufficiency.

TEST-TAKING HINT: This is an evaluation question. The key to answering this question is the test taker's ability to interpret lab values associated with pre-eclampsia. There are two levels of pre-eclampsia. Pre-eclampsia *without* severe features and pre-eclampsia *with* severe features. All but one of these findings indicates a progression of the client's condition toward pre-eclampsia with severe features, as the kidneys and liver begin to struggle with the demands of pregnancy. The test taker must read each response slowly, noting that answer #2 relates to protein in the urine and answer #3 relates to protein in the blood. See California Maternal Quality Care Initiative, p. 22 at https://pqcnc-documents.s3.amazonaws.com/cmop/cmopresources/CMQCC_Preeclampsia_Toolkit_1.17.14.pdf.

10. 1. A weight gain of 10 pounds in a 4-week period is worrisome. The recommended weight gain during the second and third trimesters is approximately 1 pound per week.
    2. The pulse rate normally increases slightly during pregnancy.

3. A slight drop in BP is normal during pregnancy.
4. The respiratory rate normally increases during pregnancy.

TEST-TAKING HINT: A weight gain above the recommended rate can be related to several things, including pre-eclampsia, excessive food intake, or multiple gestations. The midwife should be advised of the weight gain to identify the reason for the increase and to intervene accordingly.

11. 1. Discovering whether or not the client has allergies is important for the nurse to learn if medications are to be ordered, but that is not the most important information the nurse needs to learn.
2. The nurse should assess the client's blood pressure.
3. Fundal height assessment is important but not the most important information the nurse needs to learn at this time.
4. Discovering whether or not the client has stressors at work is important, but it is not the most important information the nurse needs to learn about.

TEST-TAKING HINT: Headache is a symptom of pre-eclampsia, one of the serious hypertensive diseases of pregnancy. To assist the primary healthcare provider in determining whether or not the client is pre-eclamptic, the next action by the nurse would be to assess the woman's blood pressure.

12. **1. Altered glomerular filtration leads to protein loss and, subsequently, to fluid retention, which can lead to swelling in the face and hands.**
2. Monitoring women for the appearance of swollen hands and puffy face is related to the development of pre-eclampsia, not of cardiac failure.
3. Monitoring women for the appearance of swollen hands and puffy face is related to the development of pre-eclampsia, not of hepatic insufficiency.
4. Monitoring women for the appearance of swollen hands and puffy face is related to the development of pre-eclampsia, not of altered splenic circulation.

TEST-TAKING HINT: The hypertension associated with pre-eclampsia results in poor perfusion of the kidneys. When the kidneys are poorly perfused, the glomerular filtration is altered, allowing large molecules, most notably the protein albumin, to be lost through the urine. Proteins serve as "sponges" in the circulatory system, sucking up water by osmosis from the tissues into the blood to maintain fluid in the blood. With the loss of protein, the colloidal pressure, or ability to draw fluid from the tissues, drops in the circulatory system, allowing fluid to move into the interstitial, nonfunctioning space between cells, also called "third spacing." Unaware of where that fluid has gone, the body gets the message to retain fluids, exacerbating the problem. One of the early signs of third spacing is the swelling of a client's hands and face.

13. 1. The fetus will not be assessed for signs of severe anemia.
2. The fetus will not be assessed for signs of hypoprothrombinemia.
3. The fetus will not be assessed for signs of craniosynostosis.
4. The fetus should be assessed for intrauterine growth restriction.

TEST-TAKING HINT: Perfusion to the placenta drops when clients are pre-eclamptic because the client's hypertension impairs adequate blood flow to the placental lake. It is at the placental lake, or intervillous space, where the placenta picks up oxygen and glucose from the mother's blood by osmosis and releases fetal waste products such as carbon dioxide into the mother's circulation. When the placenta is poorly perfused, the baby is poorly nourished and fetal growth is affected.

14. **1. Clients with pre-eclampsia with severe features are at high risk for seizure.**
2. Clients with pre-eclampsia with severe features should be monitored for a drop in platelets.
3. Clients with pre-eclampsia with severe features are not at risk for explosive diarrhea.
4. Clients with pre-eclampsia with severe features are not at risk for jaundice.

TEST-TAKING HINT: A client who is diagnosed with 4+ proteinuria and 4+ reflexes will likely have other symptoms that meet criteria for pre-eclampsia with severe features. As such, these clients are at high risk for becoming eclamptic. Pre-eclamptic clients are diagnosed with eclampsia once they have had a seizure. This client would likely have thrombocytopenia, a low platelet count, not a high count. Jaundice is not a part of pre-eclampsia with severe features.

15. 1. Patellar reflexes, not clonus, are assessed by striking the patellar tendon.
2. Clonus is not assessed by palpating the woman's ankle.

3. **To assess clonus, the nurse should dorsiflex the woman's foot.**
4. Clonus is not assessed by positioning the woman's feet flat on the floor.

TEST-TAKING HINT: When clients have pre-eclampsia with severe features, they are often hyper-reflexic and develop clonus. In the setting of extreme hypertension, as with pre-eclampsia with severe features, cerebral perfusion is inhibited and cerebrovascular damage occurs. The increased permeability of the blood vessels as a result of pregnancy leads to cerebral edema, ischemia and hyperreflexia. As a result, the woman has a risk of seizure and stroke, among other outcomes (Hammer & Cipolla, 2015). To assess for hyperreflexia, the nurse assesses the client's reflexes and clonus.

The test for clonus is done when the nurse dorsiflexes the foot and then releases the foot. The nurse should observe for and count any pulsations of the foot. The number of pulsations is documented. The higher the number of pulsations (beats) there are, the more irritable the woman's central nervous system is and the higher risk of seizure. More than 2 beats of clonus is abnormal (Murray & Huelsmann, 2009).

16. 1. +1 reflexes are defined as hypo-reflexic.
2. +2 reflexes are defined as normal.
3. **+3 reflexes are defined as slightly brisker than normal, or slightly hyper-reflexic.**
4. +4 reflexes are defined as much brisker than normal, or markedly hyper-reflexic.

TEST-TAKING HINT: Although a clear categorization of reflex assessment exists, the value assigned to a reflex by a clinician does have a subjective component. Therefore, it is recommended that at the change of shift both the new and departing nurses together assess the reflexes of a client who has suspected abnormal reflexes. A common understanding of the reflex assessment can then be determined.

17. 1. The nurse would expect to see high serum creatinine levels associated with pre-eclampsia with severe features.
2. The nurse would expect to see low serum protein levels with pre-eclampsia with severe features.
3. Bloody stools are never associated with pre-eclampsia with severe features.
4. **Epigastric pain is associated with the liver involvement of HELLP syndrome.**

TEST-TAKING HINT: The acronym HELLP stands for the following signs/symptoms: (H) hemolysis, (E, L) elevated liver enzymes, and (L, P) low platelets. HELLP syndrome is one of the manifestations of pre-eclampsia when the liver is involved. As a result of toxic factors from the placenta, microvessels are damaged, portal blood flow to the liver is reduced, and liver cells are damaged. This leads to liver necrosis and rising liver function tests. In response, coagulation factors are activated, which eventually diminishes the platelet count. This rapid consumption of coagulation factors can lead to disseminated intravascular coagulation (DIC).

The client's right upper quadrant (RUQ) epigastric pain is caused by deposits of large amounts of fibrin-like material obstructing sinusoids in the liver. Blood flow is further obstructed, and edema collects between the sheath-like covering of the liver, known as Glisson's capsule, and the liver. Stretching of Glisson's capsule leads to RUQ pain (Sibai, 2004).

18. 1. At 29 weeks' gestation, the normal fundal height should be 29 cm. In pre-eclampsia with severe features, the nurse may see poor fetal growth—that is, a fundal height below 29 cm.
2. **The nurse would expect to see oliguria.**
3. The nurse would expect to see hyperreflexia—that is, patellar reflexes *higher* than the normal of +2.
4. The nurse would not expect to see nystagmus.

TEST-TAKING HINT: Kidney dysfunction is associated with pre-eclampsia with severe features. In addition, the woman with this diagnosis may have reduced urine output because of third-spacing fluid. For clients receiving magnesium sulfate, oliguria can be a risk factor for magnesium sulfate toxicity due to limited excretion of the medication through the kidneys, and rising levels of magnesium sulfate throughout the woman's circulatory system. A client's respiratory rate decreases as magnesium sulfate toxicity rises. As such, it is very important for the nurse caring for a client with this diagnosis and administering magnesium sulfate to monitor intake and output and the client's respiratory rate very closely and keep the provider informed. In addition, calcium gluconate, the antidote to magnesium sulfate, should be readily available for rescue if needed.

19. 1. Bedrest for the pre-eclamptic client is not ordered so that she may conserve energy.
2. Pre-eclamptic clients rarely complain of nausea or anorexia.

3. **Bedrest, especially side-lying, helps to improve perfusion to the placenta.**
4. Although indirectly this response may be accurate, that is not the primary reason for the positioning.

TEST-TAKING HINT: This client's question requires the nurse to have a clear understanding of the pathology of pre-eclampsia. The vital organs of pre-eclamptic clients are being poorly perfused as a result of the abnormally high blood pressure and ongoing periods of vasospasm. When a woman lies on her side, blood return to the heart is improved and the cardiac output is also improved. With improved cardiac output, perfusion to the placenta and other organs is improved. At one time, the recommendation was for "strict" bedrest, meaning the client had to stay in bed. The recommendation to remain in bed is no longer a part of standard care because the risk of blood clot formation in pregnancy is increased if the woman doesn't have at least some activity. The woman is allowed to do light activities and to walk around the house as needed.

20. 1. **Headache and decreased output are signs of pre-eclampsia.**
2. Dependent edema is seen in most pregnant women. It is related to the weight of the uterine body on the femoral vessels.
3. Hemorrhoids and vaginal discharge are experienced by many pregnant women. Hemorrhoids are varicose veins of the rectum. They develop as a result of chronic constipation and the weight of the uterine body on the hemorrhoidal veins. An increase in vaginal discharge results from elevated estrogen levels in the body.
4. Backache is seen in most pregnant women. It develops as a result of the weight of the uterine body and the resultant physiological lordosis.

TEST-TAKING HINT: Although some symptoms such as puffy feet may seem significant, they are normal in pregnancy. Other symptoms such as headache, which in a non-pregnant woman would be considered benign, may be potentially very serious in a pregnant woman. The earliest that pre-eclampsia begins is after 20 weeks of pregnancy. The diagnosis is made when hypertension is found during a prenatal visit in women whose blood pressures had been normal. It is more commonly seen in nulliparous clients in the third trimester.

21. 1. **This primigravid client—age 41 and with a history of diabetes—is at very high risk for pre-eclampsia.**
2. Multigravid clients with a history of rheumatic fever are not significantly at high risk for pre-eclampsia, unless they have a history of pre-eclampsia with their preceding pregnancies, or have developed a vascular or hypertensive disease since their last pregnancy.
3. Multigravid clients with scoliosis are not significantly at high risk for pre-eclampsia, unless they have a history of pre-eclampsia with their preceding pregnancies, or have developed a vascular or hypertensive disease since their last pregnancy.
4. Multigravid clients with celiac disease are not significantly at high risk for pre-eclampsia, unless they have a history of pre-eclampsia with their preceding pregnancies, or have developed a vascular or hypertensive disease since their last pregnancy.

TEST-TAKING HINT: Pre-eclampsia is a multi-organ, vascular disease of pregnancy. Although any woman can develop the syndrome, women who are at highest risk for the disease are primigravidas, those with multiple gestations, women who are younger than 17 or older than 34, those who had pre-eclampsia with their first pregnancy, and women who have been diagnosed with a vascular disease such as diabetes mellitus or chronic hypertension. The only woman who fits this definition is the first one.

22. 1. Fatigue and nausea and vomiting are normal in clients at 10 weeks' gestation.
2. Ankle edema and chloasma are normal in clients at 26 weeks' gestation.
3. **Epigastric pain and facial edema are not normal. This client should be referred to the nurse midwife.**
4. Bleeding gums and urinary frequency are normal in clients at 37 weeks' gestation.

TEST-TAKING HINT: This question requires the test taker to differentiate between normal signs and symptoms of pregnancy at a variety of gestational ages and those that could indicate a serious complication of pregnancy.

23. 1. The vital signs are within normal limits.
2. **There has been a 10-lb weight gain in 2 weeks and a significant amount of protein is being spilled in the urine. This client should be brought to the attention of the midwife.**
3. Trace urine protein is considered normal in pregnancy. The blood pressure is within normal limits.
4. The client has had a normal 2-lb weight gain in the past 2 weeks and her vital signs are within normal limits.

TEST-TAKING HINT: There is a great deal of information included in this question. The test taker must methodically assess each of the pieces of data. The best way to do this is to assess each piece of data individually as true or false in response to the question, "Is this normal?" Important things to attend to are the timing of the appointments—2 weeks apart; changes in vital signs—it is normal for pulse and respiratory rates to increase slightly and BP to drop slightly; changes in urinary protein—trace is normal, +2 is not normal; and changes in weight—2-lb increase over 2 weeks is normal, a 10-lb increase is not normal.

24. 1. It is inappropriate for the nurse to make this statement.
2. It is inappropriate for the nurse to make this statement.
3. It is inappropriate for the nurse to make this statement.
4. **This statement is appropriate. The nurse is offering their assistance to the client.**

TEST-TAKING HINT: Clients during the first trimester are often ambivalent about pregnancy. Those who miscarry at this time express a variety of feelings from intense sorrow to joy. The nurse should offer assistance to the client without making any assumptions about the client's feelings toward the pregnancy loss. Speaking platitudes is completely inappropriate and can shut down any opportunity to support the client. It is very appropriate to say, "I can't imagine how you must feel."

25. 1. **This meal choice is high in iron and ascorbic acid. It would be an excellent lunch choice for this client who has a below-normal hematocrit and hemoglobin.**
2. Although high in calcium, this lunch choice will not help to change the client's laboratory values.
3. Although nutritious, this lunch choice will not help to change the client's laboratory values.
4. Cream cheese has little to no nutritional value. This meal choice would provide a large number of calories and is not the most nutritious choice.

TEST-TAKING HINT: The client in the scenario is anemic. Although a hematocrit of 32% in pregnancy is acceptable, it is recommended that the value not drop below that level. The nurse, having evaluated the laboratory statement, should choose foods that are high in iron. Liver and dried fruits are good iron sources. Tomatoes are high in vitamin C, which promotes the absorption of iron.

26. **Answers 3 and 5 are correct.**
1. Placenta previa is not an acute problem. It is related to the site of placental implantation.
2. Transverse fetal lie is a malpresentation. It would not be related to the auto accident.
3. **Placental abruption may develop as a result of the auto accident.**
4. Pre-eclampsia does not occur as a result of an auto accident.
5. **The woman may go into preterm labor after an auto accident.**

TEST-TAKING HINT: The fetus is well protected within the uterine body. The musculature of the uterus and the amniotic fluid provide the baby with enough cushioning to withstand minor bumps and falls. A major automobile accident, however, can cause anything from preterm premature rupture of the membranes, to preterm labor, to a ruptured uterus, to placental abruption. The nurse should especially monitor the fetal heartbeat for any variations that may signal any of these complications.

27. 1. Cervical cerclage is performed on clients with cervical insufficiency.
2. Amniocentesis is performed to obtain fetal cells to assess genetic information.
3. Nonstress testing is performed during the third trimester to monitor the well-being of the fetus.
4. **Dilation and curettage (D&C) is performed on a client with an incomplete abortion.**

TEST-TAKING HINT: This client is experiencing an incomplete abortion. The baby has died—there is no fetal heartbeat—and she has expelled some of the products of conception, as evidenced by frank vaginal bleeding. It is important for the remaining products of conception to be removed to prevent hemorrhage and infection. A D&C in which the physician dilates the cervix and scrapes the lining of the uterus with a curette is one means of completing the abortion. Another method of completing the abortion is by administering an abortifacient medication.

28. 1. **This long-term goal is appropriate.**
2. This client is not pregnant. She will not deliver a baby.
3. This client is not in intense pain. This long-term goal is not appropriate.
4. This client is not pregnant. She will not deliver a baby.

TEST-TAKING HINT: The placental tissue in a hydatidiform mole contains many small cysts

that form a mass in the uterus similar to a grape cluster. A hydatidiform mole can have serious complications such as cancer. When nurses plan care, they have in mind short-term and long-term goals that their clients will achieve. Short-term goals usually have a time frame of a week or two and often are specific to the client's current hospitalization. Long-term goals are expectations of client achievement over extended periods of time. It is important for nurses to develop goals to implement appropriate nursing interventions.

29. 1. Pain is not associated with this condition.
2. There is no fetus; therefore, there will be no fetal heart.
3. The condition is usually diagnosed after a client complains of brown vaginal discharge early in the "pregnancy."
4. Suicidal ideations are not associated with this condition.

TEST-TAKING HINT: The most important thing to remember about hydatidiform mole is the fact that, even though a positive pregnancy test has been reported, there is no "pregnancy." The normal conceptus develops into two portions—a blastocyst, which includes the fetus and amnion, and a trophoblast, which includes the fetal portion of the placenta and the chorion. In gestational trophoblastic disease (hydatidiform mole), only the trophoblastic layer develops; no fetus develops. With the proliferation of the chorionic layer, the client is at high risk for gynecological cancer.

30. Answers 2 and 3 are correct.
1. A hematocrit of 39% is well within normal limits.
2. Women with hydatidiform mole often expel grape-like clusters from the vagina.
3. Although signs and symptoms of pre-eclampsia usually appear only after a pregnancy has reached 20 weeks or later, pre-eclampsia is seen in the first trimester of pregnancy in women with hydatidiform mole.
4. A white blood cell count of 8,000 mm^3 is well within normal limits.
5. Hypertrophied breast tissue is expected early in pregnancy.

TEST-TAKING HINT: It is very important to know the normal values of common laboratory results, especially the complete blood count, and to be familiar with deviations from normal diagnostic signs and symptoms.

31. 1. Headaches are not associated with the diagnosis of placenta previa.
2. A history of thyroid cancer is rarely associated with a diagnosis of placenta previa.
3. Previous preterm deliveries are not associated with a diagnosis of placenta previa.
4. Painless vaginal bleeding is often the only symptom of placenta previa.

TEST-TAKING HINT: There are three different forms of placenta previa: low-lying placenta—one that lies adjacent to, but not over, the internal cervical os; partial—one that partially covers the internal cervical os; and complete—a placenta that completely covers the internal cervical os. There is no way to deliver a live baby vaginally when a client has a complete previa, because the placenta (the baby's oxygen tank) would need to be delivered first. However, live babies have been delivered vaginally when the clients had low-lying or partial previas, and the baby was born before the placenta while still being oxygenated through the placenta.

32. Answers 2 and 3 are correct.
1. A jogger with low body mass index is not necessarily at high risk for placenta previa.
2. A smoker is at high risk for placenta previa.
3. A woman carrying triplets is at high risk for placenta previa.
4. Registered professional nurses are not at high risk for placenta previa.
5. Police officers are not at high risk for placenta previa.

TEST-TAKING HINT: The placenta usually implants at a vascular site on the posterior portion of the uterine wall. Two of the women are at high risk for placenta previa. There are 3 placentas nourishing fraternal triplets. Because of the amount of space needed for the placentas, it is not unusual for one to implant near or over the cervical os. The uterine lining of women who smoke is often not well perfused, sometimes resulting in the placenta implanting on or near the cervical os. Women with vascular disease and grand multigravidas are also at high risk for placenta previa.

33. 1. After the embryo dies, the nurse would expect to see vaginal bleeding. Rectal bleeding would not be expected.
2. Nausea and vomiting are not characteristic of a ruptured ectopic.
3. Sharp unilateral pain is a common symptom of a ruptured ectopic pregnancy.

4. Hyperthermia is not characteristic of a ruptured ectopic.

TEST-TAKING HINT: The most common location for an ectopic pregnancy to implant is in a fallopian tube. Because the tubes are nonelastic, when the pregnancy becomes too big, the tube ruptures. Unilateral pain can develop because only one tube is being affected by the condition, but some women complain of generalized abdominal pain.

34. 1. The timing of the pregnancy test is irrelevant.
2. The date of the last menstrual period will assist the nurse in determining how many weeks pregnant the client is.
3. The woman's previous complications are irrelevant at this time.
4. The age of the woman's menarche is irrelevant.

TEST-TAKING HINT: The date of the last menstrual period is important for the nurse to know. Ectopic pregnancies are usually diagnosed between the 8th and the 9th week of gestation because, at that gestational age, the conceptus has reached a size that is too large for the fallopian tube to contain it.

35. 1. A luteinizing hormone level will not provide information on the viability of a pregnancy.
2. Endometrial biopsy will not provide information on the viability of a pregnancy.
3. Hysterosalpingogram is not indicated in this situation.
4. Serum progesterone will provide information on the viability of a pregnancy.

TEST-TAKING HINT: When a pregnant client is seen by her healthcare provider with a complaint of vaginal bleeding, it is very important to determine the viability of the pregnancy as soon as possible. One relatively easy way to determine the viability of the conceptus is by performing a serum progesterone test. Progesterone is "pro" gestation and supports pregnancy. High levels indicate a viable embryo, whereas low levels indicate a pregnancy loss. Ultrasonography to assess for a beating heart and serum human chorionic gonadotropin levels may also be performed and provide more certain information about the location of the implantation, and size of the embryo. In addition, the location of the placenta is of importance.

36. 1. Dexamethasone is a steroid. It is not an appropriate therapy for this situation.
2. Methotrexate is the likely medication.
3. Menotropin is an infertility medication. It is not an appropriate therapy for this situation.
4. Progesterone injections are administered to some clients who have a history of preterm labor. It is not an appropriate therapy for this situation.

TEST-TAKING HINT: The conceptus is a ball of rapidly multiplying cells. Methotrexate interferes with that multiplication, killing the conceptus and, therefore, precluding the need for the client to undergo surgery. Even if the test taker were unfamiliar with its use in ectopic pregnancy but was aware of the action of methotrexate, he or she could deduce its efficacy here.

37. 83.5 mg

Because the recommended dosage is written per square meters, the nurse must calculate a safe dosage level for this medication using a body surface area formula.

Standard Method:

The formula for determining the body surface area (BSA) of a client, using the English system, is:

$$\text{BSA} = \frac{\sqrt{\text{weight (lb)} \times \text{height (in.)}}}{3{,}131}$$

The nurse first calculates the BSA—The calculation in this situation is:

$$\text{BSA} = \sqrt{\frac{136 \times 64}{3{,}131}}$$

$$\text{BSA} = \sqrt{\frac{8{,}704}{3{,}131}}$$

$$\text{BSA} = \sqrt{2.779}$$

$$\text{BSA} = \sqrt{2.78}$$

$$\text{BSA} = 1.67 \text{ m}^2$$

Standard Method:

A ratio and proportion equation must then be created and solved:

$$\frac{\text{Recommended dosage}}{1\ \text{m}^2} = \frac{\text{Safe dosage}}{\text{Client's BSA}}$$

$$\frac{50}{1} = \frac{x}{1.67}$$

$$x = 83.5\ \text{mg}$$

Dimensional Analysis Method:

The dimensional analysis formula for a safe dosage BSA calculation using the English system is:

Recommended dosage	$\sqrt{\frac{\text{weight (lb)} \times \text{height (in)}}{3{,}131}}\,\text{m}^2$	Time conversion	Unit conversion	
m^2/day		(if needed)	(if needed)	= Safe dosage

The calculation for this situation is

$$\frac{50}{1}\left|\ \sqrt{\frac{136 \times 64}{3{,}131}}\right. = \text{Safe dosage}$$

$$\frac{50}{1}\left|\ \sqrt{\frac{8{,}704}{3{,}131}}\right. = \text{Safe dosage}$$

$$\frac{50}{1}\left|\ \sqrt{2.78}\right. = \text{Safe dosage}$$

$$\frac{50}{1}\left|\ 1.67\right. = 83.5\ \text{mg}$$

The nurse now knows that the maximum dosage of methotrexate that this client can safely receive is 83.5 mg.

38. 73 mg

This question resembles the preceding question, except the weight and height are written in the metric system rather than the English system.

Standard Method:

The formula for BSA using the metric system is:

$$\text{BSA} = \sqrt{\frac{\text{weight (kg)} \times \text{height (cm)}}{3{,}600}}$$

The solution in this situation is:

$$\text{BSA} = \sqrt{\frac{52\text{kg} \times 148 \text{ cm}}{3{,}600}}$$

$$\text{BSA} = \sqrt{\frac{7{,}696}{3{,}600}}$$

$$\text{BSA} = \sqrt{2.14}$$

$$\text{BSA} = 1.46 \text{ m}^2$$

A ratio and proportion equation must then be created:

$$\frac{\text{Recommended dosage}}{1 \text{ m}^2} = \frac{\text{Safe dosage}}{\text{Client's BSA}}$$

$$\frac{50}{1} = \frac{x}{1.46}$$

$$x = 73 \text{ mg}$$

Dimensional Analysis Method:

The formula for BSA using dimensional analysis is:

Recommended dosage	$\sqrt{\frac{\text{weight (kg)} \times \text{height (cm)}}{3{,}600}}\text{m}^2$	Time conversion	Unit conversion	= Safe dosage
m^2/day		(if needed)	(if needed)	

The calculation for this situation is:

50	$\sqrt{\frac{52 \times 148}{3{,}600}}$	= Safe dosage
1		

50	$\sqrt{\frac{7{,}696}{3{,}600}}$	= Safe dosage
1		

50	$\sqrt{2.14}$	= Safe dosage
1		

50	1.46	= 73 mg
1		

The maximum dosage of methotrexate that this client can safely receive is 73 mg. Note that no decimal point or zero is seen after the 73, even though the stem stated "if rounding is needed, please round to the nearest tenth." To prevent medication errors, the Joint Commission states that trailing zeroes, as well as other important medication notations, should never be used.

39. Answers 1, 2, 3, and 4 are correct.

1. **Nausea and vomiting are common side effects.**
2. **Abdominal pain is a common side effect. The pain associated with the medication needs to be carefully monitored to differentiate it from the pain caused by the ectopic pregnancy itself.**
3. **Fatigue is a common side effect.**
4. **Light-headedness is a common side effect.**
5. Breast tenderness is not seen with this medication.

TEST-TAKING HINT: Because methotrexate is an antineoplastic agent, the nurse would expect to see the same types of complaints that he or she would see in a client receiving chemotherapy for cancer. It is very important that the abdominal pain seen with the medication not be dismissed because a common complaint of women with ectopic pregnancies is pain. The source of the pain, therefore, must be clearly identified.

40.
1. Taking the client's temperature is important, but assessing for dizziness and weakness is more important.
2. Documenting the contents and timing of the client's last meal is not the most important action.
3. Obtaining urine for urinalysis and culture is not the most important action.
4. **Assessing for complaints of dizziness or weakness is most important**

TEST-TAKING HINT: The nurse must prioritize care according to the highest risk of morbidity or mortality, or of a time-dependent nature. When the question asks the test taker to decide which action is most important, all four possible responses are plausible actions. The test taker must determine which is the one action that cannot be delayed and that may indicate a serious threat to the client's well being. In this situation, the most important action for the nurse to perform is to assess for complaints of dizziness or weakness. These symptoms are seen when clients develop hypovolemia from internal bleeding. Internal bleeding will be present if the client's fallopian tube has ruptured.

41.
1. Temperature is not the highest priority in this situation.
2. **The pulse is the highest priority in this situation.**
3. The respiratory rate is not the highest priority in this situation.
4. The blood pressure is not the highest priority in this situation.

TEST-TAKING HINT: The key to answering this question is the fact that the nursing care plan is for a client with third-trimester bleeding. By the end of the second trimester, pregnant women have almost doubled their blood volume. Because of this, if they bleed, they are able to maintain their blood pressure for a relatively long period of time. Their pulse rate, however, does rise. Nurses, therefore, must carefully attend to the pulse rate of pregnant women who have been injured or who are being observed for third-trimester bleeding. A drop in blood pressure is a very late and ominous sign.

42.
1. Clients with placenta previa are often on bedrest. This is, however, a short-term goal.
2. Another short-term goal is that the baby would have a reactive NST on day 2 of hospitalization.
3. **That the client be symptom-free until at least 37 weeks' gestation is a long-term goal.**
4. Normal vital signs on admission is a short-term goal.

TEST-TAKING HINT: Each of the goals is appropriate for a client with placenta previa. Only the statement that projects the client's response into the future, however, is a long-term goal.

43.
1. This is inappropriate. The client will need to be delivered by cesarean section.
2. Clients with complete placenta previa are discouraged from ambulating extensively. Usually, they are placed on bedrest only, although they may have bathroom privileges.
3. This is inappropriate. A 25-week-gestation baby is very preterm. The pregnancy will be maintained as long as possible, ideally at least until 37 weeks.
4. **Straining at stool can result in enough pressure to result in placental bleeding.**

TEST-TAKING HINT: Clients diagnosed with complete placenta previa are usually maintained on bedrest. Because one of the many complications of bedrest is constipation, these clients must be monitored carefully. Many primary healthcare providers order docusate sodium, a stool softener, to prevent this complication.

44. Answers 1, 3, 4, and 5 are correct.

1. **The client should be assessed for tachycardia, which could indicate that the client is bleeding internally.**
2. Referred shoulder pain is a symptom seen in clients with ruptured ectopic pregnancies.

It is unlikely that this client has an ectopic pregnancy because the signs and symptoms of that complication appear earlier in pregnancy, usually at 8 to 9 weeks' gestation.

3. **This client's signs and symptoms are consistent with both spontaneous abortion and hydatidiform mole. Although this client is only at 12 weeks' gestation, if she has a hydatidiform mole, she may be exhibiting signs of pre-eclampsia, including headache and hypertension.**
4. **This client's signs and symptoms are consistent with both spontaneous abortion and hydatidiform mole. To determine whether or not the client is carrying a viable fetus, the nurse should check the fetal heart rate.**
5. **This client's signs and symptoms are consistent with both spontaneous abortion and hydatidiform mole. Although this client is only 12 weeks' gestation, if she has a hydatidiform mole, she may be exhibiting signs of pre-eclampsia, including headache and hypertension.**

TEST-TAKING HINT: It is essential that the test taker carefully read the weeks of gestation when answering pregnancy-related questions. If the client had been earlier in the first trimester of her pregnancy, the signs and symptoms would also have been consistent with an ectopic pregnancy. It would then have been appropriate to assess for referred shoulder pain as well.

45. Answers 1, 3, 4, and 5 are correct.

1. **Passive range of motion will help to decrease the potential for muscle atrophy and thrombus formation.**
2. Fluid restriction is inappropriate. To maintain healthy bowel and bladder function, the client should drink large quantities of fluids.
3. **This client is separated from family. The separation can lead to depression. Decorating the room and enabling family to visit freely is very important.**
4. **A high-fiber diet will help to maintain normal bowel function.**
5. **Deep breathing exercises are important to maintain the client's respiratory function.**

TEST-TAKING HINT: Bedrest does not come without its complications—constipation, depression, respiratory compromise, and muscle atrophy, to name a few. The nurse must provide preventive care to maintain the health and well-being of the client as much as possible.

46.

1. The client is not at high risk for oligohydramnios but rather for polyhydramnios.
2. Placenta previa is more common in dizygotic twins because there are two placentas, and one of them may encroach on the cervical os. With a monozygotic twin pregnancy, there is only one placenta.
3. Twins are usually smaller than singletons. Although malpresentation may occur, it is unlikely that cephalopelvic disproportion will occur.
4. **Twin-to-twin transfusion is a relatively common complication of monozygotic twin pregnancies.**

TEST-TAKING HINT: The key to answering this question is the fact that monozygotic twins originate from the same egg—that is, they are mono (one) zygotic (egg) twins. They share a placenta and a chorion. Because their blood supply is originating from the same source, the twins' circulations are connected. As a result, one twin may become the donor twin while the second twin may become the recipient. The donor grows poorly and develops severe anemia. The recipient becomes polycythemic and large.

47.

1. **Fundal growth is often accelerated.**
2. Vaginal bleeding is not related to twin-to-twin transfusion.
3. Vomiting is not related to twin-to-twin transfusion.
4. Congestive heart failure is not related to twin-to-twin transfusion.

TEST-TAKING HINT: Fundal growth is accelerated for two reasons: (a) With two babies in utero, uterine growth is increased and (b) the recipient twin—the twin receiving blood from the other twin—often produces large quantities of urine, resulting in polyhydramnios.

48.

1. Progesterone levels are elevated in all pregnant women.
2. This is an appropriate weight increase: approximately 3 lb during the entire first trimester and approximately 1 lb per week after that—3 (first trimester) + 10 (1 lb per week for 10 weeks) = 13 pounds.
3. **It is possible that this client is carrying twins.**
4. Low alpha-fetoprotein levels are associated with Down's syndrome pregnancies.

TEST-TAKING HINT: After 20 weeks' gestation, the nurse would expect the fundal height to be equal to the number of weeks of the woman's gestation. Because the fundal height is 4 cm above the expected 22 cm, it is likely that the woman is either having twins or has polyhydramnios.

49. Answers 2 and 3 are correct.
1. Clients who have a history of prolapsed mitral valve are not at high risk for PPROM.
2. **Clients with UTIs are at high risk for PPROM.**
3. **Clients carrying twins, whether spontaneous or post-IVF, are at high risk for PPROM.**
4. Clients with gestational diabetes are not at high risk for PPROM.
5. Clients with deep vein thrombosis are not at high risk for PPROM.

TEST-TAKING HINT: Although the exact mechanism is not well understood, clients who have urinary tract infections are at high risk for PPROM. This is particularly important because pregnant clients often have urinary tract infections that present either with no symptoms at all or only with urinary frequency, a complaint of many pregnant clients. Also, clients carrying twins are at high risk for PPROM.

50.
1. The obstetric history is high risk for preterm delivery, not of fetal death.
2. **The nurse should emphasize the need for the client to notify the office of signs of preterm labor.**
3. Dependent edema is a normal complication of pregnancy.
4. The appearance of spider veins is a normal complication of pregnancy.

TEST-TAKING HINT: The test taker must be able to interpret a client's gravidity and parity. The letter "G" stands for gravid, or the number of pregnancies. The letter "P" stands for para, or the number of deliveries. A pregnancy with twins (multiples) counts as one pregnancy and one delivery.

The delivery information is further distinguished by four separate numbers that follow the acronym TPAL. The first number refers to "T," the number of *Term* (37+ weeks) deliveries the client has had; the second number refers to "P," the number of *Preterm* deliveries the client has had; the third number refers to "A," number of *Abortions* the client has had (any pregnancy loss before 20 weeks' gestation) whether spontaneous miscarriage (including ectopic) or therapeutic abortions; and the fourth number refers to "L," the number of *Living* children that the client currently has. For a woman who has given birth to twins, etc., each of the twins is counted at this point as a separate, living child. The client in the scenario has had 8 pregnancies (she is currently pregnant) with 3 full-term deliveries, 4 preterm deliveries, and no abortions, and she currently has 6 living children. This client's history of 4 previous preterm deliveries in combination with 8 pregnancies, puts her at high risk of another preterm delivery.

51.
1. There is nothing in this scenario that implies that this client is overweight or has gained too much weight during the pregnancy.
2. **This client is at high risk for pregnancy loss. This is an appropriate long-term goal.**
3. There is nothing in this scenario that implies that this client is at high risk for gestational diabetes.
4. There is nothing in this scenario that implies that this client is at high risk for delivering babies who are either small-for-gestational or large-for-gestational age.

TEST-TAKING HINT: This question requires the test taker to know why a client may have a cervical cerclage placed—namely, because of multiple pregnancy losses from cervical insufficiency (sometimes called "incompetent cervix"). The gravidity and parity information provides an important clue to the question. The client has had four pregnancies—with two preterm births and one abortion, but she has no living children. The goal for the therapy, therefore, is that the pregnancy will go to term.

52.
1. Clients who have a cerclage placed are not at high risk for hyperthermia in the immediate post-procedure period.
2. Hypotension is not a major complication of clients who have had a cerclage placed.
3. **Preterm labor is a complication in the immediate post-procedure period.**
4. A fetal heart dysrhythmia is not a complication related to the placement of the cerclage.

TEST-TAKING HINT: A cerclage is inserted when a client has a history of recurring pregnancy loss related to a cervical insufficiency. Losses typically occur between 14 and 26 weeks' gestation. This client has had 5 pregnancies but has only one living child. Unfortunately, with the manipulation of the cervix at the time of the cerclage, the clients may develop preterm labor. In addition

to fetal heart rate monitoring, the clients should be monitored carefully with a tocometer and palpation to assess for labor contractions.

53. 1. **This is the most important statement made by the client.**
2. The age of her first child is not relevant.
3. Her exercise regimen is not relevant.
4. The date of her miscarriage is not relevant.

TEST-TAKING HINT: Preterm labor is strongly associated with the presence of a urinary tract infection. Whenever an infection is present in the body, the body produces prostaglandins, an inflammatory hormone. Prostaglandins ripen the cervix and the number of oxytocin receptor sites on the uterine body increase in response. Preterm labor can then develop.

54. 1. **Clients who are dehydrated may experience contractions that can lead to preterm labor if the dehydration is not alleviated.**
2. This statement is inappropriate. The client may actually be in true labor.
3. After being hydrated it is possible that the client's cramping will stop.
4. It is not normal for a client to have rhythmic cramping even if she works on her feet.

TEST-TAKING HINT: Preterm cramping should never be ignored. Although the literature on hydration for preterm labor is mixed, clients are encouraged to improve their hydration initially. The client is encouraged to drink about 1 quart of fluid and to lie on her side. If the contractions do not stop, she should proceed to the hospital to have her cervix assessed. If the cervix begins to dilate or efface, a diagnosis of preterm labor would be made. If the contractions stop, clients are usually allowed to begin light exercise. But if the contractions restart, the woman should proceed to the hospital to be assessed.

55. 1. **The client should be taught to observe for signs of preterm labor.**
2. The client is not at high risk for decreased urinary output.
3. The client is not at high risk for marked fatigue.
4. Puerperal complications occur postpartum.

TEST-TAKING HINT: Clients with polyhydramnios (also called hydramnios) have excessive quantities of amniotic fluid in their uterine cavities. The excessive quantities likely result from increased fetal urine production, caused by fetal hyperglycemia. When the uterus is overextended from the large quantities of fluid, these women are at high risk for preterm labor.

56. 1. **The hydramnios is likely a result of excessive fetal urination.**
2. The hydramnios is unlikely related to hypoglycemic episodes.
3. Fetal sacral agenesis can result from maternal hyperglycemic episodes during the fetal organogenic period.
4. The hydramnios is unlikely related to impaired placental function.

TEST-TAKING HINT: For the first 16 weeks of the pregnancy, most of the amniotic fluid consists of maternal plasma which passes through the placenta into the gestational sac (Beall et al., 2007). Once the fetal kidney begins working at around 16 weeks gestation, fetal urine becomes the primary source, although the fetal lungs also contribute a small amount of fluid (Brace et al., 2018). Fetuses of mothers with diabetes often experience polyuria as a result of hyperglycemia. If the mother's diabetes is not controlled, excess glucose diffuses across the placental membrane and the fetus becomes hyperglycemic. As a result, the fetus exhibits the classic sign of diabetes—polyuria. If the mother's serum glucose levels are very high during the first trimester, it is likely that the fetus will develop structural congenital defects, including heart defects and sacral agenesis.

57. 1. **Clients with type 1 diabetes mellitus (T1DM) often need less insulin toward the end of the first trimester than they did before pregnancy.**
2. The client will be at high risk for hypoglycemic episodes.
3. Polyhydramnios does not develop until the second or third trimester. This question states the nurse is teaching the client about changes in the first trimester.
4. The client will not need to be hospitalized for fetal testing during the first trimester. However, noninvasive nonstress tests (NST) may be scheduled periodically in the provider's office in the third trimester to confirm fetal well-being.

TEST-TAKING HINT: On a physiological level, changes in various hormones of pregnancy can create periods of increased insulin sensitivity alternated by periods of reduced insulin sensitivity. This can create havoc for the client with type 1 diabetes mellitus (T1DM), and periods of hypoglycemia if her blood sugars are not monitored very closely. Insulin requirements are more unstable in the first 16 weeks of pregnancy (García-Patterson et al., 2010). For the first 9 weeks, insulin requirements

increase. This is considered the *anabolic* phase of pregnancy, when the mother's body builds up her fat stores to use later in the pregnancy, when the fetal demand for glucose is higher. Between the 9th and 16th weeks of pregnancy, insulin requirements decrease as the cells become more sensitive to insulin; as a result, less insulin is needed to maintain appropriate blood sugars. As though on a roller coaster, the insulin requirements begin increasing again between weeks 16 and 37 and then remain fairly stable until delivery (Feldman & Brown, 2016). Insulin needs during the postpartum phase also resemble a roller coaster, and that will be discussed in a separate chapter.

58. 1. This statement is incorrect. All of the client's glucose results are above recommended cut values.
2. This statement is incorrect. The 75-gram OGTT is a diagnostic test for gestational diabetes. There is no need for further testing.
3. This statement is incorrect. The majority of clients with gestational diabetes are successfully treated with diet and exercise alone.
4. This statement is correct. The client should be referred to a registered dietitian for diet counseling.

TEST-TAKING HINT: The American Diabetes Association (ADA) recommends that all pregnant women not previously diagnosed with diabetes undergo a 75-gram OGTT between 24 and 28 weeks' gestation. Those whose values exceed the following cutoff values are diagnosed with gestational diabetes:

- **Fasting—92 mg/dL (5.1 mmol/L), and either**
- **1 hour—180 mg/dL (10 mmol/L), or**
- **2 hour—153 mg/dL (8.5 mmol/L)**

(ADA, 2021a, p. S28).

59. 1. This statement is incorrect. It is recommended that clients prick the side of the fingertip to prevent injuring the most sensitive part of their fingers.
2. One-hour postprandial glucose values should be 140 mg/dL (7.8 mmol/L) or lower, not less than or equal to 146 mg/dL (8.1 mmol/L).
3. It is usually recommended that blood glucose testing be performed multiple times each day, including before and after all meals.
4. This statement is correct. All blood glucose results should be kept in a log for evaluation by the nurse and primary healthcare provider. If the results are above cutoff values, the primary healthcare provider may order dietary changes or the addition of oral hypoglycemic medications to the client's therapeutic regimen.

TEST-TAKING HINT: The American Diabetes Association (ADA), has developed recommended blood glucose target levels for clients with gestational diabetes. The target values for clients testing their blood sugars daily at home are:

- **Before a meal (preprandial): 95 mg/dL (5.3 mmol/L), or less**
- **And, either 1 hour after a meal (postprandial): 140 mg/dL (7.8 mmol/L), or less**
- **Or, 2 hours after a meal (postprandial): 120 mg/dL (6.7 mmol/L) or less**

(ADA, 2021b, p. S201, 202).

It is important for the nurse to consider, however, that although the literature refers to "cutoff values" for blood sugars that may cause harm, an international study published in 2010 determined that there is no clearly demarcated disease state. In this landmark Hyperglycemia and Adverse Pregnancy Outcome (HAPO) Study (Coustan et al., 2010) researchers measured fetal insulin levels from cord blood after birth, and found that even blood sugars below the cutoff values can lead to adverse pregnancy outcomes. Their conclusion was that there is no threshold that is "safe," and providers must be aware that the risk is on a continuum. Blood glucose values even lower than the cutoff values can cause harm (Coustan et al., 2010).

In 2010, HAPO study researchers recommended by consensus that diagnostic criteria for gestational diabetes be revised. The proposed criteria for the 75 gram, 2-hour OGTT was that the diagnosis be made with a single elevated value based on at least one of the following:

- **Fasting plasma glucose 92 mg/dl (5.1 mmol/L) or higher**
- **One-hour plasma glucose 180 mg/dl (10 mmol/L) or higher**
- **Two-hour plasma glucose 153 mg/dl (8.5 mmol/L) or higher**

Although these criteria were published in early 2010 and were endorsed by the American Diabetes Association and the World Health Organization shortly after that, they have not yet been adopted by the American College of

Obstetricians and Gynecologists (ACOG), who continue to recommend a 50-gram screening test, followed by a 100-gram OGTT if necessary (ADA, 2021a; Noctor & Dunne, 2015). The ACOG decision was endorsed by a National Institute of Health Consensus Conference in 2013 (ADA, 2021a; Noctor & Dunne, 2015), but as with many standards, that decision may change in the future. The test taker is advised to review ACOG's 50-gram screening and 100-gram diagnostic criteria. These can be accessed in the appendix.

60. 1. This question is not related to the client's need for health teaching.

2. The likelihood of developing either gestational or type 2 diabetes mellitus (T2DM) is reduced when clients exercise regularly.

3. This question is not related to the client's need for health teaching.

4. This question is not related to the client's need for health teaching.

TEST-TAKING HINT: There are a number of issues that the nurse should discuss with a client who has been diagnosed with gestational diabetes. The need for exercise is one of those topics. Other topics include diet, blood glucose testing, and treatment for hypoglycemic episodes.

61. 1. There should be a minimum of 2 fetal heart accelerations in 20 minutes.

2. This result is acceptable. There should be a minimum of 1 episode of fetal rhythmic breathing in 30 minutes.

3. This result is acceptable. There should be a minimum of 1 fetal limb extension and flexion.

4. This result is acceptable. There should be a minimum of 1 amniotic fluid pocket measuring 2 cm.

TEST-TAKING HINT: The BPP is a comprehensive assessment geared to evaluating fetal health. In addition to the four items mentioned previously, the fetus should exhibit 3 or more discrete body or limb movements in 30 minutes.

62. 1. Treatment for clients with gestational diabetes generally begins with carbohydrate counting and exercise.

2. About 95% of gestational diabetic clients are managed with diet and exercise alone.

3. This would not be ordered until after everything else had been tried, or unless blood sugars were extremely elevated.

4. This is not likely necessary.

TEST-TAKING HINT: Clients with gestational diabetes are first counseled regarding proper diet and exercise as well as blood glucose assessments. The vast majority of women are able to regulate their glucose levels with this intervention. If the glucose levels do not stabilize, the obstetrician will determine whether to order oral hypoglycemics or injectable insulin. Women who have been diagnosed with gestational diabetes (GDM) have up to a 60% lifetime risk of developing type 2 diabetes mellitus (T2DM) (Noctor & Dunne, 2015). The development of gestational diabetes is a warning that the woman's pancreas is struggling to keep up with the insulin demands of pregnancy, which can be 2 to 3 times higher than the amount needed before pregnancy (see the figure in the Gestational Diabetes section of the appendix). By eating fewer carbohydrates, the client can reduce the strain on her pancreas and preserve its function. This may effectively delay the development of type 2 diabetes in the future.

63. 1. This is incorrect. Counting fewer than 10 fetal movements in an hour warrants a phone call to her primary healthcare provider.

2. A nonstress test may be warranted since the woman felt fewer than 10 counts in an hour. She should call the primary healthcare provider to discuss next steps.

3. There is no need to redo the test, and the half-hour time frame is not the standard.

4. There is no need for the client to redo the test. Furthermore, the benefit of drinking orange juice to elicit fetal movement has not been validated in the literature.

TEST-TAKING HINT: Fetal kick counting is a valuable, noninvasive means of monitoring fetal well-being. It may be suggested by the primary healthcare provider after the client has reached 28 weeks' gestation, as away to easily confirm fetal well-being. Mothers are taught to be aware of the number of times they feel their baby kicking during an hour. If concerned, they are advised to lie down on their side, or in a semi-reclined position and consciously count the numbers of times they feel their baby kick during one hour. This should be done without distractions such as watching television. If the baby kicks 10 or more times during that hour, the woman can be reassured that the baby is healthy. If the baby kicks fewer times, the woman should notify her healthcare provider, who will likely perform either a nonstress test or, in some situations, a biophysical profile, which includes an ultrasound assessment.

64. Answers 1 and 3 are correct.
   1. **Pregnant clients with diabetes are particularly at high risk for urinary tract infections.**
   2. Pregnant clients with diabetes are not at high risk for multiples
   3. **Pregnant clients with type 1 diabetes mellitus (T1DM) are at high risk for acidosis.**
   4. Pregnant clients with diabetes are at high risk for hypertension, not hypotension.
   5. Pregnant clients with diabetes are at high risk for hyperlipidemia, not hypolipidemia.

TEST-TAKING HINT: It is very important for the test taker to read each response carefully. If the test taker were to read the responses to the preceding question very quickly, they might choose incorrect answers. For example, the test taker might pick pathologic hypotension, assuming that it says "hypertension." Pregnant clients with T1DM are at high risk for UTIs because they often excrete glucose in their urine. The glucose is an excellent medium for bacterial growth. They also should be assessed carefully for acidosis because an acidotic environment can be life threatening to a fetus. Clients with T1DM whose blood sugars rise too high are at risk of diabetic ketoacidosis (DKA). See additional information on DKA in the appendix.

65. 1. The client may need to be seen, but this is not the appropriate response by the nurse at this time.
   2. **The client likely has hypoglycemia and should drink a 4-ounce glass of juice.**
   3. It is contraindicated to have the client inject herself with insulin because her blood sugar is already too low.
   4. The client may need to speak with her primary healthcare provider, but that is not the appropriate response by the nurse at this time.

TEST-TAKING HINT: The nurse must be familiar with the differences in symptoms of hyperglycemia and hypoglycemia. A client with gestational diabetes rarely experiences symptoms of hyperglycemia, which include headache, nausea, and confusion. Hyperglycemic symptoms come on slowly. In contrast, hypoglycemic symptoms of shakiness, pallor, sweating, and a racing pulse often come on suddenly, especially if a client has not eaten soon enough after injecting her insulin. Drinking 4 ounces of orange juice, or eating a cracker with peanut butter or other simple carbohydrate, will stabilize the glucose in the woman's body. Unlike a client with T1DM, the client with gestational diabetes has a working pancreas and it secretes insulin in response to high blood levels. Injectable insulin simply assists the pancreas in providing additional insulin. As such, it is important that the client avoid drinking an entire 8 ounces of orange or other fruit juice, as this will elevate her blood sugar too high and she could easily experience another drop in her blood sugar as the pancreas releases more insulin to reduce the blood sugar levels.

66. 1. Although this is an option, it is not necessary. To avoid giving the client two injections, the regular and NPH can be administered in one syringe.
   2. **This is the appropriate method. The regular insulin should be drawn up first and then the NPH insulin in the same syringe.**
   3. Regular insulin should be drawn up first.
   4. The insulins should not be mixed together in a vial.

TEST-TAKING HINT: When administering insulin, the nurse must remember the principles of insulin balance. In people without diabetes, the pancreas maintains a continuous *background* or *basal* level of insulin throughout the day and night. This is supplemented with bursts of higher insulin at mealtimes. This process is duplicated fairly well for the client with diabetes by the use of long-acting background insulin such as NPH to cover glucose rises between meals, and short-acting insulin such as regular insulin to cover glucose rises following meals. Because regular insulin acts more quickly than NPH it is important to avoid any risk of injecting regular insulin into the bottle of NPH, which could cause hypoglycemia. If regular insulin is inadvertently injected into the bottle of NPH, the bottle of NPH must be thrown away.

For this reason, insulin must be drawn up in the correct sequence: regular insulin first and NPH insulin second. Many nurses use the phrase, "clear before cloudy," or remember the initials RN, as in "Regular" before "NPH." While drawing up regular insulin in the syringe initially, the nurse can re-inject some of the insulin back into the bottle if too much is initially removed. Refer to the appendix for more information on the physiology of basal and bolus insulin.

67. 1. **The client has been hyperglycemic for the past 3 months and is within target levels today.**
   2. The client has not been normoglycemic—she has been hyperglycemic for the past 3 months even though she is within target today.
   3. The client has not been normoglycemic.
   4. The client has not been within target for the past 3 months.

TEST-TAKING HINT: It is very important for a glycohemoglobin test to be performed at the same time that a fasting glucose is done to have an idea of a diabetic client's glucose control over the past 3 months. This is compared to the results of the fasting test. When in a hyperglycemic environment, the red blood cell (RBC) becomes a compound molecule with a glucose group attached to it. Because the RBC lives for approximately 120 days, the healthcare provider can estimate the glucose control of the client over the preceding 3 months' time by analyzing the glycohemoglobin. Some providers explain this in terms of the RBC being coated with layers of glucose. When the RBC is cut in half, the laboratory can assess the average blood sugar level over the past 3 months very much like analyzing the growth rings of a tree. A reading of up to 5.5% glycohemoglobin (111 mg/dL, or 6.2 mmol/L) is considered a normal, nondiabetic A1C. The American Diabetes Association (ADA, 2020) targets for blood sugar levels in clients with diabetes are:

- A1C less than 7%
- Preprandial blood sugar of 70–130 mg/dL (3.9–7.2 mmol/L)
- Postprandial blood sugar of less than 180 mg/dL (10 mmol/L).

An HgbA1c level of 7% indicates the client has been hyperglycemic for the past 3 months with an average daily blood glucose level of 154 mg/dL (8.6 mmol/L). Because her fasting blood glucose level of 100 mg/dL (5.5 mmol/L) is within the premeal target, the nurse can deduce that the client has had poor glucose control for the past 3 months and is within target levels today.

68. 1. Estrogen does not compete with insulin.
2. Progesterone does not compete with insulin.
3. Human chorionic gonadotropin does not compete with insulin.
4. Human placental lactogen is an insulin antagonist, so the client will require higher doses of insulin as the level of placental lactogen increases.

TEST-TAKING HINT: During the first trimester, the insulin needs of a woman with type 1 diabetes are usually low. Once the diabetic client enters the second trimester, however, insulin demands increase. One of the most important reasons that insulin demands increase is the increasingly higher levels of human placental lactogen (HPL) produced by the placenta that are released into the mother's bloodstream. By increasing the insulin resistance of the mother's cells, more glucose circulates in the mother's blood, making more glucose available to cross the placenta to the fetus. This is what contributes to gestational diabetes and reveals the previously unknown existence of insulin insufficiency in these clients. For the first time, the inability of the pancreas to manufacture or store insulin appropriately, is revealed. As such, gestational diabetes can serve as a warning. Clients can learn to make permanent changes that can delay the onset of type 2 diabetes mellitus (T2DM) in the future by reducing the demands on the pancreas.

69. 1. It is unlikely that this client will need insulin injections.
2. It is unlikely that this client will need insulin injections.
3. It is unlikely that this client will need any medication.
4. It is unlikely that this client will need any medication. If the client follows her diet and exercises regularly, she will probably control the diabetes.

TEST-TAKING HINT: The client should be reminded that if she follows her diet and exercises regularly, she will likely be able to manage her diabetes without medication. She should also be encouraged to continue the diet and exercise after delivery to prevent the development of type 2 diabetes later in life.

70. 1. Hyperglycemia is most damaging to the fetus during the first trimester of pregnancy. Although it is abnormal at 38 weeks' gestation, it is not the most important finding.
2. Acidosis is fatal to the fetus. This is the most important finding.
3. Hypocapnia is abnormal, but it is not the most important finding.
4. A high glycohemoglobin is abnormal, but it is not the most important finding.

TEST-TAKING HINT: It is essential that the nurse monitor clients for situations that would put the fetus in jeopardy of being in an acidotic environment. This includes maternal hypoxia and diabetic ketoacidosis (DKA). Normal blood pH is around 7.4. This client's pH of 7.2 indicates her blood pH is at a life-threatening level for the fetus. Her history of vomiting and reported symptoms of a bladder infection put her at risk of euglycemic diabetic ketoacidosis (EDKA), a less common form of DKA with blood sugars below 200 mg/dL (11.1 mmol/L) (Muppidi et al., 2020). Because of the misleading blood glucose levels, the condition can be difficult to diagnose (Muppidi et al., 2020). Precipitating factors include infection and intractable vomiting, among others (Sibai & Viteri, 2014). The astute nurse

recognizes the cues of nausea and vomiting, noting that these conditions are not normal in the third trimester of pregnancy.

In addition to recognizing nausea and vomiting as abnormal, the nurse also recognizes that an infection can lead to abnormally high levels of metabolic acids in maternal blood. This can overwhelm the mother's acid–base balance, as noted. As a result, not only can acidosis lead to nausea and vomiting, it may also negatively affect the fetus. The force of cardiac contractions diminishes in the presence of acidemia, reducing perfusion of the placenta and starting a vicious circle of fetal hypoxia and metabolic acidemia in the fetus, as a result. The fetal heart rate must be carefully monitored for late decelerations. For more information on DKA, see the appendix.

71. 1. This client is many years past her baby's death. Grief counseling is not an immediate need for this client.

2. This client is in need of nutrition counseling.

3. The woman is not in need of infection control counseling at this time.

4. Although there may be some genetic basis to spina bifida, about 95% of affected babies are born to parents with no family history of the disease.

TEST-TAKING HINT: There is a strong association between low folic acid intake during the first trimester of pregnancy and spina bifida, a neural tube defect. It is very important that all clients, and especially clients with a family or personal history of a neural tube defect, consume adequate amounts of folic acid during their pregnancies. It is recommended that all women consume at least 600 mg of the vitamin per day. To that end, to prevent neural tube defects, it is recommended that pregnant women with no family history take a supplement of 400 mg per day, while pregnant women with a family history take a supplement that is 10 times the standard dose, or 4 mg per day.

72. 1. The criteria for a reactive NST are at least two FHR accelerations of 15 bpm lasting 15 or more seconds during a 20-minute period. During this time, the provider would also expect to see moderate baseline variability in the FHR. However, the FHR accelerations are key.

2. The maternal heart rate is not evaluated during an NST.

3. This is the definition of a reactive nonstress test—there are at least two fetal heart-rate accelerations of 15 bpm lasting 15 or more seconds during a 20-minute period.

4. The maternal heart rate is not evaluated during an NST.

TEST-TAKING HINT: A reactive nonstress test (NST) is not predictive. It is done to determine whether or not the fetus is hypoxemic at the time of the test (Preboth, 2000). A reactive NST indicates the fetus is not hypoxic at that time. Because hypoxemia due to a placenta negatively affected by diabetes mellitus, pre-eclampsia, or postdates is generally a slow process, NSTs are usually performed twice weekly. In the case of a nonreactive nonstress test, when the fetal heart fails to show 2 accelerations of 15 bpm lasting 15 or more seconds during a 20-minute period, more extensive testing, including a biophysical profile, is usually indicated.

73. Answers 1, 3, and 4 are correct.

1. Sexual intercourse has been recommended to women as a means of stimulating labor.

2. Aromatherapy is not recommended to women as a means of increasing their Bishop score.

3. Breast stimulation can be used to stimulate labor.

4. Castor oil has been used as a means of promoting contractions.

5. Aerobic exercise is not recommended to women as a means of increasing their Bishop score.

TEST-TAKING HINT: Many natural interventions have been used in obstetrics to ripen the cervix and increase women's Bishop scores and/or to stimulate labor. Because oxytocin is produced during orgasm and when the breasts are stimulated, both intercourse and breast stimulation can be used as complementary methods of stimulating labor. In addition, semen has a high concentration of prostaglandins, which can help to ripen the cervix. Castor oil stimulates the bowels and is thought to increase the irritability of the uterus, as a result. Caution must be taken before using these methods. If there is any indication that the baby may be unable to withstand labor, these means should not be employed.

74. Answers 1, 2, 4, and 5 are correct.

1. This response is correct. The woman should be maintained in the lateral recumbent position during the surgery because, if laid flat, the gravid uterus

would compress the great vessels and impede the return of blood to the heart.

2. **This response is correct. The fetal heart rate and contraction pattern should be monitored frequently after surgery by an obstetrical nurse for any signs of fetal stress and/or for preterm labor.**
3. This client is pregnant; she is not postpartum. The fundus must be monitored for signs of preterm labor, the client has no lochia.
4. **The client would be at high risk for postoperative vomiting and for postoperative gas pains for 2 reasons: Progesterone during pregnancy slows gastric motility and the stomach and intestines are displaced by the gravid uterus. In addition, nausea and vomiting are complications of general anesthesia.**
5. **This response is correct. Because pregnancy puts the client at risk of thrombi, antiembolic stockings should be placed on the client before surgery and should remain in place for the entire time that she is immobile.**

TEST-TAKING HINT: Non-obstetrical surgery is performed on a pregnant woman only when absolutely necessary. Her obstetrical provider should be included in writing pre-operative, operative, and postoperative orders related to the pregnancy. These orders must include frequency and type of fetal monitoring during and after surgery. The client's hormone levels of pregnancy, cardiovascular changes of pregnancy, and the size of the gravid uterus all place her at risk of complications. Maintenance of the pregnancy itself is at risk because of the surgery. During a nonobstetric surgical procedure on a client who is carrying a viable fetus (generally 25 weeks' gestation and beyond), obstetrical staff must be kept informed in case an emergent cesarean section becomes necessary. An obstetrical provider with operating room privileges, obstetrical nurses, and a neonatal intensive care team must be readily available. In addition, a tray of cesarean section surgical instruments and a baby warmer and resuscitation equipment must be immediately available. Postoperatively, an obstetrical nurse must remain with the client to perform obstetrical assessments. This is in addition to the post-anesthesia care unit (PACU) RN who will perform nonobstetrical post-anesthesia recovery care.

75. 1. **Vaso-occlusive crises are precipitated by hypoxia in both pregnant and nonpregnant clients with sickle cell disease.**
2. Acidosis, not alkalosis, precipitates vaso-occlusive crises.
3. Dehydration, not fluid overload, precipitates vaso-occlusive crises.
4. A hyperglycemic state does not precipitate vaso-occlusive crises.

TEST-TAKING HINT: Sickle cell disease (SCD) is an automosal recessive, inherited disease. It occurs when both parents carry the abnormal hemoglobin "S" (HbS) gene and pass it on to their offspring.

Red blood cells are normally smooth and round, and they move through the blood vessels easily, carrying oxygen for the cells. HbS can distort RBCs into the shape of a farm implement called a sickle, or the letter "C," in response to precipitating factors. These factors may include hypoxia, acidosis, dehydration, and/or a change in normal body temperature because of a fever or extreme cold (Maakaron, 2020). Sickle cell disease causes a range of acute and chronic vascular complications as a result of ongoing vaso-occlusion and hypoxia. With a sickle cell crisis, many of the cells become sticky and semi-solid, their sickle shape causing them to stick together. This can cause injury to the blood vessels and/or occlude small blood vessels. Blockage of blood flow to dependent organs and limbs causes extreme pain during a vaso-occlusive crisis. With appropriate IV fluids and oxygenation, the acidosis and hypoxia can be reversed. In addition, because sickle crises are so painful, narcotic analgesics will be required. The sickled RBCs may resume their round shape after treatment but they become fragile and are more easily destroyed, leading to anemia (Maakaron, 2020). This is a very serious state for the pregnant woman and her fetus.

76. 1. Although narcotic medications must be administered to relieve the pain of the crisis, this is not the priority action.
2. Although heat to the joints must be applied to dilate the blood vessels, this is not the priority action.
3. Although the client should be kept on bedrest to protect the joints and to prevent further sickling, this is not the priority action.
4. **Administering intravenous fluids is the priority action.**

TEST-TAKING HINT: Although this question is not directly related to pregnancy, the nurse must be able to translate information from another

medical discipline into the obstetric area. The priority action to maintain survival is to improve perfusion to the client's organs. When the client is dehydrated, the sickled red blood cells clump together, inhibiting perfusion. By providing intravenous fluids, the blood can more easily flow through the vessels and perfuse the organs, including the placenta.

77. Answers 2, 3, and 4 are correct.

1. Clients with obesity are not especially at high risk for placenta previa.
2. **Clients with obesity are at high risk for gestational diabetes.**
3. **Clients with obesity are at high risk for deep vein thrombosis.**
4. **Clients with obesity are at high risk for pre-eclampsia.**
5. Clients with obesity are not especially at high risk for chromosomal defects.

TEST-TAKING HINT: Because clients who enter pregnancy with obesity are at high risk for type 2 diabetes mellitus (T2DM), many obstetricians schedule an oral glucose tolerance test early in pregnancy rather than waiting until after 24 weeks' gestation. As a result, the diabetes complication is discovered much earlier and intervention can begin much sooner. The clients are also carefully monitored for signs and symptoms of pre-eclampsia and deep vein thrombosis.

78.

1. This statement is not true. Clients with obesity are encouraged to gain about 11 to 20 pounds during their pregnancies.
2. This statement is not true. Although clients with obesity are encouraged to eat fewer calories than clients without obesity, they are still encouraged to gain weight during their pregnancies.
3. This statement is not entirely true. Although it is true that obesity is correlated with neural tube defects, the information on weight gain is incorrect. Clients with obesity are expected to gain approximately 0.4 to 0.6 pounds per week during their second and third trimesters, or a total of 11 to 20 pounds during their pregnancies.
4. **This statement is true. Clients without obesity are encouraged to gain between 25 and 35 pounds during their pregnancies, while clients with obesity are encouraged to gain only 11 to 20 pounds.**

TEST-TAKING HINT: It is not appropriate for a client with obesity, (defined as a client whose BMI is 30 kg/m2 or more), to lose weight or to refrain from gaining weight during her pregnancy. When clients lose weight, they begin to break down fats and ketones develop. An acidic environment is unsafe for the unborn baby. Overweight women, or those whose BMI is between 25 and 29.9 kg/m2 are also recommended to gain fewer pounds than the normal weight client, that is, between 15 and 25 pounds during their pregnancies (ACOG, 2013a). It is important to maintain the client's sense of self-esteem and to tell her that the reasons for the recommendation of less weight gain are to avoid obstetrical complications of preterm birth and cesarean section, among other risks.

79.

1. **The nurse should report the positive results to the doctor. The client should not be sent home before notifying the provider of the NST result unless the provider's order states otherwise.**
2. There is no need to perform the nipple stimulation test.
3. There is no need to induce the client.
4. There is no need to administer oxygen to the client.

TEST-TAKING HINT: This client is postdates. As a result, the placenta is at risk of calcification and reduced fetal oxygenation. The NST is being performed to assess the well-being of the fetus. The reactive NST result is evidence that the fetus is well oxygenated *at this time*. Like any well-oxygenated person, the fetal heart rate increases with movement and exercise. There is no need to provide emergent care. The nurse must be aware of the provider's plan for care, which may include scheduling another NST in 2 to 3 days, sending the client home to await spontaneous labor, or scheduling an oxytocin induction for postdates before the fetus demonstrates inadequate oxygenation.

80. Answers 1, 2, 3, and 5 are correct.

1. **The client should call her primary healthcare provider if she experiences fever or chills.**
2. **Albeit rare, because the fetus or umbilical cord can be injured during an amniocentesis, the client should report either a decrease or an increase in fetal movement.**
3. **An amniocentesis can precipitate preterm labor. The client should report abdominal pain or cramping.**
4. Neither rash nor pruritus is associated with amniocentesis.

5. **The client should report any fluid loss through the vagina, whether blood or amniotic fluid. The placenta may become injured or the membranes may rupture during an amniocentesis.**

TEST-TAKING HINT: During an amniocentesis, the amniotic sac is entered with a large needle, using ultrasound for guidance. As a result of the procedure, a number of complications can develop, including infection, preterm labor, rupture of the membranes, and/or fetal injury. Although the incidence of complications is small, it is very important for the nurse to advise the client of the signs of each of these problems.

81. **Answers 1, 2, and 3 are correct.**
   1. **It would be appropriate to perform a biophysical profile (BPP).**
   2. **It would be appropriate to perform a nonstress test (NST).**
   3. **It would be appropriate to perform an umbilical artery (UA) Doppler assessment**
   4. Chorionic villus sampling (CVS) is performed during the first trimester. The results provide fetal genetic information.
   5. Human chorionic gonadotropin (HCG) testing is performed during the first trimester to confirm the pregnancy. The hormone is produced by the trophoblastic layer until approximately 13 weeks' gestation.

TEST-TAKING HINT: A fetus with IUGR is growing more slowly than expected. The restricted growth may be caused by poor placental blood flow related to poor placental health. The NST and BPP are initial tests performed to provide information regarding the health and well-being of the fetus. If they indicate concerns, a UA Doppler study may be done for more information. The umbilical artery (UA) Doppler assessment is performed to assess the blood flow through the placenta. See the appendix for more information on Doppler flow studies.

82. 1. **A BPP of 4 indicates that fetal well-being is compromised.**
   2. BPP assesses the well-being of the fetus. It does not assess maternal well-being.
   3. BPP assesses the well-being of the fetus. It does not assess maternal well-being.
   4. The BPP does evaluate the level of amniotic fluid in the amniotic sac, but the BPP cannot predict if or when the amniotic sac may rupture.

TEST-TAKING HINT: The biophysical profile (BPP) includes an ultrasound evaluation and a non-stress test (NST). It is performed when fetal well-being is a concern. Four assessments are performed via ultrasound: fetal breathing movements, gross body movements, fetal tone, and amniotic fluid volume. The fifth assessment (for fetal heartrate accelerations) is assessed through the NST by use of an external fetal heart-rate monitor. Each assessment may receive a value of 0 or 2. A total score of 0 to 10 is possible. The lower the score, the more evidence of a compromised fetus.

83. 1. The L/S ratio indicates the maturity of the fetal lungs, not the coagulability of maternal blood.
   2. **The L/S ratio indicates the maturity of the fetal lungs.**
   3. The L/S ratio indicates the maturity of the fetal lungs, not the potential for erythroblastosis fetalis.
   4. The L/S ratio indicates the maturity of the fetal lungs, not the potential for gestational diabetes.

TEST-TAKING HINT: The lecithin and sphingomyelin (L/S) ratio is an established factor to determine fetal lung maturity. Lecithin and sphingomyelin are two components of surfactant, the slippery substance that lines the alveoli and reduces the stickiness of the lungs after birth, making the work of breathing easier once the fetus is born. The fetal lungs have usually reached maturation when the ratio of the substances is 2:1 or higher. To perform the test, the obstetrician must obtain amniotic fluid during an amniocentesis. A quick test, called a shake or foam test, can also be performed on the amniotic fluid to assess fetal lung maturation. (It is important to note that even with an L/S ratio above 2:1, the lungs of fetuses of diabetic mothers are often immature.)

84. 1. **The baby is preterm.**
   2. The L/S ratio is not related to blood loss.
   3. The L/S ratio is not related to hyperbilirubinemia.
   4. The L/S ratio is not related to pre-eclampsia.

TEST-TAKING HINT: The amount of lecithin must be 2 times the amount of sphingomyelin before the provider can be assured that the fetal lungs are mature. The ratio in this scenario—1:1—indicates that the surfactant is insufficient for extrauterine respirations.

85. 1. It would be best to choose a time when the fetus is most active.
2. This is the best position for perfusing the placenta.
3. Fewer than 10 counts in 1 hour should be reported.
4. It is unnecessary to refrain from eating prior to the test.

TEST-TAKING HINT: Because the goal of fetal kick counting is to monitor fetal well-being, it is best to do the test when the baby is most active and is most likely to be well nourished and well oxygenated. Many women find that the best time for the assessment is immediately after a meal.

86. 1. Caudal agenesis is a severe birth defect that can result from maternal hyperglycemia in early pregnancy.
2. Cardiomegaly is one of the common signs of erythroblastosis fetalis.
3. The nurse would expect to see polyhydramnios, not oligohydramnios.
4. Hyperemia is not related to erythroblastosis fetalis or Rh incompatibility.

TEST-TAKING HINT: Erythroblastosis fetalis is the fetal condition that results when an Rh-negative (Rh–) mother who is sensitized to Rh-positive (Rh+) blood is pregnant with an Rh-positive (Rh+) baby. This can occur if the mother had a previous pregnancy loss, or gave birth to a baby who was Rh positive (Rh+) and did not receive Rh₀(D) immune globulin after the birth. With the next pregnancy, maternal antibodies cross the placenta and destroy the fetal red blood cells. As a result, the baby becomes severely anemic. Cardiomegaly is one of the complications that occurs as a result of the severe fetal anemia.

With anemia, the number of oxygen-carrying red blood cells (RBCs) is diminished. As a result, the fetal heart tries to compensate by pumping harder to circulate the available RBCs to the cells. Like any muscle, with increased exercise the heart becomes enlarged and thickened, a condition referred to as cardiomegaly. The word "cardio" refers to the heart; "megaly" means "abnormal enlargement." Unfortunately, this end result reduces the heart's efficiency. Heart failure is a possible outcome.

87. 1. Rh₀(D) immune globulin is administered to all Rh-negative (Rh–) mothers because fetal blood type is usually unknown.
2. Although in rare instances the Coombs test may be positive, the direct Coombs test is usually negative.
3. Although this is an important action that must be taken before the administration of any medication, it is especially critical in this situation.
4. Rh₀(D) immune globulin is not reconstituted.

TEST-TAKING HINT: Rh₀(D) immune globulin acts by suppressing the immune response of Rh-negative (Rh–) individuals to Rh-positive (Rh+) red blood cells. It is indicated only for Rh-negative (Rh–) individuals.

88. 1. Although the dosage can be administered in the gluteal muscles, the deltoid is the preferred site of the Rh₀(D) immune globulin injection.
2. Although the dosage can be administered in the gluteal muscles, the deltoid is the preferred site of the Rh₀(D) immune globulin injection.
3. Although the dosage can be administered in the vastus lateralis, the deltoid is the preferred site of the Rh₀(D) immune globulin injection.
4. Although the dosage can be administered in the gluteal muscles, the deltoid is the preferred site of the Rh₀(D) immune globulin injection.

TEST-TAKING HINT: Whenever possible, it is preferable to inject the antibodies into the recommended injection site. The antibodies are absorbed optimally from that site and, therefore, are more apt to suppress the mother's immune response.

89. 1. A varicella titer is not necessary.
2. Although the woman's obstetric history is important, it is not essential that it be assessed at this time.
3. It is essential that the woman's blood type be assessed.
4. It is not appropriate to assess the woman's cervical patency.

TEST-TAKING HINT: If the woman is found to be Rh negative (Rh–), the woman must receive a dose of Rh₀(D) immune globulin within 72 hours of the miscarriage even though the fetal blood type is unknown. If the fetus were Rh-positive (Rh+) and the woman were not to receive Rh₀(D) immune globulin, the woman's immune system might be stimulated to produce antibodies against Rh-positive (Rh+) blood. Any future Rh-positive (Rh+) fetus would be in danger of developing erythroblastosis fetalis. It is also important for the nurse to check the woman's rubella titer. If the woman is nonimmune to rubella, she should receive the MMR vaccine prior to discharge.

90. 1. The baby's Rh status cannot change.
2. That the mother produces no Rh antibodies is the expected outcome of Rh₀(D) immune globulin administration.
3. The baby will not produce antibodies.
4. The mother's Rh status cannot change.

TEST-TAKING HINT: It is important for the nurse to understand the immune response to an antigen. In this situation, the antigen is the baby's Rh-positive (Rh+) blood. It can leak into the maternal bloodstream from the fetal bloodstream at various times during the pregnancy. Most commonly it happens at the time of placental delivery. Because the mother is antigen negative—that is, Rh-negative (Rh–), when exposed to Rh-positive (Rh+) blood, her immune system develops antibodies. Rh₀(D) immune globulin is composed of Rh-positive (Rh+) antibodies. It acts as passive immunity. By acquiring these antibodies by injection, the mother's immune system does not develop antibodies via the active immune response with her next pregnancy, if the baby is Rh-positive (Rh+).

91. 1. It is unnecessary to perform a daily nitrazine assessment.
2. Breast tenderness is unrelated to PPROM.
3. This client must abstain from intercourse for the remainder of the pregnancy.
4. It is unnecessary for the client to weigh her saturated pads.

TEST-TAKING HINT: Outpatient care remains an alternative for prelabor, preterm rupture of membranes (PPROM) in the periviable pregnancy at 23 to 24 weeks gestation (ACOG, 2020b), Once the membranes are ruptured, the barrier between the vagina and the uterus is broken. As a result, the pathogens in the vagina and the external environment are potentially able to ascend into the sterile uterine body. In addition, once the membranes are ruptured, the client is at high risk for preterm labor. Both anal and vaginal intercourse must be curtailed for both of these reasons.

92. 1. A fern test is performed to assess for the presence of amniotic fluid.
2. A biophysical profile assessment is performed to assess fetal well-being, not for the presence of amniotic fluid.
3. During amniocentesis, amniotic fluid is extracted from the uterine body to perform genetic analyses or fetal lung maturation assessments as well as other analyses. It is not done to assess for rupture of the membranes.
4. The Kernig assessment is performed on clients who are suspected of having meningeal irritation. It is unrelated to pregnancy.

TEST-TAKING HINT: The fern test was so named because when amniotic fluid dries on the slide and is viewed under a microscope, it appears as a fern-like image. The image is a reflection of the high estrogen levels in the fluid that create a crystalline pattern. When the fern appears, it is likely that amniotic fluid is leaking from the amniotic sac. It is important to note, however, that ferning is not specific to amniotic fluid. Other fluids, such as blood, semen, cervical mucus, and some urine specimens can also yield a crystallized, fern pattern.

93. 1. It is not unsafe for women 18 years of age to become pregnant.
2. Cat feces are a potential source of toxoplasmosis.
3. Peanut butter is an excellent source of protein.
4. Women who work as surgeons are not especially at high risk.

TEST-TAKING HINT: The nurse must be familiar with any possible circumstances that place antepartal clients and their fetuses at high risk. Toxoplasmosis is an illness caused by a protozoan. The organism can be contracted in a number of ways, including eating rare or raw meat, drinking unpasteurized goat milk, and coming in contact with cat feces. When contracted by the mother during pregnancy, it can cause serious fetal and neonatal disease.

94. 1. The symptoms are not likely caused by *Staphylococcus aureus*.
2. The symptoms are not likely caused by *Streptococcus albicans*.
3. The symptoms are not likely caused by *Pseudomonas aeruginosa*.
4. The client is likely suffering from listeriosis, an infection caused by *Listeria monocytogenes* bacteria.

TEST-TAKING HINT: Soft cheeses and unpasteurized milk can carry listeria. Listeria infection is a serious condition that can cause miscarriages, stillbirths, and preterm labor. It also carries the risk of serious illness and death to newborns. Pregnant, Latina women are at highest risk to contract listeriosis (CDC, n.d.-e). It is important that the nurse communicate to all pregnant women the need to refrain from consuming those substances with a clear rationale for the warning.

95. **1. The symptoms of listeriosis are similar to symptoms of the flu and include fever and muscle aches.**
2. Neither rash nor thrombocytopenia is related to listeriosis.
3. Neither petechiae nor anemia is related to listeriosis.
4. Neither amnionitis nor epistaxis is related to listeriosis.

TEST-TAKING HINT: Even though the disease in nonpregnant adults is relatively mild, if listeriosis is contracted during pregnancy, it can lead to serious fetal and neonatal complications. It is important for the nurse to provide the client with needed dietary education to prevent antepartal disease.

96. 1. If treated early, there likely will be no pregnancy or fetal damage noted.
2. If the mother is treated before delivery, the baby will not be born with congenital syphilis.
3. Usually a single shot of penicillin administered to the mother will cure her and protect the baby.
4. The woman is past the first trimester when the major organ systems are developed.

TEST-TAKING HINT: Clients are assessed for sexually transmitted infections during the pregnancy—usually at the first prenatal visit and shortly before the expected date of delivery. It is important to test all women, even those who have an apparently low probability of diseases, including married women and women from the upper socioeconomic strata. Infections, including those that are sexually transmitted, can be contracted by anyone.

97. 1. Domestic birds rarely carry serious disease.
2. The client should be advised to wear gloves when gardening.
3. All meat should be cooked until well done to prevent contracting toxoplasmosis and other meat-borne bacterial illnesses.
4. Dogs rarely carry serious disease.

TEST-TAKING HINT: Clients should be advised to wear gloves when gardening because cat feces can carry the toxoplasmosis protozoa. Feral and outdoor domestic cats are non-discriminating about where they urinate and defecate. They easily could be using the vegetable garden for a cat box. As such, it is also very important for everyone, and especially pregnant women, to wash fresh fruits and vegetables before eating them.

98. **1. Rubella is a teratogenic disease. The parents should notify any pregnant friends who may have been exposed.**
2. Rubella is a virus. Penicillin will not treat it.
3. Rubella is a relatively benign illness when contracted in childhood.
4. Rubella is not a pruritic illness. Diphenhydramine is not needed.

TEST-TAKING HINT: Of all of the communicable illnesses, rubella is the most potentially teratogenic. If mothers contract the disease during the first trimester, up to 50% of the fetuses will develop congenital defects. The incidence of disease does drop with each successive week, but older fetuses are still at high risk for injury. The most common defects from rubella are deafness, cataracts, and cardiovascular disease (CDC, n.d.-g).

99. 1. This answer is incorrect. Antibiotics for GBS are not given prenatally. They are administered during labor after hospital admission.
2. This answer is incorrect. Group B strep bacteria are normal flora for this client. She need not take her temperature.
3. This answer is correct. Exposure to group B strep is very dangerous for neonates.
4. This answer is incorrect. Group B strep does not cause scarlet fever. Group A strep causes scarlet fever and strep pharyngitis.

TEST-TAKING HINT: This question does not ask whether the information is true, but whether or not the response is *appropriate* for the client. However, if the test taker first identifies which statement/s are true and which one/s are false, it makes answering the question easier by eliminating almost all of the options.

Group B strep (GBS) can cause serious neonatal disease. Babies are at high risk for meningitis, sepsis, pneumonia, and even death. Intravenous antibiotics are administered to the laboring mother every 4 hours to decrease the colonization in the mother's vagina and rectum. In addition, the antibiotics cross the placenta and act as a prophylaxis for the baby if given at least 4 hours before birth.

100. 1. There is not a high incidence of chromosomal defects in babies born to teen mothers.
2. Teens do not have an inordinately high intake of manganese and zinc.

3. Teens are prone to having preterm deliveries rather than post-term deliveries.
4. **Teens are likely to delay entry into the healthcare system.**

TEST-TAKING HINT: Late entry into prenatal care is particularly problematic for teen pregnancies. Because organogenesis occurs during the first trimester, by the time many teens acknowledge that they are pregnant and seek care, they are already past this critical period. They are likely to have consumed damaging substances or, at the very least, consumed inadequate quantities of essential nutrients such as folic acid.

101. 1. The client's heart rate is important but it is not the most important vital sign.
2. The client's respiratory rate is important but it is not the most important vital sign.
3. **The client's blood pressure is the most important vital sign.**
4. The client's temperature is important but it is not the most important vital sign.

TEST-TAKING HINT: Adolescents who are 16 years old or younger are particularly at high risk for hypertensive illnesses of pregnancy. It is especially important for the nurse and the client's primary healthcare provider to determine the client's baseline blood pressure to identify any elevations as early as possible.

102. 1. Although eating burgers with fries is not the best choice for the young woman to make, it is not the most important comment for the nurse to respond to at this time.
2. This comment is informative because the nurse learns that this client has multiple sex partners. It is not the most important comment, however.
3. **The nurse must respond to this comment. This young woman is repeatedly exposing her fetus to alcohol.**
4. This comment is important because this young woman is not completing her education, but it is not the most important comment for the nurse to respond to at this time.

TEST-TAKING HINT: The nurse must prioritize care with all clients, focusing on the highest risks for the fetus. This young woman will eventually need to be counseled regarding diet, infection control, and her education, but the fetus is at highest risk at the present time from repeated alcohol exposure. Alcohol exposure is injurious for the unborn child throughout the entire pregnancy. The nurse must discuss this with the young woman at this time.

103. 1. The teen's partner may or may not be actively engaged in the pregnancy process. If he is interested in attending prenatal appointments, he should be welcomed. If not, the nurse should help the young woman to identify other important support people.
2. The pregnant teen has the same choices that the pregnant adult has. She can decide to terminate the pregnancy, maintain the pregnancy and make a plan for adoption, or maintain the pregnancy and retain custody of the child. It is not the nurse's choice to make, although the nurse should provide the young woman with all of her options.
3. **It is important for the young woman to work toward completing the tasks of adolescence at the same time that she is engaged in maintaining a healthy pregnancy. She should continue her education.**
4. Unless a genetic anomaly is in the young woman's medical history, it is unnecessary for the client to undergo single gene analysis. All women, no matter what age, can opt to have chromosomal studies performed.

TEST-TAKING HINT: Working with adolescents can be exciting as well as challenging. The nurse is likely to be the client's most important support system during the early weeks of the pregnancy. Slowly, with the nurse's help, it is hoped that the client will make healthy choices that include eating well, refraining from drinking alcohol and using drugs, and staying in school.

104. 1. **Adolescents are at high risk for preterm labor.**
2. Lifestyle issues and ethnicity are more important high-risk predictors of GDM than age.
3. Pregnant teens are at high risk for delivering babies who are small-for-gestational age rather than macrosomic babies.
4. Pregnant teens are at high risk for anemia rather than for polycythemia.

TEST-TAKING HINT: It is very important that pregnant teens learn the telltale signs of preterm labor, such as intermittent backache, cramping, and discomfort low in the pelvic area. Because of their lifestyle choices, pregnant teens are at high risk for low-birth-weight, preterm births.

105. 1. This is an inappropriate statement. The nurse should act as a counselor, not as a decision maker.

2. **This is an excellent response. The question opens the door for the teenager to discuss her feelings and thoughts.**
3. This is a true statement, but it is inappropriate to say to a young woman who is ambivalent about her pregnancy.
4. This is an inappropriate statement. The nurse should act as a counselor, not as a decision maker.

TEST-TAKING HINT: It is very important that nurses working in the obstetric area come to terms with their role and with their own beliefs and biases. One's personal belief system should not influence the nurse's teaching and counseling roles. The nurse must be truthful and unbiased when counseling any prenatal client, including the pregnant teen.

106. 1. Pregnant adolescents usually have an excellent protein intake, although they may or may not have an adequate magnesium intake.
2. **Pregnant adolescents' diets are often deficient in calcium and iron.**
3. Pregnant adolescents usually have an excellent carbohydrate intake and zinc intake.
4. Cereals and grains are enriched with the B vitamins, and most adolescents do eat these foods.

TEST-TAKING HINT: Adolescents are in need of higher levels of both calcium and iron during their pregnancies than are adult women. These nutrients are needed because many of the teens who become pregnant have not completed their own growth. Calcium is necessary not only for the teen's own bone growth but also for the bone growth of the fetus. Similarly, iron is needed for both the teen's and the baby's hematological function.

107. 1. Striae gravidarum, stretch marks, are a normal pregnancy finding.
2. **A client who is complaining of dyspnea on exertion is likely going into left-sided congestive heart failure.**
3. It is expected for a client in the third trimester to gain approximately 1 pound per week, or 4 pounds per month.
4. Patellar reflexes of +2 is a normal finding.

TEST-TAKING HINT: Pregnancy is a significant stressor on the cardiac system. Women who enter the pregnancy with a history of cardiac problems must be monitored very carefully not only by the obstetric provider but also by an internist or cardiologist. The nurse must be vigilant in observing for signs of cardiac failure, including respiratory and systemic congestion.

108. 1. Asking about vaginal or clitoral surgery is a possible follow-up question that may be asked, but it is not the most important question that the nurse should ask.
2. Asking about genital piercings is a possible follow-up question that may be asked, but it is not the most important question that the nurse should ask.
3. Asking about genital tattoo removal is a possible follow-up question that may be asked, but it is not the most important question that the nurse should ask.
4. **Asking about forced sexual activity is an essential question for the nurse to ask.**

TEST-TAKING HINT: The nurse should question all obstetric clients about a possible history of physical abuse and/or sexual abuse. Women are especially high risk for abusive injuries during pregnancy. Any client who exhibits trauma to the genital area, therefore, must be viewed as a possible victim of sexual abuse.

109. 1. Asking about the time of day when the woman's fatigue is most severe is not a priority action.
2. Recommending a pregnancy test is not a priority action.
3. **Continuing the interview of the woman in private is the priority action. The nurse should escort the client to a location where the partner cannot follow.**
4. Offering suggestions on ways to decrease the vomiting is not a priority action.

TEST-TAKING HINT: This couple is exhibiting classic signs of an abusive relationship. The woman is subjective, looking down and allowing her partner to respond to questions. The partner is dominant and demeaning in his description of his partner. To question the woman regarding her relationship, it is important for the nurse to interview the client in private. The women's bathroom is an excellent location for the interview. Domestic abuse can also happen in a lesbian relationship, and in this situation, a private conversation in the women's bathroom is not always possible. Regardless of the location, the suggestion for a private consultation must be made without raising suspicion on the part of the partner, if at all possible. For this reason, some clinics have a policy that they visit with all clients alone initially, then invite the partner to join the client for the obstetrical portion of the

exam. This information is given in print to clients at their first prenatal visit so no suspicions are raised.

110. **Answers 3 and 4 are correct.**
1. Genetic changes in the fetal reproductive system have not been associated with smoking during pregnancy.
2. Extensive central nervous system damage has not been associated with smoking during pregnancy.
3. **The word "addiction" does not apply to a fetus, since the fetus does not purposefully seek nicotine after birth. However, a fetus may be born *dependent* on nicotine and suffer withdrawal when the level of nicotine is reduced after birth.**
4. **Smoking in pregnancy does cause fetal intrauterine growth restriction.**

TEST-TAKING HINT: Smoking results in vasoconstrictive effects throughout the body. Vasoconstriction negatively affects the blood supply in the placental lake at the placental site. As a result, placentas of women who smoke are much smaller than those of nonsmoking women, and their fetuses receive less oxygen and nutrients via the placenta. This results in fetal growth restriction (IUGR). In addition, because fetuses become dependent on nicotine before birth, the babies of women who smoked during pregnancy suffer from nicotine withdrawal after birth, especially if the mother bottle feeds. Mothers who smoke are encouraged to breastfeed their babies. It is both comforting to the baby, and may also provide a low level of nicotine to the baby to assist in reducing some of the discomforts of withdrawal (March of Dimes, n.d.).

111.
1. Replacing a light fixture in the nursery should not adversely affect the pregnancy.
2. **Sanding the paint from an antique crib is a dangerous activity because antique cribs are often painted with lead-based paint.**
3. Planting tulip bulbs in the side garden should be a safe activity as long as the client wears gloves.
4. Shoveling snow from the driveway should be safe as long as the client does not become dyspneic.

TEST-TAKING HINT: It is very important that clients stay away from aerosolized lead that can develop when lead paint is being sanded. Lead can enter the body through the respiratory tract as well as through the gastrointestinal tract. Once it is ingested, the lead enters the vascular tree and is transported across the placenta to the unborn baby. The baby, especially the baby's central nervous system, can be adversely affected by the lead.

112.
1. **Progesterone is a hormone that relaxes smooth muscle. This action leads to the delayed emptying of the gallbladder during pregnancy.**
2. Although there is a genetic tendency for people of some ethnic groups to excrete large quantities of cholesterol, a contributing factor in gallbladder disease, there is not a direct genetic link to the problem.
3. Women are more likely to have gallbladder disease than men, and older women are more prone to the disease than younger women.
4. Gallbladder disease is related to high levels of cholesterol in the diet and in the bloodstream.

TEST-TAKING HINT: The hormones of pregnancy not only maintain the pregnancy but also affect all parts of the body. High estrogen levels can lead to nosebleeds and gingivitis, and high progesterone levels can lead to constipation and gallbladder disease.

113.
1. Pedal edema is not related to pseudocyesis.
2. **There will be no fetal heartbeat when a client has pseudocyesis.**
3. Polycythemia (hematocrit above 40%) is not related to pseudocyesis.
4. Clients who have pseudocyesis state that they do feel their babies move.

TEST-TAKING HINT: Pseudocyesis is a false pregnancy. Although rare, there are some women who develop pregnancy symptoms and believe themselves pregnant even though they are not actually pregnant. This is a psychiatric illness. The women may develop many of the presumptive signs of pregnancy but there will be few, if any, probable signs and no positive signs of pregnancy.

114.
1. Although women who have had gynecological cancer and who are unable to conceive may be at high risk, those with cancers in other systems are not at high risk of pseudocyesis.
2. Women with celiac disease are not at high risk for pseudocyesis.

3. **Women who have had a number of miscarriages are at high risk for pseudocyesis.**
4. Grand multiparas are not at high risk for pseudocyesis.

TEST-TAKING HINT: **The prefix "pseudo" means "false" and "cyesis" means "pregnancy." Women who develop pseudocyesis are women who have an overwhelming desire to become pregnant. Those who have had multiple miscarriages may be so desperate that they develop signs of pregnancy but are not really pregnant.**

115. Answers 2, 3, and 5 are correct.

1. It would be inappropriate to perform contraction stress tests, as these can lead to active labor.
2. **There should be blood available in the blood bank in case the woman begins to bleed.**
3. **The nurse would expect to keep the woman on bedrest with bathroom privileges only. Passive range-of-motion exercises will help to prevent atrophy of the woman's muscles.**
4. Although important to monitor, it would be unnecessary to assess the electrolytes daily. The client is able to eat a normal diet.
5. **The nurse would expect that weekly biophysical profiles would be done to assess fetal well-being.**

TEST-TAKING HINT: **Because clients with placenta previa are at high risk for bleeding from the placental site, it is essential that their activity be limited. Blood must be readily available in the laboratory for transfusion in case of hemorrhage. In addition, they must be monitored carefully for signs of fetal well-being. It would be inappropriate to stimulate contractions because dilation of the cervix would stimulate bleeding. With placenta previa, a cesarean section is necessary since the placenta is located over the cervix and must not be delivered before the baby. To deliver the placenta before delivering the baby would mean asphyxiating the fetus, as the oxygen source—the placenta—would be delivered first, effectively suffocating the fetus.**

116.

1. This answer indicates metabolic acidosis, as evidenced by PCO2 less than 60, and bicarb less than 22. The client does not have metabolic acidosis. This would be consistent with a diagnosis of diarrhea.
2. This answer indicates respiratory alkalosis. The client does not have respiratory alkalosis. This would be consistent with a diagnosis of hyperventilation.
3. This answer indicates respiratory acidosis. The client does not have respiratory acidosis. This would be consistent with a diagnosis of respiratory distress.
4. **This answer is correct. It is consistent with a client in metabolic alkalosis. This is consistent with a diagnosis of hyperemesis gravidarum.**

TEST-TAKING HINT: **If assessed methodically, the test taker should have little trouble determining the correct answer. The first action is to remember the basics of acid–base balance. Blood pH depends on the balance of acids and base (buffers); thus, "acid/base balance." The lungs and the kidneys are the two organs responsible for maintaining the pH of the blood. Lungs blow off acidic CO2 and kidneys excrete the alkaline HCO3 as needed. This keeps the acidity of the body within the normal range of 7.35 to 7.45.**

Begin your assessment of this question by determining the expected results. If a woman is vomiting repeatedly, one would expect her to have lost acid from the stomach. This upsets the acid–base balance, and all replacement acid must equal the acid that was lost. In an attempt at homeostasis, parietal cells in the stomach create and replace the hydrochloric acid (HCL) lost through vomiting. They do this by pulling acids—hydrogen (H) and chlorine (CL) ions—from the blood. The "payment" for the acid ingredients is bicarbonate ions. For each hydrogen (H) and chlorine (CL) ion the cells pull from the venous blood to replace the HCL that was vomited, they create and "exchange" one bicarbonate (base) ion, putting it into the blood in exchange (Heitzmann & Warth, 2007). The blood now has a higher level of bicarbonate (HCO3) than normal, leading to a higher pH. The location of the parietal cells, between the stomach and the veins gives them convenient access to both the stomach and the veins. One could think of this as a "front door" to the stomach and a "back door" to the veins (or pantry) that service the stomach.

Having determined that alkalosis is an expected finding, the test taker should then look at the pH and bicarb levels. The PO2 and CO2 levels are now distractors. The expectation is that the pH will be higher than the normal of 7.35 to 7.45, and the HCO3 will be higher than the normal of 22 to 26 mEq/L. (It will be the work of the kidneys to excrete the excess HCO3 and restore homeostasis.) Only answers 2 and 4 contain a pH reading higher than 7.45. Of these two, only answer #4 has an HCO3 reading higher than 26.

117. 1. The blood count is important but it is not highest priority.
2. Starting an intravenous infusion with multivitamins takes priority.
3. An admission weight is important but is not highest priority.
4. The urinalysis is important but is not highest priority.

TEST-TAKING HINT: Clients who are vomiting repeatedly are energy depleted, vitamin depleted, electrolyte depleted, and often dehydrated. It is essential that the client receive her IV therapy as quickly as possible. The other orders should be completed soon after the IV is started.

118. **1. The nurse would expect that the baby has dysplastic kidneys.**
2. The nurse would not expect to find that the baby has coarctation of the aorta.
3. The nurse would not expect to find that the baby has hydrocephalus.
4. The nurse would not expect to find that the baby has hepatic cirrhosis.

TEST-TAKING HINT: After 20 weeks' gestation, the majority of amniotic fluid is produced by the fetal kidneys. Oligohydramnios may be caused by a number of factors. One of those factors may be fetal. As such, when a pregnancy is complicated by oligohydramnios, ultrasounds may be performed to check for defects in the fetal renal system.

119. 1. The nurse would not expect to find that the baby has pulmonic stenosis.
2. The nurse would expect to find that the baby has tracheoesophageal fistula.
3. The nurse would not expect to find that the baby has ventriculoseptal defect.
4. The nurse would not expect to find that the baby has developmental hip dysplasia.

TEST-TAKING HINT: Babies swallow the amniotic fluid while in utero. When there is a surplus of fluid, ultrasounds may be performed to check for defects in the fetal gastrointestinal system. If the fetus cannot swallow the fluid due to a tracheoesophageal fistula, the fluid builds up within the uterus.

120. 1. A bicornuate uterus will not predispose a client to infection.
2. A bicornuate uterus will not predispose a client to palpitations.
3. A bicornuate uterus will predispose a client to cramping and preterm labor.
4. A bicornuate uterus will not predispose a client to oliguria.

TEST-TAKING HINT: If the nurse is unfamiliar with the term *bicornuate*, They could break down the word into its parts to determine its meaning: *bi* means "2" and *cornuate* means "horn." A bicornuate uterus, therefore, is a uterus that has a septum down the center, creating a 2-horned fundus. Sometimes the uterus is heart-shaped and sometimes the uterus is divided in half. Because of its shape, there is often less room for the fetus to grow. The uterus becomes irritable and predisposes the client to preterm labor. However, a pregnancy may still be carried to term.

121. 1. Clients who are third spacing are often pre-eclamptic. The blood pressure, therefore, may be elevated. This is not, however, the most important sign for the nurse to assess.
2. The faces and hands of clients who are third spacing often appear puffy. The appearance, however, is not the most important sign for the nurse to assess.
3. Weight is the most important sign for the nurse to assess.
4. The client's pulse rate may change, but it is not the most important sign for the nurse to assess.

TEST-TAKING HINT: When clients third space, they are retaining fluids. Fluid is very heavy. A sudden weight increase is, therefore, the most important assessment the nurse can make to determine whether or not a client is third spacing. Clients who are being assessed for pre-eclampsia, therefore, should be weighed daily. Although the appearance of the client may change, this is a subjective assessment. Weight is an objective assessment that can be trended more precisely.

122. 1. Because it is dangerous for tongue blades to be inserted into the mouths of seizing clients, the nurse should not place a tongue blade in the client's room.
2. The side rails and the headboard should be padded in case the client has another seizure.
3. The room of an eclamptic client should be quiet. Excess stimulation can precipitate a seizure.
4. There is no reason to provide grief counseling to this client.

TEST-TAKING HINT: When a client has been diagnosed with eclampsia, she has already had at least one seizure. Not until she is medically stabilized, should the baby be delivered. The nurse, therefore, must be prepared to care for the client during another seizure that may occur before treatment has started. The most

important action during the seizure is to protect the client from injury. Padding the side rails and headboard will provide that protection.

The best place for the fetus to recover from the hypoxia associated with an eclamptic seizure is within the uterus. The fetal heart rate will often show a prolonged deceleration during the maternal seizure, but generally recovers following maternal stabilization. This client's fetus is exhibiting normal heart rate variability with late decelerations reflecting the hypoxic episode during the uterine seizure contraction. Recommended treatment following eclampsia is delivery, but not until after the client and her fetus have been stabilized (Ross, 2019). Delivery may be by oxytocin induction or by cesarean section, depending on fetal and client status.

123. 1. Hyperemesis gravidarum (HG) is characterized by excessive vomiting during pregnancy. Hypertension is not a common symptom of HG.

2. Unless the pregnant client developed chronic hypertension during her pregnancy, hydatidiform mole is the most likely cause of her high blood pressure.

3. The hypertension seen in pre-eclamptic clients rarely appears before 20 weeks' gestation. This client is exhibiting signs much earlier in her pregnancy.

4. Although hypertensive clients are at high risk for gestational diabetes, this client was normotensive until her pregnancy. In addition, clients who do exhibit diabetic symptoms early in pregnancy are diagnosed with type 2 diabetes mellitus (T2DM), not gestational diabetes.

TEST-TAKING HINT: There is no viable fetus in a pregnancy complicated by hydatidiform mole. Rather, the trophoblastic layer, that is, the portion of the fertilized ovum that should become the fetal portion of the placenta, proliferates. The hyperproliferation of the placental tissue often results in the pregnant client developing pre-eclamptic symptoms during the first trimester.

124. Answers 3 and 4 are correct.

1. Throat swabs are taken for group A strep, not group B (GBS).
2. The nipple has nothing to do with GBS
3. **The vagina and rectum are cultured for group B strep.**
4. **The vagina and rectum are cultured for group B strep.**
5. The nostrils are not cultured for GBS.

TEST-TAKING HINT: Group B strep is a normal flora that comes and goes in many women, without symptoms. Cultures are taken at approximately 36 weeks' gestation because that gives a more accurate assessment of risk at the time of delivery. Cultures taken earlier can result in false-negative findings. The bacteria can lead to severe disease in neonates, including septicemia and meningitis.

Antibiotics are administered to affected women during labor and delivery to prevent transmission to the neonate. If infected, babies can die unless they're treated aggressively. The American College of Obstetrics & Gynecology (ACOG) recommends that IV antibiotics be administered to affected women every 4 hours throughout labor (ACOG, 2020a). Labor should not be delayed or extended in order to administer antibiotics, but fetuses whose mothers have received at least 2 doses have better outcomes than those who have fewer doses (ACOG, 2020a).

125. 1. Unless there is a neurological indication, electroencephalograms are not administered to pregnant women.

2. The nurse should request an order for an oral glucose tolerance test.

3. Biophysical profiles are performed during the third trimester to assess fetal well-being.

4. Lecithin/sphingomyelin ratios are performed late in the third trimester to assess fetal lung maturity.

TEST-TAKING HINT: Clients from a number of ethnic groups, for example, Latina, Native Americans, Asian Americans, and so forth, are at high risk for type 2 diabetes mellitus (T2DM). In addition, clients with obesity are at high risk for the disease. Instead of waiting until 24 weeks' gestation to have previously-healthy pregnant clients undergo oral glucose tolerance testing, it is recommended by the American Diabetes Association that women in high-risk groups be tested early in their pregnancies. Those with abnormal results will be diagnosed with T2DM rather than gestational diabetes. They can begin taking steps early, to protect their pancreases from being overworked, by reducing their carbohydrate intake and by exercising regularly.

126. Answers 1 and 2 are correct.

1. **Preterm labor is associated with placenta previa.**
2. **An intermittent backache could indicate that the client's previous contractions are getting stronger, a common sign of early labor that must be further investigated.**

3. A heating pad is *not* contraindicated for clients with placenta previa.
4. Persistent (not intermittent) backache can be a symptom of placental abruption.
5. A vaginal exam is contraindicated for clients with placenta previa.

TEST-TAKING HINT: This client has had 3 previous preterm deliveries. This puts her at high risk of having another preterm delivery with this pregnancy. In addition, placenta previa is associated with preterm delivery, giving this client another risk factor. Any suggestion of labor must be investigated and reported to the primary healthcare provider immediately, since she will need to have a cesarean section if labor cannot be delayed or stopped.

The American College of Obstetricians and Gynecologists (ACOG) recommends a single dose of steroids for clients between 24 0/7 and 33 6/7 weeks' gestation if they are expected to deliver within 7 days (ACOG, 2017c). Because this fetus is at just 33 weeks' gestation, a course of steroids for fetal lung maturity is recommended and must be started soon if she is going into labor. It is standard of care to administer magnesium sulfate to delay the onset of labor for 48 hours until the steroids have been administered, if possible, even with placenta previa (Morfaw et al., 2018).

In addition, magnesium sulfate can help with fetal neuroprotection. The literature provides evidence that magnesium sulfate infusions to women at less than 32 weeks' to 34 weeks' gestation who are at risk of imminent birth reduces the incidence of cerebral palsy in their babies (De Silva et al., 2018). This client is at 33 weeks' gestation, so she meets criteria for both antenatal steroids and magnesium sulfate for fetal neural protection.

127. Answers 1, 2, and 4 are correct

1. **If she is in early labor, the contractions will become stronger. Since this is her fifth pregnancy, her labor will likely go very fast, once it begins in earnest, and decisions for cesarean section will need to be made swiftly.**
2. **Uterine contractions can cause increased vaginal bleeding.**
3. Intrauterine fetal death can occur if the placenta is delivered vaginally before the fetus. There is nothing in the question to suggest that an imminent vaginal delivery is likely.
4. **A cesarean section is always necessary for a client with placenta previa, since the placenta is the fetal oxygen source and must not be delivered (and disconnected from the mother) before the baby is delivered.**

TEST-TAKING HINT: If possible, the nurse must determine whether or not it seems that the client is in labor, as decisions must be made quickly if the client needs a cesarean section. By staying one step ahead of what might happen, the nurse provides the best care for this client.

128. Answers 1(b), 2(a), 3(b), 4(a), 5(a), and 6(a) are correct.

Potential Order	(a) Anticipated	(b) Nonessential
1. IV antibiotics.		X
2. Administer acetaminophen.	X	
3. Preparation for surgery.		X
4. Administer magnesium sulfate.	X	
5. Corticosteroids.	X	
6. Continuous fetal monitoring.	X	

1(b) **IV antibiotics are nonessential at this point because no decision has been made for a cesarean section. IV antibiotics are generally given within an hour of the cesarean section.**

2(a) **Acetaminophen is not contraindicated at this time, even if the client eventually needs a cesarean section, as clotting times are unaffected by this medication, should she eventually need surgery.**

3(b) **There is nothing in the question to suggest the client must be prepared for surgery. She has a backache and headache at this point.**

4(a) **The nurse may anticipate an order for magnesium sulfate for the reasons listed in the TEST-TAKING HINT for the previous question such as reduction of contractions, promotion of fetal lung maturity, and fetal neural protection.**

5(a) **The nurse may anticipate an order for steroids to accelerate fetal lung maturity.**

6(a) **Continuous fetal monitoring can be initiated without a provider's order Often the provider will order it anyway, so that nothing is overlooked. It is vital**

for assessing the FHR and contraction pattern. If the contractions are more regular, it could more strongly support the possibility of preterm labor. If the nurse has already placed the electronic fetal monitor, a report of the findings can be shared with the provider during the phone call.

TEST-TAKING HINT: This is a client who is pregnant with her 5th baby. She has had 3 preterm births previously, and has a placenta previa, two risk factors for another preterm delivery. The case study indicates the provider was notified previously of the client's irregular contractions, and a plan was made to consider an infusion of magnesium sulfate. However, no order was given to begin the infusion at that time. The additional information of an intermittent backache suggests these contractions are getting stronger. Because the client is at 33 weeks' gestation, steroids to support fetal lung maturation are an appropriate plan, and magnesium sulfate to delay contractions and cervical dilation until the doses have been administered, is prudent. Until the provider determines that the client is in active labor, or that the early labor contractions cannot be stopped and a cesarean section is necessary, orders for preoperative antibiotics and preparation for surgery are not anticipated.

129. 1. There is nothing in the question to indicate the client is anxious
2. **The primary goal at this time is to determine whether or not the client is in labor.**
3. There is nothing in the question to indicate the client is at risk of hemorrhaging at this time. There is no mention of increased or heavy bleeding. She may or may not be in labor, as that has not yet been determined.
4. **An ongoing goal of nursing in the antepartum unit is to maintain fetal well-being.**

TEST-TAKING HINT: The case study indicates that the client has back pain, which the nurse knows may indicate the start of labor, and that the fetal monitor tracing indicates fetal well being. The other answer options are not stated as issues in the case study. The client has not said she is anxious, and she is not bleeding. The test taker must take care to respond only to the information in the question stem, and not to answers that indicate general standard of care.

130. Answers 2, 3, and 4 are correct.
1. Although the client has requested medication for her backache, and reduction in pain is a valid nursing care goal, this medication does not treat a condition related to survivability. It can be completed after the other medications have been administered.
2. **Steroids can improve the fetal survival rate and reduce morbidity if the client is in labor. For the fetus, this improves survival, the first step on Maslow's hierarchy of needs, and as such it should be a priority.**
3. **Magnesium sulfate is important to administer in order to reduce contractility of the uterus and to provide fetal neuroprotection if the client does deliver. Once again, this relates to fetal survivability and reduction of morbidity.**
4. **It is important to assist the client in returning to bed and to place the electronic fetal monitor to assess contraction frequency and fetal well-being.**
5. The client's vital signs are important, but they are not one of the three most important assessments at this time since there is no suggestion that the client's vital signs are abnormal.
6. The heating pad can wait until the other orders have been completed.

TEST-TAKING HINT: The test taker is limited to 3 actions in the response. Choosing responses that connect directly to maternal or fetal survival is a prudent approach to answering test questions.

131. The correct answers are 1(b), 2(c), 3(b), 4(b), and 5(a).

Assessment Findings	(a) Improved	(b) No change	(c) Declined
1. Fetal heart rate 150 with moderate variability.		X	
2. Contractions every 10 minutes, lasting 30–45 seconds.			X
3. Contractions are mild on palpation.		X	
4. The client reports dark blood on her pad.		X	
5. Back pain 3/10	X		

1(b) The FHR assessment is unchanged. It is still reassuring.
2(c) The contraction pattern has become regular, which would indicate a declining status in that the client might be in early, preterm labor.
3(b) The finding of continued *mild* contractions versus *moderate* or *strong*, indicates there could still be some time before active labor begins. Mild contractions on palpation were a previous finding, so this is unchanged.
4(b) The report of dark blood is not a change. More frequent bleeding episodes, or heavier bleeding would indicate a less stable condition.
5(a) The client's back pain was previously 5/10, so a reduction to 3/10 is an improvement.

TEST-TAKING HINT: Placenta previa is a condition where the placental implantation covers the cervix. Bleeding is painless. When the cervix is closed, and only occasional spotting occurs, the fetus is not in immediate danger. As the cervix dilates, however, less of the placenta is attached to its uterine source of oxygen, bleeding becomes more profuse, and fetal safety is jeopardized. Delivery by cesarean section is always required for placenta previa. This client is having regular contractions, which is a change from her previous condition. In addition, the episode of dark blood indicates the uterine contractions have caused bleeding from the placental attachment site. The finding of dark blood suggests it is not acute, but "old blood." The FHR is stable, which is reassuring. It is possible the uterus will respond to magnesium sulfate once it has reached a therapeutic level and will slow down the contractions long enough to allow for steroids to improve fetal lung maturity. The provider will likely use a sterile speculum to do a cervical exam and assess for dilation and effacement as part of the client assessment.

132. 1. Although placenta previa is an obstetric complication, the hemoglobin is within normal limits. There is nothing in the question to indicate she is actively bleeding.
2. Although a client with T2DM has a high-risk condition, the blood glucose is within normal limits.
3. A placental abruption is a life-threatening situation for the fetus and possibly for the mother. It has been 15 minutes since the client was assessed. Although the FHR was within the normal range 15 minutes ago, this is the nurse's priority because the condition can deteriorate rapidly.
4. A client who is Rh-negative (Rh–) may or may not be carrying a baby who is Rh-positive (Rh+). Either way, a hematocrit of 31%, although low, is not an emergent value.

TEST-TAKING HINT: In this question, the test taker must discriminate among four situations to discern which is the highest priority. There is nothing in the stem to indicate the client with placenta previa is actively bleeding. The client with T2DM has a fasting blood glucose within normal limits. A client who has a placental abruption, however, is already in a life-threatening situation, both for her fetus and for herself. Although her abruption is considered "partial," it may be unstable. The nurse must assess the fundal tone and bleeding, and there is no report on the status of those assessments during the previous shift. The Rh negative (Rh–) client who had a cerclage yesterday is the least urgent client. She will likely be discharged home today.

133. 1. As a result of placental bleeding, the fetus can suffer significant blood loss that results in anemia, demonstrated by a sinusoidal fetal heart-rate pattern.
2. Pain-free vaginal bleeding is consistent with a diagnosis of placenta previa, not placental abruption. In addition, a client with a placental abruption might not always present with vaginal bleeding if the blood is trapped within the uterus.
3. Accelerations are a reassuring sign of a fetus with adequate oxygenation, which is not likely with placental abruptions.
4. A placental abruption is not an infectious state. The nurse would not expect to see hyperthermia.

TEST-TAKING HINT: The nurse must distinguish the differences in fetal risk and client symptomatology in placental abruption and placenta previa. If this question is read quickly, it's possible the test taker could confuse the two conditions and answer incorrectly. In a placental abruption, bleeding occurs within the uterus, on the maternal side of the placenta, as maternal vessels pull away from the placenta. As a result, a pool of blood grows between the placenta and the uterus, acting as a wedge to lift more and more of the placenta from the nourishing uterine wall. The percentage of placenta still "working" to oxygenate the fetus is reduced. Only a portion

of the placenta continues to actively exchange carbon dioxide from the baby for oxygen from the mother. Profuse maternal bleeding puts the mother's life at risk; hypoxia threatens the fetus.

134. 1. Polyhydramnios is not a risk factor for placental abruption.
2. Flu is not a risk factor for placental abruption.
3. Cancer survivors are not at risk for placental abruption.
4. Cocaine is a powerful vasoconstrictive agent. Its use at any time during pregnancy places pregnant clients at high risk for placental abruptions regardless of gestational age.

TEST-TAKING HINT: It is very important that the test taker not read into any question or response. In the preceding question, all four of the clients are in the hospital with preterm conditions. The test taker should not presume the cause of the complications when they are not stated but rather look for the answer that does absolutely place the client at high risk for the abruption.

135. 1. An order for oxytocin administration should be questioned.
2. The fetal heart rate should be assessed regularly.
3. Weighing the vaginal pads is appropriate at this time to measure bleeding.
4. Assessing the hemoglobin and hematocrit is appropriate at this time.

TEST-TAKING HINT: A placenta previa may be one of three types: (a) complete previa, where the placenta covers the entire cervical opening; (b) partial previa, where the placenta covers part of the cervical opening; or (c) marginal previa, where the placenta borders the cervix. Because the stem states that this client has symptomatic placenta previa, the test taker can conclude that the client is actively bleeding into the vagina. It would be appropriate to monitor the fetal heart rate for any signs of hypoxia, to weigh pads to determine the amount of blood loss, and to assess the hematocrit and hemoglobin to check for anemia. The nurse should question the order for oxytocin administration since the type of previa is unknown. Labor and a vaginal birth might be an option with marginal previas. However, the nurse must confirm the type of previa the client has before starting oxytocin. Generally, a client with placenta previa requires a caesarean section to deliver the baby safely.

136. 20 mL of blood

TEST-TAKING HINT: One mL of fluid weighs approximately 1 gram. The nurse can estimate, therefore, that the blood loss is:

$$24 - 4 = 20 \text{ mL of blood}$$

137. 1. Leopold's maneuvers assess for fetal positioning in utero. Placental placement cannot be assessed externally.
2. Although women can have completely concealed bleeding with an abruption, the quantity of blood loss will not differentiate between the two pathologies.
3. The most common difference between placenta previa and placenta abruption is the absence or presence of abdominal pain.
4. Maternal blood pressure is inconclusive. Women with chronic hypertension are at high risk for both problems.

TEST-TAKING HINT: Because at least some of the blood from a placental abruption is trapped behind the placenta, women with that complication usually complain of intense, unrelenting pain. In contrast, the blood from a symptomatic placenta previa flows freely through the vagina, meaning the bleeding from that complication is virtually pain free.

138. 1. Because the client will have a cesarean section with anesthesia, the client should be taught coughing and deep-breathing exercises for the postoperative period.
2. Because the client will not be going through labor, it is inappropriate to teach her about the phases of the first stage of labor.
3. Because the client will not be going through labor, it is inappropriate to teach her about Lamaze breathing techniques.
4. Because the client will not be going through labor, it is inappropriate to teach her about Leboyer hydro-birthing.

TEST-TAKING HINT: When a client has a complete placenta previa, the placenta fully covers the internal part of the cervix. If the client were to go through labor, the placenta would be forced to separate from the uterus and be delivered first, essentially cutting off life support for the fetus. The client would bleed profusely and the baby would exsanguinate and die. The only safe way to deliver the baby, therefore, is via cesarean section.

9 High-Risk Intrapartum

Although giving birth is a natural event that can be expected to progress safely and efficiently on its own without medical interventions, a number of obstetrical emergencies and medical problems do occur occasionally. These can adversely impact both the mother and the fetus during labor and delivery. As labor progresses, the risk increases.

Prenatal problems that can negatively impact labor and delivery include hypertensive illnesses, diabetes mellitus, and placental dysfunction. During labor and delivery itself, areas of risk include induction of labor, operative deliveries that include forceps and vacuum extractors, and dystocias. All of these are potentially harmful to both mother and baby. In addition, labors that begin prematurely or postmaturely can negatively impact fetal well-being.

Nurses who provide quality care are familiar with the monitoring required to identify potential and acute complications and are able to provide appropriate interventions that include timeliness in provider notification. The nurse is often the sole caregiver during labor, working in tandem with the primary healthcare provider through clinical judgment and communication. By being aware of risk factors and intervening appropriately, the nurse fosters trust from the provider and from the clients. That attitude of trust supports a sense of safety and positive outcomes in spite of the risks.

KEYWORDS

The following words include English vocabulary, nursing/medical terminology, concepts, principles, or information relevant to content specifically addressed in the chapter or associated with topics presented in it. English dictionaries, your nursing textbooks, and medical dictionaries such as *Taber's Cyclopedic Medical Dictionary* are resources that can be used to expand your knowledge and understanding of these words and related information.

Abruptio placentae (placental abruption)
Acidemia
Acidosis
Amniotic fluid embolism (AFE)
Anaphylactoid syndrome of pregnancy (ASP)
Betamethasone
Biophysical profile
Bishop score
Calcium gluconate
Cesarean section
Cord compression
Dexamethasone
Dinoprostone
Disseminated intravascular coagulation (DIC)
Eclampsia
External version
Fetal fibronectin (fFN)
Fetal heart decelerations—early, variable, late, prolonged
Forceps
General anesthesia
Grief and mourning
Group B streptococcus
Head compression
HELLP syndrome
Hepatitis B
Herpes simplex type 2
HIV/AIDS
Hyperstimulation
Hypertensive illnesses of pregnancy
Hypoxemia
Hypoxia
Induction
Magnesium sulfate
McRoberts maneuver
Misoprostol
Multigravida
Multipara
Naloxone
Nifedipine

Oxytocin
Placenta previa
Post-term labor
Pre-eclampsia
Preterm labor
Primigravida
Primipara
Prolapsed cord
Prostaglandins
Regional anesthesia (epidural and spinal)
Shoulder dystocia (turtle sign)
Tachysystole
Tetanic contraction
Terbutaline
Tocolytic
Trial of labor after cesarean section (TOLAC)
Uterine rupture
Uteroplacental insufficiency
Vacuum extraction
Vaginal birth after cesarean section (VBAC)

QUESTIONS

CASE STUDY: *The first six questions below are part of an evolving case study. All six questions follow the Next Generation NCLEX© question format of six steps:*

1. Recognize cues—What matters most?
2. Analyze cues—What could it mean?
3. Prioritize hypotheses—Where do I start?
4. Generate solutions—What can I do?
5. Take action—What will I do?
6. Evaluate outcomes—Did it help?

(National Council of State Boards of Nursing [NCSBN], 2020). For more information on the Next Generation NCLEX (NGN) question formats, see NGN quarterly newsletters at https://www.ncsbn.org.
NCLEX questions assume the nurse has a provider's order for listed interventions, unless noted otherwise.

1200: The nurse is caring for a client with an obstetrical history of G2 P1001. The client is at 41 weeks' gestation and was admitted for a labor induction with oxytocin 4 hours ago. The oxytocin was started at 2 milliunits per minute (mu/min) by pump. At that time, the nurse documented the following: cervical exam 4 cm, 75% effaced, –3 station with an intact bag of waters. Vital signs: T 100° F (37.7° C), P 82, R 20, BP 130/80. FHR 120 bpm with moderate variability. The client was examined 2 hours ago and has requested an epidural for pain. As the nurse prepares to perform another vaginal exam, the client says, "I think my water just broke."

1. **Recognize cues.** What matters most?
   Highlight the assessment findings that require immediate follow-up.
   1. Contractions every 2 minutes, lasting 60 to 80 seconds each.
   2. Spontaneous rupture of membranes.
   3. T 100.4° F (38° C).
   4. FHR 110 bpm with moderate variability.

2. **Analyze cues.** What could it mean?
Which of the following is most likely occurring, based on the information given?
1. Active labor.
2. Fetal intolerance of labor.
3. Cephalopelvic disproportion (CPD).
4. Fetal engagement.

3. **Prioritize hypotheses.** Where do I start?
Which nursing action is indicated, nonessential or contraindicated?

Nursing Action	(a) Indicated	(b) Nonessential	(c) Contraindicated
1. Vaginal Exam			
2. Maternal position change			
3. Oxygen administration by nonrebreather mask			
4. Intrauterine pressure catheter (IUPC) insertion			
5. Discontinue oxytocin			

4. **Generate solutions.** What can I do?
1400: The nurse has completed a vaginal examination. The following has been documented: cervical dilation 5 cm, 100% effaced, zero station. The client has requested an epidural and the nurse has assisted the client to the bathroom in preparation for her epidural. What are the next two priorities the nurse should address first and second?

(a) First Address:	(b) Followed by:
1. Light meconium staining of membranes	1. Light meconium staining of membranes
2. Fetal heart rate	2. Fetal heart rate
3. Maternal temperature of 100.4° F	3. Maternal temperature of 100.4° F
4. IV bolus for epidural	4. IV bolus for epidural
5. Maternal vital sign assessments	5. Maternal vital sign assessments

5. **Take action.** What will I do?
1600: The client received her epidural and is resting comfortably. The oxytocin has been increased incrementally and is now at a rate of 10 milliunits per minute. Contractions are occurring every 5 minutes, lasting 60 to 80 seconds. FHR is 120 bpm, with moderate variability. Mark an X in the box to indicate the appropriate interventions the nurse should take now, to support a successful labor and delivery of a healthy newborn for this client based on the information given. **Select all that apply.**

Nursing Interventions	Place an X in the box to indicate appropriate interventions
1. Lateral maternal positioning	
2. Increase oxytocin rate	
3. Administration of IV antibiotics	
4. Indwelling catheter insertion	
5. Oxygen administration by nonrebreather mask	
6. Apple juice intake	

6. **Evaluate outcomes.** Did it help?
1830: The nurse is completing another client assessment of labor progress. The nurse's assessment reveals the client is 6 cm, +1 station, and 100% effaced. Contractions are every 5 minutes, lasting 60 seconds. She was just catheterized for 300 mL. The FHR is 150 bpm with moderate variability, and maternal vital signs are T 100.4° F (38° C), P 88, RR 18, BP 138/76.

Place an X in the appropriate box below to indicate whether these findings indicate the nursing interventions were effective, ineffective, or unrelated to the client findings.

Nursing Action	(a) Effective	(b) Ineffective	(c) Likely Unrelated
1. Maternal position changes			
2. Oxytocin rate increase			
3. Apple juice intake			
4. Catheterization			

7. A client has been diagnosed with water intoxication after having received IV oxytocin for over 24 hours. Which of the following signs/symptoms would the nurse expect to see?
   1. Confusion, drowsiness, and vomiting.
   2. Hypernatremia and hyperkalemia.
   3. Thrombocytopenia and neutropenia.
   4. Paresthesias, myalgias, and anemia.

8. The primary healthcare provider has ordered oxytocin for induction for 4 clients. In which of the following situations should the nurse refuse to comply with the order?
   1. Primigravida with a transverse lie.
   2. Multigravida with cerebral palsy.
   3. Primigravida who is 14 years old.
   4. Multigravida who has type 1 diabetes mellitus (T1DM).

9. A client at 38 weeks' gestation with hypertension and oligohydramnios is being induced with IV oxytocin. She is contracting q 3 min × 60 to 90 seconds. She suddenly complains of abdominal pain. The nurse notices significant fetal heart rate bradycardia. Which of the following interventions should the nurse perform first?
   1. Turn off the oxytocin infusion.
   2. Administer oxygen via face mask.
   3. Reposition the patient.
   4. Call the obstetrician.

10. An oxytocin induction of a client at 42 weeks' gestation is started at 0900 at a rate of 2 milliunits per minute. The client's primary physician orders an increase of the oxytocin drip by 0.5 milliunits per minute every 10 minutes until contractions are every 3 minutes × 60 seconds. The nurse refuses to comply with the order. Which of the following is the rationale for the nurse's action?
    1. Fetal intolerance of labor has been noted when oxytocin dosages greater than 2 milliunits per minute are administered.
    2. The relatively long half-life of oxytocin can result in unsafe intravascular concentrations of the drug as ordered.
    3. It is unsafe practice to administer oxytocin intravenously to a client who is carrying a postdates fetus.
    4. A contraction duration of 60 seconds can lead to fetal compromise in a baby that is postmature.

11. A client at 40 weeks' gestation has received misoprostol for cervical ripening. The nurse would be correct in carefully monitoring for which of the following signs and symptoms?
1. Diarrhea and back pain.
2. Hypothermia and rectal pressure.
3. Urinary retention and rash.
4. Tinnitus and respiratory distress.

12. A client with an obstetrical history of G3 P1010, is receiving oxytocin via IV pump at 3 milliunits/min. Her current contraction pattern is every 3 minutes × 45 seconds with moderate intensity. The fetal heart rate is 150 to 160 bpm with moderate variability. Which of the following interventions should the nurse take at this time?
1. Stop the infusion.
2. Give oxygen via face mask.
3. Change the client's position.
4. Monitor the client's labor client.

13. A client at 40 $^{2}/_{7}$ weeks' gestation has had ruptured membranes for 15 hours with no labor contractions. Her obstetrician has ordered 10 units oxytocin to be diluted in 1,000 mL Ringer's lactate. The order reads: *Administer oxytocin IV for induction per protocol.* The protocol indicates the oxytocin is to be started at 0.5 milliunits per min. Calculate the drip rate for the infusion pump to be programmed. How many mL/hr would the pump be programmed to infuse? **Please calculate to the nearest whole number.**

_________ mL/hr

14. The nurse notes a pattern of tachysystole during a client's oxytocin induction. The nurse turns off the oxytocin infusion. Which of the following outcomes indicates that the nurse's action was effective?
1. Contraction intensity moderate.
2. Contraction frequency every 3 minutes.
3. Fetal heart rate 140 bpm4.
4. Fetal attitude flexed.

15. A nurse is monitoring the labor of a client who is receiving IV oxytocin at 10 milliunits per minute.Which of the following clinical signs would lead the nurse to stop the infusion?
1. Change in maternal pulse rate from 76 to 98 bpm.
2. Change in fetal heart rate from 128 to 102 bpm.
3. Maternal blood pressure of 150/100.
4. Maternal temperature of 102.4° F (39.1° C).

16. A client with an obstetrical history of G1 P0000 received dinoprostone for cervical ripening 8 hours ago. The Bishop score at that time was 4. The Bishop score is now 10. Which of the following actions by the nurse is appropriate?
1. Perform nitrazine analysis of amniotic fluid.
2. Report abnormal findings to the obstetrician.
3. Place client on her side.
4. Monitor for onset of labor.

17. The physician has ordered dinoprostone for four clients at term. The nurse should question the order for which of the women?
1. Primigravida with Bishop score of 4.
2. Multigravida with late decelerations.
3. Primigravida with fetal heart rate of 155 and Bishop score of 4.
4. G6 P3202 with blood pressure 140/90 and pulse 92.

18. A client with an obstetrical history of G4 P1021, has been admitted to the labor and delivery suite for induction of labor. The following assessments have been made: Bishop score of 2, fetal heart rate of 150 with moderate variability and no decelerations, T98.6° F (37° C), P 88, R 20, BP 120/80, negative obstetric history. Dinoprostone has been inserted. Which of the following findings would warrant the removal of the prostaglandin?
1. Bishop score of 4.
2. Fetal heart rate of 155
3. Respiratory rate of 24.
4. Contraction frequency of 1 minute.

19. There are four clients in active labor in the labor suite. Which of the clients should the nurse monitor carefully for a potential uterine rupture?
1. Age 15, G3 P0020, in active labor.
2. Age 22, G1 P0000, eclampsia.
3. Age 25, G4 P3003, last delivery by cesarean section.
4. Age 32, G2 P0100, first baby died during labor.

20. A client is admitted in labor with spontaneous rupture of membranes 24 hours earlier. The fluid is clear and the fetal heart rate is 120 bpm with moderate variability. Which assessment is most important for the nurse to make at this time?
1. Contraction frequency and duration.
2. Maternal temperature.
3. Cervical dilation and effacement.
4. Maternal pulse rate.

21. A client at 39 weeks' gestation with a fetal heart rate baseline at 145 bpm, tells the admitting labor and delivery room nurse that she has had to wear a pad for the past 4 days "because I keep leaking urine." Which of the following is an appropriate action for the nurse to perform at this time?
1. Palpate the client's bladder to check for urinary retention.
2. Obtain a urine culture to check for a urinary tract infection.
3. Assess the fluid with nitrazine and see if the paper turns blue.
4. Percuss the client's uterus and monitor for ballottement.

22. The nurse notes that the fetus of a laboring client is exhibiting signs of fetal intolerance of labor. Which of the following actions should the nurse take?
1. Administer oxygen via nasal cannula.
2. Place the client in high Fowler's position.
3. Remove the internal fetal monitor electrode.
4. Increase the intravenous infusion rate.

23. Four women request to labor in the hospital bathtub with waterproof fetal heart rate (FHR) monitoring devices. In which of the following situations is this contraindicated? **Select all that apply.**
1. Client during transition.
2. Client during second stage of labor.
3. Client receiving oxytocin for induction.
4. Client with meconium-stained fluid.
5. Client with a temperature of 100.4° F (38° C).

24. A full-term client, contracting every 15 min × 30 sec, has had ruptured membranes for 20 hours. Which of the following nursing interventions is contraindicated or considered high risk at this time?
1. Intermittent fetal heart auscultation.
2. Vaginal examination.
3. Intravenous fluid administration.
4. Nipple stimulation.

25. A client at 39 weeks' gestation is admitted to the labor and delivery unit with vaginal warts from human papillomavirus. Which of the following actions by the nurse is appropriate?
1. Notify the healthcare practitioner for a surgical delivery.
2. Follow standard infectious disease precautions.
3. Notify the nursery of the imminent delivery of an infected neonate.
4. Wear a mask whenever the perineum is exposed.

26. A client telephones the labor and delivery suite and states, "My bag of waters just broke and it smells funny." Which of the following responses would be essential for the nurse to make at this time?
1. "Have you notified your doctor of the smell?"
2. "The bag of waters always has an unusual odor."
3. "Your labor should start very soon."
4. "Have you felt the baby move since your water broke?"

27. A client at 40 weeks' gestation with an obstetrical history of G3 P2002 has just been admitted in early labor. She has vaginal candidiasis. Which of the following should the nurse advise the client about?
1. She may need a cesarean delivery.
2. She will be treated with antibiotics during labor.
3. The baby may develop thrush after delivery.
4. The baby will be isolated for at least one day.

28. A client who is hepatitis B surface antigen positive is in active labor. Which action by the nurse is appropriate at this time?
1. Obtain an order from the obstetrician to prepare the client for cesarean delivery.
2. Obtain an order from the obstetrician to administer intravenous penicillin during labor and the immediate postpartum.
3. Obtain an order from the pediatrician to administer hepatitis B immune globulin and hepatitis B vaccine to the baby after birth.
4. Obtain an order from the pediatrician to place the baby in isolation after delivery.

29. A client with an obstetrical history of G2 P1001 has just entered the labor and delivery suite with ruptured membranes for 2 hours, fetal heart rate of 145 bpm with moderate variability, contractions every 5 minutes $\times$ 60 seconds, and a history of herpes simplex type 2. She has no observable lesions. After notifying the doctor of the admission, which of the following is the appropriate action for the nurse to take?
1. Check dilation and effacement.
2. Prepare the client for surgery.
3. Place the bed in Trendelenburg position.
4. Check the biophysical profile results.

30. Immediately prior to an amniotomy, the external fetal heart monitor tracing shows 145 bpm with moderate variability and early decelerations. Immediately following the procedure, the tracing shows a fetal heart rate of 120 with a prolonged deceleration. A moderate amount of clear, amniotic fluid is seen on the bed linens. The nurse concludes that which of the following has occurred?
1. Placental abruption.
2. Eclampsia.
3. Prolapsed cord.
4. Succenturiate placenta.

31. Immediately after a client's membranes rupture spontaneously, the nurse notes a loop of the umbilical cord protruding from the client's vagina. Which of the following actions are essential for the nurse to perform? **Select all that apply.**
1. Put the client in the knee-chest, or Trendelenburg position.
2. Assess the fetal heart rate by palpating the cord.
3. Administer oxygen by tight face mask.
4. Telephone the primary healthcare provider with the findings.

32. A client's membranes ruptured spontaneously while the nurse was at the bedside. Which of the following factors makes her especially at high risk for having a prolapsed cord? **Select all that apply.**
1. Breech presentation.
2. Vertex presentation at –3 station.
3. Oligohydramnios.
4. Dilation 2 cm.
5. Transverse lie.

33. A nurse is triaging four clients on the labor and delivery unit. Which of the following actions should be a priority for nursing care?
1. Check the blood sugar of a gestational diabetic.
2. Assess the vaginal blood loss of a client who is recovering from a spontaneous abortion.
3. Assess the patellar reflexes of a client with pre-eclampsia without severe features.
4. Check the fetal heart rate of a client whose membranes just ruptured.

34. A delirious client is admitted to the hospital in labor. She has had no prenatal care and vials of crack cocaine are found in her pockets. The nurse monitors this client carefully for which of the following intrapartum complications?
1. Prolonged labor.
2. Prolapsed cord.
3. Abruptio placentae.
4. Retained placenta.

35. A client with a current history of illicit drug use is in active labor. She requests pain medication. Which of the following actions by the nurse is appropriate?
1. Encourage the client to refrain from taking medication to protect the fetus.
2. Notify the primary healthcare provider of her request.
3. Advise the client that she can receive only an epidural because of her history.
4. Assist the client to do labor breathing.

36. The nurse is caring for a laboring woman who is 42 weeks pregnant. For which of the following should the nurse carefully monitor this client and fetus?
1. Late decelerations.
2. Hyperthermia.
3. Hypotension.
4. Early decelerations.

37. A client with an obstetrical history of G3 P2002 is 6 cm dilated. The fetal monitor tracing shows recurrent late decelerations. The client's doctor informs her that the baby must be delivered by cesarean section. The client refuses to sign the informed consent. Which of the following actions by the nurse is appropriate?
1. Strongly encourage the client to sign the informed consent.
2. Prepare the client for the cesarean section.
3. Inform the client that the baby will likely die without the surgery.
4. Provide the client with ongoing labor support.

38. Given the fetal heart rate pattern shown below, which of the following interventions should the nurse perform first?

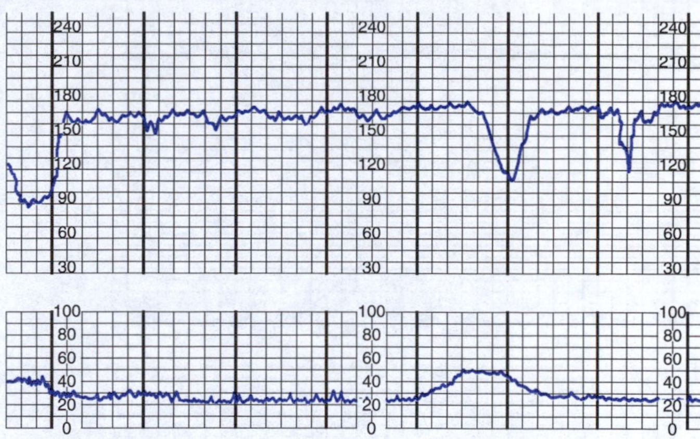

1. Increase the intravenous drip rate.
2. Apply oxygen by face mask.
3. Turn the client to her side.
4. Report the tracing to the obstetrician.

39. Which of the tracings shown below would the nurse interpret as indicative of uteroplacental insufficiency?

1. 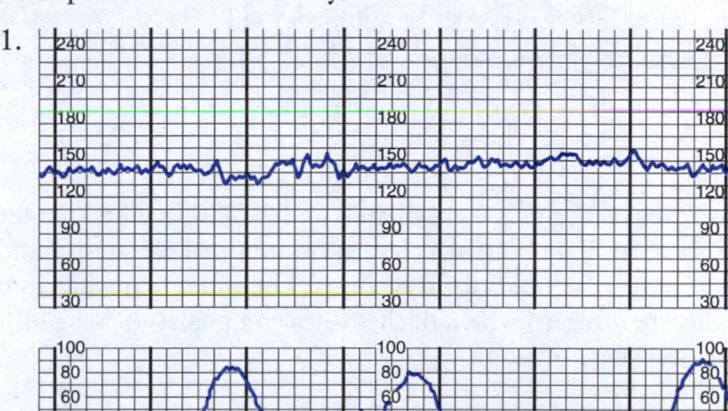

2. 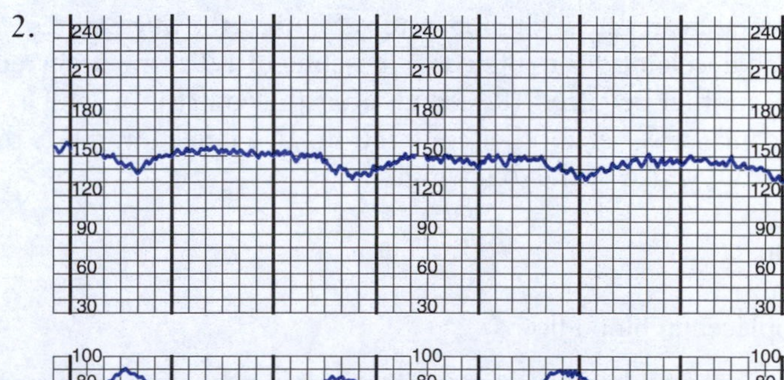

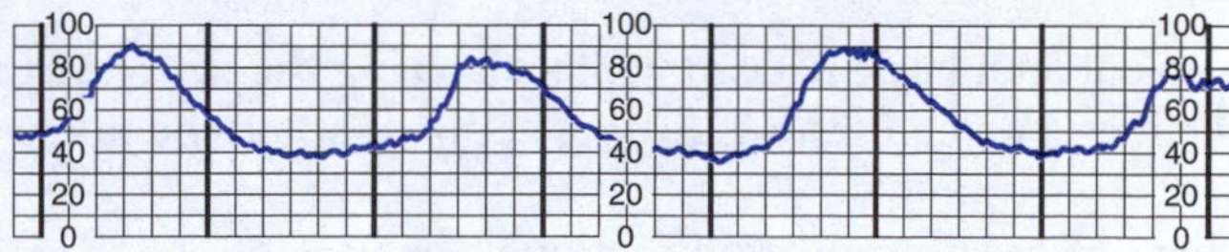

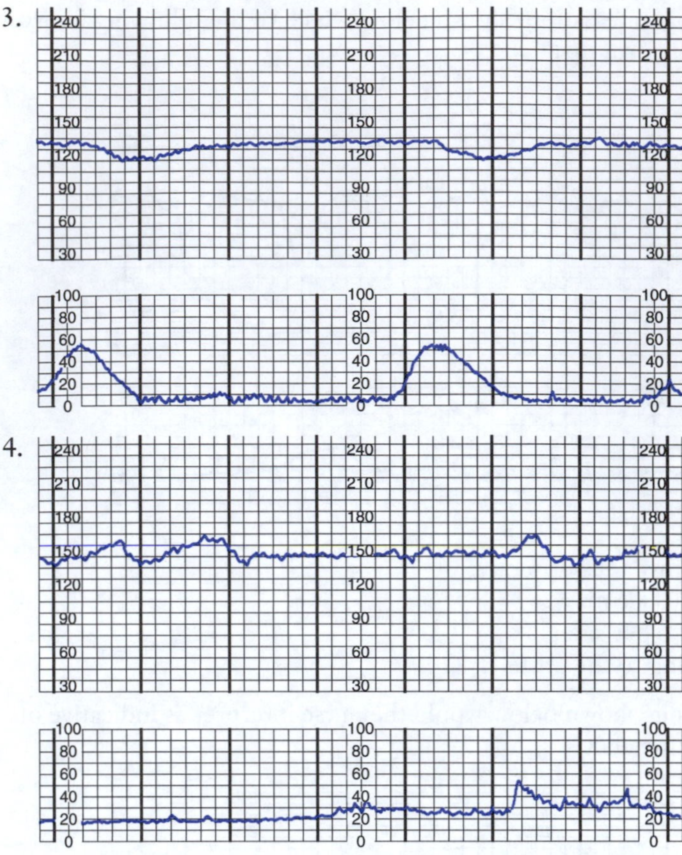

40. A client's assessments reveal that she is 4 cm dilated and 90% effaced with a fetal heart rate tracing showing recurrent late decelerations, minimal variability, and contractions every 3 minutes, each lasting 90 seconds. The nursing management of the client should be directed toward which of the following goals?
1. Completion of the first stage of labor.
2. Delivery of a healthy baby.
3. Safe pain medication management.
4. Prevention of a vaginal laceration.

41. When monitoring a fetal heart rate with moderate variability, the nurse notes V-shaped or U-shaped decelerations to 80 from a baseline of 120. One occurred during a contraction, another occurred 10 seconds after the contraction, and a third occurred 40 seconds after yet another contraction. The nurse interprets these findings as resulting from which of the following?
1. Metabolic acidosis.
2. Head compression.
3. Cord compression.
4. Insufficient uteroplacental blood flow.

42. A nurse notes a sinusoidal fetal heart pattern while analyzing the fetal heart tracing of a newly admitted client. Which of the following actions should the nurse take at this time?
1. Encourage the client to breathe with contractions.
2. Notify the primary healthcare provider.
3. Increase the intravenous infusion.
4. Encourage the client to push with contractions.

43. A client is in active labor. Which of the following assessments would warrant immediate intervention?
1. Maternal $PaCO_2$ of 40 mm Hg.
2. Alpha-fetoprotein (AFP) values of 2 times normal.
3. Three fetal heart accelerations during contractions.
4. Recurrent late decelerations with minimal variability.

44. A 35-year-old client with pre-eclampsia is being induced with oxytocin. She is contracting every 3 minutes, with each contraction lasting 30 seconds. Suddenly the client becomes dyspneic and cyanotic, and begins to have chills. Which of the following nursing interventions is of highest priority?
1. Check blood pressure.
2. Assess fetal heart rate.
3. Administer oxygen.
4. Stop oxytocin infusion.

45. Which of the following is the appropriate nursing care outcome for a client who suddenly develops anaphylactoid syndrome of pregnancy (ASP) during labor?
1. Client will be infection free at discharge.
2. Client will exhibit normal breathing function at discharge.
3. Client will exhibit normal gastrointestinal function at discharge.
4. Client will void without pain at discharge.

46. A laboring client who has developed an apparent anaphylactic syndrome of pregnancy (ASP) response is not breathing and has no pulse. In addition to calling a code, which of the following actions by the nurse, who is alone with the client, is appropriate at this time?
1. Perform cardiac compressions and breaths in a 15 to 2 ratio.
2. Provide chest compressions at a depth of at least 2 inches.
3. Compress the chest at the lower ½ of the sternum.
4. Provide rescue breaths over a 10-second time frame.

47. A client at 38 weeks' gestation is in labor and delivery with a painful, board-like abdomen. Which of the following assessments is appropriate at this time?
1. Fetal heart rate.
2. Cervical dilation.
3. White blood cell count.
4. Maternal lung sounds.

48. While waiting to conclude the third stage of labor, the obstetrician states that a client has placenta accreta. The nurse would expect to see which of the following signs/symptoms?
1. Hypertension.
2. Hemorrhage.
3. Bradycardia.
4. Hyperthermia.

49. The nurse is monitoring a client in labor with an obstetrical history of G2 P1001, at 41 weeks' gestation. See the nurse's cervical and FHR assessments from 1200 to 2200 below.

- 1200: cervix, 4 cm; 80% effaced; –3 station; FHR 124 bpm with moderate variability.
- 1700: cervix, 6 cm; 90% effaced; –3 station; FHR 120 bpm with moderate variability.
- 2200: cervix, 8 cm; 100% effaced; –3 station; FHR 124 bpm with moderate variability.

Based on the assessments, which of the following should the nurse conclude?
1. Labor is progressing well.
2. The client is likely carrying a macrosomic fetus.
3. The fetus is not tolerating labor.
4. The client will be in second stage in about five hours.

50. After a multiparous client has been in active labor for 15 hours, an ultrasound is done. The results show that the obstetric conjugate is 10 cm and the suboccipitobregmatic diameter is 10.5 cm. Which of the following labor findings is related to these results?
1. Full dilation of the cervix.
2. Full effacement of the cervix.
3. Station of –3.
4. Frequency every 5 minutes.

51. Which of the following situations should the nurse conclude is a vaginal delivery emergency?
1. Third stage of labor lasting 20 minutes.
2. Fetal heart dropping during contractions.
3. Three-vessel cord.
4. Shoulder dystocia.

52. During a vaginal delivery, the obstetrician declares that a shoulder dystocia has occurred. Which of the following actions by the nurse is appropriate at this time?
1. Administer oxytocin intravenously per doctor's orders.
2. Flex the client's thighs sharply toward her abdomen.
3. Apply oxygen using a tight-fitting face mask.
4. Apply downward pressure on the client's fundus.

53. The fetal monitor tracing of a laboring client who is 9 cm dilated shows recurrent late decelerations. The nurse notes a moderate amount of greenish-colored amniotic fluid gush from the vagina after the healthcare provider performs an amniotomy. Which of the following conditions is the client at risk for, at this time?
1. Risk for infection related to rupture of membranes.
2. Risk for fetal injury related to possible intrauterine hypoxia.
3. Risk for impaired tissue integrity related to vaginal irritation.
4. Risk for maternal injury related to possible uterine rupture.

54. In which of the following clinical situations would amnioinfusion be appropriate?
1. Placental abruption.
2. Meconium-stained fluid.
3. Polyhydramnios.
4. Late decelerations.

55. A nurse is monitoring a client who is receiving an amnioinfusion. Which of the following assessments is critical for the nurse to make to prevent a serious complication related to the procedure?
1. Color of the amniotic fluid.
2. Maternal blood pressure.
3. Cervical effacement.
4. Uterine resting tone.

56. During the delivery of a macrosomic baby, a client developed a fourth-degree laceration. The nurse has just reviewed with the client, the provider's education about the laceration. Which comment by the client indicates she understands the extent of her laceration?
1. "My laceration extended into the muscles around my anus."
2. "My laceration extended into my urinary meatus where I pee."
3. "My laceration extended through my rectal sphincter into my rectum."
4. "My laceration extended up to my clitoris."

57. Which of the following lab values should the nurse report to the physician as being consistent with the diagnosis of HELLP syndrome?
1. Hematocrit 48%.
2. Potassium 5.5 mEq/L.
3. Platelets 75,000.
4. Sodium 130 mEq/L.

58. A client who has been diagnosed as having pre-eclampsia with severe features is receiving magnesium sulfate via IV pump. Which of the following medications must the nurse have immediately available?
1. Calcium gluconate.
2. Morphine sulfate.
3. Naloxone.
4. Oxytocin.

59. Which of the following physical findings would lead the nurse to suspect that a client who has pre-eclampsia with severe features has developed HELLP syndrome? **Select all that apply.**
1. 3+ pitting edema.
2. Petechiae.
3. Jaundice.
4. 4+ deep tendon reflexes.
5. Elevated specific gravity.

60. A client is on magnesium sulfate for pre-eclampsia with severe features. The nurse must notify the attending physician regarding which of the following findings?
1. Patellar and biceps reflexes of 3+.
2. Urinary output of 30 mL/hr.
3. Respiratory rate of 16 rpm.
4. Serum magnesium level of 10 mg/dL.

61. A client with pre-eclampsia with severe features at 38 weeks' gestation, is being induced with IV oxytocin. Which of the following would warrant the nurse to stop the infusion?
1. Blood pressure 160/110.
2. Frequency of contractions every 3 minutes.
3. Duration of contractions of 130 seconds.
4. Fetal heart rate 155 bpm with early decelerations.

62. A client is in labor and delivery with a diagnosis of HELLP syndrome. The nurse notes the following blood values:

PT (prothrombin time)	99 sec (normal 60 to 85 sec).
PTT (partial thromboplastin time)	30 sec (normal 11 to 15 sec).

For which of the following signs and symptoms would the nurse monitor the client?
1. Pink-tinged urine.
2. Early decelerations.
3. Patellar reflexes +1.
4. Blood pressure 140/90.

63. The nurse observes a new staff member caring for an eclamptic client following a seizure. Which of the following actions by the staff member indicates an understanding of eclampsia?
1. Check each urine for presence of ketones.
2. Pad the client's bed rails and headboard.
3. Provide visual and auditory stimulation.
4. Place the bed in the high Fowler's position.

64. A client at 40 weeks' gestation has an admitting platelet count of 90,000 cells/mm^3 and a hematocrit of 29%. Her lab values 1 week earlier were platelet count 200,000 cells/mm^3 and hematocrit 37%. Which additional abnormal lab value would the nurse expect to see?
1. Decreased serum creatinine level.
2. Elevated red blood count (RBC).
3. Decreased aspartate aminotransferase (AST).
4. Elevated alanine aminotransaminase (ALT).

65. A nurse administers magnesium sulfate via infusion pump to a laboring client who has pre-eclampsia with severe features. Which of the following outcomes indicates that the medication is effective?
1. Client has no patellar reflex response.
2. Urinary output is 30 mL/hr.
3. Respiratory rate is 16 rpm.
4. Client has no grand mal seizures.

66. A doctor orders a narcotic analgesic for a laboring client. In which of the following situations is it essential for the nurse to hold the medication and not administer it?
1. Contraction pattern is every 3 min x 60 sec.
2. Fetal monitor tracing shows late decelerations.
3. Client sleeps between contractions.
4. The blood pressure is 150/90.

67. A client with an internal fetal spiral electrode in place has just received an IV narcotic for pain relief. Which of the following monitor tracing changes should the nurse anticipate?
1. Early decelerations.
2. Late decelerations.
3. Minimal variability.
4. Accelerations after contractions.

68. The nurse is caring for two post–cesarean section clients in the post–anesthesia suite. One of the clients had her surgery under spinal anesthesia, while the other client had her surgery under epidural anesthesia. Which of the following is an important difference between the two types of anesthesia?
1. The level of the pain relief is lower in spinals.
2. Placement of the needle is higher in epidurals.
3. Epidurals do not fully sedate motor nerves.
4. Clients with spinal anesthesia complain of nausea and vomiting.

69. To reduce possible side effects from a cesarean section under general anesthesia, clients are routinely given which of the following medications?
1. Antacids.
2. Tranquilizers.
3. Antihypertensives.
4. Anticonvulsants.

70. During intubation before general anesthesia, the anesthesia provider asks the nurse to apply cricoid pressure. Place an X on the location where the nurse should apply the pressure.

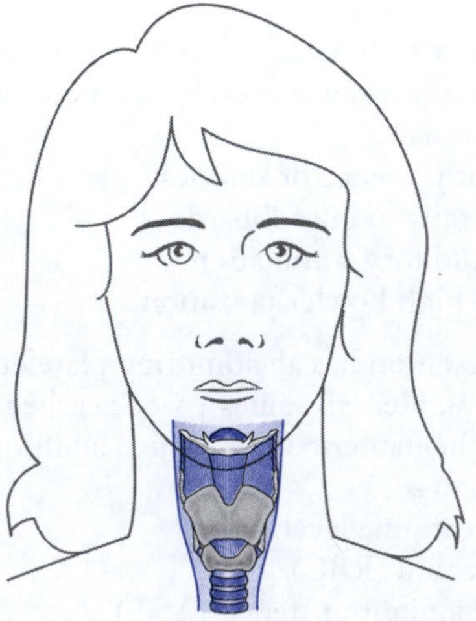

71. The nurse understands that a client undergoing an emergency cesarean section is likely experiencing a great deal of anxiety. Which of the following nursing interventions would be appropriate for this client?
1. Apply antiembolic boots bilaterally.
2. When possible, explain all procedures slowly and carefully.
3. Administer an antacid per MD orders.
4. Monitor the FHR and maternal vital signs.

72. A pregnant client with an obstetrical history of G3 P2002 had her two previous children by cesarean section. She would like to have a vaginal birth this time and requests a trial of labor after cesarean section (TOLAC). Which of the following situations would exclude a TOLAC and mandate that this delivery also be by cesarean?
1. The client refuses to have a regional anesthesia.
2. The client is postdates with intact membranes.
3. The baby is in the occiput posterior position.
4. The previous uterine incisions were vertical.

73. An anesthesiologist informs the nurse that a client scheduled for cesarean section will have the procedure under general anesthesia rather than regional anesthesia. Which of the following would warrant this decision?
1. The client has a history of drug addiction.
2. The client is allergic to morphine sulfate.
3. The client is a 13-year-old adolescent.
4. The client has had surgery for scoliosis.

74. A client is delivering a macrosomic baby. The midwife is performing a mediolateral episiotomy. Draw a line where the episiotomy is being performed.

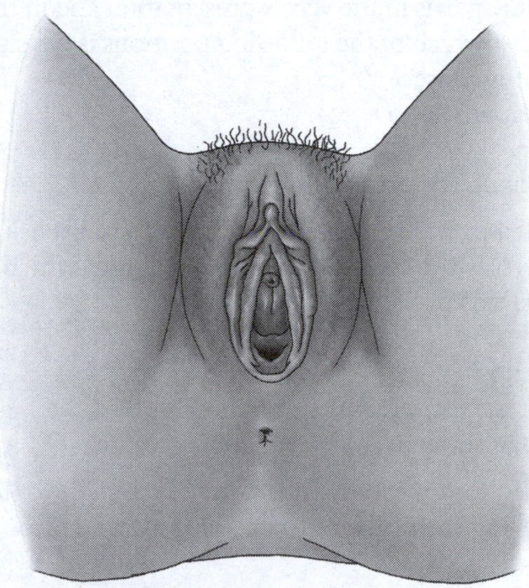

75. The nurse is triaging four full-term primigravid clients in the labor and delivery unit. The nurse requests a bedside consultation by the primary healthcare provider for which of the clients? The client who has: **Select all that apply.**
1. Cervical cerclage.
2. FHR 155 bpm with moderate variability.
3. Maternal blood pressure of 92/60.
4. Full effacement.
5. Active herpes simplex 2.

76. A client has been in the second stage of labor for 2½ hours. The fetal head is at +4 station and the fetal heart rate is showing recurrent late decelerations. The obstetrician advises the client that the baby will be delivered with forceps. Which of the following actions should the nurse take at this time?
1. Obtain a consent for the use of forceps.
2. Encourage the client to push between contractions.
3. Assess the fetal heart rate continuously.
4. Advise the client to refuse the use of forceps.

77. The charge nurse is monitoring the progress of four women who are in labor. The nurse is aware that which clients will likely need a cesarean delivery? **Select all that apply.**
1. Fetus is in the left sacral posterior (LSP) position.
2. Placenta is attached to the posterior portion of the uterine wall.
3. Fetus has been diagnosed with meningomyelocele.
4. Client is hepatitis B surface antigen positive.
5. The lecithin/sphingomyelin ratio in the amniotic fluid is 1.5:1.

78. A charge nurse is working with four nurses new to the obstetrical unit. During their shift, the fetal heart rate patterns on all four fully dilated clients shows minimal variability and late decelerations. The primary healthcare providers all request forceps to speed the deliveries. In which of the situations should the nurses be advised to refuse to provide the delivery forceps? **Select all that apply.**
1. Maternal history of asthma.
2. Right occiput posterior position at +4 station.
3. Transverse fetal lie.
4. Mentum presentation and –1 station.
5. Maternal history of cerebral palsy.

79. A client had an epidural inserted 2 hours ago. It is functioning well, the client is hemodynamically stable, and the client's labor is progressing as expected. Which of the following assessments is the highest priority at this time?
1. Assess blood pressure every 15 minutes.
2. Assess pulse rate every 1 hour.
3. Palpate the client's bladder.
4. Auscultate lungs.

80. A fetus is entering the pelvis in the vertex presentation and in the extended attitude. The nurse determines that which of the following positions is consistent with this situation?
1. LMA (left mentum anterior).
2. LSP (left sacrum posterior).
3. Dorso-superior.
4. ROP (right occiput posterior).

81. A client is scheduled to have an external version for a breech presentation. The nurse carefully assesses the client's chart knowing that which of the following is a contraindication to this procedure?
1. Station –2.
2. 38 weeks' gestation.
3. Reactive nonstress test (NST).
4. Previous cesarean section.

82. A client is scheduled for an external version. The nurse would expect to prepare which of the following medications to be administered prior to the procedure?
1. Oxytocin.
2. Methylergonovine.
3. Betamethasone.
4. Terbutaline.

83. A physician has notified the labor and delivery suite that four clients will be admitted to the unit. The client with which of the following clinical findings would be a candidate for an external version?
1. +3 station.
2. Left sacral posterior position.
3. Flexed attitude.
4. Rupture of membranes for 24 hours.

84. A client with an obstetrical history of G3 P2002 has just had an external version. The nurse monitors this client carefully for which of the following?
1. Decreased urinary output.
2. Elevated blood pressure.
3. Severe occipital headache.
4. Variable fetal heart decelerations.

85. A client at 32 weeks' gestation is contracting every 3 min, with each contraction lasting 60 sec. She is receiving magnesium sulfate intravenously by pump. For which of the following maternal assessments is it critical for the nurse to monitor the client?
1. Low urinary output.
2. Temperature elevation.
3. Absent pedal pulses.
4. Retinal edema.

86. A nurse is caring for a primiparous client at 35 weeks' gestation. The client is having uterine contractions. Which of the following confirms that the client is in preterm labor? **Select all that apply.**
1. Contraction frequency every 15 minutes.
2. Effacement 10%.
3. Dilation 3 cm.
4. Cervical length of 2 cm.
5. Contraction duration of 30 seconds.

87. The nurse in the obstetrician's office is caring for four prenatal clients with singleton pregnancies at 25 weeks' gestation. With which of the following clients should the nurse carefully review the signs and symptoms of preterm labor (PTL)? **Select all that apply.**
1. 38-year-old in an abusive relationship.
2. 34-year-old whose first child was born at 32 weeks' gestation.
3. 30-year-old whose baby has a two-vessel cord.
4. 26-year-old with a history of long menstrual periods.
5. 22-year-old who smokes 2 packs of cigarettes every day.

88. The nurse is caring for a client at 30 weeks' gestation whose fetal fibronectin (fFN) levels are positive. It is essential that she be taught about which of the following?
1. How to use a blood glucose monitor.
2. Signs of preterm labor.
3. Signs of pre-eclampsia.
4. How to do fetal kick count assessments.

89. A client at 28 weeks' gestation with intact membranes is admitted with the following findings: Contractions every 5 min × 60 sec, 3 cm dilated, 80% effaced. Which of the following medications will the obstetrician likely order?
1. Oxytocin.
2. Methylergonovine maleate.
3. Magnesium sulfate.
4. Morphine sulfate.

90. Three clients at 30 weeks' gestation are on the labor and delivery unit in preterm labor. For which of the clients should the nurse question a doctor's order for beta agonist tocolytics?
1. A client with hypothyroidism.
2. A client with breast cancer.
3. A client with cardiac disease.
4. A client with asthma.

91. A preterm labor client at 30 weeks' gestation reported rupture of membranes 4 hours ago. This was confirmed on examination. The nurse prepares to administer IM dexamethasone When the client asks why she is receiving the drug, the nurse replies:
1. "To help to stop your labor contractions."
2. "To prevent an infection in your uterus."
3. "To help to mature your baby's lungs."
4. "To decrease the pain from the contractions."

92. A client with insulin-dependent diabetes is in active labor. The physician has written the following order: Administer regular insulin 5 units per hour via IV pump. The insulin has been diluted as follows: 50 units/500 mL normal saline. At what rate should the nurse set the pump? **Please calculate to the nearest whole number.**

_________ mL/hr

93. A 30-year-old client with an obstetrical history of G2 P0010 is in preterm labor. She is receiving nifedipine. Which of the following maternal assessments noted by the nurse must be reported to the primary healthcare provider immediately?
1. Heart rate of 100 bpm.
2. Wakefulness.
3. Audible rales.
4. Daily output of 2,000 mL.

94. A client at 42 weeks' gestation with an obstetrical history of G3 P2002is admitted to the labor suite for induction. A biophysical profile (BPP) report on the client's chart indicates a BPP score of 6 out of 10. The nurse should monitor this client carefully for which of the following?
1. Maternal hypertension.
2. Maternal hyperglycemia.
3. Increased fetal heart variability.
4. A fetal heart-rate pattern of late decelerations.

95. Five minutes ago, the primary healthcare provider performed an amniotomy (ruptured the client's membranes) on a client at 40 weeks' gestation. The client's obstetrical history is G3 P1011. The fetus was at –4 station, and in ROP position at the time of the amniotomy. The fetal heart rate is now 140 bpm with a prolonged deceleration. The fluid is green tinged. The nurse concludes that which of the following situations is present at this time?
1. The fetus is post-term.
2. The presentation is breech.
3. The cord is prolapsed.
4. The amniotic fluid is infected.

96. The nurse is assessing the Bishop score on a client who is postdates. Which of the following measurements will the nurse assess? **Select all that apply.**
1. Gestational age.
2. Rupture of membranes.
3. Cervical dilation.
4. Fetal station.
5. Cervical position.

97. A client with a fetal demise is admitted to labor and delivery in the latent phase of labor. Which of the following behaviors would the nurse expect this client to exhibit?
1. Crying and sadness.
2. Talkative and excited.
3. Quietly doing rapid breathing.
4. Loudly chanting songs.

98. A physician writes the following order—Administer penicillin G, 5 million units IV x 1, then 2.5 million units q 4 h until delivery—for a newly admitted laboring client with ruptured membranes. The client had positive vaginal and rectal cultures for group B streptococcal (GBS) bacteria at 36 weeks' gestation. Which of the following is a rationale for this order?
1. The client is at high risk for chorioamnionitis.
2. The baby is at high risk for neonatal sepsis.
3. The bacterium is sexually transmitted.
4. The bacterium causes puerperal sepsis.

99. A client at 42 weeks' gestation is admitted to the labor and delivery suite with a diagnosis of acute oligohydramnios. The nurse must anticipate seeing which of the following? **Select all that apply.**
1. Variable FHR decelerations.
2. Late FHR decelerations.
3. Oliguria.
4. Tachysystole.

100. A nurse has been assigned to circulate during a cesarean section for triplets. Which of the following actions should the nurse take before the birth of the babies? **Select all that apply.**
1. Count the number of sterile sponges.
2. Document the time of the first incision.
3. Notify the pediatric or neonatal staff.
4. Perform a sterile scrub on the client.
5. Assemble the sterile instruments.

101. A client presents to the labor and delivery suite for a labor check. It is essential that the nurse note the client's status in relation to which of the following infectious diseases? **Select all that apply.**
1. Hepatitis B.
2. Rubeola.
3. Varicella.
4. Group B streptococcus.
5. HIV/AIDS.

102. The primary healthcare provider for a client at 38 1/7 weeks' gestation calls the labor and delivery suite to schedule an induction for the next day. The client is having no medical or pregnancy complications. Which of the following responses by the nurse would be appropriate?
1. "At what time would you like to begin the induction?"
2. "What is the client's Bishop score?"
3. "I am sorry but the client will not be able to be induced tomorrow."
4. "I will have the prostaglandin induction medication prepared."

103. A client whose fetus is exhibiting signs of erythroblastosis fetalis is admitted to the labor and delivery unit. The nurse would expect to see which of the following fetal heart rate monitor tracings?
1. Marked fetal heart rate variability.
2. Prolonged fetal heart rate accelerations.
3. Sinusoidal fetal heart rate pattern.
4. Periodic variable decelerations.

104. The fetal heart rate pattern of a client in active labor shows moderate variability with late decelerations. The nurse makes which of the following interpretations of the pattern?
1. Category I pattern requiring tocolytic medication administration.
2. Category II pattern requiring lateral positioning, oxygen administration via face mask, and intravenous fluid bolus.
3. Category III pattern requiring lateral positioning, oxygen administration via face mask, intravenous fluid bolus, and amnioinfusion.
4. Category IV pattern requiring immediate termination of labor.

105. A client has been diagnosed with a hypercoagulability syndrome (thrombophilia) Which of the following medications would the nurse expect the primary healthcare provider to order?
1. Heparin.
2. Warfarin.
3. Aminocaproic acid.
4. DDAVP (desmopressin acetate).

CASE STUDY: *The following case studies utilize an NGN test question format referred to as the "Bowtie." In the electronic NCLEX examination, test takers will drag and drop their answers into the appropriate boxes (NCSBN, 2021).*

The labor and delivery nurse is admitting a client in active labor. The client is at 37 weeks' gestation with an obstetrical history of G2 P0100 and a diagnosis of pre-eclampsia with severe features. Her cervical exam is 3 cm, 100% effaced, 0 station. The external fetal monitor (EFM) shows contractions every 3 minutes x 60 seconds. Fetal heart rate (FHR) is 130 bpm with periods of moderate and minimal variability and intermittent late decelerations.

106. Select a complication for which the fetus is at increased risk.
1. Cephalopelvic disproportion.
2. Hypoxia.
3. Posterior presentation.
4. Prolapsed cord.

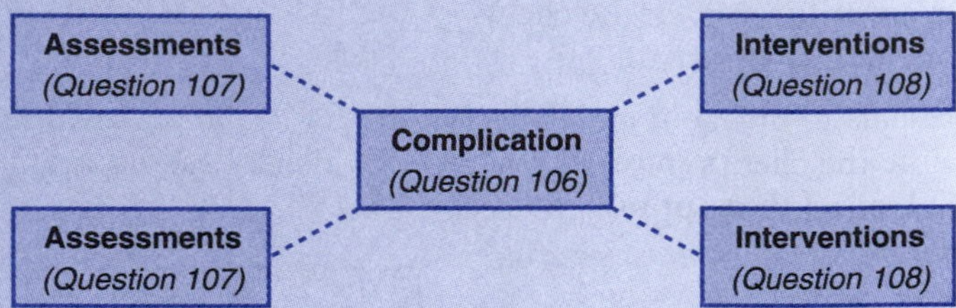

107. Which of the following assessments are important for the nurse to monitor in order to identify the complication noted in the previous question? **Select two.**
1. Variable decelerations.
2. Fetal descent.
3. Scalp stimulation response.
4. Leopold maneuvers.
5. Late decelerations.
6. Fern testing.

108. **Specify two interventions** the nurse should perform for the mother as a way to reduce the risk of the fetal complication.
1. IV bolus.
2. Lateral positioning.
3. Oxygen administration.
4. Epidural.

CASE STUDY:

The labor and delivery nurse is admitting a client in active labor. She is at 41 weeks' gestation with an obstetrical history of G5 P3013. Contractions are coming every 3 to 5 minutes x 60 seconds. FHR is 145 bpm with moderate variability. Her cervical exam is 3 cm, 100% effaced, zero station. She had a primary cesarean section 18 months ago with her last baby who weighed 9 lbs 2 oz (4139 grams) and she experienced a postpartum hemorrhage that required 6 units of blood. This baby's estimated weight is 7 lbs (3175 grams). She plans a trial of labor after cesarean section (TOLAC).

109. Select a complication for which the client is at increased risk.
1. Prolonged labor.
2. Uterine rupture.
3. Prolapsed cord.
4. Precipitous delivery.

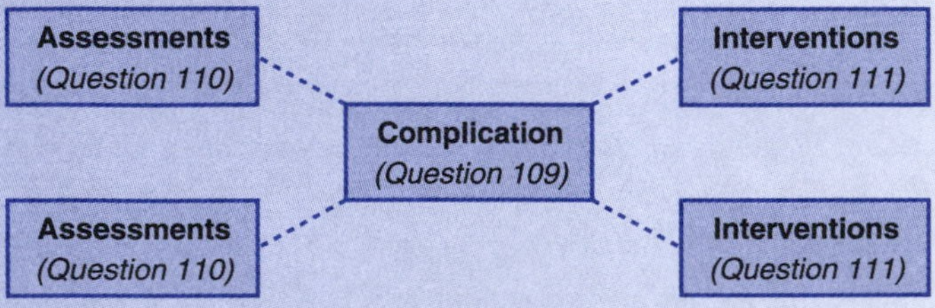

110. Which of the following assessments are important for the nurse to monitor to identify the complication? **Select two.**
1. Fetal bradycardia.
2. Unstable vital signs.
3. Late decelerations.
4. Severe headache.

111. Specify two priorities the nurse should address as a way to reduce the risk of the complication.
1. Encourage ambulation to reduce the time in labor.
2. Maintain continuous electronic fetal monitoring (EFM).
3. Insert indwelling bladder catheter.
4. Monitor labor pattern and progress.

CASE STUDY:

A client with an obstetrical history of G4 P3003 was admitted to the labor and delivery unit 9 hours ago for an oxytocin induction at 40 weeks' gestation. She has a medical history of gestational diabetes, which she has been controlling with carbohydrate counting. She has been pushing for an hour and the fetus has remained at +2 station during that time. Contractions are every 2 to 3 minutes x 60 seconds and she is pushing well with them. Oxytocin is running by pump at 10 milliunits per minute. FHR is 130 bpm with moderate variability and no decelerations (a Category 1 tracing). She has an epidural in place for pain control.

112. Select a complication for which the client is at increased risk.
1. Precipitous delivery.
2. Retained placenta.
3. Hypoglycemia.
4. Shoulder dystocia.

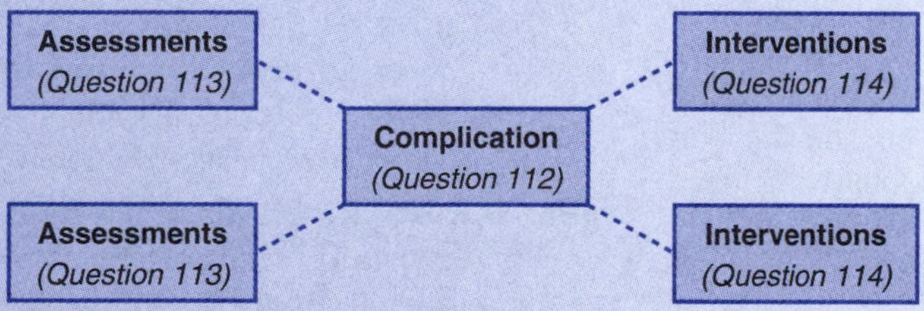

113. Which of the following assessments are important for the nurse to monitor to identify the complication? **Select two.**
1. Capillary blood glucose (CBG).
2. Time of fetal head delivery.
3. Turtle sign.
4. Uterine atony.

The fetal head delivered after four hours of pushing and the nurse noted the turtle sign before delivery.

114. Specify two interventions the nurse should perform as a way to reduce the risks of the complication.
1. Place the client in the McRoberts position.
2. Turn off the oxytocin.
3. Administer oxygen by mask at 10 L/min.
4. Provide suprapubic pressure.

ANSWERS AND RATIONALES

The correct answer number and rationale for why it is the correct answer are given in **boldface blue type**. Rationales for why the other possible answer options are incorrect also are given, but they are not in boldface type.

1. 1. Although this contraction pattern of every 5 minutes indicates the oxytocin rate should be increased to achieve the goal of contractions every 2 to 3 minutes, it does not require immediate follow-up. The duration of 60 to 80 seconds does not require immediate follow-up. It could indicate that the client's intrinsic oxytocin is being stimulated. Because the contractions are 5 minutes apart, the fetus has time between contractions to tank up on oxygen.
   2. With the fetal station previously at –3 and spontaneous rupture of membranes, immediate follow-up is required to confirm there is no prolapsed cord, since the fetus is not engaged in the pelvis as a "plug" to prevent the cord from slipping through the cervix.
   3. Her temperature has risen a bit from 100° F (37.7° C) to 100.4° F (38° C). This requires monitoring, but is not an immediate emergency.
   4. FHR 110 bpm with moderate variability is within the normal range of 110 to 160 bpm. The current FHR shows a drop in the baseline. As such, it bears watching. It's possible the fetus is sleeping. The moderate variability indicates adequate fetal oxygenation at this time.

TEST-TAKING HINT: In this step, the nurse must recognize client conditions that require immediate action, and those that can wait. This client's induction was started 4 hours ago for postdates at 41 weeks' gestation. The nurse's primary focus must be on adequate oxygenation for the fetus, since the placenta may have developed calcifications as a result of being "overdue." As a result of calcifications, less oxygen is transferred from the intervillous space to the placenta for delivery to the fetus. The nurse must be alert for symptoms of fetal hypoxia such as late decelerations. In this case, the mother's slight increase in temperature could simply be that she is a bit dehydrated from breathing through the contractions, and her metabolism is increased because of the labor contractions. Currently, the fetus is being well oxygenated as evidenced by moderate variability. The biggest risk is the rupture of membranes and the previous fetal station that could allow for a prolapsed cord.

2. **Answers 1 and 4 are the correct answers.**
   1. The client is most likely entering active labor with increased contraction strength. This has resulted in spontaneous rupture of membranes.
   2. The presence of moderate variability indicates the baby is tolerating labor.
   3. There is nothing to suggest cephalopelvic disproportion (CPD) at this time. It is not uncommon for a fetus to be at –3 station at the start of an induction before rupture of membranes.
   4. Although the nurse will complete a vaginal exam to check for prolapsed cord, it is likely that with the spontaneous rupture of membranes, the fetal head is now engaged, since the pillowy bag of waters is no longer in the way. A vaginal exam will confirm that hypothesis. The FHR does not suggest a prolapsed cord, but it is prudent to perform a vaginal exam after spontaneous rupture of membranes to confirm there is no "occult" or unseen umbilical cord near the cervix, which would guide in maternal positioning. Umbilical cord prolapse is most often accompanied by a prolonged FHR deceleration. The stem does not indicate that event has happened.

TEST-TAKING HINT: This question evaluates the test taker's ability to interpret the meaning of the clinical scenario. The nurse identifies both positive and negative hypotheses based on client events, to inform next steps. In this case, the hypotheses are only positive. In just 8% of pregnancies, spontaneous rupture of membranes occurs before labor begins (American College of Obstetricians and Gynecologists [ACOG], 2020b). Generally, for a client with contractions, spontaneous rupture of membranes indicates the beginning of active labor. The fluid, itself, can stimulate stronger contractions. As such, the nurse can assume that the client is likely now in active labor and following rupture of membranes, the fetal head can move down into the pelvis for engagement. Each response above includes the clinical judgments the nurse should make.

3. Answers 1(a), 2(a), 3(b), 4(c) and 5(b) are correct.

Nursing Action	(a) Indicated	(b) Nonessential	(c) Contraindicated
1. Vaginal Exam	X		
2. Maternal position change	X		
3. Oxygen administration by non-rebreather mask		X	
4. Intrauterine pressure catheter (IUPC) insertion			X
5. Discontinue oxytocin		X	

1(a). A vaginal exam is indicated to confirm there has been no umbilical cord prolapse. The nurse might also find that without the buoyancy of amniotic fluid, the fetal head is at a lower station and is now engaged since the membranes ruptured. Ruptured membranes can lead to active labor and secretion of endogenous oxytocin, making it necessary to turn down the rate of the oxytocin infusion to avoid or in response to tachysystole.

2(a). With the FHR of 110 bpm, a maternal change of position could wake up the fetus, if it's asleep and/or improve fetal oxygenation if that is impacting the lower FHR.

3(b). There is nothing to suggest the fetus needs supplemental oxygenation.

4(c). There is nothing to suggest an invasive IUPC is needed to monitor the strength of the contractions at this time. The spontaneous rupture of membranes can indicate an increase in the strength of the contractions. In addition, rupture of membranes releases hormones that can promote labor contractions intrinsically. The prudent nurse must remember that contraction strength must always be assessed by palpation and not just by numbers on a screen, even when an IUPC is in use.

5(b). There is no reason to discontinue the oxytocin. The contractions are only 5 minutes apart and the fetus is well-oxygenated. Instead, the oxytocin should be increased for a more active labor pattern.

TEST-TAKING TIP: Now, the nurse will prioritize hypotheses and determine which one should guide her first interventions. Each of the responses above includes appropriate clinical judgments in this step. This question reveals how the test taker has sorted through possible interventions to determine the most important next steps.

4. Answers (a)4 and (b)5 are correct answers.

(a) First Address:	(b) Followed by:
1. Light meconium staining of membranes	1. Light meconium staining of membranes
2. Fetal heart rate	2. Fetal heart rate
3. Maternal temperature of 100.4° F	3. Maternal temperature of 100.4° F
4. IV bolus for epidural	4. IV bolus for epidural
5. Maternal vital sign assessments	**5. Maternal vital sign assessments**

(a)1. Light meconium is not an unexpected finding with postdates pregnancies. The FHR is reassuring, regardless.

(a)2. The fetal heart rate is not a priority at this time.

(a)3. The maternal temperature is not a priority at this time. The mother's temp of 100.4° F (38° C) in isolation without other risk factors is not considered an infection. However, now that the membranes have ruptured, there is an increased risk of infection. Further vaginal exams should be limited and the frequency of temperature and vital sign assessments should be increased.

(a)4. The focus at this time is on client safety during the epidural insertion. The nurse should address the IV bolus first. This client will need an IV bolus of 500 to 1000 mL before the epidural insertion, to maintain her blood pressure throughout the procedure. The bolus is often started when the client gets up to empty her bladder before the procedure.

(b)5. Once the client returns to her bed for the epidural, the nurse will need to take a complete set of vital signs. Blood pressure, respirations, and pulse rate will be closely monitored at specified intervals throughout and after the procedure.

TEST-TAKING TIP: The light meconium, fetal heart rate, and maternal temperature are distractors. The test taker demonstrates a knowledge of normal findings when they identify that those three factors are not worrisome at this time, and that client care specific to the epidural takes priority. Having determined that client safety during epidural insertion is most important right now, the nurse generates solutions to accomplish that goal.

5. **Answers 1, 2, and 6 are correct.**

Nursing Interventions	Place an X in the box to indicate appropriate interventions
1. Lateral maternal positioning	X
2. Increase oxytocin rate	X
3. Administration of IV antibiotics	
4. Indwelling catheter insertion	
5. Oxygen administration by nonrebreather mask	
6. Apple juice intake	X

1. **Lateral maternal positioning allows for optimum maternal circulation and placental perfusion. For epidural efficacy, the decision for which side the client lies on will be based partly on which side is most painful for the client. She should lie on the side that is the most painful, to support bathing the nerves on that side with the pain medication. It is appropriate to encourage the client to change her position every 30 minutes in order to facilitate rotation of the fetus through the birth canal as it completes the cardinal movements of labor.**
2. **The goal for contraction frequency is generally 2 to 3 minutes apart (from the start of one contraction to the start of the next), with at least 60 to 120 seconds of rest between. This client's contractions are every 5 minutes, so it is appropriate to turn up the oxytocin as ordered, now that she is comfortable.**
3. There is no indication for this client to have antibiotics. The nurse should be aware of the standards for antibiotic use for clients who are GBS positive, those with prolonged rupture of membranes, and for those with fevers.
4. Although this client has an epidural, she may be able to use a bedpan during labor. Because the client will not likely feel the urge to void, the nurse must palpate for bladder filling at least every 1 to 2 hours. A full bladder can prevent fetal descent. Many providers' orders indicate that if a client cannot void spontaneously, a straight catheter may be inserted and removed. A common provider's order is that if a straight catheter is necessary two times, an indwelling catheter may be placed the second time.
5. There is nothing in this question to indicate the client requires oxygen.
6. **Clear liquids are appropriate for this client.**

TEST-TAKING TIP: With no worrisome clinical factors at this time, the nurse's attention returns to the over-arching goal of supporting labor progress and birth. This question evaluates the test taker's ability to identify appropriate and prudent nursing care actions. Each of the responses above is self-explanatory.

6. **Answers 1(a), 2(b), 3(c), and 4(a) are correct.**

Nursing Action	(a) Effective	(b) Ineffective	(c) Likely Unrelated
1. Maternal position changes	X		
2. Oxytocin rate increase		X	
3. Apple juice intake			X
4. Catheterization	X		

1(a). **Maternal position change was effective in assisting with fetal descent by promoting the rotation of the fetus in the pelvis. The fetus was previously at zero station and is now at +1 station.**

2(b). **Because the contractions are still 5 minutes apart, the increase in oxytocin has not yet been effective and further increases are indicated.**

3(c). **It is not likely the apple juice was related to any of the nurse's assessments. However, because labor is hard work, the apple juice provides energy and fluids, which are important.**

4(a). **The urine amount of 300 mL could have prevented fetal descent. Although it is not clear whether or not the fetus descended to +1 station before or after the catheterization, it is likely that emptying the bladder was effective in promoting fetal descent.**

TEST-TAKING HINT: In this last step of clinical judgment, the nurse evaluates outcomes to determine whether or not the interventions helped meet the goals, or not. If the goals were not met, the nurse begins again at recognizing cues that show the goals were not met, and continuing on with analysis, prioritizing hypotheses, generating solutions, taking actions, and re-evaluating those actions for success.

Although this client's cervix is dilating and the fetus is descending, the contractions are still 5 minutes apart. The nurse must weigh the risks of continuing to increase the oxytocin until contractions occur at least every 2 to 3 minutes apart, with delaying the increases and putting the client at risk of a longer labor and risk of postpartum hemorrhage as a result. At 6 cm, the client is just entering the active phase of labor and descent of the fetus will promote endogenous oxytocin release in a feedback mechanism. As a result, contractions are likely to occur closer together on their own and the nurse may actually reduce the oxytocin rate as a result. By continuing to assist the client in changing positions, monitoring the fetus, and increasing the oxytocin rate until contractions are 2 to 3 minutes apart, the nurse plays an important role in assuring a safe outcome for this client and her baby.

7. 1. **These are the classic signs of water intoxication.**
2. With water intoxication, the client would show signs of hyponatremia and hypokalemia.
3. Thrombocytopenia and neutropenia are unrelated to water intoxication.
4. Paresthesias, myalgias, and anemia are unrelated to water intoxication.

TEST-TAKING HINT: Clients who receive oxytocin over a long period of time are at high risk for water intoxication. The oxytocin molecule is similar in structure to the antidiuretic hormone (ADH) molecule so the body retains fluids in response to the medication. As such, careful monitoring of intake and output is essential when clients are induced with oxytocin.

8. 1. **Induction is contraindicated in transverse lie.**
2. When indicated, it is safe to induce a client with cerebral palsy.
3. When indicated, it is safe to induce a pregnant adolescent.
4. When indicated, it is safe to induce a client with diabetes mellitus.

TEST-TAKING HINT: A baby in the transverse lie is lying sideways and cannot enter the birth canal as a result. Whenever a vaginal birth is contraindicated, induction is also contraindicated.

9. 1. **Whenever there is marked fetal bradycardia and oxytocin is running, the nurse should immediately turn off the oxytocin drip.**
2. Oxygen should be administered, but the mask should be put on after the oxytocin has been turned off.
3. Repositioning is indicated, but should be performed after the oxytocin has been turned off.
4. The obstetrician should be called, but after the oxytocin has been turned off.

TEST-TAKING HINT: Whenever there is evidence of fetal compromise and oxytocin is being infused, the medication should be stopped immediately to allow for improved placental perfusion. Oxytocin creates strong contractions. During each contraction the blood flow to the placenta (placental perfusion) is temporarily reduced. In this question, the complaint of abdominal pain suggests a possible placental abruption, giving another reason to turn off the oxytocin.

10. 1. There is no specific dose of oxytocin that causes fetal intolerance of labor.
2. **The standard of care is to increase the dosage of oxytocin at a minimum time interval of every 30 minutes, not every 10 minutes.**
3. Although postdates babies are at higher risk for fetal intolerance of labor, it is not contraindicated to induce with oxytocin.
4. A 60-second contraction duration is normal.

TEST-TAKING HINT: The half-life (the time it takes for half of a medication to be metabolized by the body) of oxytocin is relatively long—about 15 minutes. At least 3 half-lives usually elapse (45 minutes) before therapeutic responses are noted. Increasing the infusion rate every 10 minutes, therefore, can soon lead to oxytocin levels that are higher than necessary, resulting in contractions that come too frequently (tachysystole) and consequent fetal intolerance of labor.

11. 1. **A common side effect of misoprostol is diarrhea. Back pain could be a sign of the start of labor, since labor contractions are often first felt in the back.**
2. Hypothermia and rectal pain are not associated with misoprostol administration. In fact, fever and chills are possible side effects.
3. Urinary retention and rash are not associated with misoprostol administration.
4. Tinnitus and respiratory distress are not associated with misoprostol administration.

TEST-TAKING HINT: The nurse is ultimately watching for signs of labor. Misoprostol is a synthetic prostaglandin medication approved for nonobstetric use to prevent stomach ulcers. It is used off-label in obstetrics to ripen the cervix for induction. Prostaglandins are naturally produced in the cervix and uterus. They serve as mediators of cervical ripening. When used in obstetrics for cervical ripening, prostaglandins activate collagenase, an enzyme that prepares the cervix to thin out and dilate in response to uterine contractions.

12. 1. The infusion should be maintained.
 2. There is no indication for oxygen at this time.
 3. If she is comfortable, there is no need to change the client's position.
 4. It is appropriate to monitor the client's labor.

TEST-TAKING HINT: Even if the test taker were unfamiliar with a normal contraction pattern—as seen in the stem of the question—knowing that the fetal heart pattern is normal, guides in selecting the correct answer. Three of the responses imply that the nurse should take action because of a complication. Only response 4 indicates that the nurse should continue monitoring the labor. In this situation, the one response that is different from the others is the correct answer.

13. **3 mL/hr.**

TEST-TAKING HINT:

Standard Method:

The nurse must do a number of calculations to determine the pump drip rate in this client. First, the nurse must determine how many milliunits are in 1,000 mL of fluid:

Known: 1 unit = 1,000 milliunits
Using ratio and proportion
1 unit: 1,000 milliunits = 10 units: x milliunits
x = 10,000 milliunits

Next, the nurse must determine how many milliunits are to be infused per hour (because pumps are always calibrated mL/hour):

Using ratio and proportion

0.5 milliunits: 1 minute = x milliunits = 60 minutes
x = 30 milliunits

Finally, the nurse must do a ratio and proportion to determine the mL per hour:

10,000 milliunits: 1,000 mL = 30 milliunits: x mL
x = 3 mL/hr

Formula for Dimensional Analysis Method:

Known volume	Desired dosage	Time conversion	Unit conversion	
Known dosage	Desired time	(if needed)	(if needed)	= x volume/min

1,000 mL	0.5 milliunits	60 minutes	1unit	
10 units	1 minute	1 hour	1,000 milliunits	= x volume/min

x = 3 mL/hr

14. 1. Moderate intensity of contractions can continue without oxytocin.
 2. A frequency pattern of every 3 minutes is ideal.
 3. There is nothing in the stem to indicate that the FHR was of concern.
 4. The attitude of the baby has nothing to do with tachysystole.

TEST-TAKING HINT: When a nurse intervenes, a positive outcome is expected. This question is asking the test taker to evaluate an expected outcome of reduced contraction frequency. Tachysystole is defined as more than 5 contractions in 10 minutes, averaged over a 30-minute window (Simpson, 2016). This is equivalent to contractions that are closer than every two minutes. In this situation, the nurse is determining whether or not the action has reversed the tachysystole that developed from oxytocin administration. The finding of a normal contraction frequency (every 3 minutes) is evidence of a positive outcome. (The term "hyperstimulation" has been replaced by the word "tachysystole" for legal reasons, since "hyperstimulation" implies harm as a result of medical care.) Although tachysystole may result in a FHR pattern of concern, a fetus may seem to tolerate tachysystole for a period of time. That is the case in this question, as the stem of the question does not indicate an unfavorable FHR at this time. As such, the test taker should not assume that FHR concerns are present. However, whether or not the fetus is tolerating tachysystole, the nurse must intervene to reduce the contraction frequency and promote fetal well-being.

15. 1. The pulse rate has likely increased because the client is working with her labor. It is not an indication to turn off the oxytocin.
 2. The baseline fetal heart rate is below the normal rate of 110 to 160. This finding warrants that the oxytocin be stopped.
 3. Maternal hypertension is not an indication to stop oxytocin administration. However, it warrants further assessments.
 4. Hyperthermia is not an indication to stop oxytocin administration.

TEST-TAKING HINT: The labor and delivery nurse is responsible for two clients—one they can see (the mother), and one they cannot see (the fetus). This question provides vital signs for both of these clients. The nurse must determine which client's vital signs are unsafe under the influence of oxytocin. In this case, the fetal vital signs are the most urgent. Oxytocin increases the contractility of the uterine muscle. When the muscle contracts, the blood supply to the placenta is diminished, and very little to no oxygen is supplied to the fetus during the contraction. A drop in fetal heart rate below the normal rate is indicative of poor oxygenation to the fetus and is unsafe, especially when oxytocin is being administered. The nurse is responsible to recognize this and to protect the fetus from harm.

16. 1. There is no indication in the scenario that the membranes have ruptured.
2. The Bishop score is expected to rise when dinoprostone is administered.
3. The client may rest in any position she desires, as long as she is not flat on her back.
4. **The nurse should monitor this client for the onset of labor.**

TEST-TAKING HINT: The Bishop score reflects the normal changes of the cervix at the end of the pregnancy and indicates readiness for labor. It is used to assess how likely the client's cervix will respond to an oxytocin induction and lead to a vaginal delivery. Four cervical signs are assessed—dilation, position, effacement, and consistency. In addition, the station of the fetal head within the maternal ischial spines is assessed. Each of these five assessments is scored with a value of 0, 1, 2, or 3. A total score is calculated; the maximum Bishop score is 15. A client is considered ready for oxytocin induction if the Bishop score is at least 8 or higher.

Prelabor Status Evaluation Scoring System

	Score			
	0	1	2	3
Cervical position	Posterior	Midposition	Anterior	—
Cervical consistency	Firm	Medium	Soft	—
Cervical effacement (%)	0–30	40–50	60–70	≥0
Cervical dilation (cm)	Closed	1–2	3–4	≥5
Fetal station	−3	−2	−1	+1/+2

Adapted from Bishop, E. H. (1964). Pelvic scoring for elective induction. *Obstetrics & Gynecology, 24*, 266.

17. 1. Dinoprostone is appropriate for this client. A primigravida with a Bishop score of 4 needs dinoprostone to ripen the cervix in preparation for the induction of contractions with oxytocin.
2. **Dinoprostone is not appropriate for this client. This client's fetus is already showing signs of fetal hypoxemia, as evidenced by late decelerations. An induction is contraindicated, as it would increase the risk of fetal injury by reducing available oxygen with each contraction. This client will likely need a cesarean section.**
3. Client dinoprostone is appropriate for this client. The fetal heart rate of 155 bpm is within the normal range of 110 to 160 bpm and the Bishop score is less than 8, so a dose of dinoprostone is appropriate for cervical ripening.
4. Neither a high gravidity nor an elevated blood pressure is a contraindication to dinoprostone administration.

TEST-TAKING HINT: It is important to remember that although the fetus of a pregnant client may be at term, it is not always safe for labor contractions to be stimulated. Although dinoprostone is not directly used for induction, it is an agent that promotes cervical ripening in preparation for labor. It can stimulate contractions and oxytocin may not be needed. As such, it must not be used in a situation where the fetus is exhibiting signs of poor uteroplacental blood flow and may be compromised further by the addition of labor contractions.

18. 1. The expected outcome from the administration of dinoprostone is an increase in the Bishop score and readiness for oxytocin induction. Her Bishop score has increased from 2 to 4, so the dinoprostone should be allowed to continue to stimulate cervical changes.
2. A fetal heart rate of 155 bpm is within normal limits and not significantly different from the original baseline of 150 bpm.
3. A respiratory rate of 24 is not a contraindication to the administration of prostaglandins for cervical ripening.
4. **A contraction frequency of 1 minute, even with a short duration, would warrant the removal of the medication.**

TEST-TAKING HINT: A frequency of 1 minute (an example of tachysystole), even if the duration of each contraction was 30 seconds, would mean that there were only 30 seconds when the uterine muscle was relaxed between contractions.

This short amount of time would not provide the placenta with enough time to take up adequate oxygen for the fetus. Fetal bradycardia is a likely outcome with such frequent contractions. The benefit of dinoprostone versus misoprostol is that because dinoprostone has a tail, like a tampon, it can be removed when indicated; misoprostol cannot be removed because it is a tablet or is in a capsule. Misoprostol may be administered vaginally or orally. With misoprostol use, other means of reducing contraction frequency must be used when indicated.

19. 1. Although this teenager has had two abortions, she is not markedly at high risk for uterine rupture.
2. A primigravida with eclampsia is not markedly at high risk for uterine rupture.
3. Any client who has had a previous cesarean section is at risk for uterine rupture.
4. Clients with a history of fetal death are not markedly at high risk for uterine rupture.

TEST-TAKING HINT: A vaginal birth after cesarean section (VBAC) can be performed only if the client had a low transverse uterine incision (also called a Pfannenstiel incision, or "bikini cut") in the uterus during her previous cesarean section. Scars are not elastic and do not contract and relax the way muscle tissue does. The "uterine rupture" is actually "scar failure." It happens when the uterine scar from the previous cesarean section opens under the strain of the uterine contractions.

20. 1. Contraction frequency and duration are important, but they are not the highest priority at this time.
2. Maternal temperature is the highest priority.
3. Cervical change is important, but it is not the highest priority at this time.
4. Maternal pulse rate is important, but it is not the highest priority at this time.

TEST-TAKING HINT: The vaginal vault is an unsterile space. When membranes have been ruptured over 18 hours, there is potential for pathogens to ascend into the uterine cavity and cause infection. Elevated temperature is a sign of infection and would require prompt notification of the provider. The maternal temperature is the most important assessment for this client, because if an infection is present, antibiotic treatment must be started as soon as possible to prevent maternal and fetal morbidity. Any assessment that involves maintenance of the first step of Maslow's hierarchy of needs—survival—is generally the right answer.

21. 1. It is unlikely that the client has a distended bladder.
2. Although the client may have a urinary tract infection (UTI), an order is needed for a urine culture. This is not the first action that the nurse should take.
3. The fluid should be assessed with nitrazine paper.
4. This is not the way to assess for ballottement, and assessing for ballottement is not a priority at this time.

TEST-TAKING HINT: A continuous fluid leak is not likely urine. It is more likely that this client's bag of waters has ruptured spontaneously and she could be at high risk of infection. The most convenient way to test for rupture of membranes is with nitrazine paper. Nitrazine paper is another name for litmus paper. It detects the pH of fluid. Amniotic fluid is alkaline, whereas urine is acidic. If the paper turns a dark blue, the nurse can conclude that the membranes have ruptured and that the client is leaking amniotic fluid, not urine. Nitrazine paper is often paired with a fern test for diagnosis.

22. 1. Oxygen administered during labor should be delivered via a tight-fitting, rebreather mask at 8 to 10 liters per minute, not by a nasal cannula.
2. The client should be positioned on her side, not high Fowler's position, to increase placental perfusion.
3. The best way to monitor the fetus is with an internal electrode.
4. Increasing the IV rate helps to improve perfusion to the placenta.

TEST-TAKING HINT: Because the fetus is being oxygenated via the placenta, it is essential that in cases of fetal intolerance of labor, the amount of oxygen perfusing the placenta be maximized. This requires high concentrations of oxygen to be administered via mask, blood volume to be increased by increasing the IV drip rate, and cardiac blood return to be maximized by positioning the client on her side to remove pressure from the aorta and the vena cava. These are standard nursing interventions for most situations of fetal intolerance of labor.

23. Answers 4 and 5 are correct.
1. The transition phase is an excellent time to use hydrotherapy.
2. Many clients do push during the early part of second stage in the water bath even if they don't plan on a water birth.
3. Clients undergoing induction may labor in a water bath. During induction, the

fetus should be monitored continually by waterproof electronic fetal monitoring.

4. **Meconium-stained amniotic fluid may indicate fetal intolerance of labor. Continuous electronic fetal monitoring in the bed (not in the tub) would, therefore, be indicated. If an emergency cesarean section becomes necessary, the client can be moved to the operating more quickly if she is already in her labor bed and not in the tub.**
5. **The warm water in the bath may increase the woman's temperature, leading to an increased FHR and fetal tachycardia. As such, a water bath is contraindicated for a client with a temp of 100.4° F (38° C) or above.**

TEST-TAKING HINT: Hydrotherapy is an excellent complementary therapy for the laboring clients. The warm water is relaxing and many clients find that their pain is minimized. One theory for pain relief posits that the water floats the abdominal muscles away from the uterus, reducing the burden on the contracting uterus. Like everything else, however, hydrotherapy is not recommended in all situations. For the nurse who is interested in more information on hydrotherapy in labor and birth, it is important to note other contraindications for hydrotherapy during labor and birth, as endorsed by the American College of Nurse-Midwives (ACNM) and other professional groups (ACNM, 2017, pp 121–122).

24. **Answers 1 and 2 are correct.**
    1. **Intermittent fetal heart auscultation is not appropriate at this time. With ruptured membranes for more than 18 hours, this client is at risk of chorioamnionitis and the fetus should be monitored continuously for signs of infection such as tachycardia.**
    2. **Vaginal examinations should be minimized because of the client's high risk of chorioamnionitis.**
    3. Intravenous fluid administration is appropriate at this time.
    4. Nipple stimulation is appropriate at this time. It can serve to stimulate labor and assist with delivery before too many more hours pass.

TEST-TAKING HINT: The client in this scenario is at risk of an ascending infection from the vagina to the uterine body because she has prolonged rupture of membranes. Any time a vaginal examination is performed, the chance of infection rises. Nipple stimulation is appropriate because endogenous oxytocin will be released, which would augment the client's weak labor pattern.

25. 1. Human papillomavirus is not an indication for cesarean section.
    2. **Standard precautions are indicated in this situation.**
    3. A baby born to a client with HPV receives standard care in the well-baby nursery.
    4. HPV is not airborne. A mask is not required.

TEST-TAKING HINT: Although HPV is a sexually transmitted infection and it can be contracted by the neonate from the mother, the Centers for Disease Control and Prevention do not recommend that cesarean section be performed merely to prevent vertical transmission of HPV (CDC, n.d.-d). However, if the size of the anogenital warts obstructs the pelvic outlet or if vaginal delivery would result in excessive bleeding, cesarean delivery is indicated.

26. 1. This comment is inappropriate.
    2. The amniotic fluid smells musty but it does not naturally have an offensive smell.
    3. This statement is likely true but it is not based on an accurate assessment.
    4. **The most important information needed by the nurse should relate to the health and well-being of the fetus. Fetal movement indicates that the baby is alive. The client should be advised to go to the hospital for evaluation.**

TEST-TAKING HINT: There are two concerns in this scenario: (1) the fact that the membranes just ruptured, and (2) the smell of the fluid. The nurse should, therefore, consider two possible problems: (1) possible prolapsed cord, which may occur as a result of the rupture of the amniotic sac, and (2) possible infection, which may be indicated by the smell. Normal fetal movement will give the nurse some confidence that the cord is not prolapsed. This is the first question that should be asked. Then, the client should be advised to go to the hospital to be assessed. There, she will be assessed for confirmation of ruptured membranes, for possible infection, signs of labor, and direct fetal and contraction assessment by use of electronic fetal monitoring (EFM) and palpation.

27. 1. Candidiasis is not an indication for cesarean section.
    2. *Candida* is a fungus. Antifungals, rather than antibiotics, are administered to treat *Candida*.
    3. **Thrush is the term given to oral candidiasis, which the baby may develop after delivery.**
    4. There is no need to isolate a baby born to a client with candidiasis.

TEST-TAKING HINT: *Candida* can be transmitted to a baby during delivery as well as postdelivery via the mother's hands. Initially, the baby will develop oral thrush, but eventually the mother may notice a bright pink diaper rash on the baby as well. If she is breastfeeding her baby, she may develop a yeast infection of the breast that is very painful. The mother with candidiasis should be advised to wash her hands carefully after toileting to minimize the possibility of transmission to the neonate. If the baby develops thrush or diaper rash, it will require treatment, as well, since the yeast can be transferred to the mother through breastfeeding.

28. 1. Cesarean delivery is not necessary for clients who are hepatitis B positive.
2. Ampicillin is ineffective against hepatitis B, which is a virus. Ampicillin may be administered to clients who have positive group B strep (GBS) vaginal or rectal cultures.
3. Within 12 hours of birth, the baby should receive both the first injection of hepatitis B vaccine and HBIG (hepatitis B immune globulin).
4. Babies born to clients who are hepatitis B surface antigen positive are cared for in the well-baby nursery. No isolation is needed.

TEST-TAKING HINT: Although this is a client who is in labor, the nurse must anticipate the needs of the neonate after delivery. Because it is recommended that the baby receive the medication within a restricted time frame, it is especially important for the nurse to be proactive and obtain the physician's order so that care can continue seamlessly for the newborn (Schillie et al., 2018).

29. 1. It is appropriate for the nurse to assess the client's dilation and effacement.
2. Surgical delivery is not indicated by the scenario.
3. There is no reason to place the client in the Trendelenburg position.
4. There is no indication that a BPP has been performed.

TEST-TAKING HINT: Although cesarean deliveries are recommended to be performed when a client has an active case of herpes simplex, surgical delivery is not indicated when no lesions or prodromes are present. Clients who have histories of herpes with no current outbreak, therefore, are considered to be healthy laboring clients who may deliver vaginally (CDC, n.d.-c). Because this client is in labor with her second baby, the labor is likely to progress quickly and a baseline vaginal examination is necessary, once the nurse has found no lesions present.

30. 1. There are no signs of placental abruption in this scenario.
2. The client has not had an eclamptic seizure.
3. The drop in fetal heart rate with a prolonged deceleration indicates that the cord has likely prolapsed.
4. There are no signs that this client has a succenturiate placenta.

TEST-TAKING HINT: Prolonged decelerations are caused by cord compression. A precipitous drop in the fetal heart baseline for 2 minutes or more is an indirect indication that the cord is being compressed, resulting in decreased oxygenation to the fetus. It is essential for the healthcare team to confirm or rule out a prolapsed cord and implement emergency measures as appropriate. These include a vaginal exam to manually press the fetal head back into the uterus off the cord, maternal Trendelenburg position, oxygen administration by rebreather mask at 10 L/min, and others.

31. Answers 1, 3, and 4 are correct.
1. The first action the nurse should take is to place the client in the knee-chest, or Trendelenburg position.
2. The nurse should assess the fetal heart rate but not by palpating the cord. Palpation can cause cord spasm. The EFM or Doppler should be used.
3. Oxygen should be administered.
4. The primary healthcare provider should be notified immediately.

TEST-TAKING HINT: The pressure of the fetal head on the prolapsed cord can rapidly result in fetal death by occlusion of the umbilical cord vessels. Palpation of the umbilical cord can cause cord spasm, further reducing available oxygen to the fetus. Therefore, the nurse must act quickly to relieve the pressure on the cord while avoiding cord manipulation. Actions that can take pressure off the cord include placing the client in the Trendelenburg position and pushing the fetal head off the cord with a gloved hand, or filling the bladder with sterile water to assist in lifting the fetal head from the cord. This situation is an obstetric emergency. Many helping hands are required for the best outcome.

32. Answers 1, 2, and 5 are correct.
1. When a baby is in the breech presentation, there is increased risk of prolapsed cord because the presenting part may not fully block the cervical opening.
2. The presenting part is floating, which increases the risk of prolapsed cord

because once again, even though the baby is in vertex presentation, it is at –3 station, leaving the cervical opening unblocked.

3. With a decreased quantity of amniotic fluid (oligohydramnios) there a decreased risk of prolapsed cord.
4. Dilation of 2 cm is not a situation that is at high risk for prolapsed cord. The cord is not likely to slip through such a small opening.
5. **When a baby is in the transverse lie, there is increased risk for prolapsed cord for the same reason as in the other 2 correct answers: the cervical opening is not blocked.**

TEST-TAKING HINT: In medicine, the word "prolapse" means something that slips down or falls out of place. An umbilical cord that slips down into the birth canal and protrudes beside or ahead of the presenting part of the fetus is called a "prolapsed cord." The presenting part then compresses the cord, preventing the fetus from being oxygenated. Once the membranes have ruptured, there are several situations that can increase the possibility of cord prolapse. These situations include malpresentations such as breech and shoulder presentations. A shoulder presentation is the same as a transverse lie. Additional situations that are at high risk for cord prolapse are polyhydramnios (high amounts of amniotic fluid), premature rupture of membranes (rupture of membranes before labor has started, when the fetus might not be engaged in the pelvis enough to block the cervix), and negative fetal stations.

33.
1. Although the blood glucose of a client with diabetes is important, it can wait. This client has gestational diabetes (GDM) so she doesn't likely need insulin.
2. Although the vaginal blood loss assessment of a client who has had a spontaneous abortion is important, it is usually minimal. This client is not actively miscarrying, but is recovering. She can wait. There is nothing in the question to suggest her bleeding is more than normal.
3. It is important to assess the patellar reflexes of a client with pre-eclampsia, but in pre-eclampsia without severe features, that action can wait.
4. **The priority action for this nurse is to assess the fetal heart rate of a client whose membranes have just ruptured. The nurse is assessing for prolapsed cord, which is an obstetric emergency.**

TEST-TAKING HINT: Identifying the priority action is the most difficult thing that nurses must do. The nurse must determine which of the situations is most life threatening. If the client with ruptured membranes has a prolapsed cord, it could be life threatening to the fetus. That assessment is urgent. None of the other situations, as presented in the question, is life threatening to either the mother or the fetus. The best answer relates to the finding that may require an immediate intervention.

34.
1. Prolonged labor is not associated with cocaine use. The opposite is more often seen: precipitous (rapid) labor.
2. Prolapsed cord is not specifically associated with cocaine use.
3. **Placental abruption is associated with cocaine use (Forray & Foster, 2015).**
4. Retained placenta is not specifically associated with cocaine use.

TEST-TAKING HINT: Crack cocaine is a powerful vasoconstrictive agent. Placental abruption, when the placenta detaches from the decidual lining of the uterus, is of particular concern. It is thought to occur because of the hypertensive and vasoconstrictive effect of cocaine, which causes disruption in the placental adherence to the uterine wall. Premature rupture of membranes is another side effect of cocaine (Forray & Foster, 2015).

35.
1. It is inappropriate to discourage a laboring client from taking pain medication simply because she has a dependence on drugs.
2. **The nurse should notify the primary healthcare provider of the client's request.**
3. Substance abuse is not a contraindication for analgesic medication in labor.
4. Although the client may benefit from labor breathing, she has requested pain medication and that request should be acted upon.

TEST-TAKING HINT: The nurse should be aware of two important facts: Pain is the fifth vital sign as identified by The Joint Commission (TJC), and actions must be taken to reduce the pain of those with drug dependence in the same manner that the pain of clients without drug dependence is managed. Although it is strongly discouraged for clients to take illicit drugs when pregnant, the nurse must maintain a caring philosophy and provide unbiased care to drug-dependent clients.

36. **1. This fetus is at high risk for the development of late decelerations.**
   2. Based on the scenario, neither mother nor fetus is at high risk for hyperthermia.
   3. Based on the scenario, neither mother nor fetus is at high risk for hypertension.
   4. Early decelerations are normal. They are usually seen during the first stage of labor.

TEST-TAKING HINT: The test taker must attend to all important information in the question. The gestational age of this fetus is 42 weeks. The baby and placenta, therefore, are both postdates. Placental function usually deteriorates after 40 weeks' gestation as a result of normal placental calcification at term. As such, the nurse should monitor this client carefully for signs of inadequate fetal oxygenation as evidenced by late decelerations.

37. 1. The client does have a legal right not to sign the form. To badger her about her decision is inappropriate.
   2. Practitioners who perform surgery on a client who has refused to sign a consent form can be arrested for assault and battery.
   3. It is inappropriate to scare a client into submission.
   4. At this point the appropriate action for the nurse to take is to continue providing labor support. If accepted, emergency interventions, like providing oxygen by face mask and repositioning the client, would also be indicated.

TEST-TAKING HINT: If the client's primary healthcare provider is convinced that surgery is the only appropriate intervention, a court order may be sought to mandate the client to accept surgery. The nurse's role at this point, however, is to provide the client with care in a nonthreatening, compassionate manner. The nurse must acknowledge and accept the client's legal right to refuse the surgery. Careful documentation is always important, but even more so in a situation like this, where a bad outcome is possible due to a client's refusal of care. Documenting specific words used by medical staff to explain the risk, and those used by the client in her refusal for care, is recommended.

38. 1. Increasing the IV rate is appropriate, but it is not the first action that should be taken.
   2. Applying oxygen via face mask is appropriate, but it is not the first action that should be taken.
   3. Repositioning the client is the first action that should be taken.
   4. Although the decelerations should be reported to the healthcare practitioner, this is not the first action that should be taken.

TEST-TAKING HINT: The nurse must fully understand the etiology of the decelerations. Variable decelerations—decelerations that look like a "V" or an extended "U" and that occur irrespective of the timing of contractions—occur as a result of umbilical cord compression. It is possible, therefore, that if the mother is positioned differently, the pressure on the cord will be shifted and the decelerations will resolve. If the first position change does not resolve the problem, the nurse should try additional position changes. It is also important for the nurse to do all that he or she can to resolve the problem—by administering oxygen and increasing the IV drip rate—before calling the physician. The combined information can be helpful to the provider in determining next steps for care.

39. 1. This monitor tracing shows a variable fetal heart baseline. This is a tracing of a well-oxygenated fetus.
   2. This monitor tracing shows a variable fetal heart baseline with early decelerations. Early decelerations are related to head compression. This is a normal finding during first stage labor and is considered a vagal response to head compression.
   3. This monitor tracing shows a fetal heart baseline with minimal variability and late decelerations. These decelerations are related to uteroplacental insufficiency.
   4. This monitor tracing shows a variable fetal heart baseline with accelerations. This depicts a well-oxygenated fetus.

TEST-TAKING HINT: A tracing that depicts decelerations that begin late in a contraction and return to baseline well past the time that the contraction ends are called late decelerations. Late decelerations are related to poor uteroplacental blood flow (Pillarisetty & Bragg, 2020).

40. 1. This client is only 4 cm dilated. Unless the late decelerations resolve, completion of stage 1 is not a priority.
   2. The nurse's goal at this point must be the delivery of a healthy baby.
   3. Because late decelerations and minimal variability are present, pain management is not a priority at this time.
   4. The nurse has no control over vaginal lacerations.

TEST-TAKING HINT: Nursing goals may change repeatedly during a client's labor. The nurse must assess the client's progress in relation to the health and well-being of both the mother and the fetus. As long as the fetus is responding well, the nurse's focus should relate to maternal comfort and care. Once fetal compromise is noted, however, nursing priorities often shift to more specific goals such as "improve fetal oxygenation."

41. 1. Diminished variability and late decelerations are an indication of fetal acidosis.
2. Although variable decelerations can be related to fetal descent during pushing, there is nothing in this question that indicates the mother is pushing in second stage.
3. The contractions described in the scenario (variable decelerations) result from cord compression.
4. Decelerations related to uteroplacental insufficiency (late decelerations) are spoon-shaped contractions that begin late in the contraction (after the peak), and return to baseline after the contraction ends.

TEST-TAKING HINT: Fetal heart rate tracings reflect the response of the fetal central nervous system to intrauterine hypoxia. The test taker should first assess what is reassuring about this fetal monitor tracing as described. Moderate variability and a baseline rate of 120 are both reassuring. They indicate the fetus has adequate oxygenation. This rules out answer #1, "metabolic acidosis." The description of the decelerations as (a) V-shaped, and (b) occurring in both the presence and absence of contractions indicates that these are variable decelerations which result from cord compression. They are not necessarily worrisome if combined with reassuring factors.

42. 1. Although breathing with contractions is important, it will make no difference for a sinusoidal pattern.
2. Sinusoidal patterns are related to Rh isoimmunization, fetal anemia, severe fetal hypoxia, or a chronic fetal bleed. They also may occur transiently as a result of intravenous narcotic administration for pain. Because this client has just been admitted, medication administration is not a likely cause and a more serious condition could be the cause. The primary healthcare provider must be notified immediately.
3. Increasing the intravenous fluid rate will not help to resolve any of these severe fetal problems.
4. There is no indication in the scenario that this client is fully dilated.

TEST-TAKING HINT: Sinusoidal fetal heart patterns exhibit no variability and have a uniform wave-like pattern somewhat like a crawling snake. The nurse would see no periods when the heart rate appears normal. The fetus is in imminent danger. The primary healthcare provider must be notified immediately so that appropriate interventions can begin. The client will most likely need to have a stat cesarean section.

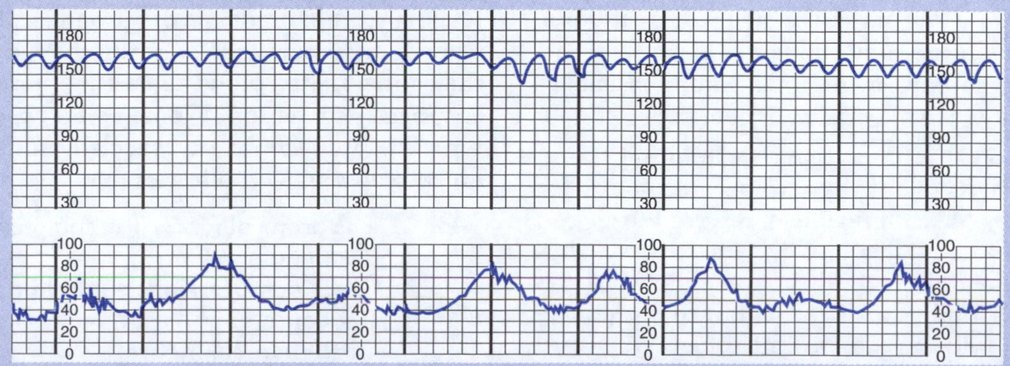

43. 1. The normal $PaCO_2$ of an adult is 35 to 45 mm Hg, so there is no need to intervene if the maternal $PaCO_2$ is 40 mm Hg.
2. Although the alpha-fetoprotein level is well above normal, high levels of AFP are indicative of spina bifida, not of an acute problem. The AFP is a prenatal finding that would not impact labor and delivery care at this point.
3. Fetal heart accelerations, especially when they occur during contractions, are indicative of fetal well-being.
4. Recurrent late decelerations with minimal variability indicate a fetus who is struggling to maintain adequate oxygenation and is at risk of metabolic acidosis. The primary healthcare provider must be notified immediately and the nurse must implement appropriate interventions such as administering oxygen, an intravenous bolus of lactated ringer's solution, and changing the maternal position immediately.

TEST-TAKING HINT: The test taker must read all four responses before choosing the best one. Although answer 2 includes a value that is not normal, it does not describe a labor and delivery situation. In addition, no medical intervention will change this value. A fetal heart rate pattern of recurrent late decelerations and minimal variability, however, is of immediate concern, and immediate medical interventions are indicated (Turner et al., 2020). By the time the nurse assesses and reports this to the primary healthcare provider, a period of at least 30 minutes has often occurred during which the nurse determines that this is not just a transient finding.

44. 1. Blood pressure assessment is important, but it is not the priority action.
2. FHR assessment is important, but it is not the priority action.
3. The nurse's priority action is to administer oxygen, which will treat both the mother and the fetus.
4. It is appropriate to stop the infusion, but that is not the priority action.

TEST-TAKING HINT: This client is exhibiting the classic signs of anaphylactoid syndrome of pregnancy (ASP), previously referred to as amniotic fluid embolism (AFE). The name change was recommended recently because the word "embolism" implies a blockage, but the response is more of a widespread, proinflammatory anaphylactic response to amniotic fluid in the mother's bloodstream. The condition can be recognized by four cardinal findings: respiratory distress, altered mental status, hypotension, and disseminated intravascular coagulation (DIC) (Barnhart & Rosenbaum, 2019). As part of the anaphylactic response to amniotic fluid, the client can develop pulmonary edema, where the alveoli are flooded and cannot take in oxygen or eliminate carbon dioxide effectively.

Fortunately, this is a very rare event. Risk factors can include maternal age over 35, pre-eclampsia, polyhydramnios, and induction, although the condition is still an enigma. When ASP occurs, the baby's health is secondary because the mother is in a life-threatening situation.

The test taker should remember that the answer to a "highest priority" question is most often related to the first step of Maslow's hierarchy of needs—basic survival. In this question, the administration of oxygen is required for survival. The blood pressure assessment, fetal heart rate assessment, and discontinuation of the oxytocin are important, but they are not initial interventions for survival. The nurse must apply oxygen and call a code immediately, since the client is at risk of a cardiopulmonary arrest. The other assessments can occur while the code team is on the way and can be shared in a bedside report.

45. 1. Infection is not directly related to the presence of ASP.
2. Because ASP begins in the lungs, the appropriate nursing care outcome is that the client survives and is breathing normally at discharge.
3. Gastrointestinal function is not related to the presence of ASP.
4. Urinary function is not related to the presence of ASP.

TEST-TAKING HINT: ASP is an enigma, but the physiology is thought to be triggered when a small amount of amniotic fluid seeps into the mother's bloodstream. The fluid may contain meconium or other foreign material such as fetal hair, which reduces the prognosis for a good outcome. Once entering the lungs, the contaminated blood causes an immediate anaphylactic reaction. Women who experience forceful, rapid labors are especially at risk for this life-threatening complication.

46. 1. The protocol for cardiac compression and breath ratio is 30 to 2.
2. Chest compressions should be delivered at a depth of at least 2 inches and no more than 2.4 inches.
3. Because of the size of the gravid uterus, the hands should be placed slightly higher

than the lower 1/2 of the sternum when delivering cardiac compressions. For a nonpregnant client, the hands are placed on the lower 1/2 of the sternum.
4. Each breath should be delivered over a 1-second time frame.

TEST-TAKING HINT: The American Heart Association frequently revises cardiopulmonary resuscitation (CPR) guidelines. The responses above reflect the 2015 guidelines. The test taker should be familiar with current protocols. In addition to the responses above, it is important for the rescuer to perform manual displacement of the uterus toward the left to decrease the compression of the gravid uterus on the aorta and vena cava (AHA, 2015, p. S502).

47. 1. **A fetal heart rate check is the appropriate assessment.**
2. Cervical dilation is not important at this time.
3. The white blood cell count is unrelated to the clinical situation.
4. Maternal lung sounds are unrelated to the clinical situation.

TEST-TAKING HINT: The clinical scenario is indicative of a placental abruption. Because the only oxygenation available to the fetus is via the placenta, the appropriate action by the nurse at this time is to determine the survival and well-being of the fetus. The nurse should also assess the client's pulse rate and blood pressure. An elevated maternal pulse rate and hypotension are indicative of marked blood loss. Bleeding is not always visible in the vagina, and may sometimes remain between the placenta and the uterus, causing a board-like uterus.

48. 1. Hypertension is not related to the diagnosis of placenta accreta.
2. **The nurse would expect the client to hemorrhage.**
3. Bradycardia is not related to the diagnosis of placenta accreta.
4. Hyperthermia is not related to the diagnosis of placenta accreta.

TEST-TAKING HINT: A placenta accreta is present when the placenta grows too deeply into the uterine wall and does not detach after the birth. In the most common type of placental attachment disorder the placenta does not penetrate the uterine muscle. Other types include (a) placenta increta, when the placenta attaches even deeper into the uterine wall, including the uterine muscle; and, the most serious, (b) placenta percreta, where the placenta penetrates through the uterus and attaches to another organ such as the maternal bladder. If undiagnosed during the pregnancy, the diagnosis is made after delivery of the baby, when the placenta does not detach from the uterus. As a result, the uterus is unable to contract adequately to prevent bleeding, and hemorrhage results. Most of these issues are discovered through ultrasounds during the prenatal period and the clients are delivered by scheduled cesarean section. It is not uncommon for a hysterectomy to also be necessary to save the client's life.

49. 1. Although dilation is progressing, the station is unchanged. The baby, therefore, is not descending into the birth canal. The nurse cannot conclude that the labor is progressing well.
2. **Because the presenting part is not descending into the birth canal, the nurse can logically conclude that the baby may be macrosomic.**
3. There is no sign of fetal intolerance of labor in this scenario.
4. This client is a multigravida. Since she was most recently 8 cm, she will likely be pushing within 15 to 20 minutes and be delivered within an hour.

TEST-TAKING HINT: The test taker must carefully analyze the results of the three vaginal examinations. The fetal heart rate is virtually unchanged: the rate is within normal limits and the variability is normal. This is all very reassuring and shows the fetus is tolerating labor very well. The dilation and effacement are changing, but the lack of progressive descent of the presenting part is unexpected. When babies are too big to fit through a client's pelvis, they fail to descend. That is the conclusion that the nurse should make from the findings.

50. 1. Cervical dilation is not related to the data in the scenario.
2. Cervical effacement is not related to the data in the scenario.
3. **A high station is consistent with the data in the scenario.**
4. Contraction frequency is not related to the data in the scenario.

TEST-TAKING HINT: The dimensions noted in the stem are consistent with a diagnosis of cephalopelvic disproportion because the anterior–posterior diameter of the pelvis (obstetric conjugate) is smaller than the diameter of the baby's head (suboccipitobregmatic). When the fetal head is larger than the maternal pelvis, the baby is unable to descend.

51. 1. The normal time frame for the third stage of labor is between 5 and 30 minutes.
2. This is a vague description of both recurrent early decelerations and recurrent variable decelerations. There is too much missing information such as the FHR, variability, etc., to call it an emergency as described.
3. A three-vessel umbilical cord is normal.
4. **Shoulder dystocia is an obstetric emergency.**

TEST-TAKING HINT: "Dystocia" means "difficult" or "obstructed delivery." A shoulder dystocia, therefore, refers to difficulty in delivering a baby's shoulders. This is an obstetric emergency because the dystocia occurs in the middle of the delivery when the head has been delivered but the shoulders remain wedged in the pelvis. The most common complications are related to nerve palsies from traction placed on the baby's head in attempts to deliver the shoulder. In addition, the baby's life is threatened because the baby is unable to breathe and umbilical cord flow is often dramatically reduced during this phase of the delivery.

52. 1. Intravenous oxytocin administration is inappropriate. This would cause the uterus to contract markedly but would not assist with the delivery of the fetal shoulders.
2. **Flexing the client's hips sharply toward her abdomen, called the McRobert's maneuver, is appropriate.**
3. Oxygen administration will not assist with the delivery of the fetal shoulders.
4. Fundal pressure is inappropriate and should never be done during a delivery.

TEST-TAKING HINT: Flexing the client's hips sharply toward her abdomen increases the diameter of the pelvic outlet and straightens the pelvic curve, both of which often enable the primary healthcare provider to successfully deliver the baby. It is especially important to note that fundal pressure at the top of the uterus is contraindicated because it may actually worsen the problem by wedging the shoulders against the pubic bone, keeping them from rotating. Suprapubic pressure, on the other hand, is often helpful in assisting with the delivery by dislodging the shoulder from behind the pubic bone. The nurse must know the difference.

53. 1. Although infection can occur with prolonged rupture of the membranes, it is not a priority diagnosis at this time because the membranes were just ruptured.
2. **Green amniotic fluid in the presence of recurrent late decelerations suggests fetal stress due to intrauterine hypoxia.**
3. Vaginal irritation from meconium-stained fluid is not a risk.
4. There is little to no risk to the mother from rupturing the membranes.

TEST-TAKING HINT: Late decelerations are related to poor uteroplacental blood flow and metabolic acidosis. As a result of the poor uteroplacental exchange, the fetus is being poorly oxygenated. The fetal anal sphincter relaxes when the body is hypoxic and meconium is expelled in utero. Amniotic fluid becomes green tinged in the presence of meconium. The nurse, therefore, must conclude that the fetus is at high risk for injury related to intrauterine hypoxia, and a newborn resuscitation team should be called to attend to the baby at delivery.

54. 1. It is inappropriate to perform amnioinfusion when a placental abruption has occurred.
2. **It would be appropriate for a primary healthcare provider to order an amnioinfusion when a client's amniotic fluid is meconium stained.**
3. Amnioinfusion would increase the fluid volume even more if it were performed when polyhydramnios is evident.
4. Late decelerations, with no other finding, would not warrant amnioinfusion. A fetus with recurrent late decelerations will often need to be delivered by cesarean section, and delaying the delivery to begin an amnioinfusion is unwarranted.

TEST-TAKING HINT: Amnioinfusion is the instillation of sterile fluid into the uterine cavity through a sterile tubing device referred to as an intrauterine pressure catheter (IUPC). Its use is warranted to promote fetal well-being in certain situations where the client is laboring. The IUPC is inserted into the uterus through the vagina. It may be used to measure the actual strength of the contractions in mm Hg (millimeters of mercury) or additionally, to dilute the concentration of meconium in the amniotic fluid. Thinning the concentration of meconium in the amniotic fluid is thought to decrease the potential for the baby to aspirate meconium below the vocal cords and to improve Apgar scores (Yellayi et al., 2017).

55. 1. The color of the amniotic fluid will change. This is not a critical assessment, however.
2. Maternal blood pressure should be monitored carefully throughout labor. The assessment is not directly related to the amnioinfusion, however.

3. The effacement of the cervix should be monitored carefully throughout labor. The assessment is not directly related to the amnioinfusion, however.
4. **The uterine resting tone should be carefully monitored with an intrauterine pressure catheter (IUPC) during amnioinfusion.**

TEST-TAKING HINT: Because fluid is being continuously instilled into the uterine cavity, there is potential for the fluid to overload the space. As a result, the uterine resting tone will increase dramatically with the potential that the uterus could rupture. The fluid is expected to flow out from within the uterus, through the vagina, and onto towels and a waterproof cover on the client's labor bed. It is critically important, therefore, that the nurse monitor the resting tone frequently throughout the procedure. In addition, the nurse must weigh and document the amount of water coming out of the vagina onto the towels to confirm that fluid is not being retained within the uterus.

56. 1. This describes a third-degree laceration, which includes musculature surrounding the anus and may include the anal sphincter.
2. This does not describe a fourth-degree laceration. A fourth-degree laceration extends down, through the rectal sphincter and into the rectum, not up to the urethra.
3. **A fourth-degree laceration extends through the rectal sphincter into the rectum.**
4. This does not describe a fourth-degree laceration.

TEST-TAKING HINT: One of the many complications that can occur with episiotomy and the delivery of a macrosomic baby is a perineal laceration (a tear) or an extension of the episiotomy. If the laceration is extensive and it extends through the rectal sphincter and anus into the rectal mucosa, it is defined as a fourth degree. As a result, this client is at high risk for the development of a vaginal-rectal fistula. First-, second-, third-, and fourth-degree tears describe the depth of tears that occur around the perineum, not the urethra or clitoris.

57. 1. A hematocrit of 48% is indicative of hemoconcentration, not of HELLP syndrome.
2. Abnormal potassium levels are not related to HELLP syndrome.
3. **Low platelets are consistent with the diagnosis of HELLP syndrome.**
4. Abnormal sodium levels are not related to HELLP syndrome.

TEST-TAKING HINT: HELLP is the acronym for a serious complication of pregnancy and labor and delivery. The letters represent the following information: H, hemolysis; EL, elevated liver enzymes; LP, low platelets. When a client has HELLP syndrome, the nurse would, therefore, expect to see low hemoglobin and hematocrit levels, high liver enzymes (aspartate aminotransferase [AST] and alanine aminotransferase [ALT] levels), and low platelets, as seen in the scenario.

58. 1. **The nurse must have calcium gluconate immediately available.**
2. Morphine sulfate should not be in the client's room. It is a controlled substance.
3. Narcan does not have to be in the client's room.
4. Oxytocin should not be in the client's room. There is no indication in the stem that the client is about to deliver and might need oxytocin after the birth. To avoid inadvertent administration of oxytocin, only those medications specifically indicated for the client should be in the client's room.

TEST-TAKING HINT: Calcium gluconate is the antidote for magnesium sulfate toxicity. It is very important for the nurse to remember that, if needed, calcium gluconate must be administered very slowly, over at least 3 minutes. If calcium gluconate is administered rapidly, the client may experience sudden convulsions.

59. Answers 2 and 3 are correct.
1. A client who has pre-eclampsia with severe features could exhibit symptoms of 3+ pitting edema without the addition of HELLP syndrome.
2. **Petechiae may develop when a client is thrombocytopenic, one of the signs of HELLP syndrome.**
3. **Hyperbilirubinemia develops when red blood cells are hemolyzed (broken down), one of the changes that may develop as a result of liver necrosis. Jaundice is a symptom of hyperbilirubinemia.**
4. Reflexes of 4+ are consistent with a diagnosis of pre-eclampsia with severe features and may be present without the addition of HELLP syndrome.

5. Elevated specific gravity is consistent with a diagnosis of pre-eclampsia with severe features and may be present without the addition of HELLP syndrome.

TEST-TAKING HINT: The test taker must be able to discriminate between symptoms of severe pre-eclampsia and HELLP syndrome. Pre-eclampsia is a high-risk condition of pregnancy in which the kidneys are primarily affected. The addition of HELLP syndrome indicates the liver is also affected. If the nurse remembers what each of the letters in HELLP stands for and the body system most likely to be involved, the nurse can determine which of the responses is correct.

60. 1. Hyperreflexia is seen in pre-eclampsia with severe features. The magnesium sulfate is being administered to depress the hyperreflexia.
2. Thirty mL/hr is a minimally acceptable urinary output. Generally, this is calculated over a 2-hour timeframe. If the output drops below 30 mL/hr it should be reported.
3. A respiratory rate of 16 rpm is within normal limits.
4. **A serum magnesium level of 10 mg/dL is dangerously high. The magnesium sulfate should be turned off and the primary healthcare provider should be notified immediately. The client's respiratory rate should be counted, as the client is at high risk of respiratory depression. A bag and mask should be available if needed before the calcium gluconate antidote can be administered or before it takes effect.**

TEST-TAKING HINT: When magnesium sulfate is being administered, the nurse should monitor the client for adverse side effects including respiratory depression, oliguria, and depressed reflexes. Because a precise therapeutic level of magnesium sulfate is unknown, providers generally target a level between 4.8 and 8.4 mg/dL (4–7 mEq/L) to prevent eclamptic seizures (Berg et al., 2013). This target would be lower, of course, for clients with kidney disease, in which magnesium sulfate is not eliminated efficiently and can rise to very toxic levels as a result. When the magnesium level is above 9.6 mg/dL (>7 mEq/L), toxic effects can be seen (Berg et al., 2013) and the client's life may be at risk.

61. 1. Oxytocin is safe to administer if a client has pre-eclampsia. However, a client with a blood pressure of this magnitude is at risk of a stroke from a hypertensive crisis.
2. The frequency is within normal limits.
3. **The duration of the contractions is prolonged. We don't know how frequently the contractions are coming, but each one is lasting 2 minutes and 10 seconds. This is called a tetanic contraction. The baby is deprived of oxygen through most of the contraction, since there is no oxygen-rich blood flow to the intervillous space for placental uptake during the peak of this long contraction.**
4. The FHR is within normal limits.

TEST-TAKING HINT: A contraction that lasts longer than 90 seconds is called a tetanic contraction and can harm the fetus. Although we are not given the frequency of the contractions in the stem, a duration of 2 minutes per contraction is too long. It deprives the fetus of access to placental oxygen, no matter how frequent or infrequent the contractions might be. Not only is this client receiving oxytocin, but she is also pre-eclamptic. Pre-eclampsia is a vasoconstrictive disease state. Any client with a systolic blood pressure reading greater than or equal to 160 mm Hg and/or a diastolic greater than or equal to 110 is experiencing a hypertensive crisis. The standard of care is to treat her with appropriate medications within 30 to 60 minutes of the first hypertensive reading (ACOG, 2020c). Magnesium sulfate is not administered to treat hypertension but to prevent seizures (eclampsia). For this client, since she's being induced at 38 weeks and has magnesium sulfate infusing, the likelihood of poor placental perfusion is already high. When the contraction duration is also prolonged, the fetus is at high risk of becoming hypoxic, since fetal oxygen reserves are no doubt less than ideal.

62. 1. **This client's prolonged PT and PTT put her at high risk of disseminated intravascular coagulation (DIC). The nurse should watch for pink-tinged urine.**
2. Early decelerations are noted normally during the first stage of labor. They are benign and unrelated to deviations in PT and PTT.
3. The reflex changes are unrelated to the lab deviations.
4. The blood pressure is consistent with pre-eclampsia without severe features.

TEST-TAKING HINT: Disseminated intravascular coagulation (DIC) is a pathologic disorder of the finely balanced blood-clotting process. Clotting factors become abnormally active and form small blood clots throughout the body, which block smaller blood vessels. Some experts

have described this to the author as "circulatory tapioca pudding." If unchecked, the multitude of tiny blood clots eventually leads to multiple organ dysfunction due to reduced blood flow and reduced organ oxygenation. Because platelets and clotting factors are depleted, excessive bleeding often occurs. The nurse must be familiar with the normal range and implications of standard blood tests like PT and PTT, remembering that they measure the length of time the client's blood takes to form a clot. Even if the nurse did not know that clients who are diagnosed with HELLP syndrome are at high risk for DIC, he or she should know that clients with prolonged PT and PTT times are at high risk for spontaneous bleeds because their blood is unable to form clots appropriately, when needed.

63. 1. Eclamptic clients should be monitored for proteinuria, not for the presence of ketones.
2. The side rails of an eclamptic client's bed should be padded.
3. Eclamptic clients should be kept in a low-stimulation environment.
4. There is no rationale for placing the head of an eclamptic client's bed in high-Fowler's position.

TEST-TAKING HINT: Eclamptic clients have had at least one seizure. To protect them from injury during any potential subsequent seizures, the nurse should pad the headboard and the side rails of the client's bed.

64. 1. The nurse would expect to see an elevated serum creatinine level, not a decreased level.
2. The nurse would expect to see a low RBC count, not an elevated one.
3. The nurse would expect to see an elevated aspartate aminotransferase (AST) level, not a decreased one.
4. The nurse would expect to see an elevated alanine aminotransaminase (ALT).

TEST-TAKING HINT: This is a challenging, critical thinking question. A client may have pre-eclampsia alone, HELLP syndrome alone, or both of them together. This client is exhibiting signs of HELLP syndrome (low platelets and hemolysis). HELLP syndrome is a life-threatening liver disorder considered to be a type of pre-eclampsia with severe features. With hemolysis, the nurse would expect to see a drop in the RBC count, and with a damaged liver, elevated liver function tests such as aspartate aminotransferase (AST) and alanine aminotransaminase (ALT).

The distinguishing feature of HELLP syndrome is that the client's liver is affected. This differs from pre-eclampsia without HELLP, in which the client's kidneys are primarily affected. Pre-eclamptic clients without HELLP have poor renal function, including elevated serum creatinine levels. If the pre-eclamptic client develops HELLP syndrome additionally, her liver function tests reveal this complication.

65. 1. Completely depressed patellar reflexes are a sign of magnesium sulfate toxicity. This is not an expected outcome.
2. A normal urinary output is important, but it is not an expected outcome related to magnesium sulfate administration.
3. A normal respiratory rate is important, but it is not an expected outcome related to magnesium sulfate administration.
4. The absence of seizures is an expected outcome related to magnesium sulfate administration.

TEST-TAKING HINT: Magnesium sulfate is ordered for pre-eclamptic clients as a prophylactic measure to prevent eclamptic seizures. An expected outcome of its administration, therefore, is that the client will not have seizures. Convulsive seizures are not only dangerous for the mother, but also for the fetus. The uterus contracts during a seizure, preventing adequate oxygen uptake by the placenta. Researchers have noted that the fetal heart rate slows during and for up to 20 minutes after a maternal convulsion, suggestive of fetal hypoxia. A cesarean section is not always indicated in response to eclampsia, but when it is, the recommendation is to allow the fetus to recover within the uterus before it is delivered (Gill et al., 2020).

66. 1. This is a normal contraction pattern. It is not a contraindication to analgesic administration.
2. Late decelerations are indicative of uteroplacental insufficiency and indicate fetal intolerance of labor. It is inappropriate to administer a central nervous system (CNS) depressant to the mother at this time.
3. Sleeping between contractions is a normal phenomenon. It is not a contraindication to analgesic administration.
4. Hypertension is not a contraindication to analgesic administration.

TEST-TAKING HINT: Analgesics are central nervous system (CNS) depressants. They not only depress the CNS of the mother, reducing her pain, but also depress the CNS of the baby. It is inappropriate to administer a depressant to a mother whose fetus is already exhibiting

signs of labor intolerance. First, the variability of the baseline would be diminished, preventing the nurse from assessing that very important indicator of fetal well-being. And if the baby were to be delivered via cesarean section, the baby would likely be depressed and in need of resuscitation. The provider should make a decision about delivery since the fetal heart rate decelerations are showing signs of intrauterine hypoxia. This client will likely be taken to the operating room for a cesarean section. After a spinal anesthetic is inserted for surgery, she will be comfortable.

67. 1. Early decelerations are related to head compression. They would not be expected as a result of narcotic administration.
2. Late decelerations are related to uteroplacental insufficiency. They would not be expected as a result of narcotic administration.
3. Minimal variability would be expected as a result of narcotic administration.
4. Accelerations occur less often when the fetus is sleeping. The nurse would expect the incidence of accelerations to diminish as a result of narcotic administration.

TEST-TAKING HINT: A fetal scalp electrode (FSE) is a very thin, spiral wire attached directly to the fetal scalp. It measures the fetal heart rate directly, unlike the external monitoring device, which depends on a Doppler effect with sound waves. Administering a narcotic to the mother can make both the mother and fetus sleepy. As a result, the nurse can expect to see fewer accelerations and minimal variability.

68. 1. The level of pain relief is similar between the two types of anesthesia.
2. The level of placement of the needle is the same in the two types of anesthesia.
3. Epidurals do not fully sedate the motor nerves of the client. Epidural clients are capable of moving their lower extremities even when fully pain free.
4. Both epidural and spinal anesthesia clients have the potential of experiencing nausea and vomiting.

TEST-TAKING HINT: The nurse must understand the physiological differences between epidural and spinal anesthesia and analgesia. The single most important difference between epidural and spinal anesthesia is the placement of the medication. Both epidural and spinal anesthesia are injected into the caudal area below the level of the spinal cord itself. Epidural anesthesia is administered between two membranes outside the spinal cord, that run parallel to the spinal cord—the "epidural space." The epidural's main effects are on nerve roots outside the spinal canal. Epidurals block pain by providing a band of numbness, or analgesia. This is unlike spinals, which provide anesthesia—a complete lack of feeling. A spinal needle is inserted into the spinal canal itself, where it works by having direct contact with the spinal nerves. This provides a deeper intensity of anesthesia and analgesia and affects not only pain receptors, but motor nerves, as well. This is why a client with spinal anesthesia cannot move her legs until the medication wears off after surgery. Clients with spinal anesthesia are paralyzed until the anesthesia is metabolized by the body.

69. 1. Antacids are routinely administered pre-surgically to cesarean section clients.
2. Tranquilizers are not routinely administered pre-surgically to cesarean section clients.
3. Antihypertensives are not routinely administered pre-surgically to cesarean section clients.
4. Anticonvulsants are not routinely administered pre-surgically to cesarean section clients.

TEST-TAKING HINT: A pregnant woman having a cesarean section with general anesthesia is at risk of vomiting and aspirating stomach acids. The risk in pregnancy is higher than for nonpregnant individuals for primarily two reasons: (a) delayed stomach emptying due to pregnancy hormones, and (b) the pressure of the enlarged uterus on the stomach. To decrease the acidity of the vomitus in case of aspiration, pregnant women are routinely given antacids before surgery.

70. An X will be placed on the cricoid cartilage.

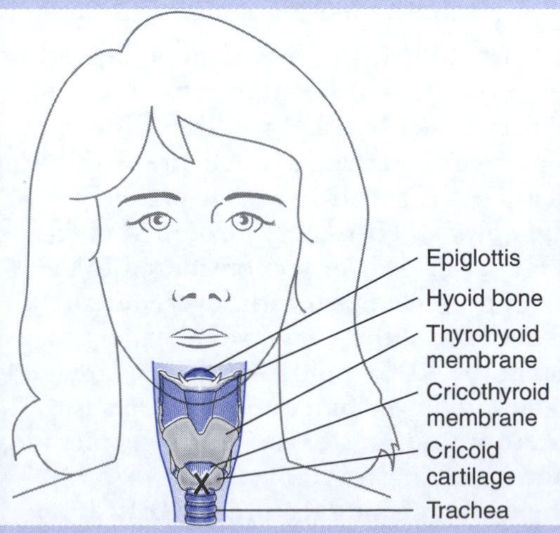

TEST-TAKING HINT: To locate the cricoid cartilage, the nurse should find the thyroid prominence, which is the largest bulge in the middle of the front of the neck. While staying in the midline, the nurse should then move the fingers lightly on the skin downward toward the chest until a gully or notch is felt. The next horizontal projection is the cricoid cartilage. With the thumb on one side of the cartilage and the index finger on the other side of the cartilage, the nurse should press firmly toward the client's back and keep pressing until the anesthesia provider advises the nurse to let go. This action presses the cricoid against the esophagus, preventing regurgitation of the stomach contents during endotracheal insertion.

71. 1. Anti-embolic stockings (sometimes called anti-embolic boots) are often applied during and after a cesarean section. However, their application is unrelated to the client's anxiety.

2. The nurse should explain all procedures slowly and carefully. An emergency cesarean section is often very traumatic for a client who had anticipated a vaginal birth. She worries not only about her own safety and the threat of surgery, but also about the baby's survival. As a result, she may not be able to understand everything that is said at the time, and needs calm reassurance as much as possible.

3. Antacid administration is warranted in this situation but is unrelated to the client's anxiety.

4. The fetal heart and maternal vital signs should be carefully monitored, but they are unrelated to the client's anxiety.

TEST-TAKING HINT: The test taker must attend to the content of each question. All of the responses are appropriate in relation to cesarean deliveries, but only response 2 is related to the client's anxiety.

72. 1. A vaginal delivery can be performed with no anesthesia.

2. A postdates pregnancy is not an absolute indication for a cesarean delivery.

3. An occiput posterior position is not an indication for a cesarean delivery.

4. The presence of vertical incisions in the uterine wall is an absolute indication for a cesarean delivery.

TEST-TAKING HINT: A previous vertical uterine incision is an absolute indicator for future cesarean delivery. The difference between a TOLAC and a VBAC is one of timing. The term TOLAC indicates "Trial Of Labor After Cesarean." The client who has had one or more cesarean sections and is laboring with hopes of having a vaginal delivery is a having a TOLAC. Once she gives birth vaginally, she has had a VBAC—a "Vaginal Birth After Cesarean."

The decision to allow a TOLAC is based on the location of the woman's previous cesarean incision. Muscle tissue that contracts during labor is located in the fundal, or top region, of the uterus. A vertical incision into the uterus cuts through fundal tissue. The scar that forms from the incision is nonelastic, putting the client at risk of uterine rupture as the contracting tissue around the scar exerts tremendous pull against it. In contrast to this, the scar of the Pfannensteil, or standard "bikini cut" incision in the lower uterine segment is pulled up and supported by the surrounding tissues during labor, much like one gathers up a sock before putting it on. A trial of labor is possible in this situation, as the scar is less likely to rupture.

It is important to note that the type of incision used previously to open the *skin* is not necessarily the type of incision used to open the *uterus*. Some clients may have a vertical *skin* incision and a low transverse Pfannensteil (bikini) *uterine* incision just above the pubic bone, or vice versa. At one time, many physicians also encouraged clients who had had low transverse (Pfannenstiel) incisions into the uterus to have all subsequent children delivered via cesarean section. However, current medical opinion holds that multiple cesarean sections bring more risks such as placenta previa and placenta accreta, than the risk of uterine rupture that a VBAC can bring. As such, TOLAC is currently encouraged if the woman's obstetrical history supports it. The topic of placenta previa risk related to cesarean births is too large to completely cover here, but the nurse is encouraged to explore the topic for further information.

73. 1. A history of drug addiction is not a contraindication for spinal anesthesia.

2. An allergy to morphine is not a contraindication for spinal anesthesia.

3. Adolescence is not a contraindication for spinal anesthesia.

4. A history of scoliosis surgery is a contraindication for spinal anesthesia.

TEST-TAKING HINT: Scoliosis is a defect in the growth of the thoracic and lumbar spine. The client's spinal surgery was performed on the vertebrae of the spinal column. As such, it is not possible to administer regional anesthesia.

74. **The test taker should have drawn an episiotomy that is about 45° from the midline. The direction in which the episiotomy is performed is usually dependent upon whether the practitioner is left-handed or right-handed.**

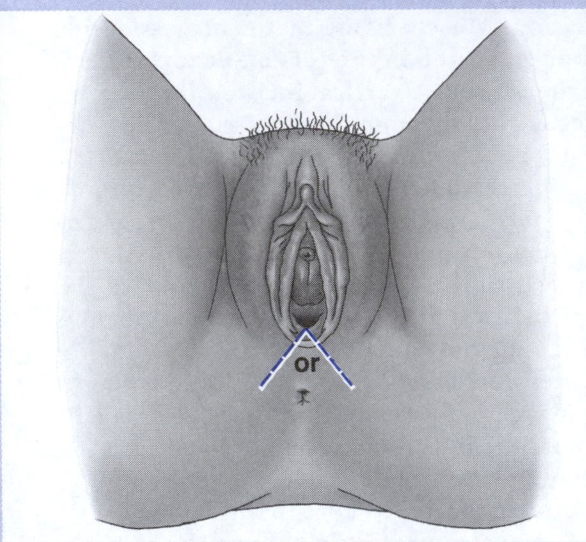

TEST-TAKING HINT: Although the nurse does not perform the episiotomy, the nurse is responsible for knowing the type of episiotomy that was performed, and for being aware of possible outcomes, assessments, and pain relief considerations that should be made during the postpartum period. Once the standard of care in the past, the mediolateral episiotomy is no longer performed as often in the United States as is a midline episiotomy. However, with a midline episiotomy and the birth of a macrosomic baby, the risk of possible extension toward or into the rectal sphincter (a third- or fourth-degree laceration) is possible.

75. **Answers 1 and 5 are correct.**
    1. **Cervical cerclage, a stitch encircling the cervix, does not rule out a vaginal delivery, but the cerclage must be removed by the provider before active labor begins.**
    2. This FHR is well within normal limits and the moderate variability is reassuring.
    3. It is unusual for a pregnant client to have a blood pressure of 92/60, but this does not indicate an emergency and does not warrant a bedside consultation as long as everything else is within normal limits.
    4. A fully effaced cervix is a sign of active labor. There is no indication for a bedside consultation by the primary healthcare provider unless the client is about to deliver. The answer does not state anything about that.
    5. **Active herpes simplex 2 is an absolute indicator for a cesarean delivery.**

TEST-TAKING HINT: The test taker must be able to differentiate in which circumstances a full-term, otherwise healthy client would be unable to deliver vaginally. There are a few absolute indicators for cesarean section: (a) maternal infection with active herpes simplex 2 and/or HIV/AIDS; (b) malpresentation—for example, horizontal lie and breech; (c) previous uterine surgery—e.g., myomectomy; (d) a vertical cesarean scar; (e) some fetal congenital anomalies—e.g., hydrocephalus and meningomyelocele; and (f) other physical conditions, including cervical cerclage in place, obstructive lesions such as fibroids in the lower gynecological system, and (g) complete placenta previa. The test taker should become familiar with each of these.

76.
    1. A consent for the use of forceps is not required. The general consent for vaginal delivery covers this possibility.
    2. Even when forceps are applied, the client should push only during contractions, adding to the force to push the baby out.
    3. **The FHR should always be assessed continuously in this situation with recurrent late decelerations. The FHR indicates fetal hypoxemia and possible hypoxia.**
    4. It is inappropriate for the nurse to advise the client to refuse the use of forceps.

TEST-TAKING HINT: This is an excellent example of a medically indicated use of forceps. The provider and nurse have determined that delivering this baby with forceps will effect delivery sooner than performing a cesarean section, taking into consideration the amount of time it will take to prepare for and complete a cesarean section versus the amount of time it will take to deliver the baby with forceps. The client is likely fatigued from pushing for over 2 hours, the presenting part is at the pelvic floor, and the baby is showing signs of fetal intolerance of labor. The use of forceps should result in a speedy delivery.

77. **Answers 1 and 3 are correct.**
    1. **The baby in the LSP position is in a breech presentation. Most breech babies are delivered by cesarean section.**

2. The placenta usually attaches to the posterior portion of the uterine wall.
3. **The meningomyelocele sac could easily rupture during a vaginal delivery. When a fetus has been diagnosed with the defect, a cesarean is usually performed.**
4. Maternal hepatitis B antigen positive status is not an indication for cesarean delivery.
5. The L/S ratio of 1.5:1 indicates that the baby's lung fields are not yet mature. This baby would benefit from a vaginal delivery.

TEST-TAKING HINT: Hepatitis B is a very serious viral disease, but vertical transmission rates are not significantly different between those babies who are born vaginally and those babies who are born by cesarean section. Although it is recommended that cesarean section be performed when a mother is affected by two viral illnesses—herpes simplex type 2 (only when active lesions are present) and HIV/AIDS—it is not recommended in the presence of other viral diseases. The fetus with an L/S ratio of 1.5:1 can benefit from a vaginal birth because contractions and birth cause a surge in endogenous fetal steroids and catecholamines which help to expel fetal lung fluid (Hillman et al., 2012).

78. Answers 3 and 4 are correct.
1. Asthmatic clients, although needing careful monitoring, are able to deliver via forceps.
2. It would be appropriate to deliver a baby whose position and station are ROP and +4 via forceps because the fetus is low in the pelvis.
3. **A baby in transverse lie is physically incapable of delivering vaginally and must be delivered by cesarean section.**
4. **It is not appropriate to deliver this baby with forceps for two reasons: (a) the baby is in a mentum position. The baby is not flexed, and the chin is presenting; (b) in addition, the fetus at –1 station is not engaged. Forceps are contraindicated for a fetus that is not low in the pelvis, regardless of the presenting part, even if the fetus is in the vertex position.**
5. Clients with cerebral palsy may be delivered with forceps.

TEST-TAKING HINT: It is unsafe to use forceps to deliver a baby when the baby's station is above +2. Until a fetus is at zero station, it is not engaged. When the baby is above that station, it is unknown whether or not there is sufficient room in the pelvis for the baby to pass through. If the fetus cannot fit through the pelvis adequately and delivery is forced with the use of forceps, very serious fetal complications could arise, including fractured skull and subdural hematoma.

79. 1. The client is hemodynamically stable. The nurse should follow the anesthesia provider's orders for vital sign frequencies, based on the unique needs of the client. Vital signs may not need to be assessed every 15 minutes after the first hour, but this is the anesthesia provider's decision to make. The client is hemodynamically stable.
2. Her pulse rate should be assessed as indicated in the provider's orders, or by unit policy.
3. **The client's bladder should be palpated.**
4. There is nothing in the scenario that implies that the client's lung fields need to be assessed.

TEST-TAKING HINT: There are three very important reasons the client's bladder should be assessed. First, clients receive at least 1 liter of fluid immediately before the insertion of an epidural. Within a 2-hour period, it is likely that the client's bladder has become full. Second, clients are unable to feel when they need to urinate with an epidural in place. Third, a full bladder can impede fetal descent.

80. 1. LMA position is consistent with the information in the stem. The chin (mentum) is anterior, in the left upper quadrant. The fetal head is hyperextended far enough that the back of the baby's head (the occiput) is in contact with the fetal spine as we would be if standing and looking straight up at the ceiling.
2. In the LSP position, the sacrum is presenting, not the vertex.
3. In the dorso-superior position, the fetus is in the transverse lie with its back up.
4. In the ROP position, the occiput is presenting so the fetal attitude is flexed toward its chest, as it should be.

TEST-TAKING HINT: The first question to ask in each of these responses is, "What is presenting?" Which fetus is vertex? In response #1, the mentum (chin) is presenting. That is one of the vertex presentations, so it's an option to consider. Response #2 is the sacrum presenting, so that's not the correct answer. The dorso-superior presentation is a transverse lie, so that's not vertex. Only responses #1 and #4 refer to a vertex (head) presentation. The next question the test taker must ask is, "Which fetus is in an extended attitude?" In the ROP position (response #4) the fetus is flexed, not extended. The fetus in an LMA position has an extended attitude with its head back. That makes response #1 the correct answer.

81. 1. Minus 2 station is not a contraindication for external version.
2. Preterm gestational age is not a contraindication for external version.
3. Reactive NST is not a contraindication for external version.
4. Previous cesarean section is a contraindication for external version.

TEST-TAKING HINT: During external version, the primary healthcare provider moves the fetus from a malpresentation—usually breech—to a vertex presentation. To accomplish the movement, the physician manually palpates the fetus externally through the mother's abdominal and uterine walls. Because significant stress is placed on the uterine body, the presence of a cesarean scar is a contraindication to the procedure. Also, because of the risk of umbilical cord entrapment, the team must be prepared to perform an emergency cesarean section if indicated.

82. 1. Oxytocin is a medication that contracts the uterus. It would not be administered prior to an external version.
2. Methylergonovine is a medication that contracts the uterus. It should never be administered prior to the delivery of the placenta.
3. Betamethasone is a steroid that is administered to the mother of a preterm infant to stimulate the maturation of the fetus's lung fields. It would not be administered prior to an external version.
4. Terbutaline is a smooth, muscle-relaxing agent. It would be administered prior to an external version to relax the uterus and prevent contractions.

TEST-TAKING HINT: It is important that the uterine muscle not impede the physician's manipulations during an external version. To facilitate the movement, therefore, a muscle relaxant is administered. Terbutaline is an example of one relaxing agent that is used by obstetricians.

83. 1. A fetus in +3 station is well engaged and likely in active labor. An external version would not be advisable or even possible.
2. LSP position is a breech presentation. It may be appropriate for a physician to perform an external version prior to this delivery.
3. A fetus in a flexed attitude is not a malpresentation.
4. Prolonged rupture of membranes is not an indication for an external version.

TEST-TAKING HINT: If a baby is in the breech presentation, the version would have to be performed before the baby has engaged in the pelvis.

84. 1. A change in urinary output after external version is unlikely.
2. An elevation in the maternal blood pressure after external version is unlikely.
3. The presence of severe occipital headache after external version is unlikely.
4. The nurse should monitor the client carefully for variable fetal heart decelerations.

TEST-TAKING HINT: The umbilical cord can become compressed during an external version. Variable decelerations are caused by umbilical cord compression. If the cord were to become compressed, the nurse would note variable decelerations on the fetal heart monitor tracing and notify the provider. The client would be monitored carefully before discharge.

85. 1. The urinary output should be carefully monitored.
2. Magnesium sulfate administration does not place clients at high risk for a temperature elevation.
3. Magnesium sulfate administration does not place clients at high risk for cessation of peripheral circulation.
4. Magnesium sulfate administration does not place clients at high risk for retinal edema.

TEST-TAKING HINT: When used for clients in preterm labor, magnesium sulfate is generally administered for just 48 hours to provide enough time for the client to receive steroids for fetal lung maturation. It has also been shown to decrease the risk of cerebral palsy and is now administered to clients at 32 weeks' gestation or less when preterm birth is anticipated (Chollat et al., 2018). Even though this client is receiving magnesium sulfate to treat preterm labor and not pre-eclampsia, prevention of toxic levels is still a nursing care goal. Magnesium sulfate is excreted through the kidneys. If the urinary output drops, the concentration of magnesium sulfate can rise in the bloodstream. If the magnesium sulfate rises to toxic levels, the client can experience respiratory depression and cardiac compromise. As such, it is very important for the nurse to carefully monitor the client's intake and output to prevent the risk of the client's retaining magnesium sulfate in her circulation.

86. Answers 3 and 4 are correct.

1. The simple presence of contractions is not diagnostic of preterm labor.
2. This could be a normal finding and does not indicate preterm labor.
3. **The dilation of 3 cm combined with contractions is indicative of preterm labor.**
4. **A cervical length of 2 cm combined with contractions is indicative of preterm labor.**
5. The presence of 30-second–duration contractions even every 5 minutes is not diagnostic of preterm labor.

TEST-TAKING HINT: Preterm labor is defined as the combination of uterine contractions and dilation of the cervix in response, prior to term gestation (between 20 and 37 weeks). The stem of the question indicates the client is contracting. Each of these answers, then, when combined with contractions, must be an indication of preterm labor. Primary healthcare providers must consider cervical change in the presence of contractions in their diagnosis of preterm labor. The diagnosis is generally made when regular uterine contractions are accompanied by a change in cervical dilation, effacement, or both, or if a client presents with regular contractions and cervical dilation of at least 2 cm (ACOG, 2016b). A cervix is generally around 2 inches in length (4 cm) before labor begins. The client with a cervical length of 2 cm is approximately 50% effaced, which is a major shortening of the cervix. This change is likely in response to the contractions.

87. Answers 1, 2, and 5 are correct.

1. **This client is high risk for PTL because she is over 35 years of age and in an abusive relationship.**
2. **A previous preterm delivery places a client at increased risk of preterm labor.**
3. The presence of a two-vessel cord does not place a client at increased risk of preterm labor.
4. A history of long menstrual periods does not place a client at increased risk of preterm labor.
5. **A client who smokes cigarettes is at high risk for preterm labor.**

TEST-TAKING HINT: Even though medical and psychosocial histories are not absolute predictors of preterm labor, there are a number of factors that have been shown to place clients at risk. These include (a) obstetrical history of multiple gestations; (b) any previous preterm delivery; (c) cigarette smoking and/or illicit drug use; (d) a number of medical conditions such as diabetes and hypertension; and (e) social issues such as adolescent pregnancy and domestic violence.

88.

1. Fetal fibronectin is not related to glucose metabolism.
2. **Positive fetal fibronectin levels are seen in clients who deliver preterm.**
3. Fetal fibronectin is not related to hypertensive conditions.
4. Fetal fibronectin is not related to fetal well-being.

TEST-TAKING HINT: Fetal fibronectin (fFN) is a substance like a glue that is created by the chorion. The nurse will recall that at the time of uterine implantation, multiple layers develop within the uterus and within the developing placenta. In the uterus, a decidual cell layer begins. This layer interfaces with the chorion, the first layer of the embryonic placenta. The next layer within the placenta is the amnion, or gestational, sac. So, the connection of the chorion to the decidual layer is essentially the fetal connection to the mom. Fetal fibronectin is the biologic glue that attaches the fetal sac to the uterine lining. Although positive results are normally seen during the first half of pregnancy, it is very rare to see positive results between 24 and 34 weeks' gestation unless the client's cervix begins to efface and dilate. It is an excellent predictor of preterm labor (PTL), indicating that the glue might not be holding and the uterus is preparing to begin preterm labor. As such, many obstetrical care providers assess the cervical and vaginal secretions of women at high risk for PTL for the presence of fFN when preterm labor is suspected. The test has a negative predictive value in that a negative fFN, indicates that just 1 woman out of 100 (1%) will begin preterm labor within the next 14 days (Jeavons, 2005). Alternately, a woman with a positive fFN can expect that preterm labor will begin.

89.

1. Oxytocin will increase the client's contractions. The administration of this medication is inappropriate at this time.
2. Methylergonovine maleate should never be administered unless the placenta is already delivered.
3. **Magnesium sulfate is a tocolytic agent. It would be appropriate for this medication to be administered at this time to stop or reduce the strength and frequency of the labor contractions.**
4. Morphine sulfate is an opioid, but is not generally used during labor because it can depress respirations, and affect the newborn respirations after the birth. This would be an additional risk factor for the newborn at the time of birth.

TEST-TAKING HINT: **The client in the scenario is exhibiting signs of preterm labor. She has regular contractions, cervical effacement, and is dilated more than 2 cm. The nurse should conclude, therefore, that a tocolytic agent (a medication used to suppress premature labor) may be ordered in this situation. The only tocolytic agent included in the choices is magnesium sulfate.**

90. 1. A history of hypothyroidism does not place a client who is to receive a beta agonist medication at risk.
2. A history of breast cancer does not place a client who is to receive a beta agonist medication at risk.
3. A history of cardiac disease would place a client who is to receive a beta agonist medication at risk because it affects the heart. The nurse should question this order.
4. A history of asthma does not place a client who is to receive a beta agonist medication at risk.

TEST-TAKING HINT: **The nurse should remember that beta agonists stimulate the "fight or flight" response. The client's heart rate will increase precipitously and there is a possibility that the potassium levels of the client may fall. These side effects place the client with heart disease at risk of heart failure and/or dysrhythmias.**

91. 1. Dexamethasone is not a tocolytic.
2. Dexamethasone is not an anti-infective.
3. Dexamethasone is a steroid that hastens the maturation of the fetal lung fields.
4. Dexamethasone is not an analgesic.

TEST-TAKING HINT: **Steroids (either IM betamethasone or IM dexamethasone) are given over a 2-day period to mothers in preterm labor, or for those with threatened preterm labor. The medications have been shown to hasten the development of surfactant in the lung fields of fetuses. Babies whose mothers have received one of these medications experience fewer respiratory complications. Surfactant is a liquid made by alveoli in the lungs. Surfactant keeps the alveoli open by reducing the surface tension, or stickiness of the alveoli. As such, this reduces the work of breathing when babies are born prematurely. At full-term, a newborn's lungs contain millions of alveoli. Premature newborns, however, have not developed enough alveoli to produce the amount of surfactant necessary for breathing comfortably. Without surfactant, they tire and may stop breathing.**

92. 50 mL/hr

Standard method:

Known units/known volume = Desired units/x volume

50 units : 500 mL = 5 units/ hr : x mL

$50x = 5 \times 500$

$50x = 2{,}500$

$x = 50$ mL/hr

Dimensional analysis method:

Known volume	Desired units	Time conversion	Unit conversion
Known units/hr		(if needed)	(if needed)

= x mL/ hr

500 mL	5 units/hr
50 min	

= x mL/ hr

$x = 50$ mL/hr

TEST-TAKING HINT: **IV pumps are always set at a mL/hr rate. There is, therefore, no need to know a drop factor when using a pump. The test taker should also note that the term "units" is written out. The Joint Commission has identified a number of unacceptable abbreviations. "U" and "mU" are unacceptable; instead, the words "units" and "milliunits" must always be written out to avoid medication errors.**

93. 1. Mild tachycardia is an expected side effect.
2. Wakefulness is an expected side effect.
3. Audible rales should be reported to the healthcare provider.
4. Daily output of 2,000 mL is within normal.

TEST-TAKING HINT: **The presence of audible rales is indicative of pulmonary edema, a serious side effect related to the medication. The pulmonary edema may be caused by the development of congestive heart failure. Whenever a client is on nifedipine, the nurse should regularly monitor the client's lung fields.**

94. 1. There is nothing in the scenario that indicates that the client is at high risk for hypertensive illness.
2. There is nothing in the scenario that indicates that the client is at high risk for hyperglycemia.
3. Increased fetal heart variability is not expected in this situation.
4. The fetal heart rate pattern is likely to show late decelerations secondary to a postmature placenta.

TEST-TAKING HINT: **A BPP below 8 may indicate that the fetus is in jeopardy. The five assessments that constitute the BPP are (a) nonstress test (NST); (b) fetal movement count; (c) fetal breathing; (d) amniotic fluid volume; and (e) fetal tone. Each assessment is given a score of 0 or 2. The total score possible is a 10.**

95. 1. The fetus is full-term. Post-term is defined 42 0/7 weeks' gestation or later.
2. The fetus is not breech; it is vertex.
3. The prolonged deceleration indicates the cord is prolapsed. This is likely because the amniotomy was performed when the presenting part was at –4 station, not yet engaged.
4. If the client were infected, the amniotic fluid would be foul smelling.

TEST-TAKING HINT: The likelihood of a prolapsed cord occurring during rupture of membranes increases when the fetal presenting part is at a negative station, unengaged. As the amniotic fluid is released from the uterus during the rupture of membranes, the cord can slip down and precede the fetus. At that time, a prolonged deceleration is seen on the electronic fetal monitor tracing because the cord is being compressed by the presenting part. This is an emergent situation. A STAT cesarean section is indicated.

96. **Answers 3, 4, and 5 are correct.**
1. Gestational age is not part of the Bishop score.
2. The status of the membranes is not part of the Bishop score.
3. Cervical dilation is part of the Bishop score.
4. Fetal station is part of the Bishop score.
5. Cervical position is part of the Bishop score.

TEST-TAKING HINT: The Bishop score is calculated to determine the inducibility of the cervix. Although gestational age and rupture of the membranes may be indications for calculating the score, neither one has a direct impact on the inducibility of the cervix.

97. **1. The nurse would expect the client to be crying and exhibiting sadness.**
2. It is unlikely that the client would be talkative and excited.
3. It is unlikely that the client would be quietly doing rapid breathing.
4. It is unlikely that the client would be loudly chanting.

TEST-TAKING HINT: A client in the latent phase of labor who is carrying a healthy fetus is likely to be talkative and excited, but a client whose fetus has died is likely to be crying and sad throughout her labor. Clients in the latent phase rarely perform slow chest breathing.

98. 1. Although the bacterium can cause chorioamnionitis, this is not the rationale for administering the antibiotic during labor.
2. Babies are susceptible to neonatal sepsis from vertical transmission of the bacteria.
3. The bacteria are not sexually transmitted. Approximately one-third of all women carry group B strep as normal vaginal and/or rectal flora.
4. Puerperal sepsis is usually caused by *Staphylococcus aureus*, or group A, strep.

TEST-TAKING HINT: At approximately 36 weeks' gestation, pregnant women are cultured for group B streptococci (GBS). If they culture positive, standard protocol is to administer a broad-spectrum antibiotic IV q 4 hours from the time they are admitted until delivery. That action markedly decreases the vertical transmission of the bacteria from the vagina into the uterus and then to the fetus.

99. **Answers 1 and 2 are correct.**
1. The nurse should carefully monitor the client for variable fetal heart rate decelerations.
2. The nurse should carefully monitor the client for late decelerations in the fetal heart rate.
3. It is unlikely the client will have oliguria.
4. Tachysystole is not a symptom associated with oligohydramnios.

TEST-TAKING HINT: Variable decelerations can occur in the presence of oligohydramnios because of insufficient fluid to cushion the umbilical cord, resulting in cord compression. In this question, the fetus is postdates at 42 weeks' gestation. The nurse would also be alert to signs of uteroplacental insufficiency such as late decelerations, because the placenta could be functioning sub-optimally due to postdates calcifications.

Amniotic fluid is present within the gestational sac at the time of implantation. As the embryo grows, most of the amniotic fluid is created by the passage of maternal plasma across the placental chorionic and amnionic tissues, into the gestational sac (Beall et al., 2007). By the time the fetal kidney is working at around 16 weeks' gestation, fetal urine begins to comprise a large part of amniotic fluid. It is worth noting that a small portion of the amniotic fluid is also derived from the lungs (Brace et al., 2018). By late gestation, fetal urine is the primary source of amniotic fluid (Brace et al., 2018). An adequate amount of fluid is necessary to cushion both the fetus and the umbilical cord, and to allow for limb movement and exercise by the fetus.

Amniotic fluid is not a stagnant pool of fluid, however; it is refreshed about every 24 hours, through intramembranous inflow and outflow controlled by the amnion at the placenta (Brace et al., 2018). Volume regulation depends on adequate swallowing and processing of the amniotic fluid by the fetus, and on the amount of urine produced by the fetus, in turn. Inadequate amniotic fluid production can be related to absent or dysfunctional fetal kidneys, obstructed urinary tract, a dysfunctional or abnormal placenta, or maternal dehydration (Dubil & Magann, 2013).

Oligohydramnios is often seen in post-term pregnancies. This is thought to be a result of sub-optimal placental function as a result of calcifications that occur naturally post-term. When the placenta begins to deteriorate, the hydration of the baby drops. In addition, if the placenta cannot deliver enough fluid to the fetus, it is likely not delivering adequate oxygen and nutrients, either.

100. Answers 1, 2, 3, and 4 are correct.

1. **The circulating nurse should participate with the surgical technician or scrub nurse in counting the sterile sponges and writing this number on the designated board for all in the room to refer to. The circulating nurse is responsible for maintaining a clear visual record of additions and totals when more sponges and needles are added to the count throughout the procedure.**
2. **The circulating nurse must also document on the designated board and in the medical record all key events that occur during the surgery, including the time of the first incision. This time is obtained from the anesthesia provider.**
3. **The circulating nurse should notify the pediatric staff in advance, allowing them time to set up for possible resuscitations. There should be one resuscitation team assembled in the delivery room for each baby that will be delivered. Each team must have appropriate equipment and personnel to care for the newborn they are responsible for.**
4. **The circulating nurse must perform a surgical site scrub on the client using sterile gloves and sterile solution before the procedure.**
5. It is not appropriate for the circulating nurse to assemble the sterile instruments because the circulating nurse is not sterile. This is the responsibility of the surgical technician or scrub nurse.

TEST-TAKING HINT: The circulating nurse is responsible for coordinating the activity in the operating room. The circulator is the only member of the team who is able to move freely throughout the room to make telephone calls, obtain needed supplies, maintain the documentation record, and the designated board often referred to as the "white board." Multiple-gestation babies are often born preterm and small-for-gestational age. The circulating nurse's primary responsibilities are for the mother and the surgical team, not the babies. There must be a resuscitation team and supplies available for each baby in case emergent care is needed.

101. Answers 1, 4, and 5 are correct.

1. **The client's hepatitis B status should be assessed.**
2. The client's rubeola status is not immediately important.
3. The client's varicella status is not immediately important.
4. **The client's group B streptococcus (GBS) status should be assessed.**
5. **The client's HIV/AIDS status should be assessed.**

TEST-TAKING HINT: There are several infectious diseases that affect care given during antepartum, intrapartum, and postpartum care, and in the newborn nursery. The answers to this question are based on the needs of the baby throughout labor and after the birth. Which diseases are most likely to threaten the baby's survival, the first level of Maslow's hierarchy of needs? The hepatitis B status is important to know so the baby can receive immune globulin in time after the birth if the mother is positive. Group B strep (GBS) status must be assessed to administer needed antibiotics to the mother during labor to protect the baby, and to guide in monitoring the baby's status after the birth. The HIV/AIDS status must be assessed to administer needed antiviral medications to the mother in labor and/or to the baby postdelivery. HIV/AIDS status will also affect the mother's decision on feeding the baby, as women who are positive for HIV/AIDS should not breastfeed. HIV/AIDS is also an indication for cesarean section delivery. A cesarean section reduces the risk of maternal–fetal transmission by delivering the baby before labor begins and before the membranes rupture. Although herpes simplex 2 lesions are not included in this question, the nurse should also

assess for the presence of active herpes lesions in the perineal area, which would be an indication for cesarean section delivery.

102. 1. It would not be appropriate for the nurse to schedule the induction for the next day because the client does not meet the standards of care for elective induction, which is no sooner than 39 weeks' gestation.
2. The client's Bishop score is irrelevant because it would be inappropriate for the client to be induced the next day.
3. The nurse should remind the provider of the policy that does not allow elective inductions to be scheduled before 39 weeks' gestation.
4. The nurse should refuse to schedule the induction for the next day.

TEST-TAKING HINT: Because this client is not even at 39 weeks, it is best if the nurse questions the order. If hospital policy does not allow for induction before 39 weeks in this situation, the nurse must follow policy.

Hospital policies and client conditions determine whether or not a provider may schedule an elective induction for the client. They are generally written in compliance with the national standards of care. The American College of Obstetricians and Gynecologists (ACOG) in agreement with the Association of Women's Health, Obstetric and Neonatal Nurses (AWHONN) has redefined full term pregnancy as 39 0/7 through 40 6/7 weeks' gestation. Pregnancies between 37 0/7 and 38 6/7 weeks' gestation are defined as early term. Unless medically indicated, and to provide the fetus with optimal intrauterine maturation, ACOG advises that inductions not be performed until pregnancies reach at least 39 weeks' gestation (ACOG, 2009). AWHONN recommends that pregnancies "Go the Full Forty."

103. 1. The nurse would not expect the fetal heart rate tracing to show marked fetal heart rate variability.
2. The nurse would not expect the fetal heart rate tracing to show prolonged fetal heart rate accelerations
3. The nurse would expect to see a sinusoidal fetal heart rate pattern.
4. The nurse would not expect the fetal heart rate tracing to show periodic variable decelerations.

TEST-TAKING HINT: A sinusoidal fetal heart rate pattern, as seen below, is an abnormal, undulating pattern. The pattern is seen when the fetus is markedly anemic as in erythroblastosis fetalis. This condition results from an Rh blood group incompatibility, where the Rh-negative mother who has previously been exposed to Rh positive blood either through miscarriage or the birth of a previous Rh-positive baby, gives birth to another Rh-positive baby without having received Rh immune globulin (RhIG) after the previous birth.

The mother's body has created antibodies to Rh-positive blood. When she is pregnant the next time, those antibodies cross the placenta and trigger an immune response against the Rh-positive fetal blood cells of the new fetus. Up to 50% of the fetal red blood cells may be destroyed, creating fetal anemia. In response, the fetal bone marrow releases low quality, immature RBCs into the fetal circulation. With fewer red blood cells to carry oxygen to fetal organs, the fetal heart is overworked. It enlarges, creating congestive heart failure. This is followed by generalized edema, a hallmark sign.

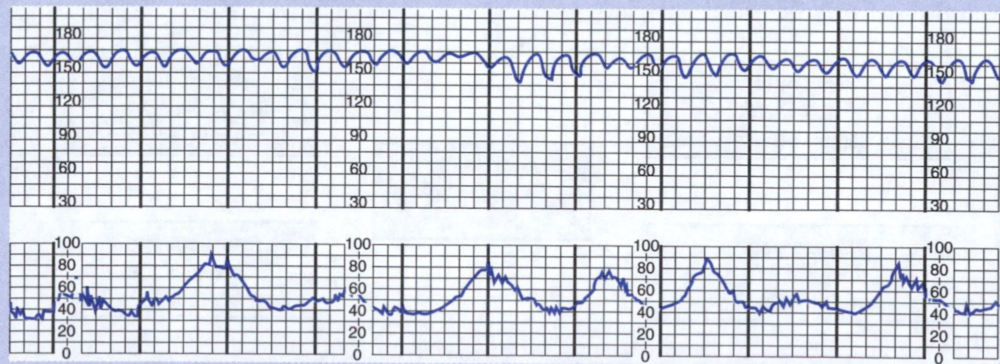

104. 1. This is not a category I pattern. Category I patterns are completely benign, i.e., normal FHR with moderate variability and no variable or late decelerations.

2. This is a category II pattern. Although there are late decelerations, the variability is moderate, indicating adequate fetal oxygenation at this time. In an attempt to correct the deceleration pattern, lateral positioning, administration of oxygen via face mask, and an intravenous fluid bolus should all be done.

3. This is not a Category III pattern. Category III patterns are ominous and are indicative of an acidotic fetus. Immediate termination of labor and moving to cesarean section is recommended.

4. There is no Category IV fetal heart pattern.

TEST-TAKING HINT: To standardize care of clients in labor and delivery, ACOG and AWHONN agreed to develop interventions based on the fetal monitoring categories defined by the National Institute of Child Health and Human Development (NICHD). Three categories were developed:

Category I—includes benign patterns that require no intervention

Category II—the "indeterminate" category includes a number of patterns including, for example, minimal variability with no late or variable decelerations and late decelerations with moderate variability. Interventions aimed at improving umbilical cord blood flow are instituted and continuous fetal heart monitoring is maintained. Fetal well-being is indeterminate with these fetal heart rate patterns and requires close monitoring and attempts to alleviate the worrisome findings.

Category III includes ominous findings indicative of severe acidosis in the fetus, i.e., absent variability with late and/or variable decelerations, bradycardia, or sinusoidal rhythm. Immediate termination of the labor and moving to cesarean section is recommended (Simpson, 2016).

105. 1. The nurse would expect the primary healthcare provider to order heparin.

2. Warfarin is contraindicated in pregnancy.

3. Aminocaproic acid is in a class of drugs known as antifibrinolytics. It is used to treat hemorrhage or to prevent hemorrhage by helping the blood to clot normally. This client's blood is already producing clots—too many of them.

4. DDAVP is administered to release blood-clotting proteins stored in the body This client already makes too many blood clots.

TEST-TAKING HINT: Clients who are hypercoagulable are clients whose blood tends to clot too quickly and/or too easily. During pregnancy, because of the increased clotting factors produced naturally under the influence of estrogen, clients with hypercoagulability are especially at high risk for heart attack and stroke. Both warfarin and heparin prevent the blood from clotting, but warfarin crosses the placenta, whereas heparin does not. To prevent complications in the fetus, heparin is the drug of choice during pregnancy.

106. 1. There is nothing to suggest cephalopelvic disproportion.

2. This fetus is at risk for hypoxia due to pre-eclampsia with severe features. The cues are intermittent late decelerations and periods of minimal variability.

3. There is nothing to suggest the fetus is in an occiput posterior position.

4. The fetus is engaged at zero station, so the cervical opening is covered by the fetal head. As such, there is nothing to suggest a prolapsed cord is a risk.

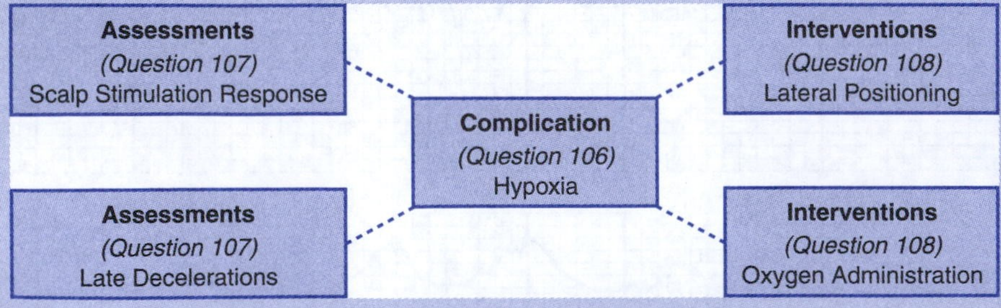

TEST-TAKING TIP: The nurse must always be thinking ahead about what might happen. In this "bowtie format," the test taker must recognize cues and analyze those cues to determine the client's most serious risk. Although the late decelerations are currently intermittent, the client's history of pre-eclampsia suggests less than optimal oxygen delivery through the placenta as a cause of these specific decelerations. The client is in early labor at 3 cm, and as the contractions increase in intensity and fetal oxygen demand increases as a result, a cesarean section might become necessary if the FHR demonstrates fetal hypoxia with recurrent late decelerations and minimal variability.

Recognizing that pre-eclampsia with severe features is a high risk condition that can lead to fetal hypoxia, the nurse connects hypoxia with the physiology of pre-eclampsia and the FHR pattern of late decelerations and periods of minimal variability that confirm the identified risk.

107. Answers 3 and 5 are correct.

1. There is nothing in the question to suggest the fetus is at risk for variable decelerations at this time.
2. Fetal descent is appropriate to assess, but it is not related to fetal hypoxia.
3. **If a fetus responds to scalp stimulation with a FHR acceleration, it indicates the fetus is not hypoxic at that time. It is important to note, however, that scalp stimulation should not be performed during a deceleration.**
4. Leopold maneuvers are important to perform at the start of labor, but they are unrelated to fetal hypoxia.
5. **Late decelerations indicate fetal hypoxia. As the fetus develops tissue hypoxia, late decelerations come first, followed by minimal variability. Recurrent late decelerations accompanied by minimal variability are an ominous sign. Recurrent late decelerations are those that occur with 50% or more of the contractions in any 20 minute window (Simpson, 2016). The nurse will monitor for that progression from *intermittent* to *recurrent* late decelerations and the absence of moderate variability. It is recommended that the fetus be delivered by cesarean section within an hour from the onset of this FHR pattern (Williams & Galerneau, 2003).**
6. Fern testing is a test to assess for rupture of membranes. It is not associated with fetal hypoxia.

TEST-TAKING HINT: Having identified hypoxia as the primary fetal risk factor, the nurse and/or test taker identifies two assessments related to that risk that would indicate a worsening condition. The Nurse must understand the differences between *hypoxemia* and *hypoxia*, and between *acidemia* and *acidosis*. The difference lies in where the condition is occurring: in the blood or in the cells. When cells are combined, they make up tissue. *Hypoxemia* means there is a decreased oxygen content in the *blood*. For the fetus, this can be reversed by administering oxygen to the mother. For the newly born baby, this can be reversed by stimulating the baby to cry lustily. This is often the treatment for respiratory acidosis.

Hypoxia means there is a decreased oxygen content in the *tissues*. This is much more serious. It is the result of prolonged hypoxemia, when the fetal cells must switch to anaerobic metabolism. As a result, the waste products of anaerobic metabolism increase the acidity of the fetal blood. If hypoxemia leads to hypoxia and the condition is prolonged, the fetus develops *metabolic acidosis*, increased concentration of hydrogen ions in tissue. This can take several days to reverse once the baby is born. If the baby is born with both hypoxia and metabolic acidosis, the baby has *asphyxia*. This is very dire.

Fetal heart rate patterns can guide the presumption of pending fetal acidemia and the nurse must intervene in a timely manner to prevent it, if possible (Cahill et al., 2012). Both late decelerations and deep variable decelerations can lead to fetal acidemia equally (Holtzmann et al., 2018). A fetal heart rate with both of these patterns in addition to tachycardia signals the highest risk of fetal acidemia (Holtzmann et al., 2015).

108. Answers 2 and 3 are correct.

1. Although an IV bolus is often appropriate for maximizing uterine blood flow, this client has pre-eclampsia with severe features. Her fluid intake is likely restricted, and a fluid bolus puts her at risk of pulmonary edema. As such, other interventions should be tried first. Because the late decelerations are intermittent and the FHR shows periods of moderate variability, the nurse can conclude that the fetus is not currently hypoxic. It follows, then, that the risks associated with an IV fluid bolus would not be prudent at this time.

2. **Lateral positioning is correct. By reducing the risk of compression of the great vessels in the abdomen, the aorta and vena cava, lateral positioning can improve maternal circulation, providing more optimal oxygenation to the placenta and from there to the fetus.**
3. **Oxygen administration at 8 to 10 L/min per rebreather mask for a few minutes can increase maternal and fetal oxygenation.**
4. Pain medication is appropriate to reduce vasoconstriction induced by pain. However, the epidural is not a procedure within the labor nurse's scope of practice.

TEST-TAKING HINT: In this question, the test taker must choose the best two interventions, even though more than one may be appropriate. Improved fetal oxygenation is the goal and can be done by maximizing uterine blood flow.

A full explanation of vascular damage related to pre-eclampsia is not possible here, and the condition continues to be researched. In a nutshell, however, experts suggest that in women with pre-eclampsia, the condition begins with the placenta (Lim & Steinberg, 2018). Upon implantation of the embryo, uterine blood vessels do not respond to hormonal signaling as they should. They do not dilate, but remain narrow, reducing the amount of blood that flows to the placenta. As a result, placental hypoxia releases free radicals related to oxidative stress (Powe et al, 2011). The free radicals damage the lining of the mother's blood vessels, the endothelium. As a result, her blood vessels become stiff, yet permeable (Enkhmaa et al., 2016). She then develops hypertension from the stiffness and edema from the permeability, as fluid leaks from the blood into the tissues. For this reason, she is at high risk of pulmonary edema with an IV bolus of fluid. Other interventions should be tried first, for maximizing uterine blood flow.

109. 1. There is nothing in the question to suggest she is at risk of a prolonged labor. This is not the first time she has given birth vaginally. Normal timeframes for a multiparous labor can be expected.
2. **Clients choosing a TOLAC are always at risk of uterine rupture during labor.**
3. The fetus is engaged at zero station, so there is no risk of a prolapsed cord.
4. Although this is her fourth baby (hopefully her third vaginal delivery), there is nothing in the question to suggest she will have a precipitous delivery. Contractions are irregular at 3 to 5 minutes apart. A precipitous delivery would be suggested if the contractions were regular, strong, and coming frequently, such as every two minutes.

TEST-TAKING HINT: There are multiple things to consider with this client's care. First, she is a multipara at 41 weeks' gestation, in spontaneous labor. Her cervix is 100% effaced, 3 cm dilated. Spontaneous labor and adequate cervical dilation are consistent factors associated with a TOLAC that leads to a successful VBAC, or vaginal birth after cesarean section (Scott, 2014). Her body is ready to give birth to this baby. Second, she has given birth vaginally two times before, so the vaginal tissues have been stretched and they will offer less resistance to the uterus and to her as she pushes. Labor should not be long. Third, this is a reasonably small baby compared to her last baby, so it should fit easily through the pelvis. Fourth, her contractions are not yet regular, but she can ambulate with a telemetry electronic fetal monitor (EFM). Walking often stimulates regular contractions. The fifth factor is of concern. Although there is just a 0.5 to 1% risk of uterine rupture in TOLAC (Scott, 2014), the closer the TOLAC is to the cesarean section, the greater the risk of rupture. Her cesarean section was just 18 months ago. Even if her uterus does not rupture, the previous scar may dehisce, and the membranes may rupture at that site, leading to an occult prolapsed cord.

However, because 20 to 40% of TOLACs are not successful for various reasons (Scott, 2014), she is at risk of needing a repeat cesarean. An IV line must be inserted on admission, and lab tests for possible cesarean section must be on the chart in case of emergency. In addition, both the anesthesia care provider and pediatric or neonatal care provider must be notified of the client's TOLAC attempt when the client is admitted, so they are aware, should an emergency cesarean become necessary.

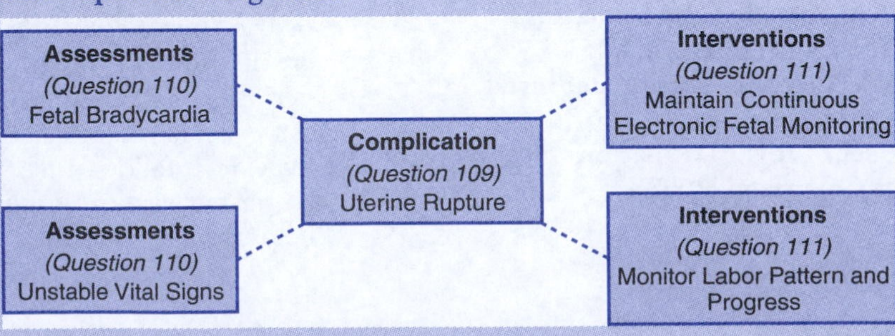

110. **Answers 1 and 2 are correct.**
   1. **Fetal bradycardia is the nonreassuring fetal heart rate tracing most indicative of uterine rupture (Scott, 2014). Sudden, significant variable decelerations are also characteristic of uterine rupture or scar dehiscence.**
   2. **Unstable vital signs suggest occult bleeding. Further assessments and notification of the primary healthcare provider are indicated.**
   3. Late decelerations are not characteristic with uterine rupture.
   4. Severe headache is not characteristic with uterine rupture. Behavior indications include anxiety, restlessness, dizziness, and shock (Scott, 2014).

TEST-TAKING HINT: Having identified the assessments of concern, the nurse will keep them in the forefront and play a proactive part in recognizing them if they occur.

111. **Answers 2 and 4 are correct.**
   1. Although ambulation may assist in improving the contraction regularity, ambulating or shortening the labor will not reduce the risk of uterine rupture.
   2. **This is a high-risk client. Continuous fetal monitoring is vital for assessing fetal well-being and may provide the first sign of uterine rupture—bradycardia.**
   3. Although this client might need a cesarean section, she does not need an indwelling catheter inserted at this time.
   4. **Close monitoring of the labor pattern and progress is necessary when caring for clients during a TOLAC. If the client has an epidural, she may not complain of pain. The nurse must look for other symptoms if that is the case. Contractions that become less frequent or less intense, loss of uterine tone (assessed by palpation), or labor progress that falls outside the expected timeframe may suggest uterine rupture and inability of the uterus to contract adequately. An assessment of fetal *ascent* back toward the uterus could be a sign of a ruptured uterus. This would be discovered when fetal station reverses from positive station to negative as though the fetus is going back into the uterus.**

TEST-TAKING HINT: It is the nurse's responsibility to consider, "What might happen?" and to be prepared to either prevent it, or to remain vigilant and intervene early and emergently when necessary. The nurse caring for a client having a TOLAC must never be lulled into a false sense of security while the client is laboring smoothly. Disasters can happen unexpectedly. However, the literature has indicated that even in the case of a uterine rupture, neurologic injury to the fetus is rare if the baby is delivered within 18 to 30 minutes of the diagnosis (Scott, 2014, p 160).

112.
   1. Although this is the client's fourth vaginal delivery and the labor has been relatively short, there is nothing to indicate she will have a precipitous delivery.
   2. Delivering at 40 weeks is not a risk factor for retained placenta.
   3. Hypoglycemia during labor is not a risk factor for a client with gestational diabetes.
   4. **The client is at risk for a shoulder dystocia. Because she is at 40 weeks' gestation and has gestational diabetes, it is possible the fetus will be on the large side. More significant, however, is the protracted length of second-stage labor. She has been pushing for 90 minutes with little descent.**

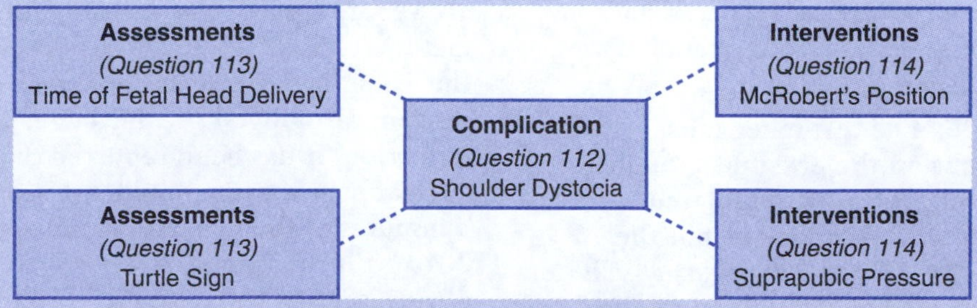

TEST-TAKING HINT: The labor nurse must recognize client medical conditions that can affect labor and delivery and must continually assess for anything that is abnormal. There is nothing in the stem to suggest a precipitous delivery or retained placenta after the birth. There is nothing to suggest the client will have hypoglycemia; in fact, with gestational diabetes, her blood sugar is likely on the high side.

A woman giving birth to her fourth baby is expected to have a shorter labor and delivery than a primiparous client will have. This client's protracted second stage is abnormal, especially for a multipara, and suggests a large baby, or fetal malpresentation such as occiput posterior, which can slow things down. What the gestational diabetes suggests, in tandem with protracted second stage, is a possible shoulder dystocia at delivery, since large, compact fetuses are often seen with clients who have diabetic conditions.

113. Answers 2 and 3 are correct.

1. Capillary blood glucose (CBG) assessments throughout labor are not indicated for this client.
2. **The nurse must document the time the fetal head was delivered, and whether or not shoulder dystocia occurs. The total time between delivery of the fetal head and delivery of the body is important for malpractice defense, should there be a shoulder dystocia or other birth injury with serious consequences.**
3. **The nurse must be alert for the turtle sign. This is identified by delivery of the fetal head, followed by retraction of the fetal head back toward the vagina.**
4. Uterine atony is not anticipated before delivery with oxytocin running during labor. However, if the baby is large, uterine atony may be an anticipated complication during the postpartum phase.

TEST-TAKING HINTS: The test taker must demonstrate a focus on the possible shoulder dystocia and nursing assessments related specifically to that risk. Whether or not the provider orders CBGs for this client, that will not affect a shoulder dystocia. A shoulder dystocia begins after delivery of the fetal head, so the precise time that the head is delivered must be documented. The nurse must watch for and identify the turtle sign, as the fetal head is drawn back toward the vaginal opening. The next important time to note is when the baby's body is delivered—the official birth time.

Uterine atony may be seen after the delivery due to the size of the baby. However, it is unrelated to nursing care for shoulder dystocia.

114. Answers 1 and 4 are correct.

1. **Placing the client in the McRoberts position with her legs tightly flexed toward her abdomen, has been thought to increase the pelvic diameter, allowing room for the fetal shoulder to slip under the symphysis pubis. More recently, studies have shown that the McRoberts maneuver actually works by allowing the pubic symphysis to lift (Desseauve et al., 2020). At the same time, the lumbar spine flattens. These two mechanical changes together—ascension of the pubic symphysis and flattening of the lumbar spine—diminish fetal trauma by releasing the anterior shoulder and reducing the stretch on the fetal brachial nerve fibers (Desseauve et al., 2020).**
2. There is no need to turn off the oxytocin. Shoulder dystocia is correlated with oxytocin but is not causal (Politi et al., 2010).
3. Although administration of oxygen could be of benefit to the fetus, the focus at this point should be on getting the baby delivered asap.
4. **Suprapubic pressure (not fundal) should be applied when indicated by the provider. The approach may be in pulses or may be continuous, and is always done from the side of the fetal back, in an attempt to rotate the fetal shoulder out from behind the maternal pubic bone into an oblique angle so it can slide out.**

TEST-TAKING HINT: Shoulder dystocia is an unpredictable and unpreventable event. There are very few predictive factors, but several risk factors (Hill & Cohen, 2016). The *risk* factors for this client include gestational diabetes, protracted descent, prolonged second stage, and oxytocin induction. It has been reported that in one study, 47% of babies with shoulder dystocia died within 5 minutes of the head being delivered (Politi et al., 2010). The goals of delivery are to avoid brachial plexus injuries and hypoxia. It is important for an obstetrical unit to participate in shoulder dystocia drills so that in the event of this emergency, caregivers know their roles and expectations, and the team works smoothly together. Birth attendants must be alert to the potential for postpartum hemorrhage after the event.

High-Risk Newborn 10

Although the vast majority of babies born in the United States are healthy and full term, there are a number of term and preterm neonates who need specialized care immediately after delivery. In 2018 the Centers for Disease Control (CDC) reported that in the United States, the rate of total preterm births rose by 3% between 2014 and 2016, from 9.57% in 2014 to 9.85% in 2016 (Martin & Osterman, 2018). The authors of these data pointed out, however, that premature births include up to 37 weeks' gestation, and the increase has been primarily in late preterm births (34 to 36 weeks) particularly in births occurring at 36 weeks (Martin & Osterman, 2018). The rate of early preterm births (before 34 completed weeks of gestation) was essentially unchanged for 2014–2016 (Martin & Osterman, 2018). Worldwide, using the definition of preterm as births before 37 weeks, the rate of preterm livebirths in 2014 (the last reported data) was 10.6% (Chawanpaiboon & Osterman, 2019). Even with the high-quality care that preterm babies receive, many of them will develop acute and chronic illnesses as sequelae to their prematurity.

This chapter will cover the nursing care of all high-risk babies, whether born prematurely, at term, and/or postmaturely (defined as more than 40 6/7 weeks' gestation). In addition, babies whose mothers have diseases such as diabetes mellitus and pre-eclampsia, and who often have neonatal problems as a result, will be discussed. Finally, a number of congenital diseases that affect babies will be included. In each situation, the nurse must possess the knowledge and expertise to provide the babies with uniquely specialized and informed care.

KEYWORDS

The following words include English vocabulary, nursing/medical terminology, concepts, principles, or information relevant to content specifically addressed in the chapter or associated with topics presented in it. English dictionaries, your nursing textbooks, and medical dictionaries such as *Taber's Cyclopedic Medical Dictionary* are resources that can be used to expand your knowledge and understanding of these words and related information.

ABO incompatibility
Acyanotic heart defects (e.g., ventricular septal defect, atrial septal defect, patent ductus arteriosus)
Appropriate for gestational age (AGA)
Arm recoil sign
Babinski reflex
Ballard scale
Beractant
Bronchopulmonary dysplasia
Café au lait spot
Chignon
Choanal atresia
Cleft lip and palate
Clubfoot
Cold stress syndrome
Conduction
Continuous positive airway pressure (CPAP)
Convection
Coombs test (direct and indirect)
Cyanotic heart defects (e.g., tetralogy of Fallot, truncus arteriosus, transposition of the great vessels)
Desquamation
Developmental dysplasia of the hip
Diaphragmatic hernia
Digoxin
Down's syndrome
Dysmaturity
Erythroblastosis fetalis
Esophageal atresia/tracheoesophageal fistula
Evaporation
Fetal alcohol syndrome (FAS)
Galactosemia

Gastroschisis
Gestational age assessment
Group B streptococcus
Hemangioma
Hemolytic jaundice
Hirschsprung disease
Hydrocephalus
Hyperbilirubinemia
Hypoglycemia
Infant of diabetic mother (IDM)
Intercostal retractions
Intrauterine growth restriction (IUGR)
Jitters
Kangaroo care
Kernicterus
Large for gestational age (LGA)
Macrosomia
Meconium aspiration syndrome
Meningomyelocele (myelomeningocele)
Methadone
Monochorionic twins
Naloxone
Necrotizing enterocolitis
Neonatal abstinence syndrome
Oligohydramnios
Opisthotonus
Ortolani sign
Phototherapy
Polyhydramnios
Popliteal angle
Port wine stain
Positive end-expiratory pressure (PEEP)
Postdates
Postmaturity
Prematurity
Radiation
Respiratory distress syndrome
Rh incompatibility
Scarf sign
Sequelae
Small for gestational age (SGA)
Square window sign
Tachycardia
Tachypnea
Talipes equinovarus
Thermoregulation
Twin-to-twin transfusion

QUESTIONS

CASE STUDY: *The first six questions below are part of an evolving case study. All six questions follow the Next Generation NCLEX© question format of six steps:*

1. Recognize cues—What matters most?
2. Analyze cues—What could it mean?
3. Prioritize hypotheses—Where do I start?
4. Generate solutions—What can I do?
5. Take action—What will I do?
6. Evaluate outcomes—Did it help?

(National Council of State Boards of Nursing [NCSBN], 2020). For more information on the Next Generation NCLEX (NGN) question formats, see NGN quarterly newsletters at https://www.ncsbn.org.
NCLEX questions assume the nurse has a provider's order for listed interventions, unless noted otherwise.

The newborn resuscitation nurse and a neonatal nurse practitioner (NNP) are attending the delivery of a baby at 41 weeks' gestation. The mother is 34 years old, a primigravida who has been in spontaneous labor for 18 hours. She has an epidural in place. Contractions were every 3 minutes throughout most of her labor until the transition stage around 5 hours ago, when she was 8 cm. Around that time, contractions came more frequently, every 2 minutes, lasting 60 seconds. She has been complete and pushing for 3½ hours. The mother has been afebrile. Estimated fetal birth weight is 7 lbs (3,175 grams).

A quick report from the labor nurse indicates the amniotic fluid has been meconium stained. The fetal heart rate (FHR) was 130 bpm with moderate variability throughout most of the labor. Intermittent late decelerations began an hour ago with periods of minimal variability. For the past 30 minutes, the FHR has been 150 bpm with recurrent late decelerations and consistent, minimal variability. The fetal heart rate is currently 90 bpm and in response, the mother has a nonrebreather mask in place with oxygen being delivered at 10 L/min.

The baby is crowning. The provider has placed the vacuum extractor on the baby's head to assist with the birth, since the mother states she is "exhausted."

1. **Recognize cues.** What matters most?
   Which of the following is of primary concern?
   1. Vacuum extractor use.
   2. Recurrent late decelerations.
   3. Contraction frequency.
   4. Gestational age 41 weeks.
2. **Analyze cues.** What could it mean?
   For each fetal assessment below, specify if the finding is consistent with the factors of postmaturity, hypoxia, or head compression. Each finding may support more than one FHR finding. Each column must have at least one response.

Fetal assessment	(a) Postmaturity	(b) Hypoxia	(c) Head compression
1. Meconium-stained amniotic fluid			
2. FHR 90 bpm			
3. Recurrent late decelerations			
4. Minimal variability			

3. **Prioritize hypotheses.** Where do I start?
   Complete the sentence below by choosing one selection from the first column and one selection from the second column.

   Note: In the NCLEX test, the test taker will have two drop-down lists to select from.

The most serious threat to the fetus is: (Choose one answer below)	As evidenced by the: (Choose one answer below)
1. Metabolic acidemia	a. Current heart rate
2. Meconium aspiration	b. Meconium stained fluid
3. Cephalohematoma	c. Minimal variability
4. Subgaleal bleed	d. Recurrent late decelerations

4. **Generate solutions.** What can I do?
The nurse is planning care for the neonate. What impacts the actions the nurse will take? **Select all that apply.**
   1. Available personnel.
   2. Newborn tone and color.
   3. Newborn heart rate.
   4. Newborn respiratory effort.

5. **Take action.** What will I do?
Which of the following interventions are most likely to be required for this baby after the birth? **Select all that apply.**
   1. Dry and stimulate the baby under the warmer.
   2. Bulb suction of mouth and nose.
   3. Assist with endotracheal intubation and suction.
   4. Assist with bag and mask ventilation.
   5. Perform chest compressions.
   6. Cord blood gas analysis.

6. **Evaluate outcomes.** Did it help?
The baby was born limp and dusky with a heart rate of 90, respiratory rate 25, and pre-ductal SpO2 of 65 after birth. The baby required ventilation with bag and mask and the heart rate rose to 110. The Apgars were 7 at 1 minute and 8 at 5 minutes. It is now 20 minutes post resuscitation. The baby is in the newborn nursery for observation and post-resuscitation care. Which of these is/are evidence of outcomes related to nursing actions? **Select all that apply.**
   1. Newborn temp is 98° F (36.6° C).
   2. Lusty cry, heart rate 150 bpm.
   3. Central cyanosis.
   4. Cord gas results: pH 7.2, CO2 65 mmhg, bicarb 20, and base deficit 12 mmol/L.

7. A 1-day-old neonate at 32 weeks' gestation is being cared for in an isolette. The nurse assesses the morning axillary temperature as 96.9° F (36.1° C). Which of the following could explain this finding?
   1. This is a normal temperature for a preterm neonate.
   2. Axillary temperatures are not valid for preterm babies.
   3. The supply of brown adipose tissue is incomplete.
   4. Conduction heat loss is pronounced in the baby.

8. Which of the following neonates is at highest risk for cold stress syndrome?
   1. Infant of diabetic mother.
   2. Infant with Rh incompatibility.
   3. Neonate that is postdates.
   4. Infant with Down's syndrome.

9. Which of the following would lead the nurse to suspect cold stress in a newborn with a temperature of 96.5° F (35.8° C)?
   1. Blood glucose of 50 mg/dL (2.8 mmol/L).
   2. Acrocyanosis.
   3. Tachypnea.
   4. Oxygen saturation of 96%.

10. Four babies are in the newborn nursery. The nurse pages the neonatologist to see the baby who exhibits which of the following?
   1. Intercostal retractions.
   2. Erythema toxicum.
   3. Pseudostrabismus.
   4. Vernix caseosa.

11. A baby is grunting in the neonatal nursery. Which of the following actions by the nurse is appropriate?
    1. Place a pacifier in the baby's mouth.
    2. Check the baby's diaper.
    3. Have the mother feed the baby.
    4. Assess the respiratory rate.

12. A nurse is preparing a 6-month-old child with a medical history of newborn kernicterus for a medical exam. Which of the following tests can the nurse anticipate will be done to determine whether or not this child has developed any sequelae to the illness?
    1. Blood urea nitrogen and serum creatinine.
    2. Alkaline phosphatase and bilirubin.
    3. Hearing testing and vision assessment.
    4. Peak expiratory flow and blood gas assessments.

13. A baby with hemolytic jaundice is being treated with fluorescent phototherapy. To provide safe newborn care, which of the following actions should the nurse perform?
    1. Cover the baby's eyes with eye pads.
    2. Turn the lights off for 10 minutes every hour.
    3. Clothe the baby in a shirt and diaper only.
    4. Tightly swaddle the baby in a baby blanket.

14. A baby is born with erythroblastosis fetalis. Which of the following signs/symptoms would the nurse expect to see?
    1. Ruddy complexion.
    2. Generalized edema.
    3. Alopecia.
    4. Erythema toxicum.

15. Which of the following laboratory findings would the nurse expect to see in a baby diagnosed with erythroblastosis fetalis?
    1. Hematocrit 24%.
    2. Leukocyte count 45,000 cells/mm^3.
    3. Sodium 125 mEq/L.
    4. Potassium 5.5 mEq/L.

16. A baby's blood type is B negative. The baby is at risk for hemolytic jaundice if the mother has which of the following blood types?
    1. Type O negative.
    2. Type A negative.
    3. Type B positive.
    4. Type AB positive.

17. A newborn admitted to the nursery has a positive direct Coombs test. Which of the following is an appropriate action by the nurse?
    1. Monitor the baby for jitters.
    2. Assess the blood glucose level.
    3. Assess the rectal temperature.
    4. Monitor the baby for jaundice.

18. An 18-hour-old baby with an elevated bilirubin level is placed under the bili lights. Which of the following is an expected nursing action in these circumstances?
    1. Give the baby oral rehydration therapy in place of all feedings.
    2. Rotate the baby from side to back to side to front every 2 hours.
    3. Apply restraints to keep the baby under the light source.
    4. Administer intravenous fluids via pump per doctor orders.

19. A neonate with jaundice must have a heel stick to assess bilirubin levels. Which of the following actions should the nurse make during the procedure?
   1. Cover the foot with an iced wrap for 1 minute prior to the procedure.
   2. Avoid puncturing the lateral heel to prevent damaging sensitive structures.
   3. Allow the site to dry after rubbing it with an alcohol swab.
   4. Firmly grasp the calf of the baby during the procedure to prevent injury.

20. A nurse is caring for a baby who is receiving phototherapy. The provider's notes read as follows: "This is a term, newborn male at 5 days of age who was admitted 24 hours ago with a total serum bilirubin (TSB) of 18 mg/dL (307.8 µmol/L) related to ABO incompatibility. Phototherapy was initiated on admission. Mother states her previous baby needed phototherapy, as well. The newborn has demonstrated an 8% weight loss since birth. Total serum bilirubin today was 15mg/dL (256.6 µmol/L). The newborn is breastfeeding and is removed from phototherapy for feedings. Elimination pattern as documented is 6 to 7 wet diapers in 24 hours."

    Which of the findings would indicate the baby's condition is not progressing as expected? **Select all that apply.**

    (Note: The paragraph above is formatted below with each sentence numbered separately. In the NGN format the test taker will be asked to highlight the statements of concern by clicking on that area.)
   1. "This is a term, newborn male at 5 days of age who was admitted 24 hours ago with a total serum bilirubin (TSB) of 18 mg/dL (307.8 µmol/L) related to ABO incompatibility."
   2. "Phototherapy was initiated on admission."
   3. "Mother states her previous baby needed phototherapy, as well."
   4. "The newborn has demonstrated an 8% weight loss since birth."
   5. "Total serum bilirubin today was 15 mg/dL (256.5 µmol/L)."
   6. "The newborn is breastfeeding and is removed from phototherapy for feedings."
   7. "Elimination pattern as documented is 6 to 7 wet diapers in 24 hours."

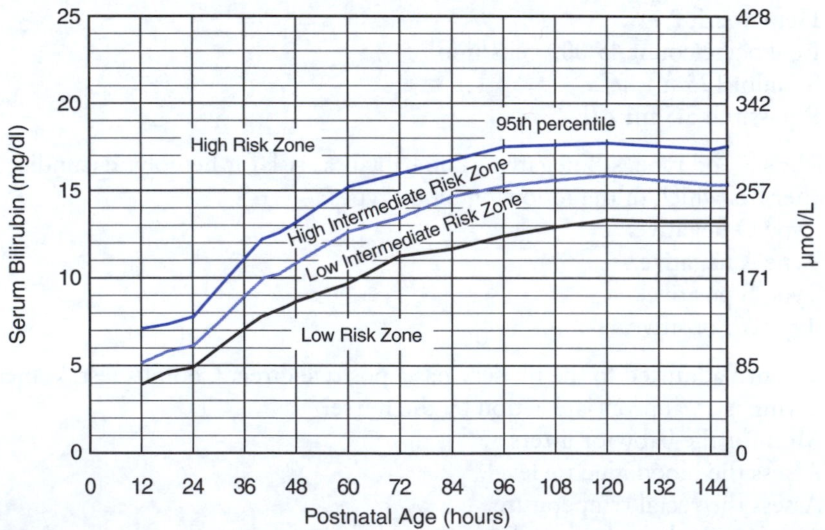

21. A newborn nursery nurse notes that a 36-hour-old baby's body is slightly jaundiced. Which of the following nursing interventions will be most therapeutic?
   1. Maintain a warm ambient environment.
   2. Have the mother feed the baby frequently.
   3. Have the mother hold the baby skin to skin.
   4. Place the baby naked by a closed sunlit window.

22. A neonate is under phototherapy for elevated bilirubin levels. The baby's stools are now loose and green. Which of the following actions should the nurse take at this time?
1. Discontinue the phototherapy.
2. Notify the healthcare practitioner.
3. Take the baby's temperature.
4. Assess the baby's skin integrity.

23. A nurse is preparing a care plan for a 5-day-old newborn under phototherapy. Which of the following client care outcomes should be included in the nursing care plan? **"During the next 24 hour period**, the baby will:
1. Have at least 6 wet diapers."
2. Breastfeed 2 to 4 times."
3. Lose less than 12% of the baby's birth weight."
4. Have an apical heart rate of 160 to 170 bpm."

24. A baby in the neonatal intensive care unit (NICU) is exhibiting signs of neonatal abstinence syndrome (NAS). Which of the following medications is contraindicated for this neonate?
1. Morphine.
2. Methadone.
3. Narcan.
4. Phenobarbital.

25. A baby whose mother was addicted to heroin during pregnancy is in the NICU. Which of the following nursing actions would be appropriate for the nurse to perform?
1. Tightly swaddle the baby.
2. Place the baby prone in the crib.
3. Provide needed stimulation to the baby.
4. Feed the baby half-strength formula.

26. A newborn in the nursery is exhibiting signs of neonatal abstinence syndrome. Which of the following signs/symptoms is the nurse seeing? **Select all that apply.**
1. Hyperphagia.
2. Lethargy.
3. Prolonged periods of sleep.
4. Hyporeflexia.
5. Persistent shrill cry.

27. Based on maternal history of alcohol abuse, a baby in the neonatal nursery is being monitored for signs of fetal alcohol syndrome (FAS). The nurse should assess this baby for which of the following?
1. Poor suck reflex.
2. Ambiguous genitalia.
3. Webbed neck.
4. Absent Moro reflex.

28. A baby born dependent on cocaine is being given oral morphine therapeutically. The nurse knows that which of the following are the main reasons for its use in newborns? **Select all that apply.**
1. Oral morphine contains no alcohol.
2. Oral morphine is nonsedating.
3. Oral morphine improves respiratory effort.
4. Oral morphine helps to control seizures.

29. A baby was born 24 hours ago to a mother who received no prenatal care. The infant has tremors, sneezes excessively, constantly roots on its hand to suck, and has a shrill, high-pitched cry. The baby's serum glucose levels are normal. For which of the following should the nurse request an order from the pediatrician?
1. Urine drug toxicology test.
2. Biophysical profile test.
3. Chest and abdominal ultrasound evaluations.
4. Oxygen saturation and blood gas assessments.

30. A nurse makes the following observations when admitting a full-term, breastfeeding baby into the neonatal nursery: 9 lb 2 oz (4,139 grams), 21 inches long, TPR: 96.6° F (35.9° C), 158, 62, jittery, pink body with bluish hands and feet, crying. Which of the following nursing actions is of highest importance?
1. Swaddle the baby to provide warmth.
2. Assess the glucose level of the baby.
3. Take the baby to the mother for feeding.
4. Administer the routine neonatal medications.

31. An infant admitted to the newborn nursery has a blood glucose level of 35 mg/dL (1.9 mmol/L). The nurse should monitor this baby carefully for which of the following?
1. Jaundice.
2. Jitters.
3. Erythema toxicum.
4. Subconjunctival hemorrhages.

32. A full-term infant admitted to the newborn nursery has a blood glucose level of 35 mg/dL (1.9 mmol/L). Which of the following actions should the nurse perform at this time?
1. Feed the baby formula or breast milk.
2. Assess the baby's blood pressure.
3. Tightly swaddle the baby.
4. Monitor the baby's urinary output.

33. A nurse is inserting a gavage tube into a preterm baby who is unable to suck and swallow. Which of the following actions must the nurse take during the procedure?
1. Measure the distance from the tip of the ear to the nose and the xiphoid process.
2. Lubricate the tube with an oil-based solution.
3. Insert the tube quickly if the baby becomes cyanotic.
4. Inject a small amount of sterile water to check placement.

34. The nurse must perform nasopharyngeal suctioning of a newborn with profuse secretions. Please place the following nursing actions for nasopharyngeal suctioning in chronological order.
1. Slowly rotate and remove the suction catheter.
2. Place thumb over the suction control on the catheter.
3. Assess type and amount of secretions.
4. Insert free end of the tubing through the nose.

35. A neonate is being given intravenous fluids through the dorsal vein of the wrist. Which of the following actions by the nurse is essential?
1. Tape the arm to an arm board.
2. Change the tubing every 24 hours.
3. Monitor the site every 5 minutes.
4. Infuse the fluid intermittently.

36. A Roman Catholic couple has just delivered a baby with an Apgar score of 1 at 1 minute, 2 at 5 minutes, and 2 at 10 minutes. Which of the following interventions is appropriate at this time?

1. Advise the parents that they should pray very hard so that everything turns out well.
2. Ask the parents whether they would like the baby baptized.
3. Leave the parents alone to work through their thoughts and feelings.
4. Inform the parents that a priest will listen to their confessions whenever they are ready.

37. The nurse assesses a newborn as follows:
Heart rate: 70
Respirations: weak and irregular
Tone: flaccid
Color: pale
Baby grimaces when a pediatrician attempts to insert an endotracheal tube
What should the nurse calculate the baby's Apgar score to be?

Apgar Scoring Grid

Sign	Score of 0	Score of 1	Score of 2
Heart Rate	Absent	Below 100 bpm	100 bpm and above
Respiratory Effort	Absent	Slow and irregular	Lusty (vigorous) cry
Muscle Tone	Flaccid	Some flexion of the extremities	Active motion or well-flexed extremities
Reflex Irritability	Absent	Grimace	Lusty (vigorous) cry
Color	Completely cyanotic or very pale baby	Pink body with cyanotic extremities (acrocyanosis)	Pink body and extremities

38. A neonate is in the neonatal intensive care nursery with a diagnosis of large for gestational age (LGA). The baby was born at 38 weeks' gestation and weighed 7 lbs 7 oz (3,500 grams). Based on this information, which of the following responses is correct? **(See the figure that follows.)**

1. The diagnosis is accurate because the baby's weight is too high for a diagnosis of average for gestational age (AGA).
2. The diagnosis is inaccurate because the baby's weight would need to be higher than 3,500 grams.
3. The diagnosis is inaccurate because the baby's weight would need to be lower than 3,500 grams.
4. The diagnosis is inaccurate because full-term babies are never large for gestational age.

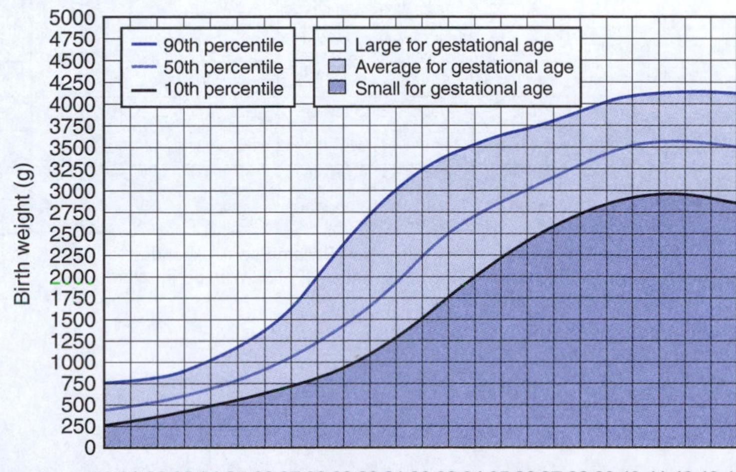

39. A neonate has been admitted to the neonatal intensive care unit with the following findings:
Completely flaccid posturing
Square window sign of 60°
Arm recoil of 180°
Popliteal angle of 160°
Full scarf sign
Heel that touches the ear
Skin that is red and translucent
Sparse lanugo
Faint red marks on the plantar surface
Barely perceptible breast tissue
Eyelids that are open but flat ear pinnae
Prominent clitoris and small labia minora
Using the Ballard scale, what is the gestational age of this neonate estimated to be?
_____ weeks.

Neuromuscular Maturity

	−1	0	1	2	3	4	5
Posture							
Square Window (Wrist)	−90°	90°	60°	45°	30°	0°	
Arm Recoil		180°	140°–180°	110°–140°	90°–110°	<90°	
Popliteal Angle	180°	160°	140°	120°	100°	90°	<90°
Scarf Sign							
Heel to Ear							

Physical Maturity

Skin	sticky; friable; transparent	gelatinous; red; translucent	smooth pink; visible veins	superficial peeling or rash, few veins	cracking; pale areas; rare veins	parchment; deep cracking; no vessels	leathery; cracked; wrinkled
Lanugo	none	sparse	abundant	thinning	bald areas	mostly bald	
Plantar Surface	heel-toe 40–50 mm:–1 <40 mm:–2	>50 mm no crease	faint red marks	anterior transverse crease only	creases ant. 2/3	creases over entire sole	
Breast	imperceptible	barely perceptible	flat areola; no bud	stippled areola; 1–2 mm bud	raised areola; 3–4 mm bud	full areola; 5–10 mm bud	
Eye/Ear	lids fused; loosely:–1 tightly:–2	lids open; pinna flat; stays folded	sl. curved pinna; soft; slow recoil	well-curved pinna; soft but ready recoil	formed and firm; instant recoil	thick cartilage; ear stiff	
Genitals (Male)	scrotum flat, smooth	scrotum empty; faint rugae	testes in upper canal; rare rugae	testes descending; few rugae	testes down; good rugae	testes pendulous; deep rugae	
Genitals (Female)	clitoris prominent; labia flat	prominent clitoris; small labia minora	prominent clitoris; enlarging minora	majora and minora equally prominent	majora large; minora small	majora cover clitoris and minora	

Maturity Rating

Score	Weeks
−10	20
−5	22
0	24
5	26
10	28
15	30
20	32
25	34
30	36
35	38
40	40
45	42
50	44

From: Ballard, J. L., Khoury, L. C., Wedig, K., et al. (1991). New Ballard Score, expanded to include extremely premature infants. *Journal of Pediatrics, 19*(3), 417-423. With permission.

40. A neonate is in the neonatal intensive care unit. The baby is 28 weeks' gestation and weighs 2 lbs 2 oz (1,000 grams). Which of the following is correct in relation to this baby's growth?
1. Weight is average for gestational age.
2. Weight is below average for gestational age.
3. Baby experienced intrauterine growth restriction.
4. Baby is large for gestational age.

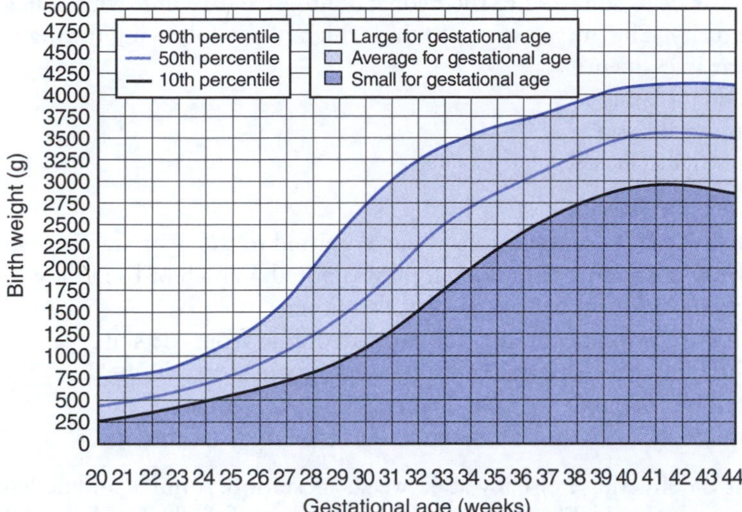

41. A neonate, 40 weeks by dates, has been admitted to the nursery. Place an X on the graph where the baby would be labeled large for gestational age.

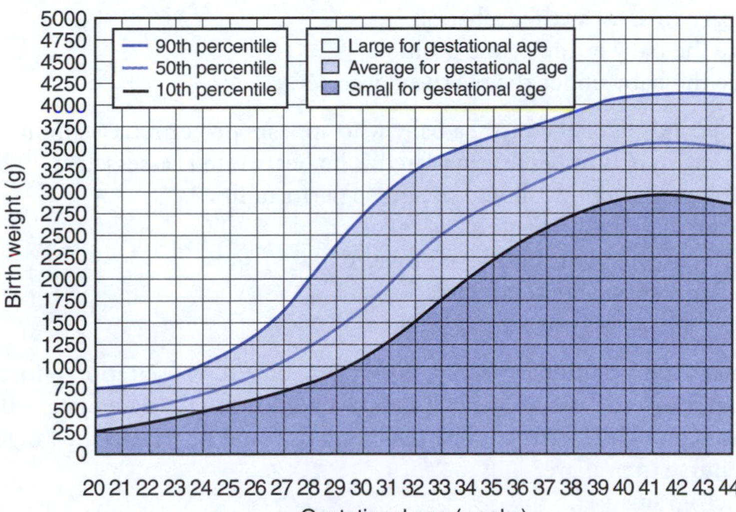

42. A baby at 42 weeks' gestation weighing 5 lbs 3 oz (2,400 grams) is admitted into the NICU. The baby's mother had no prenatal care. The neonatologist orders blood work. Which of the following laboratory findings would the nurse expect to see?
1. Blood glucose 30 mg/dL (1.7 mmol/L).
2. Leukocyte count 1,000 cells/mm^3.
3. Hematocrit 30%.
4. Serum pH 7.8.

43. A client who received an intravenous analgesic 4 hours ago has had recurrent late decelerations in labor. She will deliver her baby shortly. Which of the following is the priority action for the delivery room nurse to take?
1. Preheat the overhead warmer.
2. Page the neonatologist on call.
3. Draw up Narcan (naloxone) for injection.
4. Assemble the oral ophthalmic antibiotic.

44. A baby has been admitted to the neonatal intensive care unit with a diagnosis of postmaturity. The nurse expects to find which of the following during the initial newborn assessment?
1. Abundant lanugo.
2. Flat breast tissue.
3. Prominent clitoris.
4. Wrinkled skin.

45. A baby at 42 weeks' gestation has been admitted to the neonatal intensive care unit. At delivery, thick green amniotic fluid was noted. Which of the following neonatal care actions by the nurse is critical at this time?
1. Bath to remove meconium-contaminated fluid from the skin.
2. Ophthalmic assessment to check for conjunctival irritation.
3. Rectal temperature to assess for septic hyperthermia.
4. Respiratory evaluation to monitor for respiratory distress.

46. A client is delivering her baby at 42 weeks' gestation. A nurse and pediatrician are present at the birth. The amniotic fluid is green and thick. The baby fails to breathe spontaneously. Which of the following actions should the nurse take next? **Select all that apply.**
1. Stimulate the baby to breathe.
2. Assess neonatal heart rate.
3. Prepare to assist with intubation.
4. Place the baby in the prone position.
5. Place the baby under the overhead warmer.

47. Thirty seconds after the birth, a baby who appears preterm has exhibited no effort to breathe, even after being stimulated. The heart rate is assessed at 70 bpm. Which of the following actions should the nurse perform first?
1. Perform a gestational age assessment.
2. Inflate the lungs with positive pressure.
3. Provide external chest compressions.
4. Assess the oxygen saturation level.

48. A neonatologist requests naloxone during a neonatal resuscitation effort for a baby weighing 3 kg. The recommended dosage of naloxone for a neonate is 0.01 mg/kg to 0.1 mg/kg. Which of the following dosages would be within the range of safety for the nurse to prepare?
1. 4 micrograms.
2. 40 micrograms.
3. 4 milligrams.
4. 40 milligrams.

49. During neonatal cardiopulmonary resuscitation, which of the following actions should be performed?
1. Provide assisted ventilation at about 30 breaths per minute.
2. Begin chest compressions when heart rate is 0 to 20 beats per minute.
3. Compress the chest using the three-finger technique.
4. Administer compressions and breaths in a 5:1 ratio.

50. The staff on the maternity unit is developing a protocol for nurses to follow after a baby is delivered and fails to breathe spontaneously. Which of the following should be included in the protocol as the first action for the nurse to take?
1. Prepare epinephrine for administration.
2. Provide positive pressure oxygen.
3. Administer chest compressions.
4. Rub the back and feet of the baby.

51. A nurse in the newborn nursery suspects that a new admission, a baby at 42 weeks' gestation, was exposed to meconium in utero. What would lead the nurse to suspect this?
1. The baby is bradycardic.
2. The baby's umbilical cord is stained green.
3. The baby's anterior fontanel is sunken.
4. The baby is desquamating.

52. The birth of a baby who weighed 9 lbs 9 oz (4,500 grams), was complicated by shoulder dystocia. Which of the following neonatal complications should the nursery nurse observe for?
1. Leg deformities.
2. Brachial palsy.
3. Fractured radius.
4. Buccal abrasions.

53. During a health maintenance visit at the pediatrician's office, the nurse notes that a breastfeeding baby has thrush. Which of the following actions should the nurse take?
1. Nothing, because thrush is a benign problem.
2. Advise the mother to bottle feed until the thrush is cured.
3. Obtain an order for antifungals for both mother and baby.
4. Assess for other evidence of immunosuppression.

54. A neonate whose mother is HIV positive is admitted to the NICU. The nurse is planning care for the neonate. Which of the following interventions should the nurse include as a result of the baby's perinatal exposure to HIV/AIDS?
1. Monitor daily viral load laboratory reports.
2. Check the baby's viral antibody status.
3. Obtain an order for antiviral medication.
4. Place the baby on contact precautions.

55. A baby was just born to a mother who had positive vaginal cultures for group B streptococci (GBS). The mother was admitted to the labor room two hours before the birth. For which of the following should the nursery nurse closely observe this baby?
1. Hypothermia.
2. Mottling.
3. Omphalocele.
4. Stomatitis.

56. A baby in the newborn nursery was born to a mother with spontaneous rupture of membranes for 14 hours. The woman has *Candida* vaginitis. For which of the following should the baby be assessed?
1. Papular facial rash.
2. Thrush.
3. Fungal conjunctivitis.
4. Dehydration.

57. A baby has been admitted to the neonatal nursery whose mother is hepatitis B surface antigen positive. Which of the following actions by the nurse should be taken at this time?
1. Monitor the baby for signs of hepatitis B.
2. Place the baby on contact isolation.
3. Obtain an order for the hepatitis B vaccine and the immune globulin.
4. Advise the mother that breastfeeding is absolutely contraindicated.

58. Four full-term babies were admitted to the neonatal nursery. The mothers of each of the babies had labors of 4 hours or less. The nursery nurse should carefully monitor which of the babies for tachypnea?
1. The baby whose mother cultured positive for group B streptococci during her third trimester.
2. The baby whose mother has cerebral palsy.
3. The baby whose mother was hospitalized for 3 months with complete placenta previa.
4. The baby whose mother previously had a stillbirth.

59. Four clients at 38 weeks' gestation have just delivered. Which of the babies should be monitored closely for respiratory distress?
1. The baby whose mother has diabetes mellitus.
2. The baby whose mother has lung cancer.
3. The baby whose mother has mitral valve prolapse.
4. The baby whose mother has asthma.

60. A baby is born with caudal agenesis. Which of the following maternal complications is associated with this defect?
1. Poorly controlled myasthenia gravis.
2. Poorly controlled diabetes mellitus.
3. Poorly controlled splenic syndrome.
4. Poorly controlled hypothyroidism.

61. A macrosomic infant of a non–insulin dependent diabetic mother has been admitted to the neonatal nursery. The baby's glucose level on admission to the nursery is 30 mg/dL (1.7 mmol/L). After a feeding of the mother's expressed breast milk the baby's glucose level is 35 mg/dL (1.9 mmol/L). Which of the following actions should the nurse take at this time?
1. Nothing, because the glucose level is normal for an infant of a diabetic mother.
2. Administer intravenous glucagon slowly over 5 minutes.
3. Feed the baby a bottle of dextrose and water and reassess the glucose level.
4. Notify the neonatologist of the abnormal glucose levels.

62. A baby has just been born to a mother with type 1 diabetes mellitus (T1DM) who has retinopathy and nephropathy. Which of the following neonatal findings would the nurse expect to see?
1. Hyperalbuminemia.
2. Polycythemia.
3. Hypercalcemia.
4. Hypoinsulinemia.

63. A baby is born to a mother with type 1 diabetes mellitus (T1DM) and poor blood sugar control. If a blood sample was drawn, which of the following laboratory values would the nurse expect the neonate to exhibit during the immediate postpartum period?
1. Plasma glucose 30 mg/dL (1.7 mmol/L).
2. Red blood cell count 1 million/mm^3.
3. White blood cell count 2,000/mm^3.
4. Hemoglobin 8 g/dL.

64. A baby has just been admitted into the neonatal intensive care unit with a diagnosis of intrauterine growth restriction (IUGR). Which of the following maternal factors would predispose the baby to this diagnosis? **Select all that apply.**
1. Hyperopia.
2. Gestational diabetes.
3. Substance abuse.
4. Chronic hypertension.
5. Advanced maternal age.

65. A baby has been admitted to the NICU with a diagnosis of symmetrical intrauterine growth restriction (IUGR). Which of the following pregnancy complications would be consistent with this diagnosis?
1. Pre-eclampsia with severe features.
2. Fetal chromosomal defect.
3. Infarcts in an aging placenta.
4. Preterm premature rupture of the membranes.

66. A neonate has asymmetrical intrauterine growth restriction (IUGR) secondary to placental insufficiency. Which of the following signs/symptoms should the nurse expect to observe at delivery? **Select all that apply.**
1. Thrombocytopenia.
2. Neutropenia.
3. Polycythemia.
4. Hypoglycemia.
5. Hyperlipidemia.

67. A client is visiting the NICU to see her baby for the first time. He was born the day before at 26 weeks gestation. Which of the following methods would the nurse expect the mother to use when first making physical contact with her baby?
1. Fingertip touch.
2. Palmar touch.
3. Kangaroo hold.
4. Cradle hold.

68. A 6-month-old child is being seen in the pediatrician's office. The child was born preterm and remained in the neonatal intensive care unit for the first 5 months of life. The child is being monitored for 5 chronic problems. Which of the following problems are directly related to the prematurity? **Select all that apply.**
1. Bronchopulmonary dysplasia.
2. Cerebral palsy.
3. Retinopathy.
4. Hypothyroidism.
5. Seizure disorders.

69. A neonatologist prescribes gentamicin for a 2-day-old, septic preterm infant who weighs 1,653 grams and is 38 centimeters long. The drug reference states: *Neonatal dosage of gentamicin for babies less than 1 week of age is 2.5 mg/kg q 12–24 hours.* Calculate the safe daily dosage of this medication. **Calculate to the nearest hundredth.**

_____ mg q 24 hours

70. The neonatologist has ordered 12.5 micrograms of digoxin PO for a neonate in congestive heart failure. The medication is available in the following elixir—0.05 mg/mL. How many milliliters (mL) should the nurse administer? **Calculate to the nearest hundredth.**

_____ mL

71. A neonatologist prescribes cisplatin for a neonate born with a neuroblastoma. The baby's current weight is 3,476 grams and the baby is 57 centimeters long. The drug reference states: *Children: IV 30 mg/m² q week.* Calculate the safe dosage of this medication. **Calculate to the nearest tenth.**
_____ mg q week

72. A preterm baby is to receive 4 mg gentamicin IV every 24 hours. The medication is being injected into an IV soluset. A total of 5 mL is to be administered via IV pump over 90 minutes. The pump should be set at what rate? **Calculate to the nearest hundredth.**
_____ mL/hr

73. A mother of a preterm baby is performing kangaroo care in the neonatal nursery. Which of the following responses would the nurse evaluate as a positive neonatal outcome?
1. Respiratory rate of 70.
2. Temperature of 97° F (36.1° C).
3. Licking of mother's nipples.
4. Flaring of the baby's nares.

74. A neonate is being assessed for necrotizing enterocolitis (NEC). Which of the following actions by the nurse is appropriate? **Select all that apply.**
1. Perform hemoccult test on stools.
2. Monitor for an increase in abdominal girth.
3. Measure gastric contents before each feed.
4. Assess bowel sounds before each feed.
5. Assess for anal fissures daily.

75. A client whose baby was born at 32 weeks gestation is expressing breast milk (EBM) for the baby. The neonatologist is recommending that fortifier be added to the milk because which of the following needs of the baby are not met by the EBM?
1. Need for iron and zinc.
2. Need for calcium and phosphorus.
3. Need for protein and fat.
4. Need for sodium and potassium.

76. A 2 lb 2 oz (1,000 grams) neonate is being admitted to the neonatal intensive care unit. A surfactant has just been prescribed to prevent respiratory distress syndrome. Which of the following actions should the nurse take while administering this medication?
1. Flush the intravenous line with normal saline solution.
2. Assist the neonatologist during the intubation procedure.
3. Inject the medication deep into the vastus lateralis muscle.
4. Administer the reconstituted liquid via an oral syringe.

77. A 30-week-gestation neonate, 2 hours old, has received exogenous surfactant. Which of the following would indicate a positive response to the medication?
1. Axillary temperature 98° F (36.7° C).
2. Oxygen saturation 96%.
3. Apical heart rate 154 bpm.
4. Serum potassium 4 mEq/L.

78. For which of the following reasons would a nurse in the well-baby nursery report to the neonatologist that a newborn appears to be preterm?
1. Baby has a square window angle of 90°.
2. Baby has leathery and cracked skin.
3. Baby has popliteal angle of 90°.
4. Baby has pronounced plantar creases.

79. A full-term neonate in the NICU has been diagnosed with congestive heart failure secondary to a cyanotic heart defect. Which of the following activities is most likely to result in a cyanotic episode?
1. Feeding.
2. Sleeping in the supine position.
3. Rocking in an infant swing.
4. Swaddling.

80. The nurse is providing discharge teaching to the parents of a baby born with a cleft lip and palate. Which of the following should be included in the teaching?
1. Correct technique for the administration of a gastrostomy feeding.
2. Need to watch for the appearance of blood-stained mucus from the nose.
3. Optimal position for burping after nasogastric feedings.
4. Need to give the baby sufficient time to rest during each feeding.

81. A baby is thought to have esophageal atresia. The nurse would expect to see which of the following signs/symptoms? **Select all that apply.**
1. Frequent vomiting.
2. Excessive mucus.
3. Ruddy complexion.
4. Abdominal distention.
5. Pigeon chest.

82. The nurse is teaching a couple about the special healthcare needs of their newborn child with Down's syndrome (trisomy 21). The nurse knows that the teaching was successful when the parents state that the child will need which of the following? **Select all that apply.**
1. Yearly 3-hour glucose tolerance testing.
2. Immediate intervention during bleeding episodes.
3. A formula that is low in lactose and phenylalanine.
4. Prompt treatment of upper respiratory infections.

83. An infant in the neonatal nursery has low-set ears, single palmar creases, and slanted eyes. The nurse should monitor this infant carefully for which of the following signs/symptoms?
1. Blood-tinged urine.
2. Hemispheric paralysis.
3. Cardiac murmur.
4. Hemolytic jaundice.

84. Which of the following actions would the NICU nurse expect to perform when caring for a neonate with esophageal atresia and tracheoesophageal fistula (TEF)?
1. Position the baby flat on the left side.
2. Maintain low nasogastric suction.
3. Give small, frequent feedings.
4. Place on hypothermia blanket.

85. A nurse is assisting a mother to feed a baby born with cleft palate. Which of the following should the nurse teach the mother?
1. The baby is likely to cry from pain during the feeding.
2. The baby is likely to expel milk through the nose.
3. The baby will feed more quickly than other babies.
4. The baby will need to be fed high-calorie formula.

86. A neonate who is admitted to the neonatal nursery is noted to have a 2-vessel cord. The nurse notifies the neonatologist to request an order for which of the following assessments? **Select all that apply.**
1. Renal function tests.
2. Echocardiogram.
3. Glucose tolerance test.
4. Electroencephalogram.

87. In the delivery room, which of the following infant care interventions must a nurse perform when a neonate with a meningomyelocele is born?
1. Perform nasogastric suctioning.
2. Place the baby in the prone position.
3. Administer oxygen via face mask.
4. Swaddle the baby in warmed blankets.

88. A baby in the NICU who is exhibiting signs of congestive heart failure from an atrioventricular canal defect is receiving a diuretic. In the plan of care, the nurse should include that the desired outcome for the child will be which of the following?
1. Loss of body weight.
2. Drop in serum sodium level.
3. Rise in urine specific gravity.
4. Increase in blood pressure.

89. The nurse caring for a neonate with congestive heart failure identifies which of the following risks as highest priority?
1. Fatigue.
2. Activity intolerance.
3. Sleep pattern disturbance.
4. Altered tissue perfusion.

90. The nurse administers digoxin to a baby in the NICU who has a cardiac defect. The baby vomits shortly after receiving the medication. Which of the following actions should the nurse perform next?
1. Give a repeat dose.
2. Notify the physician.
3. Assess the apical and brachial pulses concurrently.
4. Check the vomitus for streaks of blood.

91. A baby is born with a meningomyelocele at L2. In assessing the baby, which of the following would the nurse expect to see?
1. Sensory loss in all four extremities.
2. Tuft of hair over the lumbosacral region.
3. Flaccid paralysis of the legs.
4. Positive Moro reflex.

92. When examining a neonate in the well-baby nursery, the nurse notes that the sclerae of the baby's eyes are visible above the iris of the eyes. Which of the following assessments is highest priority for the nurse to make next?
1. Babinski and tonic neck reflexes.
2. Evaluation of bilateral eye coordination.
3. Blood type and Coombs test results.
4. Circumferences of the head and chest.

93. A baby is born with a suspected coarctation of the aorta. Which of the following assessments should be done by the nurse?
1. Check blood pressures in all four limbs.
2. Palpate the anterior fontanel for bulging.
3. Assess hematocrit and hemoglobin values.
4. Monitor for harlequin color changes.

94. The nurse is developing a teaching plan for parents of an infant with tetralogy of Fallot. In which of the following positions should parents be taught to place the infant during a "blue," or "tet," spell?
1. Supine.
2. Prone.
3. Knee–chest.
4. Semi-Fowler.

95. A child has been diagnosed with a small ventricular septal defect (VSD). Which of the following symptoms would the nurse expect to see?
1. Cyanosis and clubbing of the fingers.
2. Respiratory distress and extreme fatigue.
3. Systolic murmur with no other obvious symptoms.
4. Feeding difficulties with marked polycythemia.

96. A newborn in the NICU has just had a ventriculoperitoneal (VP) shunt inserted. Which of the following signs indicates that the shunt is functioning properly?
1. Decrease of the baby's head circumference.
2. Absence of cardiac arrhythmias.
3. Rise of the baby's blood pressure.
4. Appearance of setting sun sign.

97. A neonate has just been born with a meningomyelocele. Which of the following risks should the nurse identify as related to this medical diagnosis?
1. Deficient fluid volume.
2. High risk for infection.
3. Ineffective breathing pattern.
4. Imbalanced nutrition: less than body requirements.

98. The neonatologist assesses a newborn for Hirschsprung's disease after the baby exhibited which of the following signs/symptoms?
1. Passed meconium at 50 hours of age.
2. Apical heart rate of 200 beats per minute.
3. Maculopapular rash.
4. Asymmetrical leg folds.

99. The nurse assessed four newborns admitted to the neonatal nursery and called the neonatologist for a consult on the baby who exhibited which of the following?
1. Excessive amounts of frothy saliva from the mouth.
2. Blood-tinged discharge from the vaginal canal.
3. Secretion of a milk-like substance from both breasts.
4. Heart rate that sped during inhalation and slowed with exhalation.

100. The nurse is caring for a baby diagnosed with developmental dysplasia of the hip (DDH). Which of the following therapeutic interventions should the nurse expect to perform?
1. Maintain the baby's legs in abduction.
2. Administer pain medication as needed.
3. Assist with bilateral leg casting.
4. Monitor pedal pulses bilaterally.

101. A baby has been diagnosed with developmental dysplasia of the hip (DDH). Which of the following findings would the nurse expect to see?
1. Pronounced hip abduction.
2. Swelling at the site.
3. Asymmetrical leg folds.
4. Weak femoral pulses.

102. The nurse suspects that a newborn in the nursery has a clubbed right foot because the foot is plantar flexed as well as which of the following?
1. Right foot that will not move into alignment.
2. Positive Ortolani sign on the right.
3. Shortened right metatarsal arch.
4. Positive Babinski reflex on the right.

103. The parents of a baby born with bilateral club foot ask the nurse what medical care the baby will likely need. Which of the following should the nurse tell the parents? The baby will:
1. Need a series of leg casts until the correction is accomplished.
2. Have a Harrington rod inserted when the child is about 3 years old.
3. Have a Pavlik harness fitted before discharge from the nursery.
4. Need to wear braces on both legs until the child begins to walk.

104. The nurse caring for an infant with a congenital cardiac defect is monitoring the child for which of the following early signs of congestive heart failure? **Select all that apply.**
1. Palpitations.
2. Tachypnea.
3. Tachycardia.
4. Diaphoresis.
5. Irritability.

105. The nurse assessed four newborns in the neonatal nursery. The nurse called the neonatologist for a cardiology consult on the baby who exhibited which of the following signs/symptoms?
1. Setting sun sign.
2. Generalized edema
3. Flaccid extremities.
4. Polydactyly.

106. A preterm infant has a patent ductus arteriosus (PDA). You are orienting a nurse new to the unit and are listening to the nurse's explanation of the condition to the parents. Which of the following information the nurse gives to the parents about this condition requires follow-up with the nurse and with the parents? **Select all that apply.**
1. Hole has developed between the left and right ventricles.
2. Hypoxemia occurs as a result of the poor systemic circulation.
3. Oxygenated blood is reentering the pulmonary system.
4. Blood is shunting from the right side of the heart to the left.

107. A nurse hears a heart murmur on a full-term neonate in the well-baby nursery. The baby's color is pink while at rest and while feeding. Which of the following cardiac defects is consistent with the nurse's findings? **Select all that apply.**
1. Transposition of the great vessels.
2. Tetralogy of Fallot.
3. Ventricular septal defect.
4. Pulmonic stenosis.
5. Patent ductus arteriosus.

108. Four babies are born with distinctive skin markings. Identify which marking matches its description:

1. Café au lait spot.	A. Raised, blood vessel–filled lesion.
2. Hemangioma.	B. Flat, sharply demarcated red-to-purple lesion.
3. Mongolian spots.	C. Multiple grayish-blue, hyperpigmented skin areas.
4. Port wine stain.	D. Pale tan- to coffee-colored marking.

109. A baby admitted to the nursery was diagnosed with galactosemia. Which of the following actions must the nurse take?
1. Feed the baby a specialty formula.
2. Monitor the baby for central cyanosis.
3. Do hemoccult testing on every stool.
4. Monitor the baby for signs of abdominal pain.

110. On admission to the nursery, a baby's head and chest circumferences are 39 cm and 32 cm, respectively. Which of the following actions should the nurse take next?
1. Assess the anterior fontanel.
2. Measure the abdominal girth.
3. Check the apical pulse rate.
4. Monitor the respiratory effort.

111. A neonate is found to have choanal atresia. Which of the following physiological actions will be hampered by this condition?
1. Feeding.
2. Digestion.
3. Immune response.
4. Glomerular filtration.

112. A baby is born to a mother who was diagnosed with oligohydramnios during her pregnancy. The nurse notifies the neonatologist to order tests to assess the functioning of which of the following systems?
1. Gastrointestinal.
2. Hepatic.
3. Endocrine.
4. Renal.

113. A baby is born with esophageal atresia and tracheoesophageal fistula. Which of the following complications of pregnancy would the nurse expect to note in the mother's history?
1. Pre-eclampsia.
2. Idiopathic thrombocytopenia.
3. Polyhydramnios.
4. Severe iron deficiency anemia.

114. A baby is born with a diaphragmatic hernia. Which of the following signs/symptoms would the nurse observe in the delivery room?
1. Projectile vomiting.
2. High-pitched crying.
3. Respiratory distress.
4. Fecal incontinence.

115. A woman who has recently received fentanyl, 50 mcg IV, for labor pain is about to deliver. Which of the following medications is highest priority for the nurse to prepare in case it must be administered to the baby following the delivery?
1. Oxytocin.
2. Xylocaine.
3. Naloxone.
4. Butorphanol.

116. A newborn is noted to have a chignon. The nurse concludes that the baby was born via which of the following methods?
1. Cesarean section.
2. High forceps delivery.
3. Low forceps delivery.
4. Vacuum extraction.

117. A nurse is caring for a baby born by vacuum extraction. The nurse should assess this baby for which of the following?
1. Pedal abrasions.
2. Hypobilirubinemia.
3. Hyperglycemia.
4. Cephalohematoma.

118. A macrosomic baby in the nursery is suspected of having a fractured clavicle from a traumatic delivery. Which of the following signs/symptoms would the nurse expect to see? **Select all that apply.**
1. Pain with movement.
2. Hard lump at the fracture site.
3. Malpositioning of the arm.
4. Asymmetrical Moro reflex.
5. Marked localized ecchymosis.

119. Four babies in the well-baby nursery were born with congenital defects. Which of the babies' complications developed as a result of the delivery method?
1. Clubfoot.
2. Brachial palsy.
3. Gastroschisis.
4. Hydrocele.

120. Monochorionic twins whose gestation was complicated by twin-to-twin transfusion are admitted to the neonatal intensive care unit. Which of the following characteristic findings would the nurse expect to see in the smaller twin?
1. Pallor.
2. Jaundice.
3. Opisthotonus.
4. Hydrocephalus.

121. Monochorionic twins whose gestation was complicated by twin-to-twin transfusion are admitted to the neonatal intensive care unit. Which of the following characteristic findings would the nurse expect to see?
1. Recipient twin has petechial rash.
2. Recipient twin is larger than the donor twin.
3. Donor twin has 30% higher hematocrit than recipient twin.
4. Donor twin is ruddy and plethoric.

122. A baby, born at 3,199 grams, now weighs 2,746 grams. The baby is being monitored for dehydration because of the following percent weight loss. **Calculate to the nearest hundredth.**

_____ %

123. A breastfeeding mother of a newborn states, "I was good all during my pregnancy. I stopped drinking alcohol and I quit smoking marijuana during my pregnancy. Now that I'm no longer pregnant, one of the first things I'm going to do when I get home is have a joint." Which of the following responses is appropriate for the nurse to give?
1. "I am proud of you for waiting to have those things. It must have been hard for you to abstain for so many months."
2. "You are making the best choice since marijuana is safe while breastfeeding but alcohol is contraindicated."
3. "Because the drug in marijuana does get into breast milk and can alter a baby's development, it is best not to use the drug while breastfeeding."
4. "Both alcohol and marijuana are removed from the body within about two hours. It would be best to wait that long before breastfeeding after consuming either of them."

124. A baby at 30 weeks' gestation is admitted to the neonatal intensive care unit. The mother had been treated with a tocolytic intravenous magnesium sulfate for the preceding 10 days. For which of the following laboratory findings should the nurse assess the neonate?
1. Hypocalcemia.
2. Hyperkalemia.
3. Hypochloremia.
4. Hypernatremia.

125. Intravenous magnesium sulfate has been ordered for a client at 31 weeks' gestation in preterm labor. The client's vital signs are: TPR 98.6° F (37° C), 92, 22; BP 110/70. The nurse knows that, in addition to its tocolytic action, the rationale for its administration is to prevent which of the following neonatal complications?

1. Hypoxemia.
2. Cerebral palsy.
3. Cold stress syndrome.
4. Necrotizing enterocolitis.

126. A full-term, 36-hour-old neonate's bilirubin level is 13 mg/dL (222.3 μmol/L). Which of the following signs and symptoms would the nurse expect to see? **Select all that apply.**

1. Lethargy.
2. Jaundice.
3. Polyphagia.
4. Diarrhea.
5. Excessive yawning.

127. A neonate at 37 weeks' gestation who had Apgars of 1 and 3, is admitted to the neonatal intensive care nursery. The neonatologist orders induced hypothermia to prevent which of the following complications of hypoxic-ischemic encephalopathy (HIE)? **Select all that apply.**

1. Cerebral palsy.
2. Blindness.
3. Deafness.
4. Bipolar disease.
5. Reduced intellectual disability.

128. A baby is born to a mother with a history of depression. The mother was prescribed fluoxetine to control her symptoms. For which of the following signs and symptoms should the nurse monitor the neonate in the neonatal nursery?

1. Elevated blood pressures in the upper extremities.
2. Marked systemic cyanosis.
3. Pronounced mucus production immediately after birth.
4. Flaccid tone of all musculature.

129. A baby who is receiving phototherapy for hyperbilirubinemia must have a venipuncture to obtain a blood specimen. Which of the following nursing care actions should the nurse perform at this time?

1. Provide the baby with a sucrose-covered pacifier to suck on.
2. Advise the baby's mother to leave the room while the procedure is being performed.
3. Administer oxygen to the baby via face mask throughout the procedure.
4. Remove the eye patches while the procedure is being performed.

130. In the special care nursery, a nurse is caring for preterm neonates receiving ventilatory support from a variety of different methods. Please identify which ventilation method matches its description:

1. Continuous positive airway pressure (CPAP).	A. Augments babies' spontaneous breaths.
2. Noninvasive positive airway pressure (NIPP).	B. Keeps alveoli open during exhalation.
3. Extracorporeal membrane oxygenation (ECMO).	C. Requires endotracheal tube insertion.
4. Mechanical ventilation.	D. Form of cardiopulmonary bypass.

131. An infant in the neonatal intensive care unit has had a peripherally inserted central catheter (PICC) inserted. The nurse caring for the baby carefully monitors the neonate for which of the following complications related to the procedure? **Select all that apply.**
1. Infection.
2. Tip migration.
3. Myocardial perforation.
4. Paralysis of the diaphragm.
5. Neurological complications related to scalp vein insertions.

CASE STUDY: *The next six questions are part of an evolving case study. All six questions follow the Next Generation NCLEX© question format of six steps:*

1. Recognize cues—What matters most?
2. Analyze cues—What could it mean?
3. Prioritize hypotheses—Where do I start?
4. Generate solutions—What can I do?
5. Take action—What will I do?
6. Evaluate outcomes—Did it help?

(National Council of State Boards of Nursing [NCSBN], 2020). For more information on the Next Generation NCLEX (NGN) question formats, see NGN quarterly newsletters at https://www.ncsbn.org.
NCLEX questions assume the nurse has a provider's order for listed interventions, unless noted otherwise.

In the postpartum unit, it is 1600. A nurse has just assumed care of a baby who was born 4 hours ago at 39 weeks' gestation after a precipitous delivery. The baby's mother is 24 years old. Her obstetrical history is now G2 P2002. No maternal history is available because she states she recently moved to the area and has not yet established care with a local obstetrical care provider. Her husband's seasonal work requires frequent moves. As such, the client's group B strep (GBS) status is unknown. The labor nurse reported that the client's membranes ruptured 11 hours prior to the birth.

The baby's birthweight was 5 lbs, 5 oz (2,533 grams) with Apgar scores of 8 and 9. It was reported that he was stable and pink and vital signs were within normal limits. He was offered the breast immediately after birth and latched on, but fell asleep at the breast after 10 minutes. Because the baby is small for gestational age (SGA) his capillary blood glucose (CBG) was drawn 30 minutes after his birth. The CBG was 40 mg/dL (2.2 mmol/L). It was repeated per protocol at 2 hours of age and was 36 mg/dL (1.9 mmol/L). He was offered the breast and latched on, but did not breastfeed vigorously.

Nurses notes, 1600: "Respiratory rate 68 breaths per minute with grunting respirations and chest retractions on room air. Skin color mottled, axillary temperature 96.8° F (36° C). Heart rate 165 bpm. Poor tone, did not cry with heelstick for CBG."

132. Recognize cues. What matters most?

Identify the top 2 risk factors for this newborn.
1. Male sex.
2. Hypothermia.
3. Tachypnea.
4. Small for gestational age (SGA).
5. Mottled skin.

133. Recognize cues. What matters most?

Note: Alternately, for this step, the NCLEX might ask the test taker to identify specific findings for follow-up, as in this question.

Identify the top 4 findings that would require immediate follow-up.

Note: The NGN test will ask the test taker to drag and drop the top 4 findings to the right.

Client Findings	Top 4 Findings
1. Small for gestational age (SGA)	
2. Temperature 96.8° F (36° C)	
3. Respiratory issues	
4. Lethargy (poor response to heelstick)	
5. Prior CBG 36 mg/dL (1.9 mmol/L)	
6. Mottled skin tone	

134. Analyze cues. What could it mean?

For each client finding below, click to specify if the finding is consistent with the condition of SGA, infection, or transient tachypnea. **Each finding may support more than 1 condition.**

Note: Each column must have at least 1 response option selected. In the NGN exam, the test taker will be asked to click on the boxes within each column.

Client Findings	(a) Small for gestational age (SGA)	(b) Early onset neonatal sepsis (EOS)	(c) Transient tachypnea
1. Hypothermia			
2. Respiratory issues			
3. Breastfeeding issues			
4. Mottled skin tone			
5. Glucose instability			

135. Prioritize hypotheses. Where do I start? **This question has 2 parts.** The test taker is asked to first recognize the complication with the highest risk and then support that risk with evidence in the second part of this question.

Nurses notes 1600 (cut and pasted from above): "Respiratory rate 68 breaths per minute with grunting respirations and chest retractions on room air. Skin color mottled, axillary temperature 96.8° F (36° C). Heart rate 165 bpm. Poor tone, did not cry with heelstick for CBG."

Note: In the NGN format, the test taker will be given a drop-down list of 3 to 4 options for each part.

The baby is at highest risk for developing **(Select 1)**
1. Septic shock.
2. Necrotizing enterocolitis.
3. Hyperbilirubinemia.

as evidenced by the baby's **(Select 1)**

a. Skin color.
b. Vital signs.
c. Feeding pattern.

136. Generate solutions. What can I do?

For each potential intervention below, indicate whether it is essential, nonessential, or contraindicated. **Each intervention must have just one response.**

Nurses notes 1600 (cut and pasted from above): "Respiratory rate 68 breaths per minute with grunting respirations and chest retractions on room air. Skin color mottled, axillary temperature 96.8° F (36° C). Heart rate 165 bpm. Poor tone, did not cry with heelstick for CBG."

1630 Late entry: CBG results 38 mg/dL (2.1 mmol/L). Did not breastfeed. Spoonfed 5 drops expressed colostrum.

1800: Refused expressed colostrum. Continues to be lethargic. Vital signs, 96.8° F (36° C) axillary, HR 165, respirations 70 per minute. Skin tone continues to be mottled. CBG 36 mg/dL (1.9 mmol/L).

Potential Intervention	(a) Essential	(b) Nonessential	(c) Contraindicated
1. Notify provider			
2. Request an order for oxygen supplementation			
3. Assess capillary refill time			
4. Initiate contact precautions			
5. Place baby under overbed warmer with skin probe			
6. Feed baby expressed colostrum			
7. Weigh all diapers			
8. Place pulse oximetry on baby's foot			
9. Keep hat on baby's head to conserve warmth while under warmer.			
10. Request an order to establish intravenous access			

137. Take action. What will I do?

The nurse has determined a capillary refill time of >2.5 seconds, oxygen saturation of 93%. The baby is showing signs of jitteriness. The nurse has given report to the provider and has received the following orders. What 3 orders should be performed first? **Select three.**

1. Capillary blood glucose.
2. Intravenous access.
3. Chest x-ray.
4. Blood and cerebrospinal fluid (CSF) cultures.
5. Antibiotics.
6. Oxygen by nasal prongs.

138. Evaluate outcomes. Did it help?

The nurse has completed all the provider's orders as listed above.

Nurses notes (copied from above):

1800 Refused expressed colostrum. Continues to be lethargic. Vital signs, 96.8° F (36° C) axillary, HR 165, respirations 70 per minute. Skin tone continues to be mottled. CBG 36 mg/dL (1.9 mmol/L).

Nurses notes 1930: Resting quietly under overbed warmer with skin probe in place. CBG 34 mg/dL (1.8 mmol/L). Skin tone remains mottled, Oxygen saturation remains at 93% with nasal prongs. Vital signs 98° F (36.6° C) axillary temp, HR 160, RR 65.

For each assessment finding below, indicate whether the baby's condition has improved, demonstrates no change, or has worsened or declined. **Each assessment finding must have just one response.**

Assessment Finding	(a) Improved	(b) No change	(c) Condition declined
1. CBG 34 mg/dL (1.8 mmol/L)			
2. Skin tone mottled			
3. Capillary refill >3 seconds			
4. Oxygen saturation 93%			
5. Temperature 98° F (36.6° C)			
6. Heart rate 160			
7. Respiratory rate 65			

ANSWERS AND RATIONALES

The correct answer number and rationale for why it is the correct answer are given in **boldface blue type.** Rationales for why the other possible answer options are incorrect also are given, but they are not in boldface type.

1. **Recognize cues.** What matters most?
   1. Although vacuum extractor use may be accompanied by risk to the baby, its use is not the primary concern at this point.
   2. **Recurrent late decelerations are the primary concern because they indicate fetal hypoxia. The accompanying minimal variability and the change from intermittent late decelerations to a recurrent pattern indicates a worsening fetal condition.**
   3. A contraction pattern of every 2 minutes with a duration of 60 seconds is not abnormal. Although the contraction frequency could contribute to fetal hypoxia, there is no oxytocin running and no way to reduce the frequency, so this is not the primary concern.
   4. The gestational age of 41 weeks could be correlated with fetal hypoxia and an aging, sub-optimal placenta, but that is not the primary concern at this time.

TEST-TAKING HINT: The nurse can do nothing about the vacuum extractor use. The contraction frequency is not of concern. The nurse can do nothing about the gestational age. What matters most to the nurse is the anticipated fetal condition at birth as a result of recurrent late decelerations. This fetus has likely had adequate oxygen reserves in spite of being postdates because the FHR was within normal range and demonstrated moderate variability for the majority of this labor. The late decelerations and minimal variability started within the past hour. We don't know how long the FHR has been 90 bpm, but since the fetus is crowning, it will be delivered soon; especially with the vacuum extractor assistance.

2. **Analyze cues.** What could it mean?
   Answers 1(a and b), 2(b and c), 3(a and b), and 4 (a and b) are correct.

Fetal assessments	(a) Post-maturity	(b) Hypoxia	(c) Head compression
1. Meconium-stained amniotic fluid	X	X	
2. FHR 90 bpm		X	X
3. Recurrent late decelerations	X	X	
4. Minimal variability	X	X	

1(a and b). Intrauterine meconium passage has long been recognized as a risk factor in pregnancies beyond 40 weeks' gestation, and in situations where the fetus is hypoxic (Lakshmanan & Ross, 2008; Sayad, 2020).

2(b and c). A fetus experiencing hypoxia or head compression in second stage may demonstrate bradycardia (Vintzileos & Smulian, 2016). Fetal bradycardia is defined as an FHR below 110 (National Certification Corporation, 2010; Simpson, 2016).

3(a and b). Late decelerations are correlated with both postmaturity and hypoxia. They are a demonstration of fetal hypoxia due to suboptimal fetal oxygenation due to placental insufficiency. Normal placental calcifications that occur as the pregnancy passes the due date can reduce the working surface of the placenta, as in this case study. For more information on late decelerations, see the appendix.

4(a and b). As with late decelerations, minimal variability can also reflect fetal hypoxia due to placental insufficiency. Vintzileos and Smulian (2016) have reported that "most fetuses are developing acidemia when . . . they exhibit tachycardia with decelerations and worsening variability" (p 263).

TEST-TAKING HINT: In this step of *analyzing cues*, the nurse analyzes the current clinical picture with the question, "what could it mean?" Having determined that the FHR pattern suggests poor oxygenation (hypoxia) related to placental dysfunction as the highest risk for this fetus, the nurse moves to the next step of prioritizing hypotheses.

3. **Prioritize hypotheses.** Where do I start?
   Answers 1 and d are correct.

The fetus is at highest risk of developing: (Choose one answer below)	As evidenced by the: (Choose one answer below)
1. Metabolic acidemia	a. Current heart rate
2. Meconium aspiration	b. Meconium stained fluid
3. Cephalohematoma	c. Minimal variability
4. Subgaleal bleed	d. Recurrent late decelerations

First column:

1. **The recurrent late decelerations indicate the fetus is developing metabolic acidemia, the highest risk to the newborn. Without adequate reserves of oxygen, the fetal metabolism switches to anaerobic metabolism, which releases lactic acid and ketones into the fetal blood. Metabolic acidemia means the source of the acids in circulation is due to the waste products of anaerobic cellular activity (metabolism).**
2. Although there is meconium in the amniotic fluid, it is not a given that the fetus has aspirated any of it. Meconium aspiration is more likely to occur after the delivery if the newborn cries lustily. However, routine endotracheal suctioning after delivery of the head, before delivery of the body, is no longer recommended (Wyckoff et al., 2015).
3. A second stage of 3½ hours can lead to a cephalohematoma, but that is not the highest risk to this baby's safety. There is nothing in the stem such as a boggy presenting part, to suggest this is developing.
4. A subgaleal bleed is a rare but very serious complication. Its incidence has risen along with the use of vacuum extractors (Colditz et al., 2014). Although the nurse will keep that complication in mind, at this time the provider has just placed the vacuum extractor. Fetal conditions that are favorable for vacuum extractor use include +5 station, and estimated fetal weight of 7 lbs (3,175 grams). Subgaleal bleeds are more often seen in macrosomic babies (Aberg et al., 2016) and this baby's estimated fetal weight is not in that range.

Second column:

a. The current FHR of 90 bpm is not evidence of metabolic acidemia.
b. Meconium-stained fluid is not evidence of metabolic acidemia.
c. Minimal variability can be related to metabolic acidemia, but it is not a diagnostic finding, as it can also be related to fetal sleep.
d. **Recurrent late decelerations for a period of time are diagnostic of metabolic acidemia.**

4. **Generate solutions.** What can I do?
   All of the answers are correct.
   1. **At least 2 staff members must be available to care for the newborn in a resuscitation. Generally this is an RN and a respiratory therapist or newborn primary healthcare provider. If more staff members are available, the nurse's role may change, based on the skill sets of all attending personnel.**
   2. **The newborn's tone and color are included with other assessments to guide the resuscitation efforts. Both of these can change throughout the resuscitation and determine "next steps."**
   3. **Newborn heart rate determines the need for chest compressions and gives feedback about the success of ventilation efforts.**
   4. **Newborn respiratory effort determines whether or not bulb syringe alone, or the addition of endotracheal intubation and ventilation is necessary.**

TEST-TAKING HINT: This newborn will need resuscitation. Although answers to this question include some of the factors in the Apgar score, and resuscitative efforts begin before the first minute of life (and before the first Apgar score) the test taker must not assume it is a trick question. The nurse identifies his or her role in the resuscitation, based on the available personnel in attendance and each person's skills. Throughout the resuscitation, the newborn's response to interventions, which include answers two through four, are assessed.

5. **Take action.** What will I do?
   Answers 1, 2, 4, and 6 are correct.
   1. **The first step is to dry and stimulate the baby while maintaining its temperature. Temperature maintenance is critical for stabilization of the newborn. Having been suddenly forced out of a consistently warm environment, the thermoregulatory system is forced to begin working from a disadvantaged beginning—wet skin in an often cool environment. In response, the baby's metabolic system attempts to conserve heat by cutaneous vasoconstriction. If hypothermia is prolonged, the consequences to the baby include hypoglycemia, hypoxia, and metabolic acidosis (Kumar et al., 2009).**
   2. **Bulb suction of the mouth before the nose is appropriate.**
   3. Although this baby's amniotic fluid is meconium-stained, it is no longer standard of care to routinely intubate for tracheal suctioning in the presence of meconium-stained fluid, as the risks have been shown to be greater than the benefits (Wyckhoff et al., 2015).
   4. **Positive pressure ventilation (PPV) with oxygen is the primary "medication" for newborn babies needing support. The American Heart Association Neonatal Resuscitation Program (NRP) algorithm recommends PPV for a fetus with a variety of criteria, including a heart rate between 60 and 100 at birth (Escobedo et al., 2019). Often PPV for a few seconds is all it takes before the baby cries lustily and becomes vigorous. This fetus is moments away from delivery. An FHR of 90 suggests that this baby will need PPV. Everything and everyone should be ready to begin the resuscitation immediately.**
   5. Chest compressions are initiated if the newborn's heart rate is 60 or less (Aziz et al., 2020; Wyckhoff et al., 2015). If the FHR remains at 90 bpm, chest compressions are not likely to be required.
   6. **Because the late decelerations and minimal variability suggest fetal acidosis, cord blood gas analysis is likely to be required for a complete assessment.**

TEST-TAKING HINT: The nurse is ready with possible interventions. All newborns must be dried and stimulated. The best place for this to happen is on the mother's chest, but in this situation, because the FHR is already low at 90 bpm, it may go even lower before the birth. In light of the recurrent late decelerations and minimal variability, the safest place for the provider to place the baby after the birth is in an overbed warmer for resuscitation. Bulb suction of mouth first, followed by nose, is routine. Endotracheal suction is not a routine procedure. Bag and mask ventilation will likely be necessary and will likely lead to a rise in the heart rate. Chest compressions will be necessary if the newborn's heart rate is 60 or less. The nurse must have supplies ready for receiving a clamped segment of the umbilical cord for blood gas analysis. In addition, 2 heparinized syringes with client labels on the syringes, indicating an umbilical vein sample and an umbilical artery sample should be prepared. A container of ice for transporting the syringes to the lab must also be ready. Care of the newborn must come first, before drawing blood for cord gases, and classic studies have shown that a clamped segment of the umbilical cord at room temperature can yield accurate blood gas results for up to an hour if there is a lag time before they are drawn (Duerbeck et al., 1992).

6. **Evaluate outcomes.** Did it help?
   Answers 1 and 2 are correct.
   1. **The newborn temp is normal, indicating the baby was kept warm during the resuscitation. To prevent overheating, a temperature probe must be placed on the baby's abdomen or another appropriate location as soon as possible once the baby is placed under the warmer.**
   2. **The baby is vigorous, indicating good oxygenation.**
   3. Peripheral cyanosis is common in newborns. Persistent central cyanosis beyond 5 to 10 minutes after the birth suggests a potentially life-threatening condition related to cardiac, metabolic, neurologic, infectious, and/or pulmonary disorders (Eichenwald, 2020) unrelated to nursing actions.
   4. Cord gases are not directly related to nursing actions, and reflect the intrauterine environment of the fetus before birth, not after the resuscitation. This particular cord gas sample shows a CO2 of more than 60 and a high base deficit of 12, indicating this baby had a mixed respiratory and metabolic acidosis. This would be anticipated in light of postdates contributing to placental calcifications, leading to placental insufficiency with reduced oxygen in the fetal circulation.

TEST-TAKING HINT: Placing the baby under the warmer, and providing bag and mask ventilation had a positive impact on the newborn's temperature, heart rate, and respirations. The nursing care would not be reflected in the central cyanosis or cord gases. Keeping the hypothesis of placental dysfunction in mind, the nurse's interventions are based on preserving fetal oxygen reserves and assisting with delivery of adequate oxygen to the cells as they return to aerobic metabolism after the birth. The nurse assists the newborn with external heat sources, whether from an overbed warmer, or within the mother's arms, and confirms adequate oxygen intake.

A resuscitation can be effective very quickly, which is always rewarding to parents and healthcare providers. Cord gases can be very helpful in providing a snapshot of the baby's oxygen environment before birth. This can give caregivers a predictor of the types and intensities required in post-birth care in addition to possible neurological sequelae (Saneh et al., 2020). A mixed respiratory and metabolic acidosis is most commonly seen, as the initial reduction in oxygen reserves leads to respiratory acidosis, and when it is prolonged it moves into metabolic acidosis (Saneh et al., 2020). See the appendix for more information on acid-base balance and a memory hack for quick determinations of the presenting type of acidosis.

Goals of resuscitation in the delivery room are to maintain the newborn's body temperature, stabilize the airway and provide or confirm adequate newborn oxygenation and ventilation. The resuscitation team must continually assess and reassess their resuscitation efforts based on newborn response. Good communication and teamwork are essential, as always.

7.
1. The normal temperature of a premature baby is the same as that of a full-term baby.
2. Axillary temperatures, when performed correctly, provide accurate information.
3. **Preterm babies are born with an insufficient supply of brown adipose tissue that is needed for thermogenesis, or heat generation.**
4. There is nothing in the question that would explain conduction heat loss.

TEST-TAKING HINT: It is important for the test taker not to read into questions. Even though conduction can be a means of heat loss in the neonate and, more particularly, in the premature infant, there are three other means by which neonates lose heat—radiation, convection, and evaporation. Conduction could be singled out as a cause of the hypothermia only if it were clear from the question that conduction was the cause of the problem.

8.
1. Infants of diabetic mothers are often large for gestational age, but they are not especially at high risk for cold stress syndrome.
2. Infants born with Rh incompatibility are not especially at high risk for cold stress syndrome.
3. **Postdates babies are at high risk for cold stress syndrome because while still in utero they often metabolize the brown adipose tissue for energy when the placental function deteriorates.**
4. Babies with Down's syndrome are hypotonic, but they are not especially at high risk for cold stress syndrome.

TEST-TAKING HINT: Cold stress syndrome results from a neonate's inability to create heat through metabolic means. When nourishment is sparse, as in the case of a fetus at postdates, brown adipose tissue (BAT) and glycogen stores in the liver are the primary substances used for thermogenesis. It follows that the infant who is most likely to have poor supplies of BAT and glycogen is the postdates infant who cannot generate much heat metabolically.

9.
1. Infants with cold stress exhibit hypoglycemia. A neonatal blood glucose of 50 mg/dL (2.8 mmol/L) is normal.
2. Acrocyanosis—bluish hands and feet—is normal for the neonate during the first day or two.
3. **Babies who have cold stress will develop respiratory distress. One symptom of the distress is tachypnea.**
4. The oxygen saturation is within normal limits.

TEST-TAKING HINT: The neonate exhibits physiological characteristics that are very different from the older child or adult. For example, normal blood glucose levels are lower in neonates than in the older child and adult and acrocyanosis is normal for a neonate's first day or two, but not for older children and adults.

10.
1. **Intercostal retractions are symptomatic of respiratory distress syndrome.**
2. Erythema toxicum is the normal newborn rash.
3. Pseudostrabismus is a normal newborn finding of crossed eyes that comes and goes.
4. Vernix caseosa is the cheesy material that covers many babies at birth.

TEST-TAKING HINT: **It is important for the nurse to be familiar with the signs of respiratory distress in the neonate. Babies who are stressed by cold, sepsis, or prematurity will often exhibit signs of respiratory distress. Other signs of respiratory distress in the neonate besides intercostal retractions are grunting, tachypnea, asynchronous breathing, and cyanosis. The neonatologist should be called promptly.**

11. 1. Grunting is a sign of respiratory distress. Offering a pacifier is an inappropriate intervention.
    2. Diapering is an inappropriate intervention.
    3. The baby is not hungry. Rather, the baby is in respiratory distress.
    4. **Grunting is often accompanied by tachypnea, another sign of respiratory distress.**

TEST-TAKING HINT: **If the nurse were to attempt to grunt, he or she would feel the respiratory effort that the baby is creating. Essentially, the baby is producing his or her own positive end-expiratory pressure (PEEP) to maximize his or her respiratory function. The nurse should assess the respiratory rate for more complete information.**

12. 1. Blood urea nitrogen and serum creatinine tests are done to assess the renal system. Kernicterus does not affect the renal system. It results from an infiltration of bilirubin into the central nervous system.
    2. Although alkaline phosphatase and bilirubin would be evaluated when a child is jaundiced, they are not appropriate to assess a child's sequelae to kernicterus.
    3. **Because the central nervous system (CNS) may have been damaged by the high bilirubin levels, testing of the senses as well as motor and cognitive assessments are appropriate.**
    4. The respiratory system is unaffected by high bilirubin levels.

TEST-TAKING HINT: **Kernicterus is the syndrome that develops when a neonate is exposed to high levels of bilirubin over time. The bilirubin crosses the blood–brain barrier, often leading to toxic changes in the CNS. The term *sequelae* refers to the disorders that result after an individual has experienced a disease or injury. It can be thought of as several "sequels," to use a movie term.**

13. 1. **When phototherapy is administered, the baby's eyes must be protected from the light source.**
    2. Although the lights should be turned off and the pads removed periodically during the therapy, the lights should be on whenever the baby is in his or her crib.
    3. The therapy is most effective when the skin surface exposed to the light is maximized. The shirt should be removed while the baby is under the lights.
    4. The blanket should be removed while the baby is under the lights.

TEST-TAKING HINT: **Newborns are more prone to jaundice than adults because they are born with a high level of red blood cells that are broken down after the birth to prepare the baby for life outside the womb. As noted in the appendix, bilirubin is a waste product from red blood cell breakdown. Physiologic neonatal hyperbilirubinemia is usually harmless. It typically occurs after newborns are 24 hours of age, and resolves spontaneously by 5 to 7 days. Goals of therapy include fetal hydration and adequate defecation, since bilirubin is excreted in the stool.**

It is important to note that there is a difference between phototherapy administered by fluorescent light overhead, and phototherapy administered via fiber-optic tubing in a bili-blanket. The baby in this scenario is receiving phototherapy by fluorescent light overhead. In contrast, when a bili-blanket is used, the baby can be clothed and the baby's eyes do not need to be protected.

14. 1. Babies born with erythroblastosis fetalis are markedly anemic. They are not ruddy in appearance.
    2. **Babies born with erythroblastosis fetalis are often in severe congestive heart failure and, therefore, exhibit extreme, generalized edema.**
    3. Babies with erythroblastosis fetalis are not at high risk for alopecia (hair loss).
    4. Erythema toxicum is a normal newborn rash common in many healthy newborns.

TEST-TAKING HINT: **Erythroblastosis fetalis, also called *immune* hydrops, is a hemolytic disease of the newborn. A baby with this condition has marked red blood cell destruction in utero. This results from a blood group incompatibility, where the Rh negative mother who has previously been exposed to Rh positive blood either through miscarriage or the birth of a previous Rh positive baby, becomes pregnant with another Rh positive baby without having received Rh immune globulin (RhIG) after the previous birth.**

Mothers at risk are treated prophylactically with immunoglobulin (Ig) prophylaxis. As noted in Chapter 9, question 103, if the mother is not treated prophylactically after her first exposure

to Rh positive blood, her body creates antibodies to Rh positive blood. When she is pregnant the next time, those antibodies cross the placenta. An immune response is triggered against the Rh-positive fetal blood cells of the new fetus, and up to 50% of the fetal red blood cells may be destroyed, creating fetal anemia. In response, the fetal bone marrow releases low quality, immature RBCs into the fetal circulation. With fewer red blood cells to carry oxygen to fetal organs, the fetal heart works so hard, it enlarges, creating congestive heart failure. This is followed by generalized edema.

Thanks to modern medical treatment, *immune* hydrops is currently rare. Instead, *nonimmune* hydrops, related to conditions that include cardiac issues, twin-to-twin transfusion, and alpha thalassemia, are responsible for 85% or more of all cases of fetal hydrops today (Hamdan, 2017).

15. 1. **The baby with erythroblastosis fetalis would exhibit signs of severe anemia, which is reflected by a hematocrit of 24%.**
    2. Erythroblastosis fetalis is not an infectious condition. Leukocytosis is not a part of the clinical picture.
    3. Hyponatremia is not part of the disorder.
    4. Hyperkalemia is not part of the disorder.

TEST-TAKING HINT: A normal newborn hematocrit is generally between 55% and 68% (Shiel, n.d.).

16. 1. **Significant ABO incompatibility can occur when the mother is type O and the baby is either type A or type B, regardless of Rh factor.**
    2. ABO incompatibility is a risk only if the mother's blood is type O. If the mother's blood is type A, then ABO incompatibility is not a risk. Hemolytic jaundice from ABO incompatibility is rarely seen when the maternal blood type is A, B, or AB. Note that ABO incompatibility is different from Rh incompatibility, which can occur only if the mother is Rh-negative and the baby is Rh-positive, regardless of blood type.
    3. ABO incompatibility is a risk only if the mother's blood is type O. If the mother's blood is type B, then ABO incompatibility is not a risk.
    4. ABO incompatibility is a risk only if the mother's blood is type O. If the mother's blood type is AB, then ABO incompatibility is not a concern.

TEST-TAKING HINT: When the mother's blood is type O and the baby's is not, an ABO incompatibility is common because the mother's type O blood carries antibodies to A, B, and AB blood types. The nurse must remember that ABO incompatibility is about *antibodies in the plasma*, not Rh factors. For an allegorical memory hack to remember these risks, see the allegory in the appendix.

17. 1. The direct Coombs test assesses for the presence of antibodies already attached to red blood cells in the baby's blood. The test will not predict or explain jitters in the neonate.
    2. The Coombs test will not predict or explain hypoglycemia in the neonate.
    3. The Coombs test will not predict or explain a change in temperature in the neonate.
    4. **When the neonatal bloodstream contains antibodies, hemolysis of the red blood cells occurs and jaundice develops.**

TEST-TAKING HINT: The nurse must remember that there are two types of Coombs tests: (1) the indirect Coombs, and (2) the direct Coombs. The *indirect* Coombs test is performed on the mother to detect whether or not she carries antibodies in her plasma against her fetus's red blood cells. The *direct* Coombs test is performed on the newborn's cord blood to detect whether or not antibodies have already attached to the baby's red blood cells to destroy them.

18. 1. The neonate needs nourishment with formula and/or breast milk.
    2. **Rotating the baby's position maximizes the therapeutic response because the more skin surface that is exposed to the light source, the better the results are.**
    3. It is unnecessary to restrain the baby while under the bili lights.
    4. Intravenous fluids would be administered only under extreme circumstances.

TEST-TAKING HINT: Bilirubin levels decrease with exposure to a light source, commonly referred to as "bili lights." The goal of efficient therapy is to expose as much skin surface to the light as possible. Although fluids are needed to maintain hydration and to foster stooling, the baby can be taken out from under the bili lights for breastfeeding or bottle feeding, per the mother's chosen feeding method. If necessary, the breastfeeding baby may be supplemented with formula after breastfeeding if the mother's milk supply is not yet ample. This will promote stooling, which is key to eliminating the bilirubin.

19. 1. The foot should be covered with a warm wrap to draw blood to the area for the heel stick.
2. The lateral heel is the site of choice because it contains no major nerves or blood vessels.
3. **Alcohol can irritate the punctured skin and can cause hemolysis, so it must dry first before puncturing the skin.**
4. The ankle and foot, not the calf, should be firmly grasped during the procedure.

TEST-TAKING HINT: If the posterior surface of the heel is punctured, the posterior tibial nerve and artery could be injured. Only the lateral aspects of the heel, therefore, should be punctured.

20. Answer 5 is correct.

Note: The NGN question will provide the progress notes in paragraph format; statements will not be numbered. The test taker is asked to highlight the sentences of concern.

1. This is a background statement.
2. This is a background statement.
3. This is not an assessment of progression. Jaundice in a sibling can indicate a risk factor.
4. Because this is not compared to a previous weight-loss percentage, it is not about progression. Weight loss of up to 10% in the first week of life is within normal parameters.
5. **This statement demonstrates slow progression to recovery. It is a comparison of the bilirubin level of 18 mg/dL (307.8 μmol/L) on admission, 24 hours previously. The most significant decline in bilirubin is generally seen within the first 4 to 6 hours after the start of phototherapy. The expected decline with intensive therapy is 30 to 40% after the first 24 hours of therapy (American Academy of Pediatrics [AAP], 2004, p. 315). This baby is not showing the expected decline in total serum bilirubin after 24 hours of therapy.**
6. This is not about progression to recovery, it documents the newborn's method of feeding and prudent newborn care. Babies may be removed from phototherapy to breastfeed for 20 minutes at a time.
7. This does not define the newborn's progression to recovery. Altered newborn fluid balance may contribute to a slower recovery, but this is expected elimination and indicates adequate hydration.

TEST-TAKING HINT: An understanding of newborn physiologic jaundice begins with the fact that neonates are born with a higher number of red blood cells than they need after birth (Hansen, 2017) and physiologic jaundice is evidence of their adjustment to the RBC needs of extrauterine life. If a neonate cannot keep up with the excretion of bilirubin, and this substance is deposited in the skin, phototherapy is initiated with the goal of decreasing the rising serum bilirubin to prevent its toxic accumulation in the brain, a serious, permanent neurological complication known as kernicterus. Bilirubin can rise even higher in situations where a condition such as ABO incompatibility, as in this question, leads to additional RBC breakdown.

All newborn bilirubin levels are interpreted according to the infant's age in hours, using the Bhutani nomogram. On the Bhutani nomogram below, find the neonate's age in hours on the line at the bottom. Follow that line up to where it intersects with the neonate's total serum bilirubin (TSB) results in mg/dL in the vertical list on the left (or in μmol/L on the right) to determine the neonate's risk zone. Most hospitals provide a reference to this chart in the electronic medical record. This neonate's TSB of 18 mg/dL (307.8 μmol/L) on admission at 96 hours of age was in the high-risk zone. Now, 24 hours later, at 120 hours of age, the TSB of 15 (256.5 μmol/L) is in the low intermediate risk range. The concern is that it's not falling within the expected timeframe.

The sixth step in nursing clinical judgment, "evaluate outcomes," would be to ask, "Did phototherapy help?" The answer is, "Yes, a little," and then to explore possible contributors to the slow decline, including intake and output, length of time outside of the bili lights for breastfeeding, and other factors.

For more information on physiologic jaundice, see the appendix. For a history of phototherapy and the physiology of how it works, see https://nursing.ceconnection.com/ovidfiles/00149525-201110001-00003.pdf.

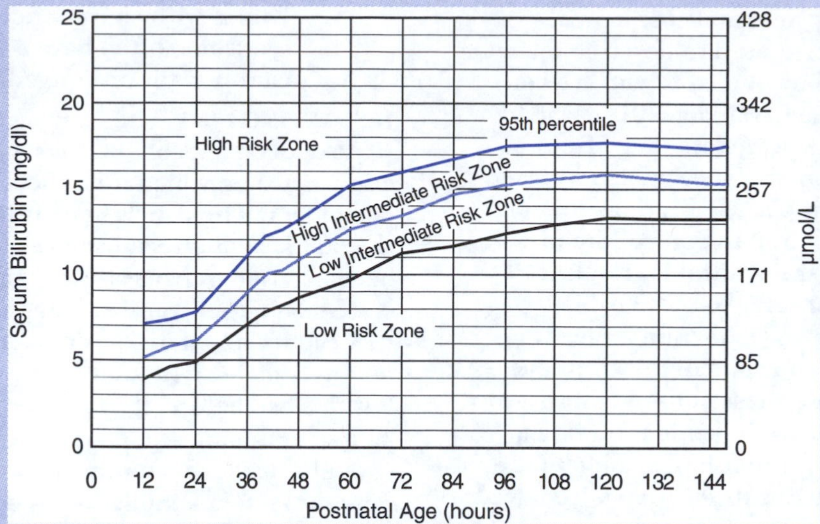

21. 1. The ambient temperature will affect the baby's temperature, but it will not affect the bilirubin level.
    2. **Bilirubin is excreted through the bowel. The more the baby consumes, the more stools he or she will produce. This is therapeutic since the more feces the baby excretes, the more bilirubin the baby will expel, and less of it will be re-absorbed.**
    3. Holding the baby skin to skin has no direct effect on the bilirubin level.
    4. The bilirubin levels of babies exposed to direct sunlight will drop. It is unsafe, however, to expose a baby's skin to direct sunlight.

TEST-TAKING HINT: This is one example of a change in practice that has occurred because of updated knowledge. In the past, babies have been placed in sunlight to reduce their bilirubin levels, but that practice is no longer considered to be safe. It is important, therefore, for the nurse to stay up to date on current practice.

22. 1. The stools are green from the increase in excreted bilirubin.
    2. There is no need to inform the healthcare practitioner. Green stools are an expected finding.
    3. Although green stools can be seen with diarrheal illnesses, in this situation, the green stools are expected and not related to an infectious state.
    4. **The stools can be very caustic to the baby's delicate skin. The nurse should cleanse the area well and inspect the skin for any sign that the skin is breaking down.**

TEST-TAKING HINT: The nurse must know the difference between signs that are normal and those that reflect a possible illness. Although green stools can be seen with diarrheal illnesses, in this situation, the green stools are expected. They are due to the increased bilirubin excreted and are not related to an infectious state.

23. 1. **Healthy, hydrated neonates saturate their diapers a minimum of 6 times in 24 hours.**
    2. To consume enough fluid and nutrients for growth and hydration, babies should breastfeed at least 8 times in 24 hours.
    3. A weight loss of over 10% is indicative of dehydration. The baby should not exceed 10% weight loss.
    4. Tachycardia can indicate dehydration.

TEST-TAKING HINT: This is an evaluation question. The test taker is being asked to identify signs that would indicate a baby who is fully hydrated. It is important for the test taker to know the expected intake and output of the neonate and to understand the evaluation phase of the nursing process.

24. 1. Morphine is an opiate narcotic. It may be administered to a baby with neonatal abstinence syndrome (NAS) to control diarrhea associated with the syndrome.
    2. Methadone may be administered to neonates who are exhibiting signs of severe NAS.
    3. **Narcan is an opiate-antagonist. If it were to be given to the neonate with neonatal abstinence syndrome, the baby would go into a traumatic withdrawal.**
    4. Phenobarbital is sometimes administered to drug-exposed neonates to control seizures.

TEST-TAKING HINT: "Neonatal abstinence syndrome" is the term used to describe the many behaviors exhibited by neonates who are born drug dependent (Kocherlakota, 2014; March of Dimes, n.d.). The behaviors range from hyperreflexia to excessive sneezing and yawning to loose diarrheal stools. Medications may or may not be administered to control the many signs/symptoms of the syndrome. Healthcare professionals do not refer to these babies as "addicted," since an "addiction" refers to intentional drug use in spite of the consequences. Babies do not choose these substances; they become physiologically dependent on them, however, when the mother has an addiction prenatally, and they can suffer from withdrawal once they are born.

25. 1. **Tightly swaddling drug-dependent babies often helps to control the hyperreflexia that they may exhibit.**
2. Placing hyperactive babies on their abdomens can result in skin abrasions on the face and knees from rubbing against the linens as they cry and writhe in pain. And, like all babies, drug-dependent babies should be placed supine during all unsupervised time periods.
3. Drug-exposed babies should be placed in a low-stimulation environment.
4. The babies should be given small, frequent feedings of either full-strength formula or breast milk.

TEST-TAKING HINT: Drug-exposed babies exhibit signs of neonatal abstinence syndrome including hyperactivity, hyperreflexia, and other signs of withdrawal. The nurse should look for nursing interventions that minimize those behaviors. Tightly swaddling the baby helps to reduce the baby's behavioral responses. It is thought to provide the baby with some security, as it resembles the close confines of the uterus before birth.

26. Answers 1 and 5 are correct.
1. **Babies with signs of neonatal abstinence syndrome repeatedly exhibit signs of hunger.**
2. Babies with neonatal abstinence syndrome are hyperactive, not lethargic.
3. Babies with neonatal abstinence syndrome often exhibit sleep disturbances rather than prolonged periods of sleep.
4. Babies with signs of neonatal abstinence syndrome are hyperreflexic, not hyporeflexic.
5. **Babies with signs of neonatal abstinence syndrome often have a shrill cry that may continue for prolonged periods.**

TEST-TAKING HINT: The baby who is exhibiting signs of neonatal abstinence syndrome is craving a substance on which it has become physically dependent. The baby's body is in distress because the highly addictive substances he or she has been exposed to have affected the central nervous system, and their removal causes a craving that cannot be filled, causing discomfort and understandable irritability. The baby has never felt this bad before; it has never before felt the pain of cramping and diarrhea. The test taker should consider symptoms that reflect central nervous system stimulation as correct responses.

27. 1. **Babies with fetal alcohol syndrome (FAS) usually have a very weak suck.**
2. Ambiguous genitalia is not a characteristic anomaly seen in FAS.
3. A webbed neck is not a characteristic anomaly seen in FAS.
4. Babies with FAS usually have an intact CNS system with a positive Moro reflex.

TEST-TAKING HINT: The characteristic facial signs of fetal alcohol syndrome— shortened palpebral (eyelid) fissures, thin upper lip, and hypoplastic philtrum (median groove on the external surface of the upper lip)—are rarely evident in the neonatal period. They typically appear later in the child's life. Rather, the behavioral characteristics of the baby with FAS, such as weak suck, irritability, tremulousness, and seizures, are present at birth.

28. Answers 1 and 4 are correct.
1. **This statement is correct. While older medications, for example, paregoric, were effective, they contained alcohol. Oral morphine does not.**
2. This statement is false. Oral morphine is sedating.
3. Oral morphine can adversely affect the neonate's respiratory effort. Some babies develop apnea spells when treated with oral morphine.
4. **This statement is correct. Oral morphine helps to control seizures.**

TEST-TAKING HINT: Oral morphine, a liquid medication, is an especially effective therapy for a baby who is experiencing severe neonatal abstinence syndrome. The narcotic relieves the cravings that the baby has for the opiate they are dependent on, and it minimizes many of the

baby's adverse symptoms such as poor feeding and seizures. Other medications that have been administered to affected neonates are methadone, phenobarbital, clonidine, and buprenorphine (Kocherlakota, 2014; Thigpen & Melton, 2014).

29. **1. The symptoms are characteristic of neonatal abstinence syndrome. A urine toxicology would provide evidence of drug exposure.**
2. Biophysical profiles are done during pregnancy to assess the well-being of the fetus.
3. There is no indication from the question that this child has any chest or abdominal abnormalities.
4. This child is not exhibiting signs of respiratory distress.

TEST-TAKING HINT: It is important for the test taker to attend to the fact that this child has normal serum glucose levels. When babies exhibit tremors, the first thing the nurse should consider is hypoglycemia. Once that has been ruled out, the nurse should consider drug exposure since the baby is exhibiting signs of drug withdrawal.

30. 1. This baby is hypothermic, but the best intervention would be to place the baby skin-to-skin with its mother or under a warmer with a skin probe rather than to swaddle the baby. In addition, the baby's glucose levels must be assessed.
2. The glucose level should be assessed to determine whether or not this baby's jitteriness is because of hypoglycemia. The glucose can be evaluated while the baby is on the mother's chest or under the warmer.
3. A feeding will elevate the glucose level if it is below normal.
4. The administration of the neonatal medicines is not a priority at this time.

TEST-TAKING HINT: The nurse should note that this baby is macrosomic and hypothermic, both of which make the baby at high risk for hypoglycemia. Jitters are a classic symptom in hypoglycemic babies. To make an accurate assessment of the severity of the problem, the baby's glucose level must be assessed.

31. 1. Jaundice is not related to blood glucose levels.
2. Babies who are hypoglycemic will often develop jitters (tremors).
3. Erythema toxicum is the newborn rash. It is unrelated to blood glucose levels.
4. Subconjunctival hemorrhages are often seen in neonates. They are related to the trauma of delivery, not to blood glucose levels.

TEST-TAKING HINT: The normal glucose level for neonates in the immediate postdelivery period is approximately 40 to 90 mg/dL (2.2 to 5.0 mmol/L). This is lower than that seen in older babies and children. Jitters are related to central nervous system irritability and are the classic symptom of hypoglycemia in the neonate.

32. **1. A baby with a blood glucose of 35 mg/dL (1.9 mmol/L) is hypoglycemic. The action of choice is to feed the baby either breast milk or formula.**
2. The baby's blood pressure is not a relevant factor at this time.
3. Tightly swaddling the baby may disguise a common finding, jitters or tremors, seen in babies who are hypoglycemic.
4. The baby's urinary output is not a relevant factor at this time.

TEST-TAKING HINT: Sugars in the milk will elevate the baby's blood values in the short term, and the proteins and fats in the milk will help to maintain the glucose values in the normal range. In the past, hypoglycemic babies were fed 5% or 10% glucose water. That is no longer standard practice because it leads to wide swings in newborn blood glucose levels as a result of high levels of endogenous insulin in response to the glucose. Breast milk or formula gives a more prolonged correction and maintenance of newborn blood sugar.

33. **1. The gavage tubing must be measured to approximate the length of the insertion.**
2. The tubing should be lubricated with sterile water or a water-soluble lubricant, not an oil-based solution.
3. If the child becomes cyanotic, the tubing should be removed immediately.
4. A small amount of air, not sterile water, should be injected into the tubing while the nurse listens with a stethoscope over the baby's stomach area. Sterile water could be hazardous if the tube is in the airway.

TEST-TAKING HINT: The placement of gavage tubing is potentially dangerous. Not only must the distance between the nose and the ear be measured but also the length from the ear to the point midway between the ear and the xiphoid process. This entire distance is the tubing insertion length. To assess placement, air, rather than water, should be injected into the tubing, because the tubing may mistakenly have been inserted into the trachea.

34. Answers 4, 2, 1, and 3 are the correct order.
   4. Inserting the free end of the tubing through the nose is the first step in nasopharyngeal suctioning process.
   2. The nurse should place a thumb over the suction control on the catheter after inserting the free end of the tubing through the nose—and before the other two steps are taken.
   1. Rotation and removal of the suction catheter should be done after the tubing has been inserted through the nose and a thumb placed over the suction control on the catheter.
   3. Assessment and documentation of the type and amount of secretions is the last step in the process.

TEST-TAKING HINT: It is important to note that once the suction control is covered, the baby is unable to take in air. It is important, therefore, to cover the suction control for very brief periods of time until the catheter is being removed.

35. 1. Neonates are incapable of controlling their movements. To maintain a patent IV site, it is essential to tape the baby's arm to an arm board. This can prevent the need to restart the IV too often.
   2. IV tubing is usually changed every 72 hours, or as needed, not every 24 hours.
   3. The IV site should be assessed regularly, at least once an hour, but it is not necessary to check it every 5 minutes.
   4. IV infusions are usually continuous, unless a medication, for example, an antibiotic, is being administered. During that time, the continuous IV infusion may be temporarily turned off.

TEST-TAKING HINT: Although restraints and arm boards are often unnecessary when caring for older children and adults, the use of restraints and/or arm boards is often necessary when caring for infants, toddlers, and other young children. This can help to keep the intravenous site intact. Skin assessments under the arm board and under the tape must be completed regularly. If possible, the arm board should be removed intermittently to allow the baby to flex the elbow, with the nurse in constant attendance.

36. 1. It is inappropriate to imply that, if a couple were to pray, their sick child will be "all right." The baby may be seriously ill and even may die.
   2. This baby's Apgar score is very low. There is a chance that the baby will not survive. Because the parents are known to be Roman Catholic, it is appropriate to ask them if they would like their baby baptized.
   3. Although it is often easier for the nurse to leave parents alone whose babies are doing poorly, it is rarely therapeutic unless the parents have requested it.
   4. It is inappropriate to assume that the parents wish to give confession, although it may be appropriate to offer to have the priest visit them.

TEST-TAKING HINT: When a baby is doing very poorly during the first minutes after delivery, there is a possibility that the baby may not survive. Couples who are Roman Catholic often wish to have their babies baptized in such situations. If a priest is not immediately available, it is appropriate for a nurse of any religious faith, to perform the baptism at that time if the parents consent.

37. The baby's Apgar score is 3.

TEST-TAKING HINT: Assessing the Apgar score is often a nursing function. The test taker, therefore, should know the criteria for the Apgar score (see the following table). The score is traditionally performed at 1 and 5 minutes after birth. A total score of 7 to 10 means that the baby is having little to no difficulty transitioning to extrauterine life. With a total score of 4 to 6, the baby is having moderate difficulty transitioning to extrauterine life. Resuscitative measures may need to be instituted. With a total score of 0 to 3, the baby is in severe distress. Resuscitative measures must be instituted.

Apgar Scoring Grid

Sign	Score of 0	Score of 1	Score of 2
Heart Rate	Absent	Below 100 bpm	100 bpm and above
Respiratory Effort	Absent	Slow and irregular	Lusty (vigorous) cry
Muscle Tone	Flaccid	Some flexion of the extremities	Active motion or well-flexed extremities
Reflex Irritability	Absent	Grimace	Lusty (vigorous) cry
Color	Completely cyanotic or very pale baby	Pink body with cyanotic extremities (acrocyanosis)	Pink body and extremities

38. 1. According to the graph, at 38 weeks' gestation, a 3,500-gram baby is between the 10th and the 90th percentiles for weight. The baby, therefore, is appropriate for gestation age.

2. A baby who is large for gestational age is defined as a baby whose weight is above the 90th percentile. According to the graph, at 38 weeks' gestation, a 3,500-gram baby is below the 90th percentile for weight. Therefore, the diagnosis is inaccurate.

3. A baby who is large for gestational age is defined as a baby whose weight is above the 90th percentile. According to the graph, at 38 weeks' gestation, a 3,500-gram baby is below the 90th percentile for weight.

4. Any baby, born at any gestational age, can be found to be large for that gestational age.

TEST-TAKING HINT: It is important for the nurse to become comfortable with reading and interpreting graphs. The following gestational age graph—with weight in grams on the *y*-axis and weeks of gestation on the *x*-axis—is cut by 3 curves. The upper curve shows the weight at the 90th percentile for babies at differing gestational ages, whereas the lower curve shows the weight at the 10th percentile for babies of differing gestational ages. Those babies who fall above the upper curve—that is, whose weights are above the 90th percentile—are defined as large for gestational age (LGA). Those babies who fall below the lower curve—those with weights that are below the 10th percentile—are defined as small for gestational age (SGA). Those babies who fall between the upper and lower curves are defined as average for gestational age (AGA). The middle curve shows the weights of babies at the 50th percentile.

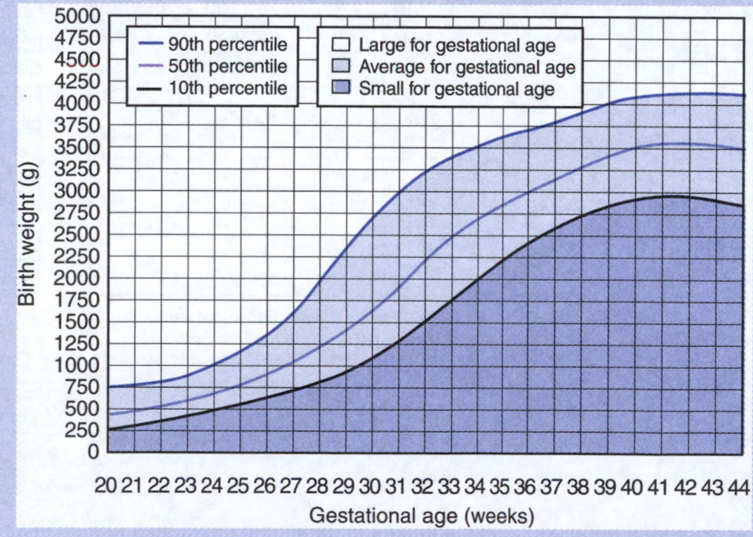

39. 24 weeks.

TEST-TAKING HINT: There are six characteristics on the neuromuscular maturity chart and six characteristics on the physical maturity chart (see the following charts). The baby is given a score for each characteristic and the scores are added together to get a total score. The total score is compared to the maturity rating chart. The baby in the question had a total score of 0, which relates to a gestational age score of 24 weeks.

Neuromuscular Maturity

	–1	0	1	2	3	4	5
Posture							
Square Window (Wrist)	-90°	90°	60°	45°	30°	0°	
Arm Recoil		180°	140°–180°	110°–140°	90°–110°	<90°	
Popliteal Angle	180°	160°	140°	120°	100°	90°	<90°
Scarf Sign							
Heel to Ear							

Physical Maturity

Skin	sticky; friable; transparent	gelatinous; red; translucent	smooth pink; visible veins	superficial peeling or rash, few veins	cracking; pale areas; rare veins	parchment; deep cracking; no vessels	leathery; cracked; wrinkled
Lanugo	none	sparse	abundant	thinning	bald areas	mostly bald	
Plantar Surface	heel-toe 40–50 mm:–1 <40 mm:–2	>50 mm no crease	faint red marks	anterior transverse crease only	creases ant. 2/3	creases over entire sole	
Breast	imperceptible	barely perceptible	flat areola; no bud	stippled areola; 1–2 mm bud	raised areola; 3–4 mm bud	full areola; 5–10 mm bud	
Eye/Ear	lids fused; loosely:–1 tightly:–2	lids open; pinna flat; stays folded	sl. curved pinna; soft; slow recoil	well-curved pinna; soft but ready recoil	formed and firm; instant recoil	thick cartilage; ear stiff	
Genitals (Male)	scrotum flat, smooth	scrotum empty; faint rugae	testes in upper canal; rare rugae	testes descending; few rugae	testes down; good rugae	testes pendulous; deep rugae	
Genitals (Female)	clitoris prominent; labia flat	prominent clitoris; small labia minora	prominent clitoris; enlarging minora	majora and minora equally prominent	majora large; minora small	majora cover clitoris and minora	

Maturity Rating

Score	Weeks
–10	20
–5	22
0	24
5	26
10	28
15	30
20	32
25	34
30	36
35	38
40	40
45	42
50	44

From: Ballard, J. L., Khoury, L. C., Wedig, K., et al. (1991). New Ballard Score, expanded to include extremely premature infants. *Journal of Pediatrics, 19*(3), 417-423. With permission.

40. 1. **The baby's weight is average for gestational age. The baby's weight of 1,000 grams (2 lb 2 oz) falls between the 10th and 90th percentile curves for 28 weeks' gestation.**
2. The baby's weight is average for gestational age.
3. Babies with intrauterine growth restriction would show weights that are below the 10th percentile for gestational age; 1,000 grams is not below the 10th percentile for a 28-week-gestation neonate.
4. Babies who are large for gestational age would show weights that are above the 90th percentile for the gestational age.

TEST-TAKING HINT: It is important for the nurse to recognize and to calculate the weights of babies that are outside the average weight for gestational age (AGA), since a variety of risk factors are associated with these babies. By noting that a baby is small for gestational age (SGA) or large for gestational age (LGA), the nurse has a head start on being proactive to monitor for expected and common conditions such as temperature instability and low blood sugar. Necessary interventions can be completed sooner, once the anticipated conditions occur, because the conditions do not come as a surprise.

41. **The test taker should locate the 40-week-gestation line on the *x*-axis and follow it up to the 90th percentile curve.**

TEST-TAKING HINT: Babies whose weights are above the 90th percentile, weighing above 4,000 grams (the white area) are labeled large for gestational age (see the figure that follows).

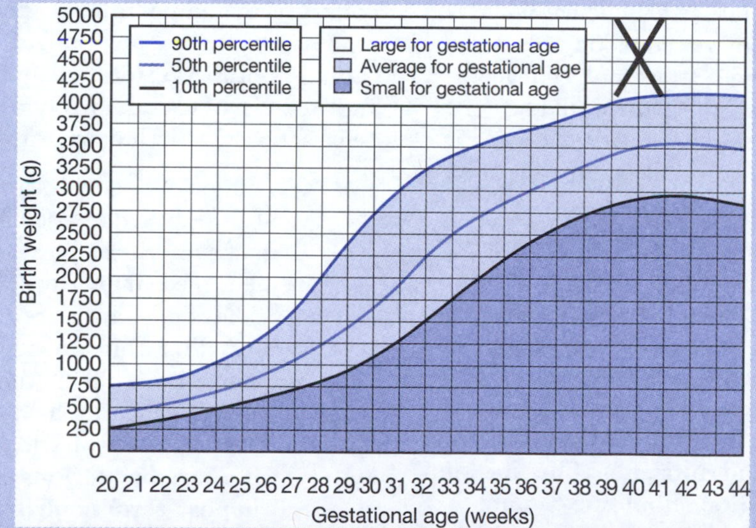

42. 1. **This baby is small for gestational age. Full-term babies (40 weeks' gestation) should weigh between 2,500 and 4,000 grams. It is very likely that this baby's placenta was less than optimal from the start of the pregnancy for any number of reasons. In addition, as the placenta aged and calcified past term, the fetus used up its glycogen stores in utero to survive, since an aging placenta is unable to deliver sufficient nutrients to the fetus. For up to 48 hours after the birth, the newborn's pancreas continues to secrete the same higher insulin levels that were required before birth, in spite of no longer receiving that amount of glucose. Having used up its glycogen stores to sustain prenatal life, and no longer receiving any glucose from the mother's blood now that it's born, the newborn is at high risk for hypoglycemia after birth.**
2. There is no indication from this scenario that this baby is leukopenic.
3. Rather than being anemic, it is likely that this baby is polycythemic to compensate for the poor oxygenation from a poorly functioning placenta. When the placenta is small, the surface area for oxygen pickup is suboptimal and the fetal hematological system creates more red blood cells so there are more oxygen carriers (polycythemia).
4. It is unlikely that this baby would be alkalotic. Rather, the baby may be acidotic from chronic hypoxemia and the metabolism of brown adipose tissue.

TEST-TAKING HINT: The test taker must attend carefully to the gestational age in any question relating to neonates. Post-term and preterm babies are at high risk for certain problems. Post-term babies are especially at high risk for hypoglycemia and chronic hypoxia because the aging placenta has not supplied sufficient quantities of oxygen and nutrients. The first step in answering this question should be to note normal lab values for each item. Then, review the physiological risks of post-term gestation to determine whether one would expect these lab values to (1) be affected by the newborn condition at all, and then (2) be high, low, or within normal limits in this scenario.

43. 1. The warmer must be preheated, but that is not the priority at this time.
2. **The neonatologist must be called to the delivery room so that he or she arrives before the baby is delivered.**
3. Narcan is not a priority at this time. The woman did receive a narcotic analgesic 4 hours ago. Although Narcan may be needed, it is not likely since she has no doubt metabolized most of the medication by this time.
4. The eye prophylaxis is not a priority at this time. It can wait until this baby is at least 1 hour old.

TEST-TAKING HINT: This is a prioritizing question. Although all of these actions may be performed by the nurse, only one is a priority. This baby is showing signs of fetal hypoxia—recurrent late decelerations. The baby may need to be resuscitated. The nurse must, therefore, page the neonatologist so that he or she is present for the birth of the baby.

44. 1. Abundant lanugo is seen in the preterm baby, not the post-term baby.
2. Absence of breast tissue is seen in the preterm baby, not the post-term baby.
3. Prominent clitoris is seen in the preterm baby, not the post-term baby.
4. **The post-term baby does have dry, wrinkled, and often peeling skin due to progressive placental deterioration and often reduced amounts of amniotic fluid.**

TEST-TAKING HINT: The test taker should be familiar with the characteristic presentations of preterm and postmature neonates. Studying the items on the New Ballard Scale and the corresponding gestational ages when the items are seen is an excellent way to associate certain characteristics with dysmature babies.

45. 1. Although the fluid is green tinged because the baby expelled meconium in utero, the bath is not a priority and may, in fact, stress the baby. The meconium may be wiped off, however.
2. The conjunctivae are not at high risk for irritation from the meconium-stained fluid.
3. There is nothing in the scenario that suggests that this baby is currently septic.
4. **Meconium aspiration syndrome (MAS) is a rare but serious complication seen in post-term neonates who are exposed to meconium-stained fluid. Respiratory distress would indicate that the baby has likely developed MAS.**

TEST-TAKING HINT: In this question, because only one answer is allowed, the test taker must select the answer that is the first of Maslow's hierarchy of needs—survival. That is answer #4. Although meconium appears black in a newborn's diaper, it is actually a very dark-green color. When diluted in the amniotic fluid, therefore, the fluid takes on a greenish tinge. Because meconium is

a foreign substance, both chemical and bacterial pneumonia can develop when meconium is aspirated by the baby.

Meconium passage occurs in utero when a fetus is postdates because of maturity of the gastrointestinal tract. Vagal stimulation during labor, whether from head compression or the forces of labor are thought to cause peristalsis and relaxation of the rectal sphincter. Meconium's presence in the amniotic fluid reduces antibacterial activity and can irritate fetal skin in cases of postmaturity. When inhaled, meconium can cause surfactant dysfunction, resulting in widespread atelectasis (Geis & Clark, 2017). In addition, substances in meconium irritate the airways and can cause widespread pneumonitis within a few hours after aspiration (Geis & Clark, 2017). Although amnioinfusion to thin down the meconium in amniotic fluid was once recommended as a routine intervention, that is no longer the case. In clinical settings with the availability of standard peripartum care and expert neonatal care, amnioinfusion has not been shown to improve outcomes in spite of thick meconium staining (Olicker et al, 2021). Routine intrapartum suctioning is also no longer recommended. Once delivered, resuscitation should be the same for newborns with clear fluid as for those with meconium-stained fluid (ACOG, 2017a; Wyckoff et al., 2015).

46. Answers 1, 2, 3, and 5 are correct.
1. Even though meconium is present in the amniotic fluid, the baby should be stimulated to breathe.
2. The baby's heart rate is a critical piece of information. If the heart rate is below 100 bpm, positive pressure ventilation and pulse oximetry should be initiated. In addition, direct ECG assessment may be appropriate.
3. Although not universally recommended, the physician may determine that intubation is needed to remove meconium-contaminated fluid from the baby's airway and/or to provide direct ventilation. It is always best to be prepared, whether or not the intervention is done.
4. The baby should be kept in a supine position, not on the belly.
5. Hypothermic neonates are at high risk of morbidity and mortality. When in need of resuscitation, they should be kept warm under an overhead heat source.

TEST-TAKING HINT: Pediatricians are not needed at every birth. In this scenario, the nurse apparently paged the pediatrician to be present at the birth once thick meconium fluid was seen. If the baby fails to breathe spontaneously, all neonatal resuscitation efforts should be instituted. It is important to note that the recommendation for intubation to remove meconium-stained fluid in all babies who fail to initiate spontaneous respirations has changed. *Routine* endotracheal intubation and suction of meconium is no longer recommended because of insufficient evidence that this was of benefit to babies born through meconium-stained fluid (Wyckoff et al., 2015). The reason for this decision was "harm avoidance" (Wyckoff et al., 2015. p. S546) as a result of insufficient evidence of the benefits of this practice. The time it took to intubate and suction led to delays in providing bag-and-mask ventilation. There were also concerns about potential harms of the procedure itself (Wyckoff et al., 2015). This is not to suggest that endotracheal intubation should never be done; the recommendation is that it should be done *selectively*, not *routinely*. The decision whether or not to intubate is currently to be determined by the resuscitating professional (Wyckoff et al., 2015).

47.
1. The gestational age assessment should be performed only after resuscitation efforts have been performed.
2. The baby's airway should be established by inflating the lungs with an ambu bag.
3. Chest compressions are begun after an airway is established and the heart rate has been assessed and is below 60 bpm.
4. Immediately after positive pressure ventilation (PPV) has been started, an oxygen saturation electrode should be placed on the baby and the values should be monitored continuously.

TEST-TAKING HINT: The steps of a neonatal resuscitation are slightly different from those for an older baby, a child, or an adult. Because the baby's survival is contingent upon the establishment of respiratory function, respiratory resuscitation must be instituted in a timely manner. If there is no spontaneous breathing and the heart rate is less than 100 bpm after birth, PPV should be begun followed immediately by continuous O2 saturation assessments and, if available, direct ECG. Cardiac compressions and intubation, if not already performed, are started if the heart rate falls below 60 bpm (Wyckoff et al., 2015).

48.
1. The 4-microgram dose is too low.
2. The 40-microgram dose is within the range of safety.
3. The 4-milligram dose is too high.
4. The 40-milligram dose is too high.

TEST-TAKING HINT: The recommended dosage for the administration of naloxone to a neonate has been cited as 0.01 mg/kg to 0.1 mg/kg. Because there are 1,000 micrograms per mg, if the dosage were written in micrograms, the dosage for a 3-kg neonate would be 30 micrograms to 300 micrograms. If the dosage were written in mg, the dosage for a 3-kg neonate would be 0.03 mg to 0.3 mg. The only choice that lies within the range of safety is 40 micrograms (Wyckoff et al., 2015).

49. 1. **Assisted ventilations should be administered at an approximate rate of 30 breaths per minute.**
2. Chest compressions should be begun when the heart rate is below 60 beats per minute.
3. Preferably, the chest should be compressed using the "2-thumb" technique. If fingers are used, 2 fingers are recommended, since 3 fingers would cover too wide an area on a neonate.
4. The compressions and ventilations should be administered in a 3:1 ratio.

TEST-TAKING HINT: The correct answer could be deduced by the test taker by remembering the normal respiratory rate of the neonate (30 to 60 breaths per minute). During a resuscitation, the nurses and other healthcare practitioners would be attempting to simulate normal functioning. Although the "2-finger" technique can be used when resuscitating infants, the "2-thumb" technique with the hands encircling the baby's chest, is the preferred technique (Wyckoff et al., 2015). It is less tiring for the professional and generates higher blood pressure for the neonate (Wyckoff et al., 2015). The most important goal of neonatal resuscitation is to work in concert with each other, providing rhythmic respiratory and cardiac support while the neonatal provider completes interventions such as umbilical line insertion and other care, as needed.

The nurse may be asked to draw blood samples from a portion of the umbilical cord after the delivery. Knowing how to differentiate the umbilical arteries from the umbilical vein is important when drawing umbilical cord blood for laboratory assessments. A sample from each vessel is important to compare the pH differences—the arteriovenous difference—between the blood from the placenta versus the blood within the umbilical artery that comes from the baby. For more information about umbilical circulation and how to differentiate between the umbilical artery and the umbilical vein, see the appendix.

50. 1. Epinephrine is administered only after other resuscitative measures have been instituted.
2. Positive pressure oxygen is administered only after initial interventions of tactile stimulation and warmth have failed.
3. Chest compressions are administered only after initial interventions have failed.
4. **The first interventions when a neonate fails to breathe include providing tactile stimulation.**

TEST-TAKING HINT: When a neonate fails to breathe, the nurse should dry the baby and provide tactile stimulation, place the child in the "sniff" position under a radiant warmer, and suction the mouth and nose with a bulb syringe, if necessary. Babies generally respond to these measures very quickly. Further intervention may be started only after these initial actions fail (Wyckoff et al., 2015).

51. 1. Bradycardia is a sign of neonatal distress but it is not related to meconium exposure.
2. **Because meconium is a dark-green color, the white tissue that makes up the umbilical cord—the Wharton's jelly—can be stained green when meconium is expelled in utero.**
3. A sunken fontanel is an indication of dehydration, not of meconium exposure.
4. A baby's skin often desquamates, or peels, when he or she is post-term. Although meconium may be expelled by a post-term baby, desquamation is not related to the meconium.

TEST-TAKING HINT: The test taker must look for cues in the question stem. The answer is not the first one because there is no mention of the baby's heart rate. Answer #2 is likely at first read because the stem indicates the fluid was meconium stained. Answer #3 has nothing to do with meconium. Answer #4 may seem likely because there is a relationship between postdates and skin peeling (also called "desquamation"). However, there is no direct relationship between meconium and peeling skin, even though meconium is a skin irritant. That leaves answer #2 as the most likely answer, since an umbilical cord may be stained green if meconium is in the amniotic fluid for a period of time.

52. 1. Limb deformities develop during pregnancy. They are not related to dystocia.
2. **During a difficult delivery with shoulder dystocia, the brachial nerve can become stretched and may even be severed. The nurse should, therefore, observe the baby**

for signs of brachial palsy, such as limited movement of the affected arm.

3. A fracture of the radius is an unlikely injury to occur even during a shoulder dystocia.
4. Buccal surfaces lie inside the cheeks. Buccal abrasions are highly unlikely injuries for the baby to sustain during a shoulder dystocia.

TEST-TAKING HINT: The key to answering this question is in understanding the terminology. A *shoulder dystocia* is a difficult delivery when the shoulder becomes stuck or fails to pass easily under the mother's pubic bone. *Deformities* are disfigurements or malformations. Although the arm and shoulder may be injured, the baby is not disfigured. A buccal abrasion would occur on the inside of the cheek. The baby with a brachial plexus injury cannot move the affected arm; the arm lays parallel to the baby's body, unlike the flexed, unaffected arm.

53. 1. *Candida* will infect both mother and baby.
2. Only under very special circumstances should a mother be advised not to breastfeed. It is safe to breastfeed when the baby has thrush.
3. ***Candida* is a fungal infection, and it is important to treat both the mother's breasts and the baby's mouth to prevent the infection from being transmitted back and forth between the two.**
4. Although immunosuppressed clients often do develop thrush, that is an unlikely cause of thrush in this situation.

TEST-TAKING HINT: It is important to avoid confusing nonobstetric pathology such as immunosuppression with common consequences of the process of birth. Thrush, which is often seen in the mouths of immunosuppressed clients, is also a common flora in the vagina. In this situation, it is not associated with an immunosuppressive disorder. The baby may have contracted the fungus in their mouth during delivery or from the mother's poorly washed hands after the delivery. Once in the baby's mouth, the fungus can be easily transferred to the mother's breast and reinfect the baby each time the baby breastfeeds if both mother and baby are not treated.

54. 1. The baby will have a positive antibody titer as a result of passive immunity through the placenta, but there will be no evidence of active viral production that early in the newborn's life.
2. There is no need to assess the antibody titer. It will definitely be positive because the mother has HIV/AIDS.
3. **The standard of care for neonates born to mothers with HIV/AIDS is to begin them on anti-AIDS medication. The mother will be advised to continue to give the baby the medication after discharge.**
4. There is no need to place the baby on contact precautions. Standard precautions in the well-baby nursery are sufficient.

TEST-TAKING HINT: The nurse must be aware that neonates must be followed after delivery because of the viral exposure in utero. The best way to prevent vertical transmission from the mother to the newborn is to administer antiviral medications to the mother during pregnancy and delivery. The most important risk factor to a neonate is the *mother's* viral load. The U.S. Department of Health and Human Services guidelines recommend that "A 4-week zidovudine (ZDV) ARV (anti-retroviral) prophylaxis regimen can be used in newborns whose mothers received ART (anti-retroviral therapy) during pregnancy and had sustained viral suppression near delivery (defined as a confirmed HIV RNA level <50 copies/mL) and for whom there are no concerns related to maternal adherence" (USDHHS, 2020, p. G-3). Treatment should be started within 6 to 12 hours after birth.

55. 1. **Hypothermia in a neonate may be indicative of sepsis.**
2. Mottling is commonly seen in neonates shortly after birth. It is considered a normal finding.
3. Omphalocele is not related to group B strep (GBS) exposure.
4. Stomatitis is not a sign associated with group B strep (GBS) exposure.

TEST-TAKING HINT: Group B streptococci (GBS) can be very serious for neonates. Before the practice of antepartum testing and intrapartum treatment for GBS status in the 1980s, the disease was often called "the baby killer." To prevent a severe infection from the bacteria, mothers with positive prenatal GBS cultures are given intravenous antibiotics every 4 hours in labor, from admission until delivery. A minimum of 2 doses is considered essential to protect the baby.

Because this client arrived only 2 hours before the delivery, there was not enough time for 2 doses to be administered, putting the neonate at higher risk. Although in older infants, children, and adults, hyperthermia is the expected temperature change when an infection is present, neonates often become hypothermic when septic (Puopolo et al., 2019).

56. 1. Although *Candida* can eventually lead to a maculopapular diaper rash, no facial rash is associated with a candidal infection.
2. Thrush is commonly seen in babies whose mothers have *Candida* vaginitis.
3. A neonatal fungal conjunctivitis is not associated with this problem.
4. Dehydration is not associated with this problem.

TEST-TAKING HINT: The nurse should be familiar with the various presentations of common fungi and bacteria. *Candida* is a fungus that is a common vaginal flora. During pregnancy, it is not uncommon for the vaginal flora to shift and for the woman to develop *Candida* vaginitis.

57. 1. Although vertical transmission of hepatitis B does occur, symptoms of the disease would not be evident during the neonatal period.
2. Standard precautions are sufficient for the care of the baby exposed to hepatitis B in utero.
3. Babies exposed to hepatitis B in utero should receive the first dose of hepatitis B vaccine as well as hepatitis B immune globulin (HBIG) within 12 hours of delivery to reduce transmission of the virus (Schille et al., 2018).
4. Breastfeeding is not contraindicated when the mother is hepatitis B positive.

TEST-TAKING HINT: Although breastfeeding is contraindicated when a mother is HIV positive, it is not contraindicated when a mother is positive for hepatitis B. Because the virus is bloodborne, the mother should take care to prevent any cracking and bleeding from her nipples and wash her hands thoroughly after changing her pad.

58. 1. Group B streptococci cause severe infections in the newborn. Neonates who are septic often develop signs of respiratory distress. Tachypnea is one sign of respiratory distress.
2. There is no relationship between cerebral palsy and respiratory distress in the neonate.
3. There is no relationship between placenta previa and respiratory distress in the neonate.
4. There is no evidence from the question that the stillbirth was related to a gestational infection.

TEST-TAKING HINT: The neonate who becomes septic will exhibit a number of what often appear to be unrelated signs and symptoms. These may include any or all of the following: hyperthermia or hypothermia, tachycardia, and any or all signs of respiratory distress such as nostril flaring, grunting, and retractions. In addition, they can have seizures, vomiting, diarrhea, and/or jaundice. It is important for caregivers to carefully review risk factors to put the puzzle together when any of these symptoms are demonstrated.

59. 1. The lung maturation of infants of diabetic mothers is often delayed. These babies must be monitored at birth for respiratory distress.
2. A maternal diagnosis of lung cancer will not affect her neonate's pulmonary function.
3. A maternal diagnosis of mitral valve prolapse does not put the baby at high risk for respiratory distress.
4. A maternal diagnosis of asthma does not put the baby at high risk for respiratory distress.

TEST-TAKING HINT: Two answers to this question relate to maternal pulmonary diagnoses, that is, lung cancer and asthma. Simply because a mother has a pulmonary problem does not mean that her neonate will have a similar problem, however. A neonate's respiratory distress is not always related to the mother's health problem. The test taker should not be swayed by this association. Babies born to diabetic mothers are at risk for delayed lung maturation (Azad et al., 2017) because higher blood sugar reduces surfactant production. These babies should be monitored for respiratory distress.

60. 1. Myasthenia gravis is not associated with caudal agenesis in the fetus.
2. Hyperglycemia associated with poorly controlled maternal diabetes mellitus is one of the most important predisposing factors for caudal agenesis in the fetus.
3. Splenic syndrome is sometimes seen in clients with sickle cell disease. It is not related to caudal agenesis in the fetus.
4. Hypothyroidism is not related to caudal agenesis in the fetus.

TEST-TAKING HINT: Women with diabetes must be in excellent glucose control before becoming pregnant. Before they become pregnant, they must understand and control their disease because fetal deformities develop during the organogenic period in the first trimester before they may even be aware they are pregnant.

61. 1. Neonatal blood glucose levels of less than 40 mg/dL (2.2 mmol/L) in the first 24 hours after birth are generally considered abnormal and require intervention (Potter & Kicklighter, 2016). A level of 35 mg/dL (1.9 mmol/L), therefore, is not normal and should be reported.

2. Glucagon may be ordered as a remedy for severe hypoglycemia. Although the glucose level is low, it is unlikely that glucagon is indicated.
3. Both breast milk and formula contain lactose. If the glucose level has not risen to normal as a result of the feeding, the nurse must notify the physician.
4. **If the glucose level has not risen to normal as a result of the feeding, the nurse should notify the physician and anticipate that the doctor will order an intravenous infusion of dextrose and water.**

TEST-TAKING HINT: Neonatal hypoglycemia must be anticipated for all macrosomic newborns and all newborns of mothers with diabetes mellitus, whether type 1 (T1DM), type 2 (T2DM), or gestational diabetes. The condition is believed to be due to fetal hyperinsulinism before birth in response to maternal hyperglycemia and high glucose levels delivered to the fetus. Although the maternal pancreas may not be able to keep up with her own high levels of glucose, the fetal pancreas is in pristine condition, and responds appropriately. Neonatal hypoglycemia is a risk factor for 4 to 7 days after birth until the neonate's own blood sugar levels are stabilized (Stanescu & Stoicescu, 2014). The target neonatal blood glucose level is 45 mg/dL, or 2.5 mmol/L (Potter & Kicklighter, 2016).

Protocols to monitor for hypoglycemia in infants of diabetic mothers exist in all well-baby nurseries and NICUs. Recommended timelines for testing neonatal blood glucose generally call for a capillary blood glucose (CBG) assessment as soon as possible after birth, followed by another test 30 minutes later, then 1 hour, 2 hours, 4 hours, 8 hours, and 12 hours after that (Potter & Kicklighter, 2016). The nurse can anticipate that plasma values of less than 20 to 25 mg/dL (1.1 to 1.4 mmol/L) require NICU admission and IV glucose (Potter & Kicklighter, 2016).

62. 1. The baby's serum protein levels should be normal.
2. **The mother's diagnoses of retinopathy and nephropathy indicate a very serious diabetic condition. As such, the placenta is likely to be functioning less than optimally. It is highly likely that the baby will be polycythemic, having increased its red blood cells to improve the oxygen-carrying capacity of the blood in utero.**
3. Rather than hypercalcemia, the nurse would expect to see hypocalcemia.
4. Rather than hypoinsulinemia, if the maternal glucose levels are higher than normal, the nurse would expect to see hyperinsulinemia in the neonate.

TEST-TAKING HINT: The nurse must be familiar with the pathology of diabetes and its effect on pregnancy. Although infants of diabetic mothers (IDMs) are usually macrosomic as a result of increased plasma glucose levels, when mothers have vascular damage, the placenta functions poorly. As a result, the fetus may be small for gestational age with intrauterine growth restriction and polycythemia from the poor nourishment and oxygenation.

63. 1. **The nurse should anticipate that the plasma glucose levels would be low.**
2. The nurse would expect to see elevated red blood cell counts rather than low red blood cell counts.
3. The white blood cell count should be within normal limits.
4. The nurse would expect to see elevated hemoglobin levels rather than low levels of hemoglobin.

TEST-TAKING HINT: The fetus, responding to the continuous supply of maternal glucose through the placenta, produces large quantities of insulin before birth. After the birth, however, the continuous supply stops, yet the pancreas continues to provide the same levels of insulin initially. It can take up to 48 hours for the baby's body to synchronize insulin production with the lower and intermittent glucose provided in breast milk or formula feedings (Abramowski et al., 2020). Until the baby makes the adjustment, he or she will exhibit hypoglycemia (less than 40 mg/dL [2.2 mmol/L]).

64. Answers 3, 4, and 5 are correct.
1. Hyperopia, another name for farsightedness, is unrelated to placental function.
2. If the mother had gestational diabetes, the nurse would expect the baby to be macrosomic, not to have IUGR.
3. **Placental function is affected by the vasoconstrictive properties of many illicit drugs as well as by cigarette smoke.**
4. **Placental function is diminished in women who have chronic hypertension.**
5. **Placental function has been found to be diminished in women of advanced maternal age.**

TEST-TAKING HINT: Any condition that inhibits the flow of blood in the mother can lead to fetal intrauterine growth restriction (IUGR)—that is, a fetus smaller than expected for the gestational period. Factors that can lead to fetal IUGR include illicit drug use, hypertension, and

cigarette smoking. The nurse must remember that IUGR is not the same as small for gestational age (SGA). The term IUGR describes a fetus that is pathologically smaller than it should be because of genetic or environmental factors. This is in contrast to the term SGA, which is simply describes a measurement of a birth weight below the 10th percentile for the newborn's gestational age.

65. 1. Pre-eclampsia with severe features is associated with asymmetrical IUGR.
 2. Chromosomal abnormalities are associated with symmetrical IUGR.
 3. An aging placenta is associated with asymmetrical IUGR.
 4. Preterm premature rupture of the membranes (PPROM) is unrelated to fetal growth.

A baby with *asymmetrical* IUGR will have a head and brain of the expected size for gestational age (called brain sparing), with thin limbs, thin body, and a very thin umbilical cord. This is seen with conditions that cause complications later in the pregnancy. Babies who are exposed to complications like pre-eclampsia or an aging placenta during the pregnancy will grow normally during the beginning of the pregnancy but start to grow poorly at the time of the insult. Their growth, therefore, will be disproportionately affected.

Conversely, babies with *symmetrical* IUGR have long-term growth restriction and all of the baby's body parts are similarly small in size. This is often seen with babies who have chromosomal defects and grow poorly from the time of conception. It may also occur if the mother has early uterine infections such as cytomegalovirus or rubella during placental development.

Postnatal risks for babies with IUGR include respiratory and feeding problems, hypothermia, hypoglycemia, and infection as well as neurological problems. This is why regular prenatal care to avoid or treat developing IUGR, if possible, is vital.

66. Answers 3 and 4 are correct.
 1. The baby will likely be born with a normal platelet count, since clotting is not an issue.
 2. The baby will likely be born with a normal white blood cell count since infection is not an issue.
 3. Babies who have lived in utero with a dysfunctional placenta usually are born with polycythemia.
 4. Babies who have lived in utero with a dysfunctional placenta will often demonstrate hypoglycemia after the birth.
 5. Rather than hyperlipidemia, babies who have lived in utero with a dysfunctional placenta may be born with hypolipidemia.

TEST-TAKING HINT: Even if the test taker were unfamiliar with the expected laboratory findings of a neonate who had been born after living with a dysfunctional placenta, deductive reasoning could assist the test taker to choose the correct responses. Dysfunctional placentas deliver less nutrition and oxygenation to the fetus. The baby's body must then compensate for these reductions by (1) metabolizing glycogen and lipid stores and burning brown fat for energy; and (2) producing increased numbers of red blood cells for adequate oxygen delivery. The neonate, therefore, is often (1) hypoglycemic and hypolipidemic; and (2) polycythemic.

67. 1. Most mothers, even those of full-term babies, usually use fingertip touch during their first physical contact with their babies.
 2. Palmar touch usually follows fingertip touch.
 3. Kangaroo hold is used in NICUs as a means of facilitating parent–infant bonding as well as promoting growth and development of the neonate.
 4. Cradle hold is the classic hold of a mother with her baby. This hold follows other touch contact.

TEST-TAKING HINT: The delivery of a preterm infant is very stressful and frightening. In fact, the appearance of the premature baby can be overwhelming to new parents. To become familiar with their baby, all parents proceed through a pattern of touch behaviors. When the baby is preterm, the procession through touch responses is often slowed but follows the same pattern.

68. Answers 1, 2, 3, and 5 are correct.
 1. Bronchopulmonary dysplasia often is a consequence of the respiratory therapy that preemies receive in the NICU.
 2. Cerebral palsy results from a hypoxic insult that likely occurred as a result of the baby's prematurity.
 3. Retinopathy is a disease resulting from the immaturity of the vascular system of the eye.

4. Hypothyroidism is one of the diseases assessed for in the neonatal screen. It is unlikely that this problem resulted from the baby's stay in the NICU.
5. **Seizure disorders can result either from a hypoxic insult to the brain or from a ventricular bleed. Both of these conditions likely occurred as a result of the prematurity.**

TEST-TAKING HINT: Many parents are of the opinion that premature babies, regardless of gestational age, will be healthy as they mature because there are so many machines to support them initially, and medications that can be given to the babies to prevent injury. Unfortunately, many babies suffer chronic problems as a result of their prematurity even when they receive excellent medical and nursing care.

69. **4.13 mg q 24 hours.**
The standard formula for calculating the safe dosage (per weight) is:

$$\frac{\text{Known dosage}}{1\text{ kg}} = \frac{\text{Needed dosage}}{\text{Weight of the child in kg}}$$

$$\frac{2.5\text{ mg}}{1\text{ kg}} = \frac{x\text{ mg}}{1.653\text{ kg}}$$

$$x = 4.13\text{ mg q 24 hours}$$

The dimensional analysis formula for calculating the safe dosage (per weight) is:

Known dosage	Child's weight in kg	Time conversion	Unit conversion	
1 kg		(if needed)	(if needed)	$= x$ dosage

2.5 mg	1.653 kg	
1 kg		$= x$

$$x = 4.13\text{ kg q 24 hours}$$

TEST-TAKING HINT: When calculating the safe dosage of a medication for a child, the nurse must first note whether the recommended dosage for the medication is written per kg or per meters squared. If the dosage is written per kg, then the denominator of the equation is in kg. If the dosage is written per m^2, the denominator of the equation is in m^2.

70. 0.25 mL.

Standard method:

Known mg : known volume = Desired micrograms : x volume

$$0.05 \text{ mg/mL} = 12.5 \text{ micrograms}/x \text{ mL}$$

(Because 1 mg = 1,000 micrograms, 0.05 mg = 50 micrograms)

$$50/1 = 12.5/x$$
$$50\,x = 12.5$$
$$x = 0.25 \text{ mL}$$

Dimensional analysis method:

$$\frac{\text{Known volume}}{\text{Known dosage}} \times \text{Desired dosage} \times \frac{\text{Time conversion}}{\text{(if needed)}} \times \frac{\text{Unit conversion}}{\text{(if needed)}} = \text{Desired volume}$$

$$\frac{1 \text{ mL}}{0.05 \text{ mg}} \times 12.5 \text{ micrograms} \times \frac{1 \text{ mg}}{1{,}000 \text{ Micrograms}} = x \text{ volume}$$

$$x \text{ mL} = 0.25 \text{ mL}$$

TEST-TAKING HINT: Digoxin is an excellent medication, but it can lead to significant side effects. It is administered in very small dosages to infants and neonates. To make sure that the calculation is accurate, nurses should always ask another healthcare practitioner to check their arithmetic.

71. 6.9 mg q week.

The standard method for calculating the safe dosage per body surface area is as follows:

$$\frac{\text{Known dosage}}{1 \text{ m}^2} = \frac{\text{Needed dosage}}{\text{Body surface area of the child (m}^2\text{)}}$$

To calculate the body surface area for this baby, the test taker must take the square root of the product of the baby's weight times its length and divided by the number 3,600.

$$\sqrt{\frac{3.476 \times 57}{3{,}600}} = 0.23 \text{ m}^2$$

(Because 1,000 g = 1 kg, 3,476 g = 3.476 kg)

Then, to calculate the safe dosage, a ratio and proportion equation must be solved.

$$\frac{30 \text{ mg}}{1\, m^2} = \frac{x \text{ mg}}{0.23 \text{ m}^2}$$
$$x = 6.9 \text{ mg q week}$$

The dimensional analysis method for calculating the safe dosage per body surface area is as follows:

$$\frac{\text{Recommended dosage}}{\text{m}^2} \times \sqrt{\frac{\text{weight(kg)} \times \text{height(cm)}}{3{,}600}} = \text{m}^2 \times \frac{\text{Time conversion}}{\text{(if needed)}} \times \frac{\text{Unit conversion}}{\text{(if needed)}} = \text{Safe BSA dosage}$$

3,476 g = 3.476 kg

$$\frac{30 \text{ mg}}{1 \text{ m}^2} \times \sqrt{\frac{3.476 \times 57}{3{,}600}} = m^2 = \text{Safe BSA dosage}$$

$$\frac{30 \text{ mg}}{1 \text{ m}^2} \left| \sqrt{\frac{198.13}{3,600}} = m^2 \right. = x \text{ mg}$$

$$\frac{30 \text{ mg}}{1 \text{ m}^2} \left| 0.23 = x \text{ mg} \right.$$

$x = 6.9$ mg q week

TEST-TAKING HINT: When calculating a safe dosage for a child using body surface area, it is important for the nurse to note whether the child's statistics are written in the metric system or the English system. If in the metric system, the divisor for the formula is the number 3,600. If the statistics are in the English system, however, the divisor is the number 3,131. In addition, it is important for the nurse to remember that neonates are weighed in grams rather than kg: 1 kg = 1,000 grams. Also, it is very easy to forget to take the square root when calculating BSA.

72. 3.33 mL/hr.

Standard method:

First, minutes must be converted to hours:

60 min = 1 hr.
90 min: x hr = 60 min : 1 hr
$x = 1.5$ hr

Next, the volume per hr must be determined:

5 mL/1.5 hours = x mL : 1 hr
$x = 3.33$ mL/hr

Dimensional analysis method:

$$\frac{\text{Known volume}}{\text{Known time}} \left| \frac{\text{Time conversion}}{\text{(if needed)}} \right. = \text{Desired volume}$$

$$\frac{5 \text{ mL}}{90 \text{ min}} \left| \frac{60 \text{ minutes}}{1 \text{ hour}} \right. = x \text{ mL/hr}$$

$x = 3.33$ mL/hr

TEST-TAKING HINT: Whenever a pump is used to deliver intravenous fluids to babies, the rate should be set in mL/hr units. Pumps should always be used to deliver IV fluids to neonates because due to their small size, they can so easily become overloaded with fluids.

73. 1. Respiratory rate of 70 is above normal. The rate should be between 30 and 60 breaths per minute.
2. Temperature of 97° F (36.1° C) is below normal. The temperature should be between 97.6° F (36.4° C) and 99° F (37.2° C).
3. The baby is showing signs of interest in breastfeeding. This is a positive sign.
4. Nasal flaring is an indication of respiratory distress, which is abnormal.

TEST-TAKING HINT: Kangaroo care, or skin-to-skin care, when mothers hold their naked babies against their own skin, is a technique that has been shown to benefit preterm infants. The vital signs of babies who kangaroo with their mothers have been shown to stabilize more quickly. The babies also have been shown to nipple feed earlier and to have shorter lengths of stay in the NICU.

74. Answers 1, 2, 3, and 4 are correct.
1. Babies with NEC have blood in their stools.
2. The abdominal girth measurements of babies with NEC increase.
3. When babies have NEC, they have increasingly larger undigested gastric contents after feeds.
4. The neonates' bowel sounds are diminished with NEC.
5. The presence of anal fissures is unrelated to NEC.

TEST-TAKING HINT: Necrotizing enterocolitis (NEC) is an acute inflammatory disorder seen in preterm babies. It appears to be related to the shunting of blood from the gastrointestinal tract, which is not a vital organ system, to the vital organs. The baby's bowel necroses with the shunting and the baby's once-normal flora become pathological. Resection of the bowel is often necessary.

75. 1. EBM is sufficient in iron and zinc.
2. Calcium and phosphorus in EBM are in quantities that are less than body requirements for the very low birth weight baby. Therefore, a fortifier may need to be added to the EBM.
3. Protein and fat are sufficient in EBM.
4. Sodium and potassium are sufficient in EBM.

TEST-TAKING HINT: Fetal brain growth in the third trimester is critical. Premature babies miss much of this benefit by being born early. Neonatal intensive care departments can help by providing supplementation of nutrients the babies would get in the womb. Unfortunately, very low birth weight babies do not receive sufficient quantities of calcium and phosphorus from the EBM. The

breast milk then is enriched with a milk fortifier that contains the needed elements (Arslanoglu et al., 2019; Underwood, 2013). Premature babies who receive breast milk have fewer complications than formula-fed babies. One of the complications seen less often in babies who receive human breast milk is necrotizing enterocolitis. Hospitals who have sought "baby friendly designation" must show that they supplement all babies in the NICU with human breast milk, whether donated or from the baby's mother (Baby Friendly USA, 2021, p. 62).

76. 1. Surfactant is not administered intravenously.
2. Surfactant is administered intratracheally. The baby must first be intubated. The nurse would assist the neonatal care provider with the procedure.
3. Surfactant is not administered parenterally.
4. Surfactant is not administered orally.

TEST-TAKING HINT: Surfactant is a slippery substance that is needed to prevent the alveoli from collapsing during expiration. It is prescribed for preterm babies who are so immature they don't have a sufficient number of alveoli to produce adequate amounts of the substance in their lung fields. The medication is used to prevent and/or to treat respiratory distress syndrome (RDS). Without surfactant, the work required of the baby for breathing has been compared to blowing up a balloon for the first time, with each breath. Surfactant reduces the resistance, making each breath more comfortable and easy. Otherwise, the baby risks alveolar collapse at the end of each respiration (Gallacher et al., 2016).

77. 1. Temperature is not related to the action of the surfactant medication.
2. A normal oxygen saturation level would be considered a positive result of the medication.
3. Heart rate is not related to the action of the medication.
4. Electrolyte levels are not related to the action of the medication.

TEST-TAKING HINT: The medication is given to provide the baby with exogenous lung surfactant. The drug is given to prevent and/or treat respiratory distress syndrome (RDS). When preterm babies have RDS, they are having respiratory difficulty that leads to poor gas exchange. When there is poor gas exchange, the oxygen saturation drops. A normal O2 saturation level, which is equal to or greater than 96%, therefore, indicates a positive outcome. Classic signs of respiratory distress include ". . . tachypnoea (respiratory rate > [greater than] 60 breaths per min),tachycardia (heart rate > [greater than] 160 beats min)nasal flaring, grunting, chest wall recessions (suprasternal, intercostal and subcostal), cyanosis and apnoea." (Gallacher et al., 2016, p. 32).

78. 1. A baby whose square window sign is 90° is preterm.
2. A baby whose skin is cracked and leathery is exhibiting a sign of postmaturity.
3. A baby whose popliteal angle is 90° is full term.
4. A baby whose plantar creases are pronounced is full term.

TEST-TAKING HINT: A number of neonatal characteristics are assessed to determine the gestational age of a neonate. Four of those characteristics are square window sign, characteristics of the skin, popliteal angle, and presence of plantar creases. The test taker should be familiar with the Ballard Scale and the many characteristics on which gestational age is measured.

79. 1. Babies who have cyanotic cardiac defects frequently feed poorly. And when they do feed, they frequently become cyanotic.
2. Sleeping is unlikely to trigger a cyanotic spell.
3. Rocking is unlikely to trigger a cyanotic spell.
4. Although the baby may be aroused when swaddled, it is unlikely to trigger a cyanotic spell.

TEST-TAKING HINT: Any activity that requires an increased oxygen demand can trigger a cyanotic spell in a neonate with a heart defect. The two activities that require the greatest amount of oxygen and energy are feeding and crying. In fact, because feeding demands that the baby be able to suck, swallow, and breathe rhythmically and without difficulty, many sick babies refuse to eat because it is such a demanding activity.

80. 1. It is not necessary to feed these babies via gastrostomy tubes.
2. Blood-stained mucus is not associated with cleft lip or palate.
3. It is not necessary to feed these babies via nasogastric tubes.
4. Cleft lip and palate babies require additional time to rest as well as to suck and swallow when being fed.

TEST-TAKING HINT: Although cleft lips and palates do affect feeding, virtually all of the affected babies are able to feed orally and some are even able to breastfeed. However, feeding from a standard bottle and/or breastfeeding may prove to be impossible for some babies with cleft lips and/or palates. In those cases, there are a number of bottles that have been designed to facilitate their feeding so that neither gastrostomy tubes nor nasogastric tubes are needed. The Haberman feeder is one example. Either expressed breast milk or formula can be put in the feeder.

81. **Answers 2 and 4 are correct.**
1. Vomiting is literally impossible.
2. **Babies with esophageal atresia would be expected to expel large amounts of mucus from the mouth because they can't swallow it into the stomach.**
3. A ruddy complexion is related to polycythemia, not esophageal atresia.
4. **Abdominal distention can be seen with esophageal atresia because air enters the stomach via the trachea.**
5. Pigeon chest is not associated with esophageal atresia.

TEST-TAKING HINT: With esophageal atresia, the esophagus ends in a blind pouch. In addition, there is usually a fistula connecting the stomach to the trachea. These babies are at high risk for respiratory compromise because they can aspirate a large quantity of oral mucus and, when a fistula is present, aspirate stomach contents. The neonatologist should be notified whenever esophageal atresia is suspected.

82.
1. There is no need for children with Down's syndrome to undergo yearly glucose tolerance testing.
2. Children with Down's syndrome are not at high risk for bleeding episodes.
3. Babies with Down's syndrome do not require special formulas. And although it can be a difficult beginning, many babies with Down's syndrome can breastfeed successfully.
4. **Because of the hypotonia of the respiratory accessory muscles, babies with Down's syndrome (trisomy 21) often need medical intervention when they have respiratory infections.**

TEST-TAKING HINT: Babies with Down's syndrome (trisomy 21) have not only a characteristic appearance but also physiological characteristics that the nurse must be familiar with. One of those characteristics is hypotonia. Because of this problem, babies with Down's syndrome are often difficult to feed during the neonatal period, have delayed growth and development, and have difficulty fighting upper respiratory illnesses.

83.
1. This baby has Down's syndrome (trisomy 21). The genetic disease is not associated with blood-tinged urine.
2. Babies with Down's syndrome (trisomy 21) are not at high risk for hemispheric paralysis.
3. **Cardiac anomalies occur much more frequently in babies with Down's syndrome (trisomy 21) than in other babies.**
4. Babies with Down's syndrome (trisomy 21) are no more at risk for hemolytic jaundice than are other babies.

TEST-TAKING HINT: Babies with Down's syndrome (trisomy 21) have the following characteristic appearance: low-set ears, single palmar creases, and slanted eyes. Because they are at high risk for internal anomalies as well, in particular cardiac defects, the nurse should carefully evaluate the babies for a heart murmur.

84.
1. Babies with a tracheoesophageal fistula (TEF) usually have the heads of their cribs elevated. The babies may be placed on one of their sides but should not be laid flat.
2. **Low nasogastric suction is usually maintained to minimize the amount of the baby's oral secretions.**
3. Babies who are born with TEF are kept NPO (nothing by mouth).
4. There is no reason to place a TEF baby on a hypothermia blanket.

TEST-TAKING HINT: Because the esophagus of a TEF baby ends in a blind pouch, he or she excretes large quantities of mucus from the mouth, placing the baby at high risk for aspiration. To decrease the potential for respiratory insult until surgery can take place, nasogastric suctioning is started and the baby's head is elevated.

85.
1. It is not painful for a baby with a cleft lip and palate to feed.
2. **It is likely that milk will be expelled from the baby's nose during feedings.**
3. Babies with clefts often take much longer to feed than do other babies.
4. Babies with clefts usually consume the same milk, either breast milk or formula, that other babies consume.

TEST-TAKING HINT: **A cleft palate condition is not visible from the outside. A baby with a cleft palate has an intact lip and cleft, or opening in the palate, the roof of the mouth. As a result, there is direct communication between the mouth and the sinuses. Because of the opening, milk is often expelled from the nose. The milk frequently enters the eustachian tubes, as well. These babies, therefore, are at high risk for ear infections.**

86. Answers 1 and 2 are correct.
   1. **Babies with 2-vessel cords are at high risk for renal defects.**
   2. **Babies with 2-vessel cords are at high risk for cardiac defects.**
   3. There is no relationship between a 2-vessel cord and glucose tolerance.
   4. Anomalies with a 2-vessel cord are primarily structural. An electroencephalogram measures brain activity, not structure.

TEST-TAKING HINT: **The umbilical cord develops in fetal life at approximately the same time as the renal and cardiac systems. Although a 2-vessel cord with just one umbilical artery (not two) and the one umbilical vein has been associated with several body systems including gastrointestinal, central nervous, and other body systems, no unique pattern of associated anomalies has been demonstrated in the literature (Akinmoladun & Olukemi, 2018). The most frequently seen anomalies are genitourinary and cardiovascular malformations (Akinmoladun & Olukemi, 2018; Hua et al., 2010). Because of this fact, when a defect is seen in the umbilical cord, both the urinary system and the cardiac systems must be assessed and monitored carefully (Akinmoladun & Olukemi, 2018).**

87.
   1. It is not routinely necessary to perform nasogastric suctioning on a baby born with a meningomyelocele.
   2. **The baby should be lain prone, on its tummy, to prevent injury to the sac.**
   3. It is not routinely necessary to administer oxygen to a baby born with a meningomyelocele.
   4. A baby born with a meningomyelocele should not be swaddled.

TEST-TAKING HINT: **The baby with meningomyelocele is born with an opening at the base of the spine through which a sac protrudes. The sac contains cerebrospinal fluid and nerve endings from the spinal cord. It is essential that the nurse not injure the sac; therefore, the baby should be placed in a prone position immediately after birth.**

88.
   1. **A diuretic will increase urinary output, which, in turn, will lead to weight loss.**
   2. A drop in sodium is not a goal of diuretic therapy.
   3. Rather than an increase in specific gravity, the nurse would expect to see a drop in specific gravity.
   4. An increase in blood pressure is not a goal of diuretic therapy.

TEST-TAKING HINT: **The heart is pumping inefficiently when a baby has congestive heart failure. Because of this pathology, the kidneys are poorly perfused, leading to fluid retention and weight gain. Diuretics are administered to improve the excretion of the fluid. When the urinary output is increased, the weight will drop and the urine will be less concentrated.**

89.
   1. Fatigue is an important risk factor for the baby with congestive heart failure, but it is not the priority risk.
   2. Activity intolerance is an important risk for the baby with congestive heart failure, but it is not the priority risk.
   3. Sleep pattern disturbance is an important risk for the baby with congestive heart failure, but it is not the priority risk.
   4. **Altered tissue perfusion is the priority risk.**

TEST-TAKING HINT: **In this question, the CAB acronym applies. When circulation is impaired, there is altered tissue perfusion. None of the other responses relates to critical physiological processes.**

90.
   1. The dose should not be readministered until it has been determined that the child's digoxin levels are within normal limits.
   2. **The nurse should notify the physician that the baby has vomited the digoxin.**
   3. This action is not needed. The apical pulse will have been assessed prior to the initial administration of the medication, and assessing the two pulses together will provide no further information.
   4. It is unlikely that the vomitus will be streaked with blood.

TEST-TAKING HINT: **Vomiting is a sign of digoxin toxicity. This baby needs to have a digoxin level drawn. Because the nurse needs an order for the test, the nurse must notify the doctor of the problem.**

91.
   1. There should not be sensory loss in all four quadrants.
   2. With a meningomyelocele there will be a sac at the base of the spine, not a tuft of hair.

3. **With a defect at L2, the nurse would expect to see paralysis of the legs.**
4. The Moro reflex will be asymmetrical because the enervation to the lower extremities is impaired.

TEST-TAKING HINT: If the test taker remembers that a sac with cerebrospinal fluid and nerves is seen at the base of the spine in a baby with meningomyelocele and that L2 innervates the motor nerves of the legs, the answer becomes obvious. This is an example of the importance of carefully studying normal anatomy and physiology and the pathophysiology of important diseases.

92. 1. Babinski and tonic neck reflexes are unrelated to the eye.
2. Pseudostrabismus is normally seen in the neonate.
3. Blood typing and Coombs testing are unrelated to the eye.
4. **The baby should be assessed for signs of hydrocephalus, especially a disparity between the circumferences of the neonatal head and the neonatal chest.**

TEST-TAKING HINT: Setting sun sign—when the sclera, the white part of the eyeball, is visible above the colored iris of the eye—is one sign of hydrocephalus. The eyes seem to be fixed downwards.

93. 1. **The blood pressures in all four quadrants should be assessed.**
2. A bulging fontanel, not coarctation of the aorta, is indicative of hydrocephalus.
3. At delivery, the hematocrit and hemoglobin will likely be the same as in a healthy baby.
4. Harlequin coloration is a normal finding.

TEST-TAKING HINT: The pathophysiology of coarctation of the aorta provides the rationale for the assessment of the blood pressures. Because the narrowing of the aorta usually occurs beyond the blood vessels that branch off to the upper body, blood is able to pass unimpeded into the upper body and the blood pressure to those body parts is strong. Further down the circulatory system, the blood has difficulty passing through the descending aorta toward the lower body. The blood pressures of the upper body, therefore, are much higher than the blood pressures in the lower extremities.

94. 1. Healthy babies should always be placed in the supine position for sleep and during unsupervised periods. For therapeutic reasons, however, sick babies may need to be placed in other positions.
2. The prone position is not the appropriate position for a baby during a "tet" spell.
3. **Parents should place an infant during a "tet" spell into the knee-chest position.**
4. The semi-Fowler position is ordinarily a safe position for a baby with tetralogy of Fallot, but during a "tet" spell, the baby should be moved to the knee-chest position.

TEST-TAKING HINT: The four defects that are present in tetralogy of Fallot— ventricular septal defect, overriding aorta, pulmonary stenosis, and hypertrophied right ventricle—create a circulatory system in which much of the blood bypasses the lungs. As a result, a baby with tetralogy is predisposed to cyanotic, or "tet," spells. When a baby is placed in a squatting or knee-chest position, the femoral arteries are constricted, decreasing the amount of blood perfusing the lower body. This leads to improved perfusion to the upper body and the vital organs. With this action, the cyanotic spell will likely resolve. Toddlers often assume a squatting position on their own during a spell.

95. 1. Cyanosis and clubbing are seen in children suffering from severe cyanotic defects but are not likely to develop with a small VSD.
2. These symptoms will unlikely develop with a small VSD.
3. **This response is correct. The nurse can expect to hear a systolic murmur with no other obvious symptoms**
4. Feeding difficulties and polycythemia are seen in children suffering from severe cyanotic defects.

TEST-TAKING HINT: The VSD—an opening between the ventricles of the heart—is the most common acyanotic heart defect seen. The defect leads to a left-to-right shunt because the left side of the heart is more powerful than the right side of the heart after birth. As blood swishes through the ventricular defect from the left to the right side between beats, one can hear an audible sound called a murmur. This sound is related to the turbulence of the blood as it passes through the VSD, sometimes described as similar to water running over rocks in a stream, between beats. It is a holosystolic (aka pansystolic) murmur, meaning it occurs throughout systole. It begins with the first heart sound (S1, or "lub") and may be heard until the second heart sound (S2, or "dub"). Small VSDs rarely result in severe symptoms and, in fact, often close over time without any treatment.

96. **1. Ventriculoperitoneal (VP) shunts are inserted for the treatment of hydrocephalus. A positive finding, therefore, would be decreasing head circumferences.**
2. VP shunts are not inserted for the treatment of cardiac arrhythmias or cardiac anomalies.
3. VP shunts are not inserted for the treatment of hypertension.
4. Setting sun sign is a sign of hydrocephalus. Appearance of setting sun sign would indicate that the shunt is functioning improperly.

TEST-TAKING HINT: Cerebrospinal fluid (CSF) is produced continuously by structures in the ventricles of the brain. Normally, it flows through the ventricles, bathing the brain and spinal cord before being eventually absorbed into the blood. Hydrocephalus occurs when more CSF is produced than the bloodstream can absorb. In the newborn, it can be caused by abnormal development of the structures in the central nervous system that obstruct the flow. These may include spina bifida, bleeding within the ventricles as a result of prematurity, or a maternal infection such as syphilis or rubella before birth that causes meningitis and swelling of fetal brain tissue (Tully & Dobyns, 2014).

One of the first signs of hydrocephalus in the neonate is increasing head circumferences. Because the fetal head is unfused, excess fluid in the brain forces the skull to expand. Once the diagnosis of hydrocephalus has been made, a VP shunt is usually inserted. The shunt is designed to remove excess cerebrospinal fluid from the ventricles of the brain, draining it into the abdominal cavity, where the body absorbs it. With the reduction in fluid, the size of the baby's head decreases.

97. 1. The baby is not suffering from a fluid volume deficit.
2. If the fragile sac is injured, the baby is at very high risk for infection.
3. The defect is below the respiratory nerves. The baby is not at high risk for respiratory difficulties.
4. Although babies with meningomyelocele must be fed in the prone position, they are able to eat without difficulty.

TEST-TAKING HINT: Babies with meningomyelocele, a form of spina bifida, are at very high risk for infection in the central nervous system until the defect is corrected. The vast majority of babies with meningomyelocele (also known as myelomeningocele) also have hydrocephalus for which they will receive a ventriculoperitoneal (VP) shunt. In addition, the most common problem associated with VP shunts is infection. Nurses, therefore, must care for these affected babies using strict aseptic technique.

98. **1. Babies who have delayed meconium excretion may have Hirshsprung's disease.**
2. Tachycardia is not associated with Hirshsprung's disease.
3. Rashes are not associated with Hirshsprung's disease
4. Asymmetrical leg folds are related to developmental dysplasia of the hip, not to Hirshsprung's disease.

TEST-TAKING HINT: Hirshsprung's disease is defined as a congenital lack of parasympathetic innervation to the distal colon. Peristalsis, therefore, ceases at the end of the intestine. Because of the absence of peristalsis, the passage of meconium is delayed.

99. **1. Excessive amounts of frothy saliva may indicate that the child has esophageal atresia.**
2. Blood-tinged vaginal discharge is a normal finding in female neonates.
3. Milk-like secretion from the breast is a normal finding in neonates.
4. It is normal for a baby's heart rate to speed slightly during inhalation and slow slightly during exhalation.

TEST-TAKING HINT: If the test taker is familiar with the characteristics of the normal neonate, the answer to this question is obvious. A baby whose esophagus ends in a blind pouch is unable to swallow his or her saliva. Instead, the mucus bubbles and drools from the mouth. Healthy babies, on the other hand, swallow without difficulty.

100. **1. To treat developmental dysplasia of the hip (DDH), babies' legs are maintained in a state of abduction.**
2. DDH is not painful. Pain medication is not indicated.
3. Casting is only done in cases where splinting is ineffective.
4. There is no need to assess pedal pulses. They are unaffected in babies with DDH.

TEST-TAKING HINT: Developmental dysplasia of the hip can vary in severity. Because the pathology of DDH is related to laxity of the ligaments of the hip joint, the rationale for

therapy is to maintain physiological positioning of the hip joint until the ligaments strengthen and mature. A cause of DDH can be related to the breech position, where the ligaments are over-stretched. After the birth, keeping the legs in a state of abduction, with the upper legs at right angles to the body, points the ball of the femur into the socket, the acetabulum. As the acetabulum grows, it deepens and the ligaments tighten up to hold the "ball and socket" joint in place. At one time, breech babies were double-diapered, relying on the diaper padding to keep the hips wide open. Currently, more reliable therapies are available such as the Pavlik harness, which a baby wears for 23 hours a day for up to 6 months. In this harness, the hip joint is maintained with the trochanter centered in the acetabulum to promote normal hip and ligament development.

101. 1. With developmental dysplasia of the hip (DDH) there is reduced hip abduction.
2. DDH is not associated with swelling at the site.
3. The leg folds of the baby, both anteriorly and posteriorly, are frequently asymmetrical.
4. Femoral pulses are unaffected by DDH.

TEST-TAKING HINT: Because of the subluxation (partial dislocation) of the hip, the gluteal and thigh folds of the baby usually appear asymmetrical. In addition to this finding, the nurse would expect to see reduced abduction of the hip and/or asymmetrical knee heights when the legs are flexed.

102. 1. During the neonatal physical assessment, the nurse is unable to move a clubfoot into proper alignment.
2. A positive Ortolani sign indicates the presence of developmental dysplasia of the hip.
3. A shortened metatarsal arch is not diagnostic of clubfoot.
4. The Babinski reflex is positive in all neonates.

TEST-TAKING HINT: In the most common form of clubfoot, the baby's foot is in a state of inversion and plantar flexion (toes are pointed down, as though planting seeds in the garden with the toes). It is important for the nurse to distinguish between positional clubfoot, which occurs from the baby's position in utero and resolves spontaneously, and a pathological condition that requires orthopedic therapy.

103. 1. The initial treatment plan for clubfoot (also called *talipes equinovarus*) usually includes a series of casts that slowly move the foot into proper alignment.
2. Harrington rod insertion has been used to treat scoliosis, not club foot
3. Pavlik harness is a therapy for a baby with developmental dysplasia of the hip.
4. Long-term bracing is not a common therapy for clubfoot.

TEST-TAKING HINT: This is an example of a question that may include a term that the test taker is unfamiliar with. If the test taker slowly breaks down the words into their component parts, the meaning of the term will become clear. The word "bilateral," of course, means that "both sides" of the body are affected. The word "talipes" is a word that contains two roots: "talis," meaning "ankle" and "pes," meaning "foot." The word, therefore, refers to a deformity of the foot and ankle—clubfoot. The term "equinovarus" specifically defines the type of clubfoot but because the therapy is the same no matter which type of clubfoot the child suffers from, further analysis is not necessary to answer this question. (Talipes equinovarus clubfoot refers to a foot that is plantar flexed and turned inward.)

104. Answers 2, 3, and 4 are correct.
1. Palpitations are not an early sign of congestive heart failure (CHF).
2. No matter whether a baby or an adult were developing CHF, the client would be tachypneic.
3. No matter whether a baby or an adult were developing CHF, the client would be tachycardic.
4. No matter whether a baby or an adult were developing CHF, the client would be diaphoretic.
5. Irritability is not an early sign of CHF.

TEST-TAKING HINT: The term that is most descriptive in the phrase "congestive heart failure" is the word "congestive," referring to "congestion." The condition develops as a result of serious intravascular and tissue congestion related to fluid retention (Boorsma et al., 2020). It is more of a collection of symptoms than a discrete diagnosis and in newborns, it is most commonly related to structural heart problems (Satou & Halnon, 2019).

If the nurse remembers that the condition occurs when the heart has to work harder than it should to circulate blood, the symptoms can be easily anticipated. Due to a congenital heart condition,

too much blood might be pumped to the lungs as with VSD and truncus arteriosus. The heart strains to push blood against the lung pressures. Like any other muscle, the heart walls thicken and stiffen with overuse. This may cause the heart muscle to "fail." This doesn't mean the heart stops working. Rather, it's less efficient than normal.

With poor circulation, a backup of blood and fluid occurs in the veins, leading to edema. Edematous lung tissue causes more strain on the heart and leads to symptoms such as difficulty breathing (retractions), rapid breathing, and increased heartrate (if each pump is inefficient, a higher number of pumps is necessary). The baby has difficulty sucking because breathing is difficult. Sweating may be present as a result of an increased cardiac workload. The blood pressure may rise due to the pressure of the tissue edema against the blood vessels. The baby may be lethargic as a result of all this extra work.

Treatments generally include surgical repair of the congenital anomaly, antidiuretics to reduce the fluid volume, ace inhibitors or beta blockers to reduce the blood pressure, medications to improve cardiac contractility, and nasogastric feedings to reduce the burden of sucking and to provide adequate nutrition (Satou & Halnon, 2019).

105.
1. Setting sun sign is a symptom of hydrocephalus. It is not a symptom of cardiac disease.
2. **Anasarca refers to overall, systemic edema. It is seen in severe cardiovascular disease. A cardiac consult would be appropriate for this baby as would, perhaps, a renal consult.**
3. A baby with flaccid extremities is exhibiting a neurological or musculoskeletal problem, not a cardiac problem.
4. A baby with polydactyly has more than 5 digits on the hands or feet. The finding has nothing to do with cardiac problems.

TEST-TAKING HINT: Although each of the answer options is abnormal, there is only one option that describes a symptom of a cardiac disease. The test taker must carefully discern what is being asked in each question to choose the one answer that relates specifically to the stem.

106. Answers 1, 2, and 4 require follow-up.
1. **A hole between the left and right ventricles is called a ventricular septal defect (VSD), not a PDA.**
2. **Unless the baby is decompensating, this defect rarely results in cyanosis. The blood is being oxygenated and, although there is mixed blood, the baby is sufficiently oxygenated.**
3. This is correct information. Some of the oxygenated blood in the aorta is forced back down into the pulmonary artery through the PDA after birth, resulting in oxygenated (left side) blood reentering and mixing with the oxygen-depleted blood going to the pulmonary system. When used in this way, the term "left to right" shunt can be interpreted as "oxygenated blood shunting to oxygen-depleted" blood.
4. **This is referring to the foramen ovale, not a PDA. The foramen ovale is a normal shunt in fetal circulation, in order for most of the oxygenated blood entering the right atrium from the umbilical vein to bypass the lungs. A physical right-to-left shunt is normal in the fetal heart, but when the term is used to refer to a newborn's heart condition, it is not always a literal reference to left and right sides of the heart. For example, the ductus arteriosus is outside of the heart, and not on either the left or the right side. See the appendix for more information.**

TEST-TAKING HINT: The ductus arteriosus is a short blood vessel unique to fetal circulation that connects the pulmonary artery to the aorta, effectively shunting most of the oxygenated blood past the lungs. Before birth, the fetal lungs are filled with amniotic fluid and the lungs don't need to oxygenate the blood, since that function is handled by the placenta. This contributes to higher pressures in the fetal atrium, since it is the right side of the heart that is pumping the oxygenated blood throughout the body during fetal life. After birth, the left side takes over this task, so it becomes stronger with higher pressures. After the baby's birth, a reference to a "left-to-right" shunt is not a literal, physical shunt. It simply means that oxygenated blood leaks or is shunted into oxygen-depleted blood. For more information on fetal circulation, see the appendix.

107. Answers 3 and 5 are correct.
1. Transposition of the great vessels is a cyanotic defect that, if it stands alone, is incompatible with life.
2. Tetralogy of Fallot is a cyanotic defect characterized by four defects: VSD, pulmonic stenosis, overriding aorta, and right ventricular hypertrophy.

3. Ventricular septal defect (VSD) is the most common cardiac defect in neonates. It is an acyanotic defect with a left to right shunt. Already oxygenated blood reenters the right ventricle. This extra blood is pumped back into the lungs, forcing both the heart and lungs to work harder.
4. Pulmonic stenosis is characterized by a narrowed pulmonic valve. The blood, therefore, is restricted from entering the pulmonary artery and the lungs to be oxygenated.
5. Patent ductus arteriosus (PDA) is a very common cardiac defect in preterm babies. It is an acyanotic defect with a left to right shunt. Already oxygenated blood reenters the pulmonary system through the ductus arteriosus.

TEST-TAKING HINT: The names of cardiac defects are very descriptive. Once the test taker remembers the pathophysiology of each of the defects, it becomes clear how the blood flow is affected. Of the choices in this question, the defects that are acyanotic defects, that is, defects that allow blood to enter the lungs to be oxygenated, are the VSD and the PDA.

108. The term in column 1 is matched to the description in column 2.
1. Café au lait spot matches with **D. A café au lait spot is a pale tan- to coffee-colored skin marking.**
2. Hemangioma matches with **A. A hemangioma is a raised blood vessel–filled lesion.**
3. Mongolian spot matches with **C. Mongolian spots are multiple grayish-blue, hyperpigmented skin areas.**
4. Port wine stain matches with **B. A port wine stain is a flat, sharply demarcated red-to-purple lesion.**

TEST-TAKING HINT: This is simply a matching question. The test taker is asked to match the lesion that is seen in neonates with the description of the lesion. In the NCLEX-RN exam, this would be a drag-and-drop type of question. The test taker will be asked to drag the corresponding definition and drop it next to the name of the lesion.

109. 1. Galactosemia is one of the few diseases that is a contraindication for the intake of breast milk or any milk-based formula.
2. Galactosemia is a metabolic defect. There is no cardiovascular component.
3. Diarrhea and other malabsorption symptoms will be seen over time, but bloody stools would not be seen in the nursery.
4. Although vomiting and diarrhea do occur, the baby is unlikely to have abdominal pains.

TEST-TAKING HINT: There are many genetic metabolic diseases that may affect the neonate. Galactosemia, an autosomal recessive disease, is characterized by an inability to digest galactose, a by-product of lactose digestion. Because breast milk and milk-based formulas are very high in lactose, affected babies must be switched to a soy-based formula.

110. 1. Because the head circumference is significantly larger than the chest circumference, the nurse should assess for another sign of hydrocephalus. A markedly enlarged or bulging fontanel is one of those signs.
2. Abdominal girth does not change when a child has hydrocephalus.
3. Hydrocephalus is not a cardiovascular problem.
4. Hydrocephalus is not a respiratory problem.

TEST-TAKING HINT: The head circumference should be approximately 2 cm larger than the chest circumference at birth. When the head circumference is markedly larger than expected, there is a possibility of hydrocephalus. The nurse should assess for other signs of the problem, such as enlarged fontanel size, setting sun sign, and bulging fontanels.

111. 1. Choanal atresia will affect the baby's ability to feed.
2. Digestion is unaffected by choanal atresia, which is a structural defect.
3. The immune response is unaffected by choanal atresia, which is a structural defect.
4. The renal system is unaffected by choanal atresia, which is a structural defect.

TEST-TAKING HINT: Choanal atresia, a congenital narrowing of the nasal passages, seriously affects babies' ability to feed. Babies are obligate nose breathers. This enables them to suck-swallow-breathe in a rhythmic manner during feeding. If their nares are blocked, as with choanal atresia, they are unable to breathe through their nose and, therefore, must stop feeding to breathe.

112. 1. A blockage in the gastrointestinal system may lead to polyhydramnios rather than oligohydramnios.
2. Oligohydramnios is not related to a defect in the hepatic system.

3. Oligohydramnios is not related to a defect in the endocrine system. Pregnancies of mothers with diabetes often are complicated by polyhydramnios.
4. **Some defects of the renal system can lead to oligohydramnios.**

TEST-TAKING HINT: A portion of the amniotic fluid is made of plasma that seeps from the mother's blood through intramembranous inflow and outflow controlled by the amnion at the placenta (Beall et al., 2007; Brace et al., 2018). Amniotic fluid volume is regulated by the digestive and urinary systems of the fetus, whose swallowing and voiding releases substances that may call for an increase or decrease of plasma (Dubil & Magann, 2013). Some of the maternal plasma is absorbed through the fetal skin, and is processed by the cells, eventually becoming urine (Brace et al., 2018). As such, most of the amniotic fluid is urine, produced by the fetal kidneys after approximately 16 to 20 weeks gestation. If there is a defect in the renal system, there may be a resulting decrease in the amount of fetal urine produced. Oligohydramnios would then result.

113. 1. Pre-eclampsia is not associated with esophageal atresia.
2. Idiopathic thrombocytopenia is not associated with esophageal atresia.
3. **Polyhydramnios, also called hydramnios, is often seen in pregnancies complicated by a fetus with a digestive blockage.**
4. Severe anemia is not associated with esophageal atresia.

TEST-TAKING HINT: Polyhydramnios can be related to both maternal and fetal conditions. This question concerns polyhydramnios relating to the fetus. Amniotic fluid levels are regulated by fetal urination and fetal lung liquid production (Dubil & Magann, 2013; Hamza et al., 2013). Regulation and reduction of amniotic fluid is accomplished through fetal swallowing, and both intramembranous and intravascular absorption through the placenta (Hamza et al., 2013). When there is a blockage in the digestive system, and the fetus is unable to swallow the fluid, or when the fetus creates larger amounts of urine than normal due to hyperglycemia, polyhydramnios can develop (Hamza et al., 2013). The nurse will recall that water (H20) is a waste product of glucose metabolism, making up a large part of urine.

114. 1. Digestive symptoms are not associated with a congenital diaphragmatic hernia.
2. High-pitched cries are associated with prematurity and some retardation syndromes.
3. **The baby will develop respiratory distress very shortly after delivery.**
4. Fecal incontinence is not associated with diaphragmatic hernia.

TEST-TAKING HINT: With a congenital diaphragmatic hernia, one or more abdominal organs moves up through a hole, or defect in the diaphragm, into the chest. This takes up the space intended for the lungs, and can cause underdevelopment of the lungs known as pulmonary hypoplasia. The newly delivered baby, therefore, is unable to breathe effectively. Fortunately, only one lung is commonly affected. Surgical treatment is necessary to repair the defect.

115. 1. Oxytocin is administered to the mother, not to the baby.
2. Xylocaine is an anesthetic agent. It would not be administered in this situation.
3. **Naloxone is an opiate antagonist. It may be administered to a depressed baby at delivery.**
4. Stadol is a synthetic opioid. It would not be administered in this situation.

TEST-TAKING HINT: It is important for the nurse to anticipate the needs of his or her clients. In this situation, because the mother has recently received an opioid analgesic, it is possible that the baby will experience central nervous system depression. In anticipation of this problem, the nurse should have the opioid antagonist available for administration if the neonatologist should order it.

116. 1. Babies born via cesarean section usually have round, unmolded heads.
2. High forceps are not used in obstetrics today. High forceps, applied to babies' heads that are not well descended, are no longer used because of the high incidence of fetal damage that results. Instead, babies who fail to descend are now delivered via cesarean section.
3. Low forceps are applied when engagement is +2 or greater (using +3 station as crowning). The baby may develop forceps marks but would not develop a chignon.
4. **Babies born via vacuum extraction often do develop chignons.**

TEST-TAKING HINT: In common language, a chignon is a hairstyle that is characterized by a bun or knot of hair worn on the back of the head

or nape of the neck. In obstetrics, a chignon is a round, bruised caput seen on the crown of the baby's head. It results from the pressure exerted on the scalp during a vacuum-assisted delivery.

117. 1. Vacuum-assisted deliveries result in injuries to the head and scalp, not to the feet.
2. The babies are at high risk for hyperbilirubinemia, not hypobilirubinemia.
3. Babies born via vacuum are not at high risk for hyperglycemia.
4. Babies born via vacuum are at high risk for cephalohematoma.

TEST-TAKING HINT: During birth, some trauma may occur to the neonate's head and scalp. This can happen with or without the use of vacuum extractors or forceps, although the injuries are more common when these instruments are used. The nurse must remember the differences between the three most common conditions that may occur to the baby's head during birth. All of the injuries occur between the scalp and the skull. These conditions are 1) caput succedaneum, 2) cephalohematoma, and 3) subgaleal hemorrhage. The difference is in the depth of the bleeding location or edema, the volume of bleeding that is possible, and whether or not the bleeding crosses suture lines.

Caput is fairly common. It is a finding of poorly defined edema that may cross the suture lines of the skull. It is not serious and resolves on its own after a few days (Nicholson, 2007). Cephalohematoma is another minor condition. A cephalhematoma develops as a result of injury to superficial blood vessels in the subcutaneous space above the periosteum—the membrane covering the skull. The bleeding is gradual, and may not be noticeable immediately. An important distinction is that a cephalohematoma has defined margins and does not cross the suture lines (Nicholson, 2007; Raines, 2020). A subgaleal bleed may have the appearance of a benign caput initially. However, it has a high mortality and morbidity rate (Fakih, 2014). The bleeding occurs under the periosteum, and consists of damage to large veins. Mortality is related to severe, unrecognized hypovolemia and coagulopathy (Fakih, 2014). Babies born by either vacuum extractor or forceps are at high risk for all three conditions. The nurse should remember that babies born with any of these conditions are at high risk for hyperbilirubinemia.

118. **Answers 1, 2, 3, and 4 are correct.**
1. The baby will demonstrate pain when the site is touched.
2. If not in the immediate period after the injury, within a few days there may be a palpable lump on the bone at the site of the break.
3. Because of the break, the baby is likely to position the arm in an atypical posture.
4. Because of the injury to the bone, the baby is unable to respond with symmetrical arm movements.
5. It is very rare to see ecchymosis at the site of the break.

TEST-TAKING HINT: Clavicle breaks are a fairly common injury seen after a difficult delivery. They usually result from a disproportion between the sizes of the maternal pelvis and the fetal body. In some cases of shoulder dystocia, birth attendants may purposefully break a baby's clavicle to enable the baby to be born as rapidly as possible since shoulder dystocia is an obstetric emergency, threatening the life of the baby.

119. 1. Clubfoot is a defect that usually develops from the positioning of the baby in utero.
2. Brachial palsy can result from either a traumatic vertex or breech delivery.
3. Gastroschisis, when skin does not cover the abdominal wall and the abdominal contents are exposed, develops during fetal development and is often related to poor maternal folic acid ingestion during organogenesis.
4. Congenital hydrocele, an accumulation of fluid in the testes of the male, develops when a membrane fails to develop between the peritoneal cavity and scrotal sac.

TEST-TAKING HINT: When babies are born with unexpected findings, the nurse must be familiar not only with the implications of the anomalies but also with an understanding of the etiology of the anomalies. If the anomaly were a result of birth trauma, the nurse must be able to clearly and accurately communicate to the parents the source of the birth injury without communicating an opinion on any potential blame for the problem.

120. **1. In twin-to-twin transfusion, the smaller twin has "donated" part of his or her blood supply to the larger twin. As a result, the smaller twin may show pallor.**
2. The smaller twin is hypovolemic, so the likelihood of jaundice is small.
3. Opisthotonus is defined as a full-body spastic posture. This is unrelated to twin-to-twin transfusion.
4. Hydrocephalus is unrelated to twin-to-twin transfusion.

TEST-TAKING HINT: **Twin-to-twin transfusion may occur in monochorionic twins because they share the same placenta. The blood from one twin, therefore, may be "transfused" into the cardiovascular system of the second twin. The donor develops intrauterine growth restriction and becomes anemic as a result, because of decreased oxygenation and nourishment. Conversely, the recipient grows much larger and becomes hyperemic. The recipient twin may suffer from heart failure because of the circulatory system overload. The larger twin is the twin at highest risk for injury because of the potential for formation of thrombi and/or hyperbilirubinemia.**

121. 1. The recipient twin's appearance is not characterized by the development of a rash.
2. The recipient is likely to be larger than the donor twin.
3. The recipient, rather than the donor, will have an elevated hematocrit.
4. The recipient, rather than the donor, will be ruddy and plethoric.

TEST-TAKING HINT: **The word "plethoric" refers to a red coloration. Because the recipient twin receives a "transfusion" from the donor, the recipient's skin color becomes dark pink, especially when crying. The donor, on the other hand, is pale and small.**

122. 14.16%.

The formula for percentage of weight loss is: Original weight minus current weight divided by original weight. The value is then multiplied by 100 to convert the number into a percentage:

3,199 – 2,746 = 453

453/3,199 = 0.1416 × 100 = 14.16%

TEST-TAKING HINT: **Unless otherwise noted, the test taker should carry the math to the nearest hundredth place when performing calculations for infants and children. Because babies are very small, a fraction of a milligram (mg) or a kilogram (kg), can make a significant difference.**

123. 1. This statement is incorrect. It is recommended that marijuana not be consumed when breastfeeding and even though alcohol may be consumed, the mother should either breastfeed immediately before drinking, or wait at least 2 hours after drinking before breastfeeding.
2. This statement is incorrect. It is recommended that marijuana not be consumed when breastfeeding.
3. This statement is appropriate. Because the drug in marijuana does get into breast milk and can alter a baby's development, it is best not to use the drug while breastfeeding.
4. This statement is incorrect. There is too little information regarding marijuana use during breastfeeding.

TEST-TAKING HINT: **LactMed (National Institutes of Health, n.d.-a). is an excellent resource for healthcare professionals working with breastfeeding clients. Practitioners can input the names of any medications or other substances that women might consume while breastfeeding into the search engine, and recommendations regarding use are provided. As can be seen from the Web address, the site is maintained by the NIH and, therefore, is a reliable site for information. The site recommends that marijuana use be curtailed while breastfeeding. In addition, because alcohol does enter breast milk in approximately the same concentration as in the maternal bloodstream, it is highly recommended that a baby be breastfed before drinking, or at least 2 hours after consumption by which time the alcohol has been metabolized. (It is important to note that the time is multiplied by the number of drinks the mother consumes.)**

124. 1. The neonate should be monitored for signs and symptoms of hypocalcemia.
2. The neonate is not at high risk for hyperkalemia.
3. The neonate is not at high risk for hypochloremia.
4. The neonate is not at high risk for hypernatremia.

TEST-TAKING HINT: **Neonates of mothers who have received magnesium sulfate for more than 5 to 7 days are at high risk for hypocalcemia (Mechcatie, 2013). In addition, prematurity itself is a risk factor for hypocalcemia because of hypoparathyroid functioning. Symptoms of the syndrome are similar to those seen in babies with hypoglycemia, for example, hypotonia, jitters, and seizures .**

125. 1. The goal of administering IV magnesium sulfate to the mother is not to prevent hypoxemia in the neonate.
2. The goal of administering IV magnesium sulfate to the mother is to prevent cerebral palsy in the neonate.
3. The goal of administering IV magnesium sulfate to the mother is not to prevent cold stress syndrome in the neonate.

4. The goal of administering IV magnesium sulfate to the mother is not to prevent necrotizing enterocolitis in the neonate.

TEST-TAKING HINT: Preterm babies born to mothers who have received at least 48 hours of intravenous magnesium sulfate prior to the birth are at reduced risk of developing cerebral palsy (Chollat et al., 2018). Cerebral palsy is one of the most common sequalae to prematurity. Whether during pregnancy, labor and delivery, or postdelivery, premature babies are at risk of developing cerebral palsy secondary to cerebral hypoxemia. When the motor centers of the brain are deprived of oxygen, the chronic illness—cerebral palsy—can result. Other neurodevelopmental complications can also result.

126. Answers 1 and 2 are correct.

1. **Babies who have hyperbilirubinemia are usually very lethargic.**
2. **Babies who have hyperbilirubinemia are jaundiced.**
3. Babies who have hyperbilirubinemia usually feed poorly.
4. Because babies who have hyperbilirubinemia feed poorly, they stool less frequently. They do not exhibit diarrhea.
5. Babies who have hyperbilirubinemia do not exhibit excessive yawning. Babies who are withdrawing from narcotic addiction exhibit excessive yawning as well as other signs and symptoms of withdrawal.

TEST-TAKING HINT: Kernicterus is the syndrome that results when babies' brains are exposed to high levels of bilirubin over time. When the bilirubin level rises, the babies initially exhibit signs of lethargy and hypotonia, including difficulty in awaking for feeds and poor suck. When exposure is prolonged or when levels rise significantly, the symptoms of spasticity develop, including high-pitched cry and seizures. In addition, the marked exposure can lead to permanent damage to the brain, including developmental disabilities, learning disabilities, and sensory losses. When a neonate is jaundiced, the nurse should consult the Bhutani nomogram to determine the likelihood of the bilirubin rising (Stanford School of Medicine, n.d.).

127. Answers 1, 2, 3, and 5 are correct.

1. **Induced hypothermia is administered to prevent neurodevelopmental complications such as cerebral palsy.**
2. **Induced hypothermia is administered to prevent or reduce blindness.**
3. **Induced hypothermia is administered to prevent or reduce deafness.**
4. Induced hypothermia is not administered to prevent psychiatric illnesses like bipolar disease.
5. **Induced hypothermia is administered to prevent or reduce limited intellectual disability.**

TEST-TAKING HINT: Induced hypothermia is an intervention that, as the name implies, entails dropping the neonate's temperature well below normal. It is currently the standard of care for babies at risk who are at least 36 weeks' gestational age (Peliowski-Davidovich & Canadian Paediatric Society, Fetus and Newborn Committee, 2012). The intervention is conducted to minimize the damage to the brain resulting from marked hypoxia at birth, resulting in the delivery of an asphyxic newborn. Neonatal brain damage is caused by ischemia or bleeding in the brain that initiates neurotoxic processes in the brain cells. For more information on induced hypothermia, including how it works, see the appendix.

128.

1. Elevated blood pressures in the upper extremities are a characteristic sign of coarctation of the aorta, a cardiac anomaly.
2. **Marked systemic cyanosis is a sign of persistent pulmonary hypertension of the newborn (PPHN), a complication seen in babies exposed to selective serotonin reuptake inhibitors (SSRIs), especially during the third trimester.**
3. Pronounced mucus production immediately after birth is a characteristic of esophageal atresia.
4. Flaccid tone of all musculature is noted in babies who are markedly hypoxic in utero but is not related to SSRIs.

TEST-TAKING HINT: PPHN is a serious complication seen in babies exposed to SSRIs during pregnancy. The problem arises when the neonate's circulation fails to convert from an intrauterine blood flow to an extrauterine blood flow. The blood flow remains a right-to-left shift (see the appendix for more information on right-to-left shift). Echocardiography is the most common diagnostic test performed when PPHN is suspected (Brown University Psychopathology Update, 2013; Huybrechts et al., 2015).

129.

1. **The nurse should provide the baby with a sucrose-covered pacifier, frequently called "sucrose soothies," to suck on.**

2. Unless the mother prefers to be absent, there is no need for her to leave the room while the procedure is being performed. Some mothers prefer to breastfeed their babies during painful procedures, instead of providing the baby with a sucrose soothie.
3. There is nothing in the stem to indicate that the baby requires oxygen.
4. There is no need to remove the eye patches while the procedure is being performed.

TEST-TAKING HINT: Venipuncture is a painful procedure. There is research to show that oral sucrose given to babies during a number of painful procedures, including venipuncture, decreases their pain responses (Stevens et al., 2016). Alternatively, if the mother prefers, she may breastfeed during the procedure to provide comfort to the baby.

130. The term in column 1 is matched to the description in column 2.
1. Continuous positive airway pressure (CPAP) matches with **B. Keeps alveoli open during exhalation.**
2. Noninvasive positive airway pressure (NIPP) matches with **A. Augments babies' spontaneous breaths.**
3. Extracorporeal membrane oxygenation (ECMO) matches with **D. Form of cardiopulmonary bypass.**
4. Mechanical ventilation matches with **C. Requires endotracheal tube insertion.**

TEST-TAKING HINT: The many forms of neonatal ventilatory support are used at distinctly different times. Initially, when a baby is having respiratory difficulty, oxygen is administered to the baby via face mask, oxyhood, or nasal canulla. When that is insufficient and additional support is needed, NIPP or CPAP is the next step. NIPP is used primarily when a baby has apnea spells since it supplements the baby's own respiratory efforts. CPAP is often needed by preterm babies because of the work required for breathing without adequate endogenous pulmonary surfactant. The positive airway pressure prevents the alveoli from collapsing during each exhalation. Mechanical ventilation and ECMO are employed when more sophisticated methods for oxygenation are needed.

131. Answers 1, 2, 3, and 4 are correct.
1. **Catheter-related bloodstream infection is the most common complication associated with PICCs.**
2. **Tip migration is a common complication. The catheter, either spontaneously or as a result of external manipulation, can move in the body either farther inward or outward.**
3. **Myocardial perforation can occur at any time. It most commonly occurs 3 days after the PICC was inserted.**
4. **Although relatively rare, paralysis of the diaphragm can occur when the PICC is inserted into the subclavian vein.**
5. Neurological complications related to scalp vein insertions are virtually nonexistent. PICCs inserted via a leg or femoral vein can lead to neurological complications.

TEST-TAKING HINT: PICCs are frequently employed in the NICU for the administration of fluids and medications. Although an essential procedure, PICC insertions and their maintenance require highly technical nursing care actions and vigilance. Even when a PICC has been inserted with care and precision, there are many complications that can occur. The nurse must be meticulous in his or her care in order to identify as well as to prevent the complications (Pettit & Wykoff, 2007).

132. Answers 1 and 3 are correct.
1. **Male sex is a risk factor for mortality in most countries (Pongou, 2013).**
2. Hypothermia is a symptom, not a risk factor.
3. Tachypnea is a symptom, not a risk factor.
4. **Small for gestational age (SGA) is a risk factor for several conditions including hypothermia, hypoglycemia, and poor feeding.**
5. Mottled skin is a symptom, not a risk factor

TEST-TAKING HINT: This question requires the nurse to start with a wide view of risk factors for this newborn before narrowing the focus to specific symptoms that require interventions. It is an example of some of the NGN questions that require the nurse to make a distinction between *symptoms* and *risk factors*. Other questions may ask the test taker to distinguish between nursing *interventions* such as temperature taking, and nursing *actions* such as administering a medication. Merriam-Webster defines a *risk factor* as "something that increases . . . *susceptibility*," and a *symptom* as "subjective *evidence* of disease or physical disturbance" (italics supplied by author).

In planning care for a newborn, a nurse must include prenatal factors, including preterm birth and birth weights that determine babies who are small for gestational age (SGA), who have intrauterine growth restriction (IUGR), and those that are large for gestational age (LGA), in guiding assessments postnatally. These factors serve as indicators for ongoing monitoring of the

newborn, even before an official medical diagnosis is determined. In this way, nurses can optimize the neonate's extrauterine life and limit or prevent morbidities such as hypoglycemia, hypothermia, respiratory distress syndrome, and sepsis.

133. Answers 2, 3, 4, and 6 are correct.

1. Being small for gestational age is a risk factor, not a symptom.
2. **A low temperature is a symptom (a finding) that can lead to a diagnosis and intervention. A concern related to hypothermia is that oxygen release to tissues is reduced with hypothermia (Zanelli et al., 2011).**
3. **Tachypnea, chest retractions, and grunting respirations are findings of immediate concern, as they indicate a problem with oxygenation.**
4. **Lethargy is a symptom of concern, as it is not a normal reaction to a heel stick.**
5. The prior CBG of 36 mg/dL (1.9 mmol/L) is trending down very slightly, and could be transitional hypoglycemia. There is nothing in the question to indicate the baby has symptomatic hypoglycemia such as tremors. Diagnosis and treatment should be focused on the most current assessments, not the CBG from 2 hours ago.
6. **Mottled skin is not normal for a newborn at 39 weeks' gestation and could indicate illness. If the baby is ill, the most likely organism is GBS, even though the client's water was broken for only 11 hours. The baby's mother would not have been given antibiotics in labor, since the CDC guidelines indicate that in the context of unknown GBS, antibiotics should be given in labor if the water is broken for 18 hours or more before birth.**

TEST-TAKING HINT: **In recognizing the most important findings, the nurse begins to narrow down where the interventions should start. The most life-threatening conditions must be treated first. This baby is showing signs of illness as evidenced by a low temperature and respiratory issues, which must be addressed first, in addition to the objective symptoms of lethargy, and mottled skin. As to the previous CBG reading of 36 mg/dL (1.9 mmol/L), the American Academy of Pediatrics recommends that babies with *symptomatic* hypoglycemia and a CBG of less than 40 mg/dL (2.2 mmol/L) who are late preterm and/or term with SGA, those who are LGA, and those with mothers on insulin should have a continuous intravenous glucose infusion (AAP, 2011). This baby is not showing symptoms of hypoglycemia, such as tremors, indicating the low blood sugar could be transitional and normal. Because the symptoms of neonatal hypoglycemia are nonspecific and overlap with symptoms of other conditions (Abramowski et al., 2020), it is difficult at this point to determine whether this baby's symptoms of lethargy, grunting respirations, and hypothermia are related to SGA, transitional hypoglycemia, or infection. The question indicates the nurse has just collected a third specimen for a current CBG. Those findings could help in determining the seriousness of the low blood sugar.**

134. Answers 1(a and b), 2(b and c), 3(b and c), 4(b), and 5(a and b) are correct.

Client Findings	(a) Small for gestational age (SGA)	(b) Early onset neonatal sepsis (EOS)	(c) Transient tachypnea
1. Hypothermia	X	X	
2. Respiratory issues		X	X
3. Breastfeeding issues		X	X
4. Mottled skin tone		X	
5. Glucose instability	X	X	

1(a and b). Low temperature is commonly seen with SGA and with illness. For SGA infants, limited fat stores, reduced brown fat, thin dermis, and increased surface area to body mass ratio put them at risk of hypothermia. With an illness such as GBS, a newborn may exhibit either high or low temperature in response to the infection.

2(b and c). Respiratory issues can occur with illness. Transient tachypnea is a self-limited condition that generally resolves within 6 hours after birth. It occurs as the result of a delay in clearing fluid from the lungs immediately after birth (Jha et al., 2020). An SGA baby generally has no respiratory issues, in spite of its size.

3(b and c). Poor breastfeeding can occur with illness, due to lethargy. If the baby has transient tachypnea, poor breastfeeding can occur due to difficulties in breathing. An SGA baby may breastfeed very well in spite of its size.

4(b). A baby with an infection may have mottled, pink, or cyanotic skin due to vascular constriction related to the infection. Babies with transient tachypnea may be cyanotic, but their skin is not generally mottled. A baby with SGA has no skin discoloration.

5(a and b). An SGA baby may have hypoglycemia due to lower glycogen stores and increased metabolic demands related to hypothermia. A baby with an illness may be hypoglycemic due to increased metabolic demands of the infection.

TEST-TAKING HINT: This question requires the nurse to recognize the symptom similarities and differences between babies with these three conditions. This is the first step in sorting through the cues to determine a priority hypothesis. The nurse is not diagnosing the baby's condition, just recognizing patterns that often go with a diagnosis. This differentiation is vital in determining the appropriate nursing interventions in order to collect and organize data points in preparation for communicating with the primary healthcare provider. It is obvious in this question that symptoms are often vague and overlap more than one possible diagnosis. However, sometimes one condition begins to stand out as the most likely cause of the baby's nonspecific collage of symptoms.

The test taker should take each condition separately (SGA, early onset neonatal sepsis, and transient tachypnea) and determine each symptom as a true/false question. If it's "true," an X is placed in the box (or in the test, the symptom is dragged into the box).

Sources are as follows: Late preterm standards (Baker, 2015); SGA (McGuire, 2017; Polin et al., 2014); Early onset neonatal sepsis (Boettiger et al., 2017); transient tachypnea (Jha et al., 2020).

135. Answers 1 and b are correct.

1. **The baby is at highest risk for developing septic shock as a result of early onset (neonatal) sepsis (EOS) infection (within 0 to 6 days of age) with group B streptococcus (GBS) bacteria. EOS can occur with or without risk factors such as maternal testing positive for GBS, ruptured membranes for at least 18 hours, maternal fever, fetal tachycardia. The only risk factor in this case study is no prenatal care leading to unknown maternal GBS status. Almost half of all culture-confirmed early onset disease among term infants is GBS (Puopolo et al., 2019). Generalized, mottled skin tone is highly suggestive of an infectious process.**
2. The baby is not at risk of necrotizing enterocolitis (NEC). Risk factors include premature birth and formula feeding. The baby in this case study is not premature and has not had formula.
3. Although SGA babies may have polycythemia and a higher risk of hyperbilirubinemia, or jaundice as a result, there is nothing in the question to suggest this baby is currently developing jaundice.

a. The baby's mottled skin tone is of concern, but skin tone is a *symptom*, not a *contributor* to septic shock.

b. **The baby's temperature is low and the heart rate is 165 bpm. Respiratory rate is 68. Septic shock should be diagnosed by clinical signs that include tachycardia, tachypnea, hypothermia, and lethargy (Davis et al., 2017). A heart rate of less than 90 bpm or greater than 160 bpm is considered a "threshold" for an increased risk of mortality in neonates, whether critically ill or septic (Davis et al., 2017, p. 1067).**

c. The baby's feeding pattern does not suggest any of the listed risks. In fact, the recommendation is that babies who are ill should be NPO (Davis et al., 2017).

TEST-TAKING HINT: "Septic shock should be suspected in any newborn with tachycardia, respiratory distress, poor feeding, poor tone, poor color, tachypnea, diarrhea, or reduced perfusion" (Davis et al., 2017, p. 1080).

136. The correct answers are 1(a), 2(a), 3(a), 4(b), 5(a), 6(c), 7(a), 8(a), 9(c), 10(a).

Potential Intervention	(a) Essential	(b) Nonessential	(c) Contraindicated
1. Notify provider.	X		
2. Request an order for oxygen supplementation.	X		
3. Assess capillary refill time.	X		
4. Initiate contact precautions.		X	
5. Place baby under overbed warmer with skin probe.	X		
6. Feed baby expressed colostrum.			X
7. Weigh all diapers.	X		
8. Monitor pulse oximetry on baby's foot.	X		
9. Keep hat on baby's head to conserve warmth while in warmer.			X
10. Request an order to establish intravenous access.	X		

1(a). The newborn's condition has changed since birth and the nurse needs specific orders for the change in condition. The provider must be notified immediately. This baby's condition is becoming serious. Early onset septicemia can become fulminant very quickly and lead to infant mortality, so every second counts and antibiotics should be started as soon as possible.

2(a). Based on the baby's respiratory assessments, he will need oxygen supplementation and possibly intubation with mechanical ventilation.

3(a). The goal of treatment for shock is to maintain organ perfusion. A capillary refill of greater than 2 minutes suggests neonatal hypotension (Davis et al., 2017, p. 1080) with associated reduction in organ perfusion. Every hour with hypotension and a capillary refill of less than 3 seconds increases the baby's risk of mortality (Davis et al., 2017).

4(b). Standard precautions should be followed as for every baby in the nursery. Additional contact precautions are not necessary with GBS.

5(a). To lessen the metabolic work of keeping himself warm, this baby should be placed in a bed with an overbed warmer with a skin probe in place. If he is not intubated, he should be on his back. A Cochrane Review found that babies *who are intubated and are on continuous monitoring* benefit by increased oxygen saturation when placed in the prone position for 5 to 48 hours at a time (Gillies et al., 2012).

6(c). Babies who are ill should be kept NPO (Davis et al., 2017).

7(a). Intake and output is essential to maintaining fluid balance. Intake and output also gives insight into organ perfusion, as it reflects kidney function.

8(a). Oxygen saturation is an important assessment, as it guides the decision for intubation and mechanical ventilation. A 95% oxygen saturation or higher is the target (Davis et al., 2017).

9(c). Once under the warmer, the baby should not be covered. Dressing or covering the baby prevents the overbed warmth to reach the baby's skin.

10(a). Once airway and breathing issues have been addressed, the providers' attention moves to circulation. Intravenous access must be readily established before blood and other bodily fluid samples are collected.

TEST-TAKING HINT: Unlike the CABs (circulation, airway, breathing) for adults, all neonatal emergencies begin with the ABCs of airway, breathing, and circulation (Balest, 2021; Wyckoff et al., 2015; Wynn & Wong, 2010). If the hospital does not have a protocol for respiratory distress that includes oxygen administration, a provider's order is required. "Supplemental or high-flow nasal cannula oxygen is the first choice for respiratory support. The decision to intubate and ventilate is based on clinical diagnosis of increased work of breathing or inadequate respiratory effort, or marked hypoxemia" (Davis et al., 2017, p. 1082).

137. Answers 2, 4, and 6 are correct

1. A repeat capillary blood glucose is important, and the development of jitteriness suggests the blood sugar is much lower than before, but stabilizing the baby comes first.
2. **Establishing intravenous access is part of stabilizing both the hypoglycemia and the circulatory system. It should be done as soon as possible. Once the IV line is established, the baby can receive intravenous fluids with glucose if necessary.**
3. A chest x-ray is a study that is important, but only after the baby is stabilized.
4. **Cultures must be drawn before antibiotics can be administered, and antibiotics should be administered as soon as possible. On the list of given interventions here, drawing body fluids for directed studies is one of the three orders that should be performed first. It would be done third, after the oxygen was administered and after the intravenous access was established.**
5. IV antibiotics are important to help the baby fight this infection before it overwhelms and leads to organ dysfunction, but this is not one of the first 3 orders that should be completed first. Because this baby is SGA, his immune system may not be as robust as a baby who is of average size. Group B streptococcus (GBS) is a leading pathogen in babies during the first week of life (Borghesi et al., 2017). Until GBS bacteria are demonstrated in blood or cerebrospinal fluid, empiric treatment with broad spectrum antibiotics is recommended, but is not started until after blood and/or cerebrospinal fluid is drawn for cultures (Benitz et al., 2015).
6. **Oxygen delivery by nasal prongs is a first step in treatment (Davis et al., 2017). If the baby cannot maintain a satisfactory oxygen saturation, mechanical ventilation will be necessary. (See the test-taking hints for the previous question for more information.)**

TEST-TAKING HINT: All of these orders are important to complete. The steps in neonatal resuscitation are to first recognize that the infant is in trouble. The second step is stabilization, such as establishing IV access, and providing oxygen supplementation or intubation. Once that is accomplished, directed testing, such as drawing blood and cerebrospinal fluid, chest x-rays, and other studies are done (Chapman, 2016).

138. The following answers are correct: 1(c), 2(b), 3(c), 4(b), 5(a), 6(a), 7(a)

Assessment Finding	(a) Improved	(b) No change	(c) Condition declined
1. CBG 34 mg/dL (1.8 mmol/L)			X
2. Skin tone mottled		X	
3. Capillary refill > 3 seconds			X
4. Oxygen saturation 93%		X	
5. Temperature 98° F (36.6° C)	X		
6. Heart rate 160	X		
7. Respiratory rate 65	X		

1(a). The baby's blood glucose continues to drop. With this steady decline, it is not likely transitional hypoglycemia. It is no doubt related to sepsis, and the provider will likely order a continuous intravenous glucose drip.

2(b). The baby's mottled skin, a sign of sepsis, continues, which is expected, since the antibiotics have not had enough time to make an improvement.

3(c). The capillary refill time is longer, which can indicate further progression of hypotension. The baby will likely need medication to maintain adequate blood pressures.

4(b). At 93%, the oxygen saturation is unchanged, but is still below the target of 95%. In correlation with the continued mottled skin tone and the respiratory rate above normal, the baby will likely need mechanical ventilation.

5(a). The baby's temperature has risen, most likely as a result of the overbed warmer.

6(a). The baby's heart rate has come down by 5 beats per minute, putting it at the threshold of higher mortality risk, and indicating the degree of illness.

7(a). The respiratory rate of 65 is improved, but is still higher than normal and is above the threshold of higher mortality risk.

TEST-TAKING HINT: The test taker's answers to these assessments demonstrates clinical judgments and decision making, a vital skill in guiding next steps. The nurse must always consider whether or not the client's condition is stable. If the client's condition has improved, additional clinical judgments must be made about whether or not these improvements are being made in the appropriate timeframes. Conversely, if the client's condition has worsened, the nurse must determine if the interventions have contributed to the client's worsening condition or not. A return to clinical judgments with additional hypotheses and decision making may be necessary.

11 High-Risk Postpartum

As with the antepartum and intrapartum periods, there are several complications that can occur during the postpartum period. The questions in this chapter will enable nurses to determine their preparedness in caring for complicated postpartum clients. The nurse will note that the most common complications in the postpartum phase are related to excess blood loss, hypertensive illnesses, and infection. The nurse must be familiar with the precipitating factors that place a client at risk for these complications as well as the signs and symptoms of the problems and how to intervene effectively in each of the situations. Additional problems that the nurse may encounter are related to psychological responses of new mothers, breastfeeding problems, surgical complications, complications associated with chronic illnesses, and blood sugar changes before and during pregnancy.

KEYWORDS

The following words include English vocabulary, nursing/medical terminology, concepts, principles, or information relevant to content specifically addressed in the chapter or associated with topics presented in it. English dictionaries, your nursing textbooks, and medical dictionaries such as *Taber's Cyclopedic Medical Dictionary* are resources that can be used to expand your knowledge and understanding of these words and related information.

Antidepressants (selective serotonin reuptake inhibitors [SSRIs] such as sertraline and aroxetine)
Blocked milk duct
Blood transfusion
Breast abscess
Breast enlargement
Breast reduction
Carboprost
Cesarean section
Child abuse
Child neglect
Congenital defect
Coombs test
Cracked nipples
Deep vein thrombosis (DVT)
Dehiscence
Diphenhydramine
Eclampsia
Engorgement
Epidural anesthesia
Fetal demise
Forceps delivery
General anesthesia
Gestational diabetes mellitus (GDM)
Grief and mourning
Hematoma
Heparin HIV
Hydralazine
Infanticide
Lanolin breast cream
Macrosomia
Magnesium sulfate
Mastitis
Methylergonovine
Metoclopromide
Morphine sulfate
Ondansetron
Paralytic ileus
Patient-controlled analgesia (PCA)
Promethazine
Placental anomalies (accreta, battledore, circumvallate, succenturiate, velamentous cord insertion)
Postpartum blues
Postpartum depression
Postpartum hemorrhage
Postpartum psychosis
Pre-eclampsia
Premature rupture of the membranes

Prochlorperazine
Puerperal infection
Puerperium
Rh immune globulin (RhIG)
Rubella vaccine
Secobarbital
Self–breast milk expression
Spinal anesthesia
Substance abuse
Titration
Type 1 diabetes mellitus (T1DM)
Type 2 diabetes mellitus (T2DM)
Uterine atony
Warfarin

QUESTIONS

CASE STUDY: *The first three questions utilize an Next Generation NCLEX© (NGN) test question format referred to as the "Bowtie." In the electronic NCLEX examination, test takers will drag and drop their answers into the appropriate boxes (National Council of State Boards of Nursing [NCSBN], 2021).*

NCLEX questions assume the nurse has a provider's order for listed interventions, unless noted otherwise.

A client with an obstetrical history of G1 P1001 and a diagnosis of pre-eclampsia with severe features delivered vaginally 3 hours ago. She had an epidural in labor. The baby weighed 7 lbs 9 ounces (3,430 grams). The labor nurse reports the client is on antibiotics for an intrapartum fever of 103° F (39.4° C) in labor and suspected chorioamnionitis. Acetaminophen 500 mg was given after the delivery. Her total quantitative blood loss after the delivery was 450 mL. Her fundus was firm just before transfer. She has been transferred to the postpartum unit with the baby. She was catheterized for 350 mL 1 hour ago following 3 hours of immediate postpartum care on the labor and delivery unit.

A magnesium sulfate solution is infusing by pump at 2 grams/hour in her right arm. In her left arm, a primary infusion of lactated ringer's is running with a piggyback of 20 units of oxytocin in 1,000 mL lactated ringer's infusing by pump at 125 mL/hour. The postpartum nurse is documenting the client's initial assessments following the handover: T 101° F (38.3° C), BP 140/90, P 100 bpm, RR 20 breaths per minute. Heavy flow, boggy fundus, 1 fingerbreadth above umbilicus, massaged to firm. Pad changed, dark clots, weight 100 mL (100 grams).

1. Select a complication for which the client is at increased risk.

Note: In the NCLEX examination the test taker will drag the selected complication to the center of the "bowtie" graph below.

1. Eclamptic seizure.
2. Postpartum hemorrhage.
3. Magnesium sulfate toxicity.

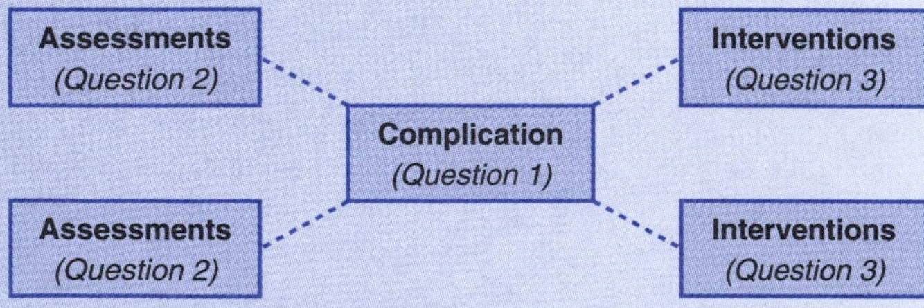

2. Which of the following assessments are important for the nurse to monitor to identify the identified complication? **Select two.**
   1. Fundal tone.
   2. Quantitative blood loss (QBL).
   3. Vital signs.
   4. Urinary output.

3. **Specify two interventions** the nurse should perform as a way to reduce the risks of the identified complication.
   1. Order magnesium sulfate level.
   2. Encourage breastfeeding.
   3. Pad the bedrails.
   4. Encourage voiding.

CASE STUDY: *The next six questions below are part of an evolving case study. All six questions follow the Next Generation NCLEX© question format of six steps:*

1. Recognize cues—What matters most? What are the red flags I see?
2. Analyze cues—What could it mean?
3. Prioritize hypotheses—Where do I start?
4. Generate solutions—What can I do?
5. Take action—What will I do?
6. Evaluate outcomes—Did it help?

(National Council of State Boards of Nursing [NCSBN], 2020). For more information on the Next Generation NCLEX (NGN) question formats, see NGN quarterly newsletters at https://www.ncsbn.org.

A client with an obstetrical history of G3 P1203 and a diagnosis of pre-eclampsia with severe features was delivered 3 hours ago by cesarean section at 36 weeks' gestation. General anesthesia was used, due to the client's diagnosis of scoliosis. The baby weighed 4 lbs 10 ounces (2,097 grams). The baby is in the NICU for observation.

The client has just been transferred from the PACU to the postpartum unit after 2 hours in recovery. The labor nurse reports that throughout the recovery period, the client's temp was 100° F (37.7° C), pulse 72 bpm, respirations 14 per minute, BP 110/70. In addition, the client has developed a moist cough. The client has been on magnesium sulfate for 48 hours for seizure prophylaxis and preterm labor, and the medication is currently infusing at 2 gm/hr by pump. She has a patient-controlled analgesia (PCA) pump for pain but has not used it yet because the labor nurse administered 4 mg IV morphine, just 30 minutes prior to the transfer.

Total quantitative blood loss after the delivery was 850 mL (850 gm by weight) with an additional 200 mL (200 gm) in the PACU. Her fundus has remained firm throughout the recovery stage. The client has an indwelling catheter in place. The labor nurse reported emptying 80 mL of clear urine from the catheter bag just before transfer to postpartum. As the client is transferred to the postpartum bed, she appears flaccid, and moans softly.

4. **Recognize cues. What matters most?** What are the red flags? Identify the four top findings that would require follow-up. **Select four.**
   1. Vital signs.
   2. Urinary output.
   3. Reflexes and clonus.
   4. Breath sounds.
   5. Surgical dressing.
   6. Uterine tone.

5. **Analyze cues. What could it mean?**
   The nurse has completed her assessments, including DTRs of 2+ and 1 beat of clonus. For each client finding, indicate with an X if the finding is consistent with impaired renal function, pain medication, magnesium sulfate side effects, or pulmonary edema. Each finding may support more than one condition. **Each column must have at least one response option.**

Client findings	(a) Consistent with impaired renal function	(b) Consistent with pain medication	(c) Consistent with magnesium sulfate	(d) Consistent with pulmonary edema
1. Respiratory rate				
2. Blood pressure				
3. Urinary output				
4. Muscle flaccidity				
5. Sleepiness				
6. Moist cough				

6. **Prioritize hypotheses. Where do I start?**
   Which of the following is likely happening or is at risk to happen, based on the findings above? **Select 1 from each column.**

At risk to happen (Select one, below)	As evidenced by . . . (Select one, below)
1. Hypoxia	a. Respiratory assessment
2. Eclamptic seizure	b. Urinary output assessment
3. Magnesium sulfate toxicity	c. Neurologic assessment
4. Pulmonary embolism	d. Vital signs

7. Generate solutions. What can I do?
An hour later the client's husband runs to the nurses' desk and says urgently, "My wife doesn't look right." When the nurse enters the room, the client is pale and diaphoretic, and difficult to awaken. Respiratory rate is 10, pulse 80, BP 110/70. The nurse calls for help and requests immediate provider notification.

For each potential nursing intervention, select the appropriate box to specify whether the intervention is essential, nonessential, or contraindicated for the care of this client. Interventions are not given in the order in which they should be performed. **Each column must have a response.**

Potential intervention	(a) Essential	(b) Nonessential	(c) Contraindicated
1. Turn off magnesium sulfate			
2. Check lochial flow			
3. Check client's pupils			
4. Assess DTRs and clonus			
5. Administer naloxone			
6. Tally 24-hour intake and output			

8. Take action. What will I do?
The pulse oximeter indicates an oxygen saturation of 93%. The provider is at the bedside examining the client, and finding absent DTRs and no clonus. Breath sounds are clear, and urinary output has been 20 mL in the past hour. The provider gives the nurse verbal orders. **Select 3 that the nurse should perform right away.**
1. Deep tendon reflexes and clonus checks hourly until stable.
2. Administer oxygen at 10 L/min per nonrebreather mask.
3. Draw blood sample for magnesium sulfate level.
4. Administer antidote of calcium gluconate 1 g IV over 3 minutes.
5. IV fluid bolus of 300 mL lactated ringer's solution.

9. Evaluate outcomes. Did it help?
The nurse completed all of the provider's orders as listed above, 1 hour ago. The magnesium sulfate level was 9 mg/dL. The 24-hour output was greater than intake, so the client received a 300 mL fluid bolus. The nurse is now reassessing the client. For each assessment finding below, select the appropriate box to specify if the finding indicates that the nurse's interventions of oxygen administration, calcium gluconate administration, and IV fluid bolus were effective, ineffective, or unrelated to the current findings. **Each column must have at least one selection.**

Assessment finding	(a) Effective	(b) Ineffective	(c) Unrelated
1. Temp 101.2° F (38.4° C)			
2. Respirations 18 per minute, BP 120/82			
3. Urine output 20 mL			
4. DTRs 2+, 1 beat clonus			
5. Asking to see baby			
6. Pulse oximetry 95%			

10. A client with gestational diabetes who delivered yesterday is currently on the postpartum unit. Which of the following statements is appropriate for the nurse to make at this time?
1. "Monitor your blood glucose 5 times a day until your 6-week checkup."
2. "I will teach you how to inject insulin before you are discharged."
3. "Daily exercise can help to prevent diabetes in the future."
4. "Your baby should be assessed every 6 months for signs of juvenile diabetes."

11. A client is receiving a blood transfusion after the delivery of her baby. The delivery was complicated by a placenta accreta and hysterectomy. Which of the following complaints by the client would warrant immediately discontinuing the infusion?
1. "One side of my back hurts all of a sudden."
2. "My hands feel so cold."
3. "I feel like my heart is beating fast."
4. "I feel like I need to have a bowel movement."

12. A client has just received carboprost because of uterine atony not controlled by IV oxytocin. For which of the following side effects of the medication will the nurse monitor this client? **Select all that apply.**
1. Hyperthermia.
2. Diarrhea.
3. Hypotension.
4. Palpitations.
5. Anasarca.

13. A client who is 2 weeks postpartum calls her obstetrician's nurse and states that she has had very little bleeding for 1 week but that today she is "bleeding and saturating a pad about every ½ hour." Which of the following is an appropriate response by the nurse?
1. "That is normal. You are starting to menstruate again."
2. "You should stay on complete bedrest until the bleeding subsides."
3. "Pushing during a bowel movement may have loosened your stitches."
4. "The physician should see you. Please go to the emergency department."

14. The nurse is performing a postpartum assessment on a client who delivered 4 hours ago. The nurse notes a firm uterus at the umbilicus with heavy lochial flow. Which of the following nursing actions is appropriate?
1. Massage the uterus.
2. Notify the obstetrician.
3. Administer an oxytocic as ordered.
4. Assist the client to the bathroom.

15. For the past 12 hours, a client has been receiving magnesium sulfate for pre-eclampsia with severe features. Her reflexes are absent and her respiratory rate is 10. Which of the following situations could be a precipitating factor in these findings?
1. Apical heart rate 104 bpm.
2. Urinary output 240 mL/12 hr.
3. Blood pressure 160/120.
4. Temperature 100° F. (37.3° C)

16. A client received general anesthesia during her cesarean section 4 hours ago. Which of the following postpartum nursing interventions is important for the nurse to make?
1. Place the client flat in bed.
2. Assess for dependent edema.
3. Auscultate lung fields.
4. Check patellar reflexes.

17. The nurse is developing a standard care plan for the post–cesarean section client. Which of the following should the nurse plan to implement?
   1. Maintain the client in left lateral recumbent position.
   2. Teach sitz bath use on second postoperative day.
   3. Perform active range-of-motion exercises until ambulating.
   4. Assess central venous pressure during first postoperative day.

18. A post–cesarean section client in the post-anesthesia recovery room received IV morphine sulfate 30 minutes ago. The nurse has administered diphenhydramine to the client who experienced itching. Which of the following actions should the nurse perform following administration of the drug?
   1. Monitor the urinary output hourly.
   2. Supervise while the woman holds her newborn.
   3. Position the woman slightly elevated on her left side.
   4. Ask any visitors to leave the room.

19. The nurse should suspect puerperal infection when a client exhibits which of the following?
   1. Temperature of 100.2° F (37.8° C).
   2. White blood cell count of 14,500 cells/mm^3.
   3. Diaphoresis during the night.
   4. Malodorous lochial discharge.

20. A breastfeeding client who is rubella nonimmune, has just received the rubella vaccine. Which of the following side effects should the nurse warn the client about?
   1. The baby may develop a rash a week after the shot.
   2. The baby may temporarily reject the breast milk.
   3. The mother's milk supply may decrease precipitously.
   4. The mother's joints may become painful and stiff.

21. In the lactation clinic, a nurse is caring for a client who delivered 3 weeks ago and has recently started treatment for postpartum depression. This is the client's third child. The nurse should expect to observe which behavior?
   1. Feelings of infanticide.
   2. Difficulty with breastfeeding latch.
   3. Feelings of failure as a mother.
   4. Concerns about sibling jealousy.

22. Which symptom would the nurse expect to observe in a postpartum client with a vaginal hematoma?
   1. Pain.
   2. Bleeding.
   3. Warmth.
   4. Redness.

23. A breastfeeding woman calls the pediatric nurse with the following complaint: "I woke up this morning with a terrible cold. I don't want my baby to get sick. Which kind of formula should I have my husband feed the baby until I get better?" Which of the following replies by the nurse is appropriate at this time?
   1. "Any formula brand is satisfactory, but it is essential that it be mixed with water that has been boiled for at least 5 minutes."
   2. "Don't forget to pump your breasts every 3 hours while the baby is being fed the prescribed formula."
   3. "The best way to keep your baby from getting sick is for you to keep breastfeeding him rather than switching him to formula."
   4. "In addition to giving the baby formula, you should wear a surgical face mask when you are around him."

24. A woman who wishes to breastfeed advises the nurse that she had a breast reduction one year earlier. Which of the following responses by the nurse is appropriate?
1. Advise the woman that unfortunately she will be unable to breastfeed.
2. Examine the woman's breasts to see where the incision was placed.
3. Monitor the baby's daily weights for excessive weight loss.
4. Inform the woman that reduction surgery rarely affects milk transfer.

25. The nurse is caring for a postoperative cesarean section client. The woman is obese and has insulin-dependent diabetes. For which of the following complications should the nurse carefully monitor this client?
1. Failed lactogenesis.
2. Dysfunctional parenting.
3. Wound dehiscence.
4. Projectile vomiting.

26. A nurse who is called to a client's room notes that the client's cesarean section incision has separated. The client points to loops of bowel at the opening. Which of the following actions is the highest priority for the nurse to perform?
1. Cover the wound with sterile wet dressings.
2. Notify the surgeon.
3. Elevate the head of the client's bed slightly.
4. Flex the client's knees.

27. The nurse notes the following vital signs of a postoperative cesarean section client during the immediate postpartum period: 100° F (37.7° C), P 68, R 12, BP 130/80. Which of the following is a correct interpretation of the findings?
1. Temperature is elevated, a sign of infection.
2. Pulse is too low, a sign of vagal pathology.
3. Respirations are too low, a side effect of medication.
4. Blood pressure is elevated, a sign of pre-eclampsia.

28. The nurse is discharging five Rh-negative clients from the maternity unit. The nurse knows that the teaching was successful when the clients who had which of the following deliveries state that they understand why they must receive a Rh immune globulin (RhIG) injection? **Select all that apply.**
1. Abortion at 10 weeks' gestation.
2. Amniocentesis at 16 weeks' gestation.
3. Fetal demise at 24 weeks' gestation.
4. Birth of Rh-negative twins at 35 weeks' gestation.
5. Delivery of a 40-week-gestation, Rh-positive baby.

29. In which of the following situations should a nurse report a possible deep vein thrombosis (DVT)?
1. The woman complains of numbness in the toes and heel of one foot.
2. The woman has cramping pain in a calf that is relieved when the foot is dorsiflexed.
3. The calf of one of the woman's legs is swollen, red, and warm to the touch.
4. The veins in the ankle of one of the woman's legs are spider-like and purple.

30. A woman at 26 weeks' gestation, has just delivered a stillborn baby after a fetal demise. Which of the following nursing actions is appropriate at this time?
1. Remind the mother that she will be able to have another baby in the future.
2. Dress the baby in a tee shirt and swaddle the baby in a receiving blanket.
3. Ask the woman if she would like the doctor to prescribe a sedative for her.
4. Remove the baby from the delivery room as quickly as possible.

31. A client with an obstetrical history of G1 P1001 has given birth to a baby boy after a normal, spontaneous, vaginal delivery. The baby had Apgar scores of 5 and 6. Because the client exhibited tremors and restlessness on admission, a urine toxicology assessment was performed with the client's permission. The results were positive for alcohol and cocaine. Which of the following interventions is appropriate for the nurse to perform for this postpartum client? **Select all that apply.**
   1. Support the client in breastfeeding her baby.
   2. Reprimand the mother for causing her baby to become addicted.
   3. Suggest that the nursery nurse feed the baby in the nursery.
   4. Provide the client with supervised instruction on baby-care skills.
   5. Recommend that the mother feed the baby formula.

32. A client delivered a 9 lb 9 oz (4,500 gm) baby 10 minutes ago with a forceps assist. The physician performed a right mediolateral episiotomy during the delivery. The baby has a cleft lip. Which of the following is the highest priority at this time?
   1. Breastfeeding education.
   2. Preventing postpartum hemorrhage.
   3. Preventing infection.
   4. Treating pain.

33. A nurse is performing a postpartum assessment on a client on postpartum day one. The nurse notes the following four signs/symptoms. The nurse should report which of the signs/symptoms to the client's healthcare practitioner?
   1. Foul-smelling lochia.
   2. Engorged breasts.
   3. Cracked nipples.
   4. Cluster of hemorrhoids.

34. A client is 36 hours post–cesarean section. Which of the following assessments would indicate that the client may have a paralytic ileus?
   1. Abdominal striae.
   2. Oliguria.
   3. Omphalocele.
   4. Absent bowel sounds.

35. A client on her first day after delivery is being monitored carefully after a significant postpartum hemorrhage. Which of the following should the nurse report to the obstetrician?
   1. Urine output 200 mL for the past 8 hours.
   2. Weight decrease of 2 pounds since delivery.
   3. Drop in hematocrit of 2% since admission.
   4. Pulse rate of 68 beats per minute.

36. A nurse has administered methylergonovine 0.2 mg PO to a grand multiparous client who delivered vaginally 30 minutes earlier. Which of the following outcomes indicates that the medication is effective?
   1. Blood pressure 120/80.
   2. Pulse rate 80 bpm and regular.
   3. Fundus firm at umbilicus.
   4. Increase in prothrombin time.

37. A nurse on the postpartum unit is caring for two postoperative cesarean section clients. One client had spinal anesthesia for the delivery, and the other client had an epidural. Which of the following complications will the nurse monitor the spinal client for, knowing the risk is lower for the epidural client?
   1. Pruritus.
   2. Nausea.
   3. Postural headache.
   4. Respiratory depression.

38. A postpartum woman has been diagnosed with postpartum psychosis. Which of the following signs/symptoms would the client exhibit?
1. Hallucinations.
2. Polyphagia.
3. Induced vomiting.
4. Weepy sadness.

39. The nurse is providing discharge counseling to a woman who is breastfeeding her baby. What should the nurse advise the woman to do if she should palpate tender, hard nodules in her breasts? **Select all that apply.**
1. Gently massage the areas toward the nipple, especially during feedings.
2. Apply warmth to the areas during feedings.
3. Alternate bottle feedings with breast feedings.
4. Apply lanolin ointment to the areas after each feeding.
5. Feed from the affected breast first.

40. A woman states that all of a sudden her 4-day-old baby is having trouble feeding. On assessment, the nurse notes that the mother's breasts are firm, red, and warm to the touch. The nurse teaches the mother to manually express a small amount of breast milk from each breast. Which observation indicates that the nurse's intervention has been successful?
1. The mother's breasts are soft to the touch.
2. The baby swallows after every fifth suck.
3. The baby's pre- and post-feed weight change is 20 grams.
4. The mother squeezes her nipples during manual expression.

41. A client's vital signs and reflexes were normal throughout pregnancy, labor, and delivery. Four hours after delivery the client's vitals are 98.6° F (37° C), P 72, R 20, BP 150/100, and her reflexes are 4+. She has an intravenous infusion running with 20 units of oxytocin added to 1,000 mL of lactated ringer's solution. Which of the following actions by the nurse is appropriate?
1. Do nothing, because the results are normal.
2. Notify the obstetrician of the findings.
3. Discontinue the intravenous infusion immediately.
4. Wait, and reassess the client after 15 minutes.

42. A nurse is caring for a client on postpartum day 2, who is preparing to go home with her infant. The nurse notes that the client's blood type is O– (negative), the baby's type is A+ (positive), and the direct Coombs test is negative. Which of the following actions by the nurse is appropriate?
1. Advise the client to keep her physician appointment at the end of the week to receive her Rh immune globulin (RhIG) injection.
2. Make sure that the client receives an Rh immune globulin (RhIG) injection before she is discharged from the hospital.
3. Notify the client that because her baby's Coombs test was negative she will not receive an injection of Rh immune globulin (RhIG).
4. Inform the client's physician that because the woman is being discharged on the second day, the Rh immune globulin (RhIG) could not be given.

43. The nurse is caring for a couple who is in the labor and delivery room immediately after the delivery of a stillborn baby who exhibited visible birth defects. Which of the following actions by the nurse is appropriate?
1. Discourage the parents from naming the baby.
2. Advise the parents that the baby's defects would be too upsetting for them to see.
3. Transport the baby to the morgue as soon as possible.
4. Give the parents a lock of the baby's hair and a copy of the footprint sheet.

44. During a cesarean section, the physician states that it appears the client has a placenta accreta. Which of the following maternal complications would be consistent with this diagnosis?
1. Blood loss of 2,000 mL.
2. Blood pressure of 160/110.
3. Jaundiced skin color.
4. Shortened prothrombin time.

45. Cloxacillin 500 mg by mouth 4 times per day for 10 days has been ordered for a client with a breast abscess. The client states that she is unable to swallow pills. The oral solution is available as 125 mg/5 mL. How many mL of medicine should the woman take per dose? **Calculate to the nearest whole.**

______ mL per dose.

46. A serum electrolyte report for a client the day after a cesarean section for eclampsia, has just been received by the nurse. The client is consuming nothing by mouth (NPO) and is receiving an intravenous solution of 5% dextrose in ½ normal saline IV at 125 mL/hr and magnesium sulfate 2 g/hr IV via infusion pump. Which of the following values should the nurse report to the surgeon?
1. Magnesium 7 mg/dL.
2. Sodium 136 mg/dL.
3. Potassium 3 mg/dL.
4. Calcium 9 mg/dL.

47. The home health nurse is visiting a client with HIV who is 6 weeks postpartum. Which of the following findings would indicate that client teaching by the nurse in the hospital was successful?
1. The client is breastfeeding her baby every two hours.
2. The client is using a diaphragm for family planning.
3. The client is taking her temperature every morning.
4. The client is seeking care for a recent weight loss.

48. A postpartum client has been diagnosed with deep vein thrombosis (DVT). For which of the following additional complications is this client at high risk?
1. Hemorrhage.
2. Stroke.
3. Endometritis.
4. Hematoma.

49. A client with an obstetrical history of G6 P6006, is 15 minutes postpartum. Her baby weighed 10 lbs 13 ounces (4,595 grams) at birth. For which of the following complications should the nurse monitor this client?
1. Seizures.
2. Hemorrhage.
3. Infection.
4. Thrombosis.

50. A client who received spinal anesthesia for her cesarean delivery is complaining of pruritus and has a macular rash on her face and arms. Which of the following medications ordered by the anesthesiologist should the nurse administer at this time?
1. Metoclopromide.
2. Ondansetron.
3. Prochlorperazine.
4. Diphenhydramine.

51. A woman with postpartum depression has been prescribed sertraline 50 mg daily. Which of the following should the client be taught about the medication?
1. Chamomile tea can potentiate the effect of the drug.
2. Therapeutic effect may be delayed 4 to 6 weeks.
3. The medication should only be taken whole.
4. A weight gain of up to 10 pounds is commonly seen.

52. A breastfeeding woman has been diagnosed with retained placental fragments 4 days postdelivery. Which of the following breastfeeding complications would the nurse expect to see?
1. Engorgement.
2. Mastitis.
3. Blocked milk duct.
4. Low milk supply.

53. The nurse assesses a postpartum, breastfeeding client two days after the delivery. The nurse notes blood on the mother's breast pad and a crack on the mother's nipple. Which of the following actions should the nurse perform at this time?
1. Advise the woman to wash the area with soap to prevent mastitis.
2. Provide the woman with a tube of topical lanolin.
3. Remind the woman that the baby can become sick if he drinks the blood.
4. Request an order for a topical anesthetic for the mother.

54. A client just delivered the placenta pictured below. The nurse will document that the client delivered a placenta with which of the following characteristics?

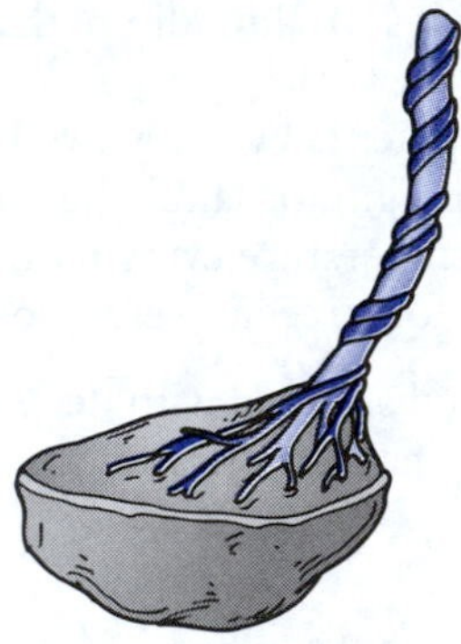

1. Circumvallate placenta.
2. Succenturiate placenta.
3. Placenta with velamentous cord insertion.
4. Battledore placenta.

55. The nurse administers Rh immune globulin (RhIG) to a postpartum client. Which of the following is the goal of the medication?
1. Inhibit the mother's active immune response.
2. Aggressively destroy the Rh antibodies produced by the mother.
3. Prevent fetal cells from migrating throughout the mother's circulation.
4. Change the maternal blood type to Rh-positive.

56. Which of the following comments suggest that a client whose baby was born with a congenital defect is in the bargaining phase of grief?
1. "I hate myself. I caused my baby to be sick."
2. "I'll take him to a specialist. Then he will get better."
3. "I can't seem to stop crying."
4. "This can't be happening."

57. A client delivered her baby by cesarean section with spinal anesthesia 1 day ago. Even though the nurse advised against it, the client has had the head of her bed in high-Fowler's position since delivery. Which of the following complications would the nurse expect to see in relation to the client's action?
1. Postpartum hemorrhage.
2. Severe postural headache.
3. Pruritic skin rash.
4. Paralytic ileus.

58. A client is receiving IV heparin for deep vein thrombosis. Which of the following medications should the nurse obtain from the pharmacy to have on hand in case of heparin overdose?
1. Vitamin K.
2. Protamine.
3. Vitamin E.
4. Mannitol.

59. A client who had no prenatal care, delivers a 10 lb 13 oz baby boy (4,595 gm) whose serum glucose result 1 hour after delivery was 20 mg/dL (1.1 mmol/L). Based on these data, which of the following tests should the mother have at her 6-week postpartum checkup?
1. Glucose tolerance test.
2. Indirect Coombs test.
3. Blood urea nitrogen (BUN).
4. Complete blood count (CBC).

60. A client with placenta previa has delivered by cesarean section. She is to receive a blood transfusion after significant blood loss following the birth. Which of the following actions by the nurse is critical prior to starting the infusion? **Select all that apply.**
1. Look up the client's blood type in the chart.
2. Check the client's arm bracelet.
3. Check the blood type on the infusion bag.
4. Obtain an infusion bag of dextrose and water.
5. Document the time the infusion begins.

61. A nurse is caring for the following 4 postpartum clients. Which clients should the nurse be prepared to monitor closely for signs of postpartum hemorrhage (PPH)? **Select all that apply.**
1. G1 P0100, delivered a fetal demise at 29 weeks' gestation.
2. G2 P2002, prolonged first stage of labor.
3. G2 P1011, delivered by cesarean section for failure to progress.
4. G3 P3003, delivered vaginally at 42 weeks, a 4 lb 8 oz (2200 grams) neonate.
5. G4 P4004, with a succenturiate placenta.

62. A client is 3 days post–cesarean section for eclampsia. The client is receiving hydralazine 10 mg, 4 times a day by mouth. Which of the following findings would indicate that the medication is effective?
1. The client has had no seizures since delivery.
2. The client's blood pressure has dropped from 160/120 to 130/90.
3. The client's postoperative weight has dropped from 154 to 144 lb.
4. The client states that her headache is gone.

63. A home care nurse is visiting a breastfeeding client who is 2 weeks postdelivery of a 7 lb (3,175 grams) baby girl over a midline episiotomy. Which of the following findings should take priority?
1. Lochia is serosa.
2. Client cries throughout the visit.
3. Nipples are cracked.
4. Client yells at the baby for crying.

64. A client who is post–cesarean section for pre-eclampsia with severe features is receiving magnesium sulfate per IV pump and morphine sulfate through a patient-controlled anesthesia (PCA) pump. The nurse enters the room on rounds and notes that the client is not breathing. Which of the following actions should the nurse perform first?
1. Give two breaths.
2. Discontinue medications.
3. Call a code.
4. Check the carotid pulse.

65. A breastfeeding client is being seen in the emergency department with a hard, red, warm nodule in the upper outer quadrant of her left breast. She states the baby cries at the breast. Her vital signs are T 104.6° F (40.3° C), P 100, R 20, and BP 110/60. She has a recent history of mastitis and is crying in pain. Which of the following conditions is the highest priority?
1. Ineffective breastfeeding.
2. Infection, as suggested by hyperthermia.
3. Emotional distress.
4. Pain.

66. A client is receiving an IV heparin drip at 16 mL/hr via an infusion pump for a diagnosis of deep vein thrombosis. The label on the ½ liter bag of D5W indicates 25,000 units of heparin have been added. How many units of heparin is the client receiving per hour? **Calculate to the nearest whole.**

______ units per hour.

67. A nurse massages the uterus of a postpartum woman after making a hypothesis of uterine atony. Which of the following outcomes would indicate that the client's condition had improved?
1. Heavy lochial flow.
2. Decreased pain level.
3. Stable blood pressure.
4. Fundus firm at or below the umbilicus.

68. Intermittent positive pressure boots have been ordered for a client who had an emergency cesarean section. Which of the following is the rationale for that order?
1. Postpartum clients are at high risk for thrombus formation.
2. Post-cesarean clients are at high risk for fluid volume deficit.
3. Postpartum clients are at high risk for varicose vein development.
4. Post-cesarean clients are at high risk for footdrop.

69. A client who received an epidural for her operative delivery has vomited twice since the surgery. Which of the following prn medications ordered by the anesthesiologist should the nurse administer at this time?
1. Metoclopromide.
2. Meperidine.
3. Secobarbital.
4. Diphenhydramine.

70. A client has just had a low forceps delivery. For which of the following should the nurse assess the woman during the immediate postpartum period?
1. Infection.
2. Bloody urine.
3. Heavy lochia.
4. Rectal abrasions.

71. A postpartum client has been diagnosed with postpartum psychosis. Which of the following is essential to be included in the family teaching for this client?
1. The client should never be left alone with her infant.
2. Symptoms rarely last more than one week.
3. Clinical response to medications is usually poor.
4. The client must have her vitals assessed every two days.

72. A postoperative cesarean section client who was diagnosed with pre-eclampsia with severe features in labor and delivery is transferred to the postpartum unit. The nurse is reviewing the client's doctor's orders. Which of the following medications that were ordered by the doctor should the nurse question?
1. Methylergonovine.
2. Magnesium sulfate.
3. Ibuprofen.
4. Morphine sulfate.

73. A couple accompanied by their 5-year-old daughter has been notified that their fetus, at 32 weeks' gestation, is dead. The father is yelling at the staff. The mother is crying uncontrollably. The 5-year-old is banging the head of her doll on the floor. Which of the following nursing actions is appropriate at this time?
1. Tell the father that his behavior is inappropriate.
2. Sit with the family and quietly communicate sorrow at their loss.
3. Help the couple to understand that their daughter is acting inappropriately.
4. Encourage the couple to send their daughter to her grandparents.

74. The nurse is caring for a client with an obstetrical history of G3 P3003, whose newborn has been diagnosed with a treatable birth defect. Which of the following is an appropriate statement for the nurse to make?
1. "Thank goodness. It could have been untreatable."
2. "I'm so happy that you have other children who are healthy."
3. "These things happen. They are the will of God."
4. "Tears are understandable at a time like this."

75. A client has given birth to a baby girl with a visible birth defect. Which of the following maternal responses would lead the nurse to suspect poor mother–infant bonding?
1. The mother states, "I'm so tired. Please feed the baby in the nursery for me."
2. The mother states, "Her eyes look like mine, but her chin is her dad's."
3. The mother says, "We have decided to name her Sarah after my mother."
4. The mother says, "I breastfed her. I still need help swaddling her, though."

76. A client who has been diagnosed with deep vein thrombosis has been ordered to receive 12 units heparin/min. The nurse receives a 500-mL bag of D5W with 20,000 units of heparin added from the pharmacy. At what rate in mL/hr should the nurse set the infusion pump? **Calculate to the nearest whole.**

______ mL/hr.

77. A client is being discharged on warfarin because of developing a pulmonary embolism after a cesarean section. Which of the following laboratory values indicates that the medication is effective?
1. Prothrombin time (PT): 12 sec (normal is 10 to 13 seconds).
2. International normalized ratio (INR): 2.5 (normal is 1 to 1.4).
3. Hematocrit 55%.
4. Hemoglobin 10 g/dL.

78. The pre-prandial blood glucose of a client with type 1 diabetes mellitus (T1DM) 12 hours after delivery is 96 mg/dL (5.3 mmol/L). The client has received no insulin since delivery. The drop in serum levels of which of the following hormones of pregnancy is responsible for the glucose level?
1. Estrogen.
2. Progesterone.
3. Human placental lactogen (hPL).
4. Human chorionic gonadotropin (hCG).

79. A breastfeeding woman, 6 weeks postdelivery, must go into the hospital for a hemorrhoidectomy. Which of the following is the best intervention regarding infant feeding?
1. Have the woman wean the baby to formula.
2. Have the baby stay in the hospital room with the mother.
3. Have the woman pump and dump her milk for two weeks.
4. Have the baby bottle-fed milk that the mother has stored.

80. A couple has delivered a 28-week stillborn baby. Which of the following nursing actions are appropriate to take? **Select all that apply.**
1. Swaddle the baby in a baby blanket.
2. Discuss funeral options for the baby.
3. Encourage the couple to try to get pregnant again in the near future.
4. Ask the couple if they would like to hold the baby.
5. Advise the couple that the baby's death was probably for the best.

81. A client is being discharged on warfarin after developing a pulmonary embolism following a cesarean section. Which of the following should be included in the client teaching?
1. Take only ibuprofen for pain.
2. Avoid overeating dark green, leafy vegetables.
3. Drink grapefruit juice daily.
4. Report any decrease in urinary output.

82. A client just delivered the placenta pictured below. For which of the following complications should the nurse carefully observe the woman?

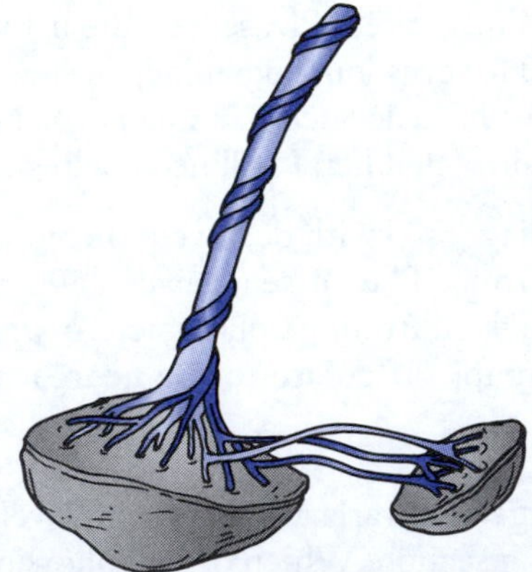

1. Endometrial ischemia.
2. Postpartum hemorrhage.
3. Prolapsed uterus.
4. Vaginal hematoma.

83. A woman has just had a macrosomic baby after a 12-hour labor. For which of the following complications should the woman be carefully monitored?
1. Uterine atony.
2. Hypoprolactinemia.
3. Infection.
4. Mastitis.

84. On admission to the labor and delivery suite, the nurse assesses the discharge needs of a primipara who will be discharged home 3 days after a cesarean section. Which of the following questions should the nurse ask the client?
1. "Have you ever had anesthesia before?"
2. "Do you have any allergies?"
3. "Do you scar easily?"
4. "Are there many stairs in your home?"

85. A woman is receiving paroxetine for postpartum depression. To prevent a drug–food interaction, the client must be advised to refrain from consuming which of the following?
1. Alcohol.
2. Grapefruit.
3. Milk.
4. Cabbage.

86. A nurse is assessing a postpartum client on the day after she delivered. She had a spontaneous vaginal delivery over an intact perineum. The fundus is firm at the umbilicus, lochia moderate, and perineum edematous. One hour after receiving ibuprofen 600 mg PO, the client is complaining of perineal pain at level 9 on a 10-point scale. Based on this information, which of the following is an appropriate conclusion for the nurse to make about the client?
1. She should be assessed by her doctor.
2. She should have a sitz bath.
3. She may have a hidden laceration.
4. She needs a narcotic analgesic.

87. A breastfeeding mother calls the obstetrician's office with a complaint of pain in one breast. Upon inspection, a diagnosis of mastitis is made. Which of the following nursing interventions is appropriate?
1. Advise the woman to apply ice packs to her breasts.
2. Encourage the woman to breastfeed frequently.
3. Inform the woman that she should wean immediately.
4. Direct the woman to notify her pediatrician as soon as possible.

88. A woman who wishes to breastfeed advises the nurse that she has had breast augmentation surgery. Which of the following responses by the nurse is appropriate?
1. Breast implants often contaminate the milk with toxins.
2. The glandular tissue of women who need implants is often deficient.
3. Babies often have difficulty latching to the nipples of women with breast implants.
4. Women who have implants are often able to breastfeed exclusively.

89. A breastfeeding client calls her obstetrician stating that her baby was diagnosed with thrush and that her breasts have become infected as well. Which of the following organisms has caused the baby's and mother's infection?
1. *Staphylococcus aureus.*
2. *Streptococcus pneumoniae.*
3. *Escherichia coli.*
4. *Candida albicans.*

90. A client on the postpartum unit has been diagnosed with deep vein thrombosis. The following titration schedule is included in the client's orders:
If INR is less than 1: administer 7,500 units heparin subcutaneously.
If INR is 1.1 to 2: administer 5,000 units heparin subcutaneously.
If INR is 2.1 to 3: administer 2,500 units heparin subcutaneously.
If INR is greater than 3: administer 0 units heparin subcutaneously.
The client's INR is 2.6. How many mL of heparin will the nurse administer if the available concentration of heparin is 5,000 units per 0.2 mL? **Calculate to the nearest tenth.**

______ mL.

91. A client who delivered vaginally, 26 hours ago, has asked for her prn oxycodone pain medication every 3 hours. Her baby is exhibiting the following symptoms: jitters, high-pitched cry, and very loose stools. Which of the following actions would be appropriate for the nurse to make at this time?

1. Immediately report the family to the local child abuse agency.
2. Advise the mother's and baby's healthcare providers regarding the behaviors.
3. Request the client's primary healthcare provider to change the medication order.
4. Advise the client to take the oxycodone less frequently.

92. A 12-year-old girl is in the postpartum unit after a vaginal delivery. Which of the following actions is appropriate for the nurse to make at this time?

1. Ask the young woman when her boyfriend will be visiting her in hospital.
2. Report the young woman to the local child protective agency.
3. Strongly advise the young woman always to use birth control in the future.
4. Advise the young woman that she is much too young to be having sex.

93. A primipara who delivered vaginally the day before, received magnesium sulfate in labor for pre-eclampsia with severe features. Which of the following healthcare referrals is the provider likely to recommend for the client? Referral to:

1. Cardiologist.
2. Gastroenterologist.
3. Hepatologist.
4. Immunologist.

94. A nurse is performing a postpartum assessment on a client who delivered at 30 weeks' gestation. Her baby is in the neonatal intensive care unit (NICU). The woman states, "The baby's doctor tells me that I should pump my breast milk for the baby, but I really don't want to breastfeed." Which of the following responses is appropriate for the nurse to make?

1. "You have the right to determine which type of feeding method you wish for your baby."
2. "Since you hadn't planned to breastfeed, you might not be aware of the benefits of breast milk for preterm babies when they are fed breast milk instead of formula."
3. "Mothers who pump milk for their babies seem to be ready to take their babies home sooner than those who bottle feed."
4. "You will be charged less money for your baby's care if you pump because your breast milk is free."

95. A client on the postpartum unit is preparing to breastfeed her baby, who was born with Down's syndrome. Which of the following actions by the nurse is appropriate at this time?

1. To prevent the baby from becoming obese, educate the mother to allow the baby to breastfeed for only 30 minutes at each feeding.
2. Provide the mother with the same breastfeeding advice that the nurse gives to all breastfeeding mothers and assume the baby will breastfeed well.
3. Assist the mother to latch her baby to the breast and educate her regarding how to assess for effective milk transfer.
4. To prevent the baby from becoming anemic, remind the mother to administer iron supplements to the baby every day.

96. A woman has just delivered a set of twins. As soon as the babies are born the mother says, "I wanted so much to breastfeed them but I know that is no longer a possibility." Which of the following statements by the nurse is appropriate at this time?

1. "It would be hard to breastfeed them both, but you could bottle feed one and breastfeed the other."
2. "It will be much easier for you to bottle feed them both. You can breastfeed your next baby if you want that experience. "
3. "What about switching off days. Bottle feed one baby and breastfeed the other one day then switch babies the next day."
4. "I can show you a number of ways to breastfeed both babies and you can make plenty of milk for both of them."

ANSWERS AND RATIONALES

The correct answer number and rationale for why it is the correct answer are given in **boldface blue type.** Rationales for why the other possible answer options are incorrect also are given, but they are not in boldface type.

CASE STUDY: *In the NGN format, test takers will be asked to drag and drop the selected answer into the appropriate box. Note that the primary complication, question 1, is in the center box.*

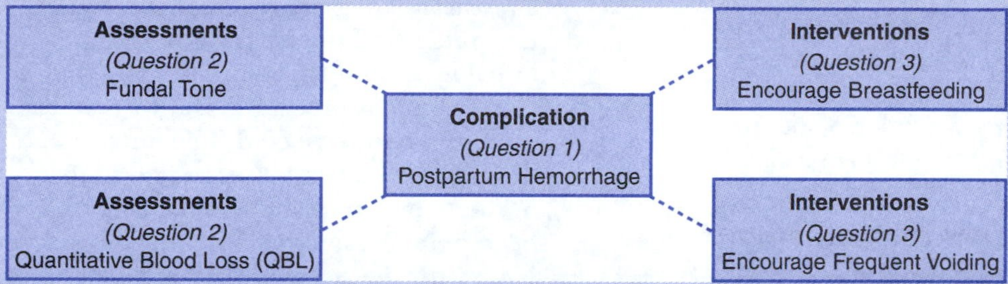

1. 1. Although all clients with pre-eclampsia with severe features are at risk for eclamptic seizures, there is nothing in the stem to suggest this particular client is at increased risk for seizure because the magnesium sulfate infusion is protective against seizures.
   2. **This client is at increased risk of postpartum hemorrhage (PPH) because of chorioamnionitis and the magnesium sulfate infusion, both of which reduce uterine tone.**
   3. Although all clients with magnesium infusions are at risk for magnesium sulfate toxicity, there is nothing in the stem to suggest this client is at increased risk. Her urine output of 350 mL after 3 hours in labor and delivery calculates to approximately 115 mL per hour, well above the minimum output of 30 mL/hour for adequate magnesium sulfate excretion.

TEST-TAKING HINT: The nurse must make a distinction between risks in general and specific risks for each client, based on that client's unique risk factors.

2. **Answers 1 and 2 are correct.**
   1. **Fundal tone was reported as firm before transfer. Because the fundus is now boggy and requires the nurse to massage it to firm, the prudent nurse would monitor the fundus closely, at least every 15 minutes initially, to prevent postpartum hemorrhage even though the client is past the *immediate* postpartum phase. Both magnesium sulfate and chorioamnionitis put this client at increased risk for hemorrhage. The length of labor and second stage are not given in the case study. The prudent nurse will review those time frames for additional information on the postpartum hemorrhage risks.**
   2. **The average blood loss with a vaginal delivery is under 500 mL. Traditionally, any amount over 500 mL with a vaginal delivery is considered a postpartum hemorrhage (Smith, 2018) and requires intervention. In 2017 the American College of Obstetrics and Gynecology (ACOG) redefined postpartum hemorrhage as a cumulative blood loss of 1000 mL regardless of birth type (vaginal or cesarean section) accompanied by signs and symptoms of hypovolemia (Wormer et al., 2019). This client's measured blood loss after the delivery was 475 mL, and with the additional 100 mL at this time (575 mL total), the client has had an excessive bleeding amount that could eventually meet one of the new criteria for a postpartum hemorrhage (1,000 ml within 24 hours).**
   3. Vital signs are important to assess. However, vital signs that would indicate hypovolemia are *late* symptoms of postpartum hemorrhage. As such, other signs must be monitored closely, to avoid vital sign indicators, which indicate serious progression of the condition. Because pregnant women have 30 to 50% more blood volume than

non-pregnant women (Aguree & Gernand, 2019), hemodynamic stability evidenced by vital signs remains relatively stable while a client hemorrhages. If a nurse waited until the vital signs indicated hemorrhage before intervening, it could be too late. In a postpartum client, objective evidence of bleeding is of primary importance, in order to prevent symptomatology that would include vital sign changes.

4. This question is not asking about risk factors for bleeding, but about assessments the nurse will make to determine that the client is bleeding too much. Although a full bladder can contribute to uterine bleeding by preventing adequate contraction of the uterus, the volume of urine output will not indicate whether or not the client is hemorrhaging.

TEST-TAKING HINT: Reading the stem of the question carefully to understand what is being asked is very important. In this question, the test taker is asked to identify assessments that help to "identify the . . . complication" of PPH selected in the previous question. Read the question too fast, and one might assume that *risk factors* for postpartum hemorrhage are the right answer. Certainly, a full bladder can be a *risk factor* for postpartum hemorrhage. However, the question does not ask for risk factors, but for assessments that *identify* the complication of postpartum hemorrhage.

3. Answers 2 and 4 are correct.

1. There is nothing in the stem to suggest the client has magnesium sulfate toxicity.
2. **Breastfeeding should be encouraged, as it promotes the release of endogenous oxytocin, which stimulates uterine tone, effectively reducing or preventing further bleeding.**
3. There is nothing in the stem to suggest the client is at risk of a seizure.
4. **This client has lost more than 500 mL of blood (575 mL total) and her fundus has required massage. A full bladder can contribute to postpartum hemorrhage. Due to changes of pregnancy, however, postpartum clients may not feel the sensation to void unless they are standing up. For this reason, the client should be encouraged to ambulate to the bathroom, or to use the commode, to keep the bladder empty. If the client continues to bleed and meets criteria for a postpartum hemorrhage as noted above, the California Maternal Quality Care Collaborative (2015) recommends that the bladder be emptied with a straight catheter, or that an indwelling catheter with a urimeter be considered. This would be essential if the bleeding is difficult to control and surgery might be necessary.**

4. Answers 1, 2, 3, and 4 are correct.

1. **Vital signs are part of the CABs of circulation, airway, and breathing, which are priority assessments for every client. In addition, several other factors are present with this client, to make vital signs a priority. These include general anesthesia, the recent administration of morphine, and the magnesium sulfate infusion. A blood pressure of 110/70 in a client who has pre-eclampsia with severe features is not expected. The nurse must sort these out. There is nothing in the question to suggest the client has been hemorrhaging or that there is an issue with the surgical dressing. Those assessments are important but are not among the top four priorities.**
2. **The client's PACU urinary output of 80 mL in 2 hours is within normal, but is on the low side, at approximately 40 mL per hour. As such, it becomes one of the four most important findings to follow up on for this client. Kidney malfunction could lead to magnesium sulfate toxicity, resulting in a threat to the CAB's of circulation, airway, and breathing.**
3. **The client's muscle flaccidity makes reflexes and clonus among the top four important findings to assess. Magnesium sulfate toxicity can be a threat to breathing.**
4. **The client's moist cough makes breath sounds among the top four findings to assess. Pulmonary edema is a risk in a client who has pre-eclampsia with severe features. The condition can be a threat to the CAB's of circulation, airway, and breathing.**
5. The surgical dressing is important, but it is not one of the top four findings, as there is nothing in the question to suggest there is a problem with it. Its condition would not be life-threatening.
6. Uterine tone is an important finding to assess, but although the client lost 1,050 mL of blood in total, there is nothing in the question to suggest she has had issues with uterine tone. Routine fundal checks should be adequate.

TEST-TAKING HINT: Clinical judgment begins with noticing what's not normal and quickly determining what assessments to make first. The

abnormal things to notice with this client include her temperature of 100° F (37.7° C), respiratory rate on the low end at 14, blood pressure on the low end at 110/70, urinary output on the low end at 80 mL/2 hours, and muscle flaccidity. Each of these things requires further assessments to determine the possible cause. The nurse begins with the symptoms that could indicate or lead to a life-threatening condition.

5. The correct answers are 1(b and c), 2(b and c), 3 (a), 4(c), 5(b and c), and 6(d).

Client findings	(a) Consistent with impaired renal function	(b) Consistent with pain medication	(c) Consistent with magnesium sulfate	(d) Consistent with pulmonary edema
1. Respiratory rate		X	X	
2. Blood pressure		X	X	
3. Urinary output	X			
4. Muscle flaccidity			X	
5. Sleepiness		X	X	
6. Moist cough				X

1(b and c). Both morphine sulfate and magnesium sulfate can depress the respiratory rate.
2(b and c). A low respiratory rate can be associated with both morphine sulfate and magnesium sulfate.
3(a). Low urinary output can be associated with impaired renal function.
4(c). Muscle flaccidity can be associated with magnesium sulfate.
5(b and c). Sleepiness can be associated with morphine sulfate and with magnesium sulfate.
6(d). The moist cough can be a symptom of pulmonary edema.

TEST-TAKING HINT: Having identified four conditions that could be related to the client's symptoms (recognizing cues), the nurse now sorts the client's symptoms by probable cause to determine, "What do these symptoms mean?" As indicated by the table, the majority of the symptoms—four—are correlated with magnesium sulfate administration. This leads the nurse to the priority hypothesis in the next question.

6. Answers 3 and b are correct.

At risk to happen (Select one, below)	As evidenced by . . . (Select one, below)
1. Hypoxia	a. Respiratory assessment
2. Eclamptic seizure	**b. Urinary output assessment**
3. Magnesium sulfate toxicity	c. Neurologic assessment
4. Pulmonary embolism	d. Vital signs

1. The client is breathing adequately at 14 breaths per minute, so neither pulmonary edema nor hypoxia is likely. Symptoms of pulmonary edema include wheezing, anxiety, shortness of breath, and other symptoms. The question does not indicate the client is experiencing these symptoms.
2. The client's reflexes and clonus are normoflexic, so an eclamptic seizure is not likely.
3. Magnesium sulfate toxicity is *at risk to happen* if the urinary output decreases to 30 mL/hour or less over 2 hours. This is the amount required for adequate excretion of magnesium sulfate to avoid magnesium toxicity.
4. The client is not at risk of a pulmonary embolism.

All of the responses in the second column are evaluated in light of their correlation with the answer selected in the first column.

a. The respiratory assessment of a moist cough is not definitive for magnesium sulfate toxicity. It could be related to pulmonary edema at the worst, or it may simply be related to irritation from the endotracheal tube during general anesthesia. It certainly bears watching.

b. The urinary output of 80 mL in 2 hours of PACU care bears watching. A client is oliguric if the urinary output is less than 30 mL per hour over 2 hours (Archer & Champagne, 2013). Because magnesium sulfate is not adequately excreted from the body in amounts less than 30 mL/hour over 2 hours (Nick, 2006), the client is then at increased risk for magnesium sulfate toxicity. Many women with pre-eclampsia have a short period of up to 6 hours after delivery during which they may be slightly oliguric (Kim & Steinberg, 2019). This must be sorted out to confirm whether their urine output is within normal range, or indicates risk.

c. The client's DTRs of 2+ and 1 beat of clonus are normoreflexic, which is the goal of magnesium sulfate therapy.

d. The client's vital signs are not suggestive of magnesium toxicity at this time.

TEST-TAKING HINT: The nurse has narrowed down the assessment of highest client risk and determined it is the risk of magnesium toxicity. The test taker must remember the three reasons that clinical assessments are performed on clients with pre-eclampsia. The first reason a nurse completes clinical assessments is to determine the central nervous system (CNS) irritability and the need for magnesium sulfate to prevent seizures. This was done at the client's admission to the hospital before the infusion was started. The second reason for clinical assessments comes during medication administration, when clinical assessments assist with confirming the efficacy of the medication to keep the client's reflexes and vital signs within the normal range. This is continuous. The third reason is to be alert for signs that could indicate the client is at risk for magnesium sulfate toxicity as a result of retention of the medication above safe levels.

Perinatal experts have created several tools for safe magnesium sulfate administration. One of these is from the Agency for Healthcare Research and Quality (AHRQ), which lists the following signs of magnesium toxicity: "respiratory depression (less than 12 respirations/minute), prolonged expiration, severe chest heaviness or shortness of breath, a significant decrease in the level of consciousness, the absence of deep tendon reflexes, and a significant decrease in the patient's pulse or blood pressure" (AHRQ, n.d., p. 15).

A triad of three indicators for safe magnesium sulfate administration has been suggested for the nurse to keep in mind: normal DTR response, normal respiratory rate, and adequate urinary output. When all three of those are normal, the nurse and provider can be reassured that the magnesium sulfate dose is within therapeutic levels (Nick, 2006). For this client, her DTRs are normoflexic, her respiratory rate is above 12, and her urinary output is above 30 mL/hour over 2 hours at this time. This indicates the magnesium sulfate is currently within therapeutic levels, although the urine output is on the low side. The nurse must remain alert to the risk of magnesium sulfate toxicity.

7. **Answers 1(a), 2(b), 3(b), 4(a), 5(c), and 6(b) are correct.**

Potential intervention	(a) Essential	(b) Nonessential	(c) Contraindicated
1. Turn off magnesium sulfate	X		
2. Check lochial flow		X	
3. Check client's pupils		X	
4 Assess DTRs and clonus	X		
5. Administer naloxone			X
6. Tally intake and output		X	

1(a). It is essential to turn off the magnesium sulfate. The client is showing signs of hypermagnesemia, also referred to as magnesium toxicity.
2(b). It is nonessential to check the client's lochia at this time. She is not showing signs of hemorrhage and the assessments related to the airway and breathing are of higher priority right now.
3(b). It is nonessential to check the client's pupils. Her blood pressure is not in the stroke or seizure range, and her condition is most likely related to hypermagnesemia, not stroke.
4(a). Deep tendon reflexes and clonus are essential assessments. Clinical signs are often considered a better indicator of magnesium sulfate toxicity than serum levels (Nick, 2006).
5(c). Naloxone is contraindicated. The client's symptomatology is not related to opioid overdose. Instead, the nurse should prepare to administer calcium gluconate, the magnesium sulfate antagonist.
6(b). Although the client's total fluid balance is important, the urine output over the previous 2 hours is more important. However, that total can be delayed until after the client is stabilized. The tally is not part of the basic circulation, airway, and breathing assessments.

TEST-TAKING HINT: The nurse has previously determined that this client is at risk of hypermagnesemia, also referred to as magnesium sulfate toxicity. When the nurse enters the room, he or she recognizes cues that validate this possibility: Where this client's assessments previously showed a respiratory rate of 14, which was near the risk level of 12 breaths per minute, the nurse now sees a respiratory rate of 10 and a noticeable decrease in consciousness. Additional nursing assessments of DTRs, clonus, and urinary output over the past hour will give further information. Loss of patellar reflexes is the first sign of magnesium sulfate toxicity and is often seen with magnesium sulfate levels of 9 to 12 mg/dL (da Costa et al., 2020). Decisions about next steps must be made quickly and must be prioritized according to the CABs of circulation, airway, and breathing.

8. **Answers 2, 3, and 4 are correct.**
   1. The provider is completing DTRs and clonus checks. The next assessments do not need to be done right away, but can wait for an hour or as ordered.
   2. **The client's oxygen saturation of 93% indicates she needs supplemental oxygen at this time. This is one of the 3 CABs.**
   3. **In order to confirm magnesium sulfate toxicity physiologically, a blood sample must be drawn and sent to the lab before the calcium gluconate antidote is given. As such, this must be done right away.**
   4. **The client has all three symptoms that indicate she is in the danger zone for magnesium sulfate toxicity. Her respiratory rate is 10, DTRs are absent, and urinary output has been 20 mL over the past 2 hours. Once the blood work is drawn, the calcium gluconate antidote must be given as ordered. Many preprinted magnesium sulfate order sets include an order to draw some blood and send it to the laboratory for a magnesium sulfate level when magnesium sulfate toxicity is suspected. If so, the nurse could have completed that order while the provider was on the way to the room. The nurse does not wait to turn off the**

magnesium sulfate until the blood is drawn or the lab results are returned. Turning off the magnesium sulfate should be the *first* action that is done.

5. An IV fluid bolus is not a time-sensitive intervention. It is often ordered as a therapeutic treatment for oliguria to test kidney function. As discussed in option 4, above, the client has all three symptoms that indicate she is in the danger zone of magnesium sulfate toxicity.

   Unlike blood loss, the volume of urine in the urimeter does not *contribute to* organ damage. Rather, the urine output serves as *confirmation* that due to kidney dysfunction, as evidenced by low urinary output, the differential diagnosis of magnesium sulfate toxicity is likely, since magnesium sulfate cannot be excreted adequately at 30 mL/hour urinary output. As a result, magnesium sulfate levels in the blood rise beyond therapeutic levels and the client experiences hypermagnesemia, also called magnesium sulfate toxicity.

TEST-TAKING HINT: The test taker will notice that the correct answers are time-dependent. The client needs oxygen now, the blood sample must be drawn now, and the calcium gluconate must be given now. The other orders, such as DTRs and giving a fluid bolus can be done after the time-dependent orders have been completed. For this client, an intravenous fluid bolus could be of benefit, but it also might need to be questioned. Oliguria is defined as less than 30 mL/hour over 2 hours. This client's output had been 40 mL per hour on admission to the unit. With the addition of 20 mL in the past hour, the total urinary output over 2 hours is 60 mL, putting her at 30 mL/hour over 2 hours. Urinary output ranges are not rocket science, however, and need not be exact before a nurse or provider takes action. They are given as reference points.

Before giving the IV fluid bolus, the nurse must calculate the total oral and intravenous fluids and urinary output up to this point in time. Intravenous fluid boluses are not appropriate for pre-eclamptic clients who have greater input than output. However, some carefully-selected clients whose output exceeds their input can benefit from measured fluid challenges until urinary output is restored or fluid balance has been established (Anthony & Schoeman, 2013). A tally of this client's 24-hour intake and output will be invaluable for clinical decision-making. The nurse must question the provider's order for an IV fluid bolus if the client's output does not equal or exceed input.

9. **Answers 1(c), 2(a), 3(b), 4(a), 5(a), and 6(a) are correct.**

Assessment finding	(a) Effective	(b) Ineffective	(c) Unrelated
1. Temp 101.2° F (38.4° C)			X
2. Respirations 18 per minute, BP 120/82	X		
3. Urine output 20 mL		X	
4. DTRs 2+, 1 beat clonus	X		
5. Asking to see baby	X		
6. Pulse oximetry 95%	X		

1(c). **The client's temperature is unrelated to the magnesium sulfate and is a new finding. The temperature leads the nurse to another set of clinical judgments relating to infection.**

2(a). **The respiratory rate and BP are improved, indicating the calcium gluconate administration was effective in reversing the effects of hypermagnesemia.**

3(b). **The urinary output of 20 mL over the past hour indicates the intravenous fluid bolus was ineffective in improving urinary output and magnesium sulfate excretion. This leads to another set of clinical judgments and assessments focused on prevention of pulmonary edema if the fluid bolus resulted in fluid overload.**

4(a). **The DTRs and clonus are now normo-reflexive, indicating effectiveness of treatment.**

5(a). **The client is awake enough to ask to see her baby, indicating effectiveness of treatment.**

6(a). **The client's respiratory rate is adequate to keep her oxygen saturation in the normal range, indicating that the magnesium sulfate, calcium gluconate, and oxygen interventions were effective.**

TEST-TAKING HINT: This question requires the nurse to understand the expected actions of calcium gluconate, oxygen administration, and the IV fluid bolus. By noticing which interventions were ineffective, the nurse moves to a new process of analyzing cues, prioritizing hypotheses, etc., related to those focused areas of concern.

10. 1. This is unnecessary. Unless they have developed type 2 diabetes mellitus (T2DM) during pregnancy, clients with gestational diabetes need not assess their blood glucose levels during the postpartum period.
2. This is unnecessary. Unless they have developed type 2 diabetes mellitus (T2DM) during pregnancy, clients with gestational diabetes need not inject insulin during the postpartum period.
3. **This is an appropriate statement to make. During exercise, muscle cells take in glucose without needing insulin. This can prevent strain on the pancreas and possibly delay or prevent future diabetes.**
4. This is not appropriate. Babies rarely develop diabetes before age 2. Plus, "juvenile diabetes" is now referred to as type 1 diabetes mellitus (T1DM).

TEST-TAKING HINT: Women who develop gestational diabetes are at high risk for developing type 2 diabetes mellitus (T2DM). They should be encouraged to eat healthy foods and to exercise to prevent or delay the onset of the chronic disease.

11. 1. **Sudden flank pain is a sign of a transfusion reaction.**
2. This is not a sign of a transfusion reaction. The client may be nervous about receiving the blood.
3. This is not a sign of a transfusion reaction. The client may be nervous about receiving the blood.
4. This is not a sign of a transfusion reaction. The client is likely having a normal bowel movement.

TEST-TAKING HINT: If the client is receiving the wrong type of blood or is allergic to the blood, she will develop flank or kidney pain. Antibodies in the client's blood are likely destroying the donated blood. The transfusion should be stopped immediately and the reaction reported to the physician and to the blood bank.

12. Answers 1 and 2 are correct.

1. **Carboprost can cause nausea, vomiting, diarrhea, and hyperthermia.**
2. **Carboprost can cause nausea, vomiting, diarrhea, and hyperthermia.**
3. Hypotension is not associated with carboprost
4. Palpitations are not associated with carboprost
5. Anasarca (extreme, generalized edema) is not associated with carboprost.

TEST-TAKING HINT: Carboprost is a type of prostaglandin that acts on the myometrial tissue of the uterus. After the birth it acts directly at the site of placental separation to stop uncontrolled bleeding. Because of the very unpleasant side effects, it is often used last, when other medications have been ineffective. It is contraindicated for clients who have asthma.

13.
1. This response is not appropriate. It is not likely that this client is menstruating at 2 weeks postpartum.
2. This response is not appropriate. This client needs to be evaluated.
3. This response is not appropriate. This is an unlikely explanation for the bleeding.
4. **This is the correct response. This client needs to be evaluated.**

TEST-TAKING HINT: The quantity of lochial discharge is usually described as scant, moderate, or heavy. A heavy discharge is described as a discharge that saturates a pad in 1 hour or less. Because this client's lochia has already become scant, it is especially concerning that she is now experiencing a heavy lochia rubra (reddish) flow.

14.
1. The uterus is contracted. Massaging the uterus will not remedy the problem of heavy lochial flow.
2. **It is important for the nurse to notify the physician. The client is bleeding more than she should after the delivery.**
3. An oxytocic agent promotes contraction of the uterine muscle. The muscle is already contracted.
4. The uterus is at the umbilicus. It is unlikely that it is displaced from a full bladder.

TEST-TAKING HINT: The nurse must act as a detective to determine the cause of the client's symptoms. When the client has heavy bleeding in spite of a firm fundus at the expected location, a laceration or hematoma is suspected. Both of these require a provider's evaluation. In this scenario, the uterus is contracted and is firm at the umbilicus, which is expected. The lochia flow, however, is heavy. The nurse must notify the practitioner for assistance because the bleeding may be due to a cervical or vaginal tissue laceration. There is no additional nursing action the nurse can take at this time.

15.
1. It is unlikely that an apical heart rate of 104 is responsible for the client's changes.
2. **The urinary output is the likely cause of the client's changes.**
3. It is unlikely that a blood pressure of 160/120 is responsible for the client's changes.
4. It is unlikely that a temperature of 100° F (37.7° C) is responsible for the client's changes.

TEST-TAKING HINT: This client is exhibiting signs of magnesium toxicity. Even though the dose may be low, the client's kidney function is likely impaired, due to pre-eclampsia with severe features. As a result, the client's kidneys are not clearing the magnesium sulfate adequately. The nurse must calculate the hourly urine output, which is 20 mL/hr. This is well below the minimum therapeutic urinary output of 30 mL/hr. Because the medication is excreted via the kidneys, when a client's output is low, the concentration of the medication can increase to toxic levels in the bloodstream. In a nutshell, the client has reduced kidney function, as evidenced by low urinary output, which has resulted in magnesium sulfate toxicity.

16.
1. The client should not be placed flat in bed now that she is awake. Her bed should be placed in the semi-Fowler's position to enable her to breathe well. She can also hold her baby better in that position.
2. There is nothing in the scenario that suggests that this client is at high risk for dependent edema.
3. **As with any postoperative client, it is important for the nurse to auscultate the client's lung fields every 4 hours to assess for rales.**
4. There is nothing in the scenario that suggests that this client is at high risk for an alteration in reflex response.

TEST-TAKING HINT: A client who is recovering from a cesarean section is both a postoperative client and a postpartum client. The nurse must perform needed physiological assessments for both of these conditions. Because this client had general anesthesia during her surgery, she is at high risk for pulmonary complications, including atelectasis and pneumonia. Since it is now

4 hours past her surgery, she is no doubt awake and does not need to remain flat. In addition, because she did not have spinal anesthesia, there is no risk for a spinal headache.

17. 1. Postoperative cesarean section clients should turn or change positions at least every 2 hours to prevent stasis of their lung fields.
2. Sitz baths are rarely ordered for post–cesarean section clients.
3. Active range-of-motion exercises will help to prevent thrombus formation in post–cesarean section clients. In addition, intermittent positive pressure boots can help during the time the client is in bed after surgery.
4. Central venous pressure is rarely assessed in post–cesarean section clients.

TEST-TAKING HINT: Postsurgical clients, whether they have intermittent positive pressure boots ordered or not, should be advised to move their legs actively at least a few times each hour. Postpartum clients, especially, are prone to blood clot formation because of the hematologic changes of pregnancy. If the client prevents pooling of blood in her extremities, she will be much less likely to develop deep vein thrombosis.

18. 1. It is unnecessary to monitor the client's hourly urinary output.
2. It is appropriate to supervise while the woman holds her newborn.
3. It is unnecessary for the client to be placed in this position.
4. It is unnecessary for visitors to leave the client's room.

TEST-TAKING HINT: Diphenhydramine is an antihistamine. One of the common side effects of both diphenhydramine and morphine is sedation. It is very likely that this client will fall asleep while holding the baby. The nurse, therefore, should supervise the mother while she holds her baby.

19. 1. Puerperal infection is defined as a temperature of 100.4° F (38° C) or higher after 24 hours postpartum.
2. Although clients who develop endometritis will have significantly elevated white blood cell counts, a WBC count of 14,500 is normal for a postpartum client.
3. Clients who develop infections may perspire profusely. However, diaphoresis is normally seen in postpartum clients and is not in itself indicative of postpartum infection.
4. A malodorous lochial flow is a common sign of a puerperal infection.

TEST-TAKING HINT: "Puerperium" is another word for "postpartum." Although a client may have a slight temperature elevation, an elevated white blood cell count, and/or be diaphoretic, all three symptoms are normally seen in the postpartum client without an infection. The only finding that would make a nurse suspect infection is the malodorous lochial flow. The other findings are well within normal range for a postpartum woman.

20. 1. The mother, not the baby, may develop a macular rash after receiving the injection. The baby will be unaffected.
2. There is no evidence to suggest that babies whose mothers have received the rubella vaccine reject their mother's breast milk.
3. There is no evidence to suggest that the mother's breast milk supply will drop.
4. One out of 4 women complains of painful and stiff joints after receiving the injection.

TEST-TAKING HINT: Even though the benefits of receiving immunizations far outweigh the side effects of the medicines, anyone who receives a vaccine should be advised of the potential complications. It is especially important for newly delivered mothers to receive anticipatory guidance regarding these changes and reassurance that the baby's health will not be compromised.

21. 1. Feelings of infanticide are rare in clients diagnosed with postpartum depression.
2. Difficulty latching babies to the breast is an independent, common problem unrelated to postpartum depression. Many mothers with depression still breastfeed successfully.
3. Mothers who experience postpartum depression often feel like failures because they anticipate euphoria and confidence. They are surprised by the anxiety and incompetence they feel in their new role.
4. Concerns about sibling rivalry are not related to postpartum depression.

TEST-TAKING HINT: If a mother who is diagnosed with postpartum depression does have difficulty latching her baby to the breast, she may view this as yet another example of her poor parenting skills. The difficulty itself, however, is unrelated to the diagnosis of postpartum depression.

22. 1. The client would be expected to complain of pain.
2. The nurse would not expect to see bleeding.
3. The nurse would not expect to note warmth.
4. The nurse would not expect to see redness.

TEST-TAKING HINT: A hematoma is a collection of blood under the skin. In the postpartum client, the hematoma is often at the vaginal opening. Although hematomas are usually simple bruises, large collections of blood can occur. A client can be silently hemorrhaging into a hematoma without obvious, outward symptoms except for unstable vital signs. Because the blood is trapped under the skin, the most common symptom is pain from the blood pressing on the pain sensors.

23. 1. This response is inappropriate. The client should not be advised to switch to formula.
2. This response is inappropriate. The client should not be advised to switch to formula.
3. This response by the nurse is appropriate.
4. This response is inappropriate. The client should not be advised to switch to formula.

TEST-TAKING HINT: The nurse can help reduce the mother's anxiety by pointing out that the baby has already been exposed to the mother and will continue being exposed to her even if she switches to formula. More important, however, is the fact that the mother will produce antibodies that will be consumed by the baby in the breast milk. The baby will, therefore, be more protected by continuing to breastfeed than by switching to formula, because formula contains no protective properties.

24. 1. This may be true, but it's not always a given. The mother may be able to breastfeed successfully, depending on the surgical approach.
2. This action can be helpful, but the placement of the incision will not necessarily determine the client's ability to breastfeed. The nurse cannot definitely confirm that the mother can make adequate milk for the baby, based on the location of an incision, since the nurse knows nothing about the procedural details.
3. This action is very important, at least initially, and is the safest approach.
4. This information is not accurate. Breast reduction surgery can affect a woman's ability to breastfeed.

TEST-TAKING HINT: During breast reduction surgery, fat tissue is removed from the breast. Because the breast is much smaller as a result, the nipple must be moved to a new location. During these procedures, the client's mammary ducts may be ligated. If the ducts are severed, the woman will not be able to transfer the milk produced in her glandular tissue to the baby. The most objective means of assessing milk transfer is by closely monitoring the baby's weights, at least initially. Pre-feed and post-feed weights as well as daily weights should be monitored to confirm adequate weight gain.

25. 1. There is nothing in this client's history that would indicate that she could not produce breast milk.
2. There is nothing in this client's history that would indicate that she is at high risk for dysfunctional parenting.
3. This client is at high risk for wound dehiscence. Her wound healing may be impaired because of her diabetes and because of her obesity.
4. There is nothing in this client's history that would indicate that she is at high risk for projectile vomiting.

TEST-TAKING HINT: Wound dehiscence is a complication for any postoperative client with obesity and insulin-dependent diabetes. The fact that this client has had a cesarean section is irrelevant.

26. 1. After the surgeon has been notified, the nurse should stay with the client while another staff member gathers supplies, including a suture removal kit and personal protective equipment as well as sterile saline solution and a large syringe.
2. The highest priority action is to notify the surgeon. This can be done in the room while a colleague gathers supplies for covering the intestines, etc.
3. After the surgeon has been notified, the nurse should elevate the client's head slightly to prevent pulling on the incision.
4. After the surgeon has been notified, the nurse should flex the client's knees slightly to prevent pulling on the incision.

TEST-TAKING HINT: Because arrival of the surgeon can take time, notification should be the highest priority. While waiting for the surgeon, positioning of the client is important because the nurse wants to take as much stress off the incision as possible. If the surgeon is delayed and the dehiscence is significant, the nurse must keep the intestines moist by placing sterile dressings saturated with sterile saline over the area (Beattie, 2007). The client will likely need to return to the operating room for wound repair. She should also be NPO.

27. 1. This temperature elevation does not indicate infection. Postpartum fever is defined as a temp greater than 100.4° F (38° C) on any 2 of the first 10 days postpartum, or as any temperature of 101.6° F (38.7° C) or greater during the first 24 hours (Wong & Rosh, 2019).
2. A low pulse rate is expected in the early postpartum period.
3. The respiratory rate of 12 is well below normal. Peripartum clients' respiratory rates average 20 breaths per minute. This client's respiratory rate could be related to pain medication in PACU, or to magnesium sulfate.
4. Although the systolic pressure is slightly elevated, a BP of 130/80 is within normal limits.

TEST-TAKING HINT: Even though explanations are provided for each of the signs, the test taker must be able to determine which explanation is correct and which are erroneous. A suggested approach is to consciously stop to think about each of the signs independently and *recognize cues*—determine whether the description is accurate or not. For example, is a temp of 100° F (37.7° C) considered to be elevated? Is a pulse of 68 considered to be too low? Are the respirations too low? And, is the blood pressure elevated? Then look at the explanations and determine if they are in alignment with the given description as you *analyze the cues* and make sense of them. By taking this action, the test taker is less likely to be swayed by a wrong answer.

28. Answers 1, 2, 3, and 5 are correct.
1. The client should receive an Rh immune globulin (RhIG) injection after a spontaneous abortion since the fetal blood type is unknown.
2. The client should receive an Rh immune globulin (RhIG) injection after an amniocentesis since the baby's blood type is unknown.
3. The client should receive an Rh immune globulin (RhIG) injection after the delivery of a fetal demise since the baby's blood type is unknown.
4. The client does not need an Rh immune globulin (RhIG) injection after the delivery of Rh-negative twins.
5. The client should receive an Rh immune globulin (RhIG) injection after the birth of an Rh-positive baby.

TEST-TAKING HINT: Rh immune globulin (RhIG), is administered to Rh negative clients in several situations: 1) prophylactically at 28 weeks' gestation; 2) after any invasive procedure such as an amniocentesis; 3) after a preterm disruption of a pregnancy such as an abortion or placenta previa bleed; and 4) after the delivery of an Rh-positive infant. Each of these scenarios carries the risk of maternal/fetal blood mixing and exposing the mother to Rh-positive blood from the baby. This exposure can trigger the mother's body to produce antibodies that could harm the next baby if it is Rh-positive. Because Rh-negative infants carry no Rh antigen, it is unnecessary to administer Rh immune globulin (RhIG) to their Rh-negative mothers.

29. 1. These findings are not consistent with a diagnosis of deep vein thrombosis (DVT). They may be due to a resolving epidural anesthesia.
2. These findings are normal. Many women complain of leg cramping.
3. These findings—swelling, redness, and warmth—indicate the possible presence of a DVT.
4. These findings are normal. Many women develop spider veins during their pregnancies.

TEST-TAKING HINT: During the daily postpartum assessment, the nurse should assess for signs of thrombosis: pain, warmth, redness, and edema. The signs are usually unilateral, meaning they're generally on just one leg. It is especially important for the nurse to refrain from palpating the calf too deeply or dorsiflexing the foot because those actions may dislodge a clot and cause a pulmonary embolism.

30. 1. This response is inappropriate. The client is not thinking about a future pregnancy at this time.
2. This response is correct. The baby should be dressed as if they were a viable baby.
3. This response is not appropriate. A sedative will make the client sleepy and she could miss the opportunity to see and remember the baby if she would like to do so.
4. This response is not appropriate. The nurse should ask the client if she would like to see or hold the baby.

TEST-TAKING HINT: The nurse should treat this baby with care and concern. Even though the baby has died, it is still a valued child to the parents. The parents should be asked whether they would like to see or hold their baby. If they choose to do so, the nurse should help the parents to see the normalcy in their request and stay with them if they choose.

31. **Answers 1 and 4 are correct.**
   1. **Breastfeeding was once contraindicated when the mother used illicit drugs. However, it should not be dismissed as a newborn feeding option for such clients. Breastfeeding is now approved in many cases for mothers with a past or current history of substance use disorder (ACOG, 2015).**
   2. This action is inappropriate. The nurse should not scold the mother for her behavior. A woman who has a history of illicit drug use should not be criminalized for breastfeeding her infant.
   3. This action is inappropriate. Rather, the nurse should encourage mother/baby interaction and provide the mother with parenting education.
   4. **Providing instruction on baby-care skills is a very important action for the nurse to perform.**
   5. It is not necessary for the mother to feed the baby formula, since breastfeeding may reduce the severity of neonatal abstinence syndrome.

TEST-TAKING HINT: Regardless of the mother's history of illicit drug use, if the mother shows an interest in caring for her baby, she must be supported in doing that as long as this does not put the baby at risk. At the same time, the nurse must refer the client to the social work department in the hospital, or report the family to child protective services for evaluation.

Because babies who have developed dependence on illicit drugs in utero often have very disorganized behavior patterns, the baby will no doubt exhibit symptoms of withdrawal and may be difficult to care for. However, breastfeeding has been shown to reduce neonatal abstinence syndrome (ACOG, 2015). The nurse must provide guidance for the mother regarding care of her infant. This also provides an opportunity for the nurse to observe the mother for any behaviors that may put the baby at risk. Such behaviors must be reported to the primary healthcare providers and to the social worker assigned to the case even though the information may affect whether or not the baby is discharged to the mother's care.

32. 1. Because the baby has a cleft lip, this is an appropriate priority, but it is not the highest priority at this time.
   2. **This is the nursing priority at this time. Because the baby is macrosomic, the client is at high risk for uterine atony that could lead to heavy vaginal bleeding, possibly resulting in fluid volume deficit.**
   3. Although the client is at high risk for infection, it is not highest priority. Infections take time to develop and this client is only 10 minutes postdelivery.
   4. Although the client is at high risk for pain, especially from the episiotomy, this is not the highest priority.

TEST-TAKING HINT: If the test taker remembers CAB as taught in CPR class—circulation, airway, breathing—it is a reminder that the client's fluid volume (circulation) must take precedence.

33. 1. **Foul-smelling lochia is a sign of endometritis.**
   2. The nurse can assist the client with actions to relieve breast engorgement.
   3. The nurse can assist the client with actions to relieve cracked nipples.
   4. The nurse can assist the client with actions to relieve hemorrhoid pain.

TEST-TAKING HINT: Some nursing actions are dependent functions. For example, nurses are able to administer antibiotics only after receiving a order. Other actions, however, are independent actions. Assisting a breastfeeding client with engorged breasts and cracked nipples and providing a sitz bath for a client with hemorrhoids are independent actions that often are addressed in protocols or preprinted order sets because they are commonly seen. Because foul-smelling lochia is an uncommon finding that could represent an infection, the provider must be notified for a decision on antibiotics.

34. 1. Abdominal striae are stretch marks. They are a normal side effect of pregnancy.
   2. Oliguria is a complication that may develop after surgery, but it is not a symptom of paralytic ileus.
   3. An omphalocele is a herniation of the intestines into the umbilical cord. It is sometimes seen in newborns.
   4. **An absence of bowel sounds may indicate that a client has a paralytic ileus.**

TEST-TAKING HINT: One of the complications of surgery and/or anesthesia is a paralytic ileus, the cessation of intestinal peristalsis. Clients may complain of nausea, bloating, and abdominal pain. Some studies have shown that gum-chewing provides a "sham" feeding that may stimulate the intestines to resume peristalsis (Cagir, 2018). Other than that, the client should be given nothing by mouth until the bowels begin moving. Among other interventions, a nasogastric

tube may be inserted to provide relief. Nursing interventions may include the suggestion to reduce the amount of narcotics taken for pain, and use nonsteroidal anti-inflammatory drugs (NSAIDs) instead, as this can reduce the inflammation that may contribute to paralytic ileus (Cagir, 2018).

35. 1. **This output is below the accepted minimum for 8 hours.**
2. This weight decrease following delivery is within normal limits.
3. A 2% drop in hematocrit is within normal limits.
4. This pulse rate is within normal limits.

TEST-TAKING HINT: The nurse must calculate the hourly urine output by dividing the amount of urine output by the number of hours. The output in the scenario is equal to 25 mL/hr. This is below the therapeutic output of 30 mL/ hr. Because this is a postpartum client, the nurse would expect high urinary outputs since diuresis is expected to have begun at this time. Postpartum clients often have slowed heartbeats, so the heart rate is within normal limits.

36. 1. One side effect of the medication is an elevation in blood pressure. This blood pressure shows that no adverse side effects have resulted from the administration of the medication.
2. Pulse rate is unrelated to the administration of the medication.
3. **The fundal response indicates that the medication was effective in contracting the uterus.**
4. The prothrombin time is unrelated to the administration of the medication.

TEST-TAKING HINT: A "grand multip" is a woman who has had 5 or more births at 20 weeks' gestation or more, whether live or stillborn. These clients are at high risk of uterine atony after the birth. Methylergonovine is an oxytocic agent. It is administered after delivery if the uterus is atonic or if the client is at high risk for uterine atony. When the uterus is noted to be well contracted and at the appropriate position in the abdomen, the nurse can conclude that the medication action was effective.

37. 1. Both the spinal anesthesia and the epidural anesthesia clients are at high risk for developing pruritus.
2. Both the spinal anesthesia and the epidural anesthesia clients are at high risk for developing nausea.
3. **The client who has had the spinal anesthesia is much more likely to develop a postural headache than a client who had epidural anesthesia.**
4. Both the spinal anesthesia and the epidural anesthesia clients are at high risk for developing respiratory depression.

TEST-TAKING HINT: Both spinal anesthesia and epidural anesthesia are forms of regional anesthesia. The same medication is used and it is placed at the same vertebral level in both instances. Both spinal and epidural anesthesia can cause a spinal headache, although the risk is higher with spinal anesthesia. With epidural anesthesia, medication is injected just outside the dura, the covering of the spinal cord. The medication passes through the dura to the nerves by osmosis, to produce pain relief. With an epidural, the dura may be unintentionally nicked before the epidural space is located.

With spinal anesthesia, the needle is passed through the dura and medication is injected into the cerebrospinal space, itself. Although the hole made by the needle is exceptionally small, the cerebrospinal fluid (CSF) sometimes leaks out after a spinal.

If the dura is nicked during an epidural, or if CSF leaks out after a spinal, the severe headache that follows when the client is upright is thought to be from traction on the meninges and meningeal vessels due to the loss of CSF and the reduction in brain cushioning (Agerson & Scavone, 2012). A blood patch, where the anesthesia provider injects some of the client's own blood into the space to form a clot and block the site of leakage (a procedure much like the original spinal or epidural), is often helpful to stop the headache.

38. 1. **The client with postpartum psychosis will experience hallucinations.**
2. Clients with diabetes mellitus, not postpartum psychosis, are polyphagic.
3. Clients with bulimia induce vomiting.
4. Clients with postpartum blues and/or postpartum depression are weepy and sad.

TEST-TAKING HINT: Clients who have been diagnosed with postpartum psychosis have a psychiatric disease. They experience hallucinations, usually auditory, including voices that may tell them to kill their babies. They should never be left alone with their babies.

39. Answers 1, 2, and 5 are correct.
1. **This answer is correct. She should gently massage the area toward the nipple.**

2. **The woman should apply warm soaks to the breast during feedings.**
3. The woman should be advised to feed her baby frequently at the breast. She should not be advised to bottle feed.
4. The woman should apply lanolin to sore or cracked nipples. It will not help prevent nodules.
5. **To promote emptying of the nodules, she should be advised to feed from the affected side first. This is because the baby's initial breastfeeding efforts are more vigorous than they may be toward the end of the feeding as the baby becomes sated and sleepy.**

TEST-TAKING HINT: A client who palpates a tender, hard nodule in her lactating breast is experiencing milk stasis. The stasis may be related to a blocked milk duct. It is very important that the woman gently massage the nodule while applying warm soaks and while feeding her baby to prevent mastitis from developing. She should not skip breastfeedings but rather should breastfeed frequently.

40. 1. **If the woman has manually removed milk from her breasts, her breasts will soften to the touch.**
2. If the baby is latched well, he should swallow after every suck.
3. The nurse would expect the baby to transfer 60 mL or more at the feeding.
4. The mother should not squeeze her nipple. The area behind the areola should be gently compressed.

TEST-TAKING HINT: This client is complaining of engorgement. The baby is having difficulty latching because the breast is swollen and inflamed, making the nipple tense and short. When the woman manually removes a small amount of the foremilk, the breast becomes softer and the nipple becomes easier for the baby to grasp. As a result, the milk ejection reflex is stimulated and the baby transfers more milk successfully.

41. 1. The results are not normal. This client's blood pressure is markedly elevated and the client is hyperreflexic.
2. **The nurse should notify the physician of the signs of pre-eclampsia.**
3. There is no need to discontinue the intravenous infusion.
4. The findings are consistent with signs of pre-eclampsia. It would be inappropriate to wait 15 minutes to verify the results before notifying the provider.

TEST-TAKING HINT: The hypertensive illnesses of pregnancy can develop at any time after 20 weeks' gestation through about 2 weeks postpartum. This client is exhibiting a late onset of pre-eclampsia—markedly elevated blood pressure and hyperreflexia. The physician should be notified as soon as possible of the changes. The American College of Obstetricians & Gynecologists (ACOG) defines hypertension as a systolic BP (SBP) of 140 mm Hg or greater, or a diastolic BP (DBP) of 90 mm Hg or greater on 2 occasions, 4 hours apart (ACOG, 2013b). It is important to note that a client is diagnosed with hypertension if either the SBP or DBP is high, as an independent reading; both of them do not need to be elevated for the diagnosis of hypertension. Severe hypertension is defined as an SBP of 160 mm Hg or greater, or a DBP of 110 mm Hg or greater (ACOG, 2013b). It is further recommended that every obstetrical unit develop a protocol for hypertensive emergencies, in which there is a preprinted order for the nurse to administer an antihypertensive medication immediately if a client's blood pressure remains in the severe hypertensive range for more than 15 minutes (ACOG, 2013b).

42. 1. This response is incorrect. Rh immune globulin (RhIG) must be administered within 72 hours of delivery to prevent the formation of antibodies.
2. **This response is correct. The nurse should not discharge an Rh– (negative) client whose baby was Rh+ (positive) until the client has received her Rh immune globulin (RhIG) injection.**
3. This response is incorrect. A negative direct Coombs test means that no maternal antibodies were detected in the baby's circulatory system, indicating the baby is not currently at risk due to Rh incompatibility. The nurse would expect to detect a negative direct Coombs test.
4. This response is unacceptable. Rh– (negative) clients should receive their Rh immune globulin (RhIG) injection before 72 hours postpartum or by discharge, whichever is earlier.

TEST-TAKING HINT: The administration of Rh immune globulin (RhIG) is the only way to prevent an Rh– (negative) client's body from mounting a full antibody response to the delivery of an Rh+ (positive) baby at some point in the future. It is malpractice for a nurse to discharge the client before she receives her injection or to delay the injection beyond the 72-hour deadline.

43. 1. This is inappropriate. Naming the baby is a means of acknowledging both the existence and the death of the baby.
2. This is inappropriate. Clients' imaginings of what the baby looks like are often much worse than the reality.
3. This is inappropriate. The couple should be provided time to be with their baby before transporting the baby to the morgue.
4. This is appropriate. The small mementos will provide the couple with something tangible to remember the pregnancy and baby by.

TEST-TAKING HINT: The experience of birth is very difficult for parents who have delivered a stillborn baby. The only contact they have had with the baby is through the pregnancy. Small mementos, such as a picture, a lock of hair, or the baby's bracelet, provide the parents with tangible remembrances of the baby. In addition, even when physical defects are present, the parents should be offered the option of viewing and holding their baby. They may still recognize family resemblances, which will help them with bonding.

44. 1. The client with a placenta accreta is at high risk for a large blood loss.
2. Placenta accreta is not related to a hypertensive state.
3. Placenta accreta is not related to the development of jaundice.
4. The nurse would not expect to detect a shortened prothrombin time when a client has a placenta accreta.

TEST-TAKING HINT: A placenta accreta's chorionic villi burrow through the endometrial lining into the myometrial lining. Separation of the placenta from the uterine wall is severely hampered. Clients often lose large quantities of blood, and it is not uncommon for the physician to have to perform a hysterectomy to control the bleeding. Clients who have had multiple uterine scars are especially at high risk for this problem. If the test taker were unfamiliar with placenta accreta, they could deduce the answer because the placenta is highly vascular and only one answer referred to a vascular issue. The average blood loss during a cesarean delivery is 1,000 mL.

45. 20 mL per dose.
Standard formula:

$$\frac{\text{Known dosage}}{\text{Known volume}} = \frac{\text{Desired dosage}}{\text{Desired volume}}$$

$$\frac{125 \text{ mg}}{5 \text{ mL}} = \frac{500 \text{ mg}}{x \text{ mL}}$$

$$125x = 5 \times 500$$
$$125x = 2{,}500$$
$$x = 20 \text{ mL per dose}$$

Dimensional analysis formula:

Dimensional analysis method for calculating the volume of medication to be administered:

$$\frac{\text{Known volume}}{\text{Known dosage}} \bigg| \frac{\text{Desired dosage}}{} = \text{Desired volume}$$

$$\frac{5 \text{ mL}}{125 \text{ mg}} \bigg| \frac{500 \text{ mg}}{} = x \text{ mL}$$

$x = 20$ mL per dose

TEST-TAKING HINT: The nurse must remember that a dose is defined as the quantity of medication that is administered to a client at one time. The client, then, is to receive 500 mg, or 20 mL, of the medication at each administration.

46. 1. A magnesium level of 7 mg/dL is therapeutic. This is an expected level.
2. The serum sodium level is normal.
3. The serum potassium is below normal. The nurse should report the finding to the physician.
4. The serum calcium is normal.

TEST-TAKING HINT: The nurse should be familiar with the normal values of commonly tested electrolytes. Although the normal magnesium level is 1.8 to 3 mg/dL, magnesium sulfate is being administered to raise the level in the client's bloodstream to a therapeutic level in order to prevent further seizures. The potassium level, however, is below the normal level of 3.5 to 5 mg/dL.

47. 1. Breastfeeding is contraindicated when a mother is HIV positive.
2. It is recommended that HIV-positive clients use condoms for family planning.
3. It is unnecessary to take her temperature every morning. If she should develop a fever, she should seek medical assistance as soon as possible, however.
4. The client should seek care for a recent weight loss. This may be a symptom of AIDS.

TEST-TAKING HINT: Although obstetric clients who enter the hospital are usually aware of their HIV status, the nurse must still review the actions that clients should take after discharge. These actions include taking all medications, bottle feeding rather than breastfeeding, using condoms during intercourse, and reporting any changes in health, such as weight loss or the appearance of thrush.

48. 1. When a client has DVT she is clotting excessively. She is not at high risk for hemorrhage.
2. The client is at high risk for stroke if a clot should travel to the brain through the vascular tree.
3. The client is not at high risk for endometritis if she has DVT.
4. The client is not at high risk for hematoma if she has DVT.

TEST-TAKING HINT: The test taker could deduce the answer to this question by determining the etiology of each of the problems. The only complication that is caused by a clot, which is the same etiology as the DVT, is a stroke.

49. 1. This client is not especially at high risk for seizures.
2. The client should be monitored carefully for signs of postpartum hemorrhage.
3. This client is not especially at high risk for infection.
4. This client is not especially at high risk for thrombosis.

TEST-TAKING HINT: An average sized baby weighs 2,500 to 4,000 grams. The baby in the scenario is macrosomic. As a result, the mother's uterus has been stretched beyond its expected capacity. In addition, this client is a "grand multipara" or a woman who has delivered 5 or more babies. The client is at high risk for uterine atony, which could result in a postpartum hemorrhage.

50. 1. Metoclopromide is an antiemetic. It is not the appropriate medication for this client.
2. Ondansetron is an antiemetic. It is not the appropriate medication for this client.
3. Prochlorperazine is an antiemetic. It is not the appropriate medication for this client.
4. Diphenhydramine is an antihistamine. It is the drug of choice for this client who has pruritus and a rash.

TEST-TAKING HINT: To answer this question, the test taker must first determine what the client's clinical problem is and then determine which medication will relieve that problem. The test taker, therefore, must be familiar with the actions of major medications. The client is exhibiting signs of an allergic response. Diphenhydramine is the only choice that will inhibit the client's immune response.

51. 1. Chamomile tea has not been shown to potentiate the effect of sertraline, but St. John's wort has been shown to have that effect.
2. The therapeutic effect of selective serotonin reuptake inhibitors (SSRIs) such as sertraline is delayed about 4 to 6 weeks from the time the medication is initiated.
3. This response is incorrect. The medication can be crushed.
4. A 10-lb weight gain is not associated with the medication.

TEST-TAKING HINT: Clients who receive medications for emotional problems as well as for physiological complaints expect to experience resolution of their symptoms in a timely fashion. If clients with postpartum depression are not forewarned of the delay of the therapeutic effects, they may stop taking the medications prematurely, believing that the medicines are useless.

52. 1. The nurse would not expect to see engorgement.
2. The nurse would not expect to see mastitis.
3. The nurse would not expect to see a blocked milk duct.
4. The nurse would expect that the woman would have a low milk supply.

TEST-TAKING HINT: The placenta produces the hormones of pregnancy, including estrogen and progesterone. When placental fragments are retained, those hormones are still being produced. Estrogen inhibits prolactin, which is the hormone of lactogenesis, or milk production. Women who have retained placental fragments, therefore, often complain of an insufficient milk supply for their babies. Women with retained placental fragments are also at high risk for postpartum hemorrhage and intrauterine infection.

53. 1. The woman should not wash with soap. Soaps destroy the natural lanolins produced by the body.
2. A small amount of lanolin should be applied to the nipple after each feeding.
3. The baby will not become sick from the blood. The woman should be warned that he may spit up digested and/or undigested blood after the feeding, however.

4. Topical anesthetics are not used on the breasts. The woman could receive an oral analgesic, however.

TEST-TAKING HINT: Using lanolin on the breasts is a type of moist wound healing. The lanolin is soothing and allows the nipple to heal without a scab developing on the surface of the nipple. Mothers are often very concerned about their babies swallowing the blood. Ingesting the blood does not adversely affect the babies unless, of course, the mother is HIV positive or carries another bloodborne virus. Other approaches to assist in nipple healing include gel coverings for the nipples so they do not rub against the bra.

54. 1. A circumvallate placenta is a placenta with an inner ring created by a fold in the chorion and amnion. Clients with this type of placenta are at high risk for antepartal complications like preterm labor.
2. A succenturiate placenta is characterized by one primary placenta that is attached via blood vessels to satellite lobe(s). Clients with this type of placenta are at high risk for postpartum hemorrhage.
3. A placenta with a vellamentous insertion has an umbilical cord that is formed a distance from the placenta. Because the vessels are unsupported between the placenta and the cord, hemorrhage may result if one or more of the vessels tears.
4. The battledore placenta is characterized by an umbilical cord that is inserted on the periphery of the placenta. Clients with this type of placenta are at high risk for preterm problems like preterm labor and hemorrhage.

TEST-TAKING HINT: There are a number of placental variations. The test taker should become familiar with each of the variations and the high-risk nature of each.

55. **1. The goal of the injection of Rh immune globulin (RhIG) is to inhibit the mother's immune response.**
2. Immune globulin is composed of antibodies. When a client receives Rh immune globulin (RhIG), she receives passive antibodies to inhibit her immune response.
3. Passive antibodies cannot prevent the migration of fetal cells throughout the mother's bloodstream.
4. A client's blood type is determined by her DNA. Rh immune globulin (RhIG) cannot change a client's DNA.

TEST-TAKING HINT: When a client receives Rh immune globulin (RhIG), she receives passive Rh antibodies. If any Rh antigen is circulating in the mother's bloodstream, the injected antibodies will destroy it. As a result, there will be no antigen in the mother's body to stimulate her mast cells to have an active antibody response. In essence, therefore, Rh immune globulin (RhIG) is injected to inhibit the client's immune response and to prevent her body from "seeing" and producing her own antibodies against that antigen in the future. It is given after each possible exposure to Rh positive blood.

56. 1. The client who states "I hate myself. I caused my baby to be sick" is voicing anger at herself.
2. The client who states "I'll take him to a specialist. Then he will get better" is exhibiting the bargaining stage of grief.
3. The client who states, "I can't seem to stop crying" is exhibiting signs of depression.
4. The client who states "This can't be happening" is exhibiting denial.

TEST-TAKING HINT: Although clients do not go through the stages of grief linearly, they do express the many stages of grief while they mourn the loss of their child of fantasy. Bargaining is a particularly vulnerable time for parents. Unscrupulous practitioners can make a great deal of money from couples who believe that their child can be cured from "special medicines" or "procedures."

57. 1. This client in high-Fowler's position is no more at high risk for postpartum hemorrhage than a spinal anesthesia client who has been kept flat after surgery.
2. The nurse would expect the client to complain of a severe postural headache.
3. This client is no more at high risk for a pruritic rash than a spinal anesthesia client who has been kept flat after surgery.
4. This client is no more at high risk for paralytic ileus than a spinal anesthesia client who has been kept flat after surgery.

TEST-TAKING HINT: Postpartum hemorrhage, pruritic rash, and paralytic ileus are complications seen in post–cesarean section clients, whether they received general anesthesia, epidural anesthesia, or spinal anesthesia. Clients who received spinal anesthesia and sit upright soon after surgery are especially at risk for postural headaches as explained in question #37.

58. 1. Vitamin K is the antidote for warfarin overdose, not for heparin overdose.
2. Protamine is the antidote for heparin overdose.
3. Vitamin E is not correct.
4. Mannitol is not correct.

TEST-TAKING HINT: When heparin is administered, clients must be monitored carefully for signs of hemorrhage. Protamine is the antidote for heparin overdose. Conversely, the antidote for warfarin, another medication often administered to clients with DVT, is vitamin K.

59. **1. The client should have a glucose tolerance test done at about 6 weeks postpartum. Women who give birth to hypoglycemic and/or macrosomic babies may have had undiagnosed gestational diabetes and are at increased risk of developing type 2 diabetes mellitus (T2DM).**
2. There is no indication in the scenario of Rh incompatibility that would require that an indirect Coombs test be done.
3. There is no indication in the scenario that this client has impaired kidney function and should have a BUN done.
4. There is no indication in the scenario that this client should have a CBC done. There is no indication of anemia or infection.

TEST-TAKING HINT: The baby born to this mother is macrosomic and hypoglycemic. The most common cause of these two neonatal complications is maternal diabetes. It is recommended that mothers who develop diabetes during pregnancy and are diagnosed with gestational diabetes, be assessed for type 2 diabetes mellitus (T2DM) at about 6 weeks postpartum. These clients must be made aware that because of their pancreatic insufficiency, women diagnosed with gestational diabetes have a 19% probability of developing T2DM within 9 years after the initial diagnosis (Feig et al., 2008). See the appendix for more information on diabetes.

60. **Answers 1, 2, 3, and 5 are correct.**
1. The nurse must check the client's blood type.
2. The nurse must check the client's name by checking the bracelet and asking the client her name.
3. The nurse must compare the client's blood type with the blood type on the infusion bag.
4. The nurse must obtain an infusion of normal saline, not dextrose and water.
5. The time the infusion begins and ends must be documented.

TEST-TAKING HINT: The potential for blood transfusion incompatibility is very real. It is essential, therefore, that the client's vital signs are checked first for a baseline. Then, two healthcare practitioners independently confirm everything related to the unit of blood to make sure that the client is receiving the correct blood. This means the first nurse doesn't simply read out the information to the second nurse, but each nurse takes the time to confirm the information independently. A special filtered infusion set must be used. If any sign of a reaction should develop, the transfusion should be stopped immediately and steps taken to inform both the provider and the lab.

Only normal saline solution is used as a solution immediately before or after blood administration. Dextrose in water is not used. It will hemolyze the red blood cells. Intravenous solutions containing calcium, such as Lactated Ringers's solution, may contribute to clot formation.

61. **Answers 2 and 5 are correct.**
1. Preterm labor clients are not especially at high risk for postpartum hemorrhage.
2. Clients who have had a prolonged first stage of labor are at high risk for postpartum hemorrhage (PPH).
3. Cesarean section clients are not especially at high risk for PPH.
4. Postdates clients who deliver small babies are not especially at high risk for PPH.
5. Clients with a succenturiate placenta are at high risk for PPH.

TEST-TAKING HINT: The muscles of the uterus of a client who has experienced a prolonged first stage of labor are fatigued. As a result, in the postpartum period the uterus may fail to contract fully enough to control bleeding at the site of placental separation. A succenturiate placenta is characterized by one primary placenta that is attached via blood vessels to satellite lobe(s). These clients are at risk for retained placental fragments and as a result, they must be monitored carefully for postpartum hemorrhage.

62. 1. Hydralazine is administered as an antihypertensive, not as an antiseizure medication. Magnesium sulfate is the drug administered as an anticonvulsant to women with eclampsia.
2. Hydralazine is an antihypertensive. The change in blood pressure indicates that the medication is effective.
3. The weight loss is secondary to fluid loss.
4. The hydralazine is not administered to treat a headache.

TEST-TAKING HINT: Hydralazine is an antihypertensive medication. Antihypertensive medications are administered to pre-eclamptic and eclamptic women. In the past, magnesium sulfate was thought by some to both lower the blood pressure and to prevent seizures. That was only partially correct, since the goal of magnesium sulfate is focused only on preventing seizures. The goal of antihypertensives is to lower the blood pressure. A change in BP from 160/120 to 130/90 is evidence of a therapeutic effect.

63. 1. Lochia serosa at 2 weeks postpartum is unusual, but it does not put the client or her baby in imminent danger.
2. This client is exhibiting signs of postpartum depression. This is a problem that must be remedied, but it does not put the client or her baby in imminent danger.
3. The client's cracked nipples do need intervention, but they do not put the client or her baby in imminent danger.
4. The client is exhibiting inappropriate behavior when she yells at the baby for crying. The nurse must make additional assessments to determine whether there is any other evidence of abuse or neglect.

TEST-TAKING HINT: The baby is the most vulnerable member of the mother–infant dyad. Because the baby is completely dependent on the care of the mother, if the nurse discovers any behavior or other evidence that makes him or her suspicious of child abuse or neglect, the nurse is obligated both morally and legally to report the situation. Clients who are experiencing postpartum depression usually perform baby care competently, and hostile behavior toward the baby is not a symptom of depression.

64. 1. The nurse should call a code before beginning rescue breathing.
2. The nurse should call a code first and then discontinue the medication.
3. The nurse should call a code first to shorten the time before the team arrives.
4. The nurse should call a code before checking the carotid pulse.

TEST-TAKING HINT: Nurses should call a code as soon as they discover a client who is nonresponsive. Immediately after calling the code, the nurse should stop the medications, begin rescue breathing, and provide chest compressions if necessary, until the code team arrives. The nurse cannot resuscitate the client alone. Precious time can be lost if the nurse begins interventions before calling for assistance.

Calcium gluconate is the antidote to magnesium sulfate toxicity. It should be administered only if an order for the medication has been given by a primary healthcare provider, or in specific situations as indicated on the provider's orders.

65. 1. Infection, as suggested by hyperthermia, is the priority condition, not ineffective breastfeeding.
2. Infection, as suggested by hyperthermia, is the priority condition. A temperature of 104.6° F (40.3° C) as well as the client's other signs/symptoms should immediately suggest the presence of infection.
3. Infection, as suggested by hyperthermia is the priority condition, not emotional distress.
4. Infection, as suggested by hyperthermia, is the priority condition, not pain.

TEST-TAKING HINT: This client has a breast abscess. Although all of the conditions are important, the highest priority is the infection. A serious infection can lead to sepsis, which can be life threatening. As such, treatment of the infection is the highest priority since it can affect client survival. It is the only one of the four conditions that is related to the acute problem of fever and pain. Ineffective breastfeeding contributed to the development of the infection. Because of the infection, the client is in pain and is in emotional distress. Once the abscess is drained and the antibiotics have been administered, the other three diagnoses will be on the road to being resolved.

66. 800 units/hour.

The standard formula to determine the number of units that the client is receiving per hour is:

total number of units : mL of IV solution = x units : flow rate

First, ½ liter must be converted to mL:

$$1{,}000 \text{ mL} : 1 \text{ liter} = x : \tfrac{1}{2} \text{ liter}$$
$$x = 500 \text{ mL}$$
$$25{,}000 \text{ units} : 500 \text{ mL} = x \text{ units} : 16 \text{ mL/hr}$$
$$500 \text{ mL } x = 25{,}000 \text{ units} \times 16 \text{ mL/hr}$$
$$x = \frac{25{,}000 \times 16}{500}$$
$$x = 800 \text{ units/hr}$$

The dimensional analysis formula to determine the number of units that the client is receiving per hour is:

$$\frac{\text{Known dosage}}{\text{Known volume}} \times \frac{\text{Desired volume/hr}}{} \times \frac{\text{Unit conversion}}{\text{(if needed)}} \times \frac{\text{Time conversion}}{\text{(if needed)}} = \text{Desired dosage/hr}$$

$$\frac{25{,}000 \text{ units}}{\tfrac{1}{2} \text{ liter}} \times \frac{16 \text{ mL/hr}}{} \times \frac{1 \text{ liter}}{1{,}000 \text{ mL}} = x \text{ units per hr}$$

$$x = \frac{25{,}000}{500 \text{ mL}} \times 16$$

$$x = 800 \text{ units/hr}$$

TEST-TAKING HINT: To calculate the amount correctly, the test taker can label each number and cancel to make sure that the result is in the units requested. As can be seen in the formula, the mLs drop out and the values that are left are units/hr.

67. 1. A heavy lochial flow would indicate that the action was unsuccessful.
2. Decreased pain is not an expected outcome of uterine massage for uterine atony.
3. A stable postpartum blood pressure is not directly related to the action of uterine massage.
4. **The expected outcome would be a well-contracted uterus at or below the umbilicus.**

TEST-TAKING HINT: Expected outcomes relate to specific hypotheses that are developed after making an assessment. This client's uterine muscle was boggy, also referred to as atonic. The nursing action taken—the massage—related directly to the nursing assessment and hypothesis—an atonic uterus. The outcome of a well-contracted uterus indicates the action was successful. It is important to assess outcomes based on their connection to the intended goal of the intervention.

68. 1. **This rationale is correct. Because of an elevation in clotting factors, all postpartum clients are at high risk for thrombus formation.**
2. The intermittent positive pressure boots improve blood return to the heart by preventing pooling of blood in the extremities. They are not applied to treat hypovolemia.
3. The rationale for the use of intermittent positive pressure boots is not related to varicose vein development. Varicose veins would, however, increase a client's potential for developing deep vein thrombosis.
4. The rationale for the use of intermittent positive pressure boots is not related to a client's potential for footdrop.

TEST-TAKING HINT: The client in the scenario is post–cesarean section. The surgeon has ordered intermittent positive pressure boots for her because she is at high risk for thrombus formation for two reasons: She is on bedrest and there is a proliferation of clotting factors in all pregnant and postpartum women. Clients who deliver vaginally do not need the boots, because they are able to ambulate immediately after delivery and, therefore, rarely experience pooling of blood in their extremities.

69. **1. Metoclopromide is an antiemetic. It is one of the drugs that may be administered to a client who is vomiting after surgery.**
2. Meperidine is a narcotic analgesic. It is not the appropriate medication for this client.
3. Secobarbital is a sedative. It is not the appropriate medication for this client.
4. Diphenhydramine is an antihistamine. It is not the appropriate medication for this client.

TEST-TAKING HINT: This client is exhibiting a common side effect of regional anesthesia: nausea and vomiting. Antiemetics are the medications of choice for this problem. Many prn medications are ordered for postsurgical clients. The nurse must become familiar with the actions and the uses of each of them.

70. 1. The nurse should monitor the client for signs of infection after the first 24 hours have passed.
2. The client is not at high risk for bloody urine.
3. **The client should be monitored carefully for heavy lochia.**
4. The client is not at high risk for rectal abrasions.

TEST-TAKING HINT: The key to answering this question is the time frame stipulated in the stem of the question—"the immediate postpartum period." There are two main maternal complications associated with forceps use: hemorrhage and infection. Hemorrhage after forceps delivery usually occurs early, secondary to cervical, vaginal, or perineal lacerations that occur during the forceps use. Infection usually develops later in the postpartum period secondary to contamination of the uterine cavity during the application of the forceps.

71. **1. It is essential that the client never be left alone with her baby.**
2. The statement is untrue. There is no set time frame for the resolution of the symptoms of postpartum psychosis.
3. Clinical response to medications is usually quite good.
4. The client's vital signs need not be assessed frequently.

TEST-TAKING HINT: Clients who have been diagnosed with postpartum psychosis have been known to have homicidal and suicidal ideations. Because the baby and other children are vulnerable, the mother should always be supervised when in their presence. In addition, if she exhibits suicidal behaviors, she should be supervised at all times.

72. **1. Methylergonovine is contraindicated for this client.**
2. Magnesium sulfate is the drug of choice for the treatment of pre-eclampsia with severe features.
3. Ibuprofen is a nonsteroidal anti-inflammatory drug (NSAID). It is an appropriate medication for the treatment of postpartum cramping. It is not contraindicated for this client.
4. Morphine sulfate is a narcotic analgesic. It is an appropriate medication for the treatment of postsurgical pain. It is not contraindicated for this client.

TEST-TAKING HINT: Methylergonovine is an oxytocic agent. It acts directly on the myofibrils of the uterus. Secondarily, it also contracts the muscles of the vascular tree. As a result, clients' blood pressures tend to rise when they receive this medication. Methylergonovine should not be administered to a client whose blood pressure is 130/90 or higher. Although this client's blood pressures are not given, the nurse must be aware that hypertension is part of the diagnosis for a client with pre-eclampsia with severe features. As such, methylergonovine is never appropriate for these clients.

73. 1. This father is grieving. His anger is appropriate at this time, even though his behavior is disconcerting.
2. **This action is appropriate. The nurse is acknowledging that every member of the family is grieving the loss.**
3. Five-year-old children do not understand death. They do, however, respond to their parents' unusual behaviors.
4. This is not the nurse's decision to make. Even though it is very difficult for the parents to deal with their own grief while caring for their daughter, the young girl may feel abandoned if sent unexpectedly to her grandparents.

TEST-TAKING HINT: Each member of a family will grieve differently. One of the important actions for the nurse is to help the members of the family to communicate with one another. Children do not understand the finality of death until about age 9, but pre–school age children often feel guilty when bad things happen. It is important for the nurse to communicate clearly that the child was not responsible for the death of the fetus.

74. 1. Stating, "Thank goodness. It could have been untreatable," inappropriate. Any defect is devastating for the parents to accept.
2. Stating, "I'm so happy that you have other children who are healthy" is inappropriate. *This* child is affected. That is all that matters.
3. Stating, "These things happen. They are the will of God," is inappropriate. The nurse must not impose personal beliefs on the couple.
4. Stating, "Tears are understandable at a time like this," is appropriate. It gives the client permission to express her grief.

TEST-TAKING HINT: Nurses must be very careful how they speak with and care for clients who have had a baby with a chronic condition. Everyone expects to have a "perfect baby." When a baby is born with a condition that requires special treatment, the couple must grieve their perfectly normal "baby of fantasy" while they bond with and accept their "baby of reality." It is important to understand that their grief may also include the pain and suffering they anticipate for their child.

75. 1. If the mother states, "I'm so tired. Please feed the baby in the nursery for me," it may be a true statement, but it may also communicate the mother's difficulty with accepting her baby.
2. If the mother states, "Her eyes look like mine, but her chin is her dad's," it indicates positive maternal bonding.
3. If the mother states, "We have decided to name her Sarah after my mother," it indicates positive maternal bonding.
4. If the mother states, "I breastfed her, but I still need help swaddling her," it indicates positive maternal bonding.

TEST-TAKING HINT: Babies with defects are more likely to be victims of child abuse and neglect than are healthy, normal babies. Nurses must evaluate the bonding between the mother and her baby. If the nurse is concerned about the bonding relationship, the mother's care must be monitored and, if necessary, the family must be referred for a home-care nurse evaluation and/or to child protective services.

76. 18 mL/hour.

The standard formula for determining the flow rate is:

Total number of units : mL of IV solution = Units/min : x flow rate
20,000 units : 500 mL = 12 units/min : x mL/hr

Because the order is written in units/min, the test taker must determine how many units the client is receiving per hour:

(12 units/min × 60 min/hr = 720 units/hr)
20,000 units : 500 mL = 720 units/hr : x
20,000 x units = 500 mL × 720 units/hr

$$x = \frac{500 \text{ mL} \times 720 \text{ units/hr}}{20{,}000 \text{ units}}$$

$$x = 18 \text{ mL/hr}$$

The dimensional analysis formula for determining the flow rate is:

Known volume	Desired dosage/min	Unit conversion	Time conversion	
Known dosage		(if needed)	(if needed)	= Volume/hr

500 mL	12 units/min	60 min	
20,000 units		1 hr	= x units per hr

$$x = \frac{360{,}000}{20{,}000}$$

$$x = 18 \text{ mL/ hr}$$

TEST-TAKING HINT: The test taker must remember that pumps are always programmed in mL/hr. Because the question included a rate of units/min, to calculate the pump rate, units/min had to be converted to units/hr. In addition, it must be remembered that per a Joint Commission on Accreditation of Hospitals directive, the word "units" must always be written out fully—that is, not abbreviated as "U."

77. 1. The PT is normal; it should be longer when a client is taking warfarin. For someone taking warfarin, the PT time should be prolonged 1.5 to 2 times normal.

2. Normal INR is 1 to 1.4. A therapeutic range following pulmonary embolism is between 2 and 3. An INR of 4 puts a person at risk of hemorrhage.

3. The hematocrit is elevated. It should be within normal limits.

4. The hemoglobin is below normal. It should be within normal limits.

TEST-TAKING HINT: The PT and/or INR are monitored during warfarin treatment to determine whether the dose of medication is effective. Warfarin is a vitamin K antagonist, meaning it interferes with the clotting of blood. This can be helpful in certain situations such as pulmonary embolism, when further clot formation must be slowed or prevented.

A prothrombin time (PT) is a test specifically made to test the effectiveness of warfarin. It measures the therapeutic effectiveness of the dose by the number of seconds it takes for a person's blood to form a blood clot. Normal time for a person not on warfarin is between 10 to 13 seconds. For a client on warfarin, the therapeutic time is 1½ to 2 times normal, or at least 15 to 20 seconds to form a clot. If the PT is more than 2 times normal or the international normalized ratio (INR) is over 3, the client is at high risk for hemorrhage.

Because various reagents are used for this test and can alter the PT times, the World Health Organization introduced an international normalized ratio (INR) to calculate from the PT result. This allows standardization of results, regardless of the reagent that was used. Often, just the INR is reported, not the PT value.

78. 1. The drop in estrogen is not related to the glucose level.

2. The drop in progesterone is not related to the glucose level.

3. The drop in human placental lactogen (hPL) is related to the glucose level.

4. The drop in human chorionic gonadotropin (hCG) is not related to the glucose level.

TEST-TAKING HINT: It is not uncommon for the glucose levels of clients with type 1 diabetes mellitus (T1DM) to be within normal limits for a day or so after delivery, as seen in this client. The hormone hPL is an insulin antagonist produced by the placenta throughout pregnancy. As the placenta grows and the hPL levels rise, the mother's body becomes more and more insulin resistant, causing her blood sugar to rise. Because her cells resist insulin's effects, they begin to use stored fats for energy and less glucose. The glucose is effectively transferred to the fetus through the placenta. This contributes to fetal growth and development.

Throughout pregnancy, the insulin needs of clients with T1DM rise incrementally as the levels of hPL in the bloodstream rise. Once the placenta is delivered, the levels of hPL drop precipitously and the cells become more sensitive to insulin. The client with T1DM may see that her glucose levels are within normal limits for hours or days after delivery and she may not initially need insulin injections (Achong et al., 2014). Experts are not certain of all the factors involved, but have suggested that the sudden reduction in insulin resistance could play a role in prolonging the pharmacological action of the insulin the client received during the intrapartum phase, especially related to long- and intermediate-acting insulin (Achong et al., 2014).

The nurse must be aware that clients with diabetes are at risk of hypoglycemia during the postpartum period as insulin is reintroduced. Hypoglycemia can also occur during breastfeeding, and the client needs education about this before discharge.

79. 1. It is unnecessary to wean the baby to formula.

2. Optimally, the baby should stay in the hospital room with the mother.

3. It is unnecessary for the mother to pump and dump for 2 weeks.

4. Although the baby could drink milk stored by the mother, this is not the best solution.

TEST-TAKING HINT: Other than the period of time that the mother is in the surgical suite, it is unlikely that anything would warrant separating the mother from her baby. The surgeon and anesthesiologist should be able to prescribe medicines that are compatible with breastfeeding. The client can easily breastfeed her baby while lying in a comfortable, side-lying position. The client should be admitted to a private, post-surgical hospital room with a crib or bassinet for the newborn. Many hospitals require the 24-hour presence of a family member or friend

with exclusive responsibility for the baby, until the mother can assume total care. The family is also expected to bring their own supplies for baby care, since the baby is not a client of the hospital.

80. Answers 1, 2, and 4 are correct.

1. **Swaddling the baby in a baby blanket is an appropriate action. The baby should be handled with respect as any living baby would be.**
2. **Discussing funeral options for the baby is an appropriate action toward the end of the family's time with their baby. Funerals provide a means for clients and their community of family and friends to celebrate the baby's short life and to support the parents in acknowledging the baby's death.**
3. It is inappropriate to encourage the couple to try to get pregnant again in the near future. This is none of the nurse's business. The couple must grieve the loss of this child.
4. **It is appropriate to ask the couple if they would like to hold the baby. Although there are some clients who will decline to hold their babies, the action is very important for those who accept the opportunity.**
5. It is inappropriate to advise the couple that the baby's death was probably for the best. This is very demeaning and unfeeling. It suggests to the client that she should not grieve her loss.

TEST-TAKING HINT: Clients must be encouraged and assisted through the process of grieving and mourning their babies. In addition, because most women will remain on the obstetric unit, there must be a mechanism to communicate the family's loss to every hospital employee interacting with the client, from nursing to housekeeping to dietary services. Some hospitals attach a specific icon on the woman's door to indicate that the client has suffered a fetal death. If a baby is placed in a tissue refrigerator initially, the baby should be warmed briefly under a warmer and wrapped in a warm blanket before being returned to the mother to hold.

Although a discussion about funeral arrangements may seem inappropriate on the day of delivery, time is of the essence. Many parents take pictures of just certain parts of the baby, such as the baby's hand around their fingers, their hands cradling the baby's feet, and so forth. Companies such as Now I Lay Me Down to Sleep (NILMDTS) based in Colorado, and often connected with local photographers, offer free services of photographers to take professional pictures of families with their babies as mementoes.

81.

1. Ibuprofen is an NSAID. It can exacerbate the action of warfarin and prolong bleeding times. The client should be encouraged to take acetaminophen, if needed, for pain.
2. **This action is correct. Dark green, leafy vegetables contain vitamin K. The vitamin would decrease the anticoagulant effect of warfarin.**
3. The client should be advised to avoid drinking grapefruit juice. It may increase the action of warfarin, leading to risk of hemorrhage.
4. Decreased urinary output would not be expected in a client taking warfarin. However, the client should be advised to report signs of internal bleeding, such as hematuria.

TEST-TAKING HINT: Education is essential when clients are discharged on powerful medications like warfarin. The nurse must consider all aspects of the client's daily life, including diet (see item #2 regarding dark green, leafy vegetables); herbs taken regularly (some, such as ginkgo biloba and ginger, can increase the action of the medication); and activities (clients should avoid playing contact sports, and using razors for shaving because of the risk of bleeding). Because common polymorphisms, that is, genetic variations in the human genome, can impact warfarin response, the provider may recommend genetic assessment of the client to determine her likely response to the medication, especially if a therapeutic response is difficult to achieve.

82.

1. Endometrial ischemia is not a complication of a succenturiate placenta.
2. **The nurse should carefully monitor this client for signs of postpartum hemorrhage.**
3. The client is not especially at high risk for a prolapsed uterus.
4. The client is not at high risk for a vaginal hematoma.

TEST-TAKING HINT: Because a succenturiate placenta has extra lobe(s), the client is at high risk for hemorrhage from the retention of one or more of the lobes within the uterus. The healthcare professional who performed the delivery may have noted one lobe but may not

have realized that an additional lobe is still in utero.

83. 1. **This client is at high risk for uterine atony.**
2. The client is not at high risk for hypoprolactinemia.
3. The client is not at high risk for infection.
4. The client is not at high risk for mastitis.

TEST-TAKING HINT: The uterus of a woman who delivers a macrosomic baby has been stretched beyond the usual pregnancy size. The muscle fibers of the myometrium have been overstretched. After delivery the muscles are often unable to contract effectively to stop the bleeding at the placental separation site.

84. 1. Asking the client if she has had anesthesia before is important, but it is unrelated to her discharge needs.
2. Asking the client about her allergies is important, but it is unrelated to her discharge needs.
3. Asking the client if she scars easily is not a priority question, and it is unrelated to her discharge needs.
4. **Asking the client about stairs in her home is important in discharge planning. The client will have had major surgery. She will need some assistance when she returns home, especially if she has a number of stairs to climb as she goes about her activities of daily living. Providers generally advise postoperative cesarean section clients to avoid going up or down stairs regularly for the first week after surgery. It can be risky for her to go up and down the stairs with the baby in her arms, especially if she is taking pain medication, which can cause drowsiness.**

TEST-TAKING HINT: Discharge care must begin on admission to the hospital. Cesarean section clients will need some assistance after discharge, especially if they must climb up and down stairs.

85. 1. **Clients should be warned about consuming alcohol when taking paroxetine.**
2. Grapefruit is not contraindicated for clients who have been prescribed paroxetine.
3. Milk is not contraindicated for clients who have been prescribed paroxetine.
4. Cabbage is not contraindicated for clients who have been prescribed paroxetine.

TEST-TAKING HINT: Paroxetine is an antidepressant. Although the concurrent use of alcohol and paroxetine has not been shown to adversely affect clients' abilities, it is advised that alcohol not be consumed while taking the medication.

86. 1. **The client should be assessed by her healthcare practitioner.**
2. The client may need a sitz bath but should be assessed first.
3. It is unlikely that this client has a hidden laceration as her lochial flow is normal.
4. The client may benefit from a narcotic but should be assessed first.

TEST-TAKING HINT: This client is complaining of an excessive amount of pain after having received a relatively large dose of ibuprofen. Because the perineum is edematous, the lochial flow is normal, and the pain level is well above that expected, the nurse should suspect that the client has developed a hematoma. The client should be assessed by her healthcare provider. The nurse must assess how quickly the pain has developed to a level of 9, as that can suggest the rate of bleeding and the acute nature and risk to the client. A current assessment of the client's vital signs will be helpful for the provider.

87. 1. Advising the woman to apply ice packs to her breasts is inappropriate. The woman should apply warm soaks to the breast, instead.
2. **Encouraging the woman to breastfeed frequently is appropriate.**
3. The woman should be discouraged from weaning.
4. It is unnecessary for the client to notify the pediatrician. The baby's health is not in jeopardy

TEST-TAKING HINT: The breasts contain 15 to 20 lactiferous ducts, very similar to primary grape cluster stems, that carry milk from the mammary glands (aka lobules) to the nipples when a woman is breastfeeding. Mastitis is a breast infection that usually affects only one duct system, or one "grape stem" and its connected "grapes," (lobules), that hold the milk. The milk is not infected, just the mother's breast tissue.

The mother should feed her baby frequently, using warm soaks to promote milk flow, and notify her obstetrician. If the client has a fever, antibiotics are usually prescribed to eradicate the bacteria. In addition, the client can massage the

tender area during breastfeeding to encourage emptying of the lobules. If the mother were to wean abruptly, milk stasis would occur, the bacteria would proliferate, and a breast abscess is likely to develop.

88. 1. This response is incorrect. The implants usually do not leach toxins into the surrounding tissue.
2. The glandular tissue of most women who choose to have breast augmentation surgery is normal.
3. This information is incorrect. Implants usually do not affect a baby's ability to latch.
4. This information is true. Women who have had augmentation surgery are usually able to breastfeed effectively.

TEST-TAKING HINT: Most mothers are able to produce milk after breast or nipple surgery, although they may not be able to produce a full milk supply. Successful milk production depends on several factors, including the location of the breast implants and surgical incisions involving the areolae and nipples, since milk supply depends on nerve stimulation of the areolae and nipples. In general, if a breast implant is placed behind the muscle, milk production is more likely to be successful because the milk ducts are rarely affected. In addition, surgical techniques that do not completely detach the areolae and nipples are more favorable to milk production. Daily weights of babies whose mothers have had breast enlargements should be monitored as a precaution, but most of these mothers do produce sufficient quantities of breast milk (CDC, n.d.-a).

89. 1. *Staphylococcus aureus* is the most common bacteria to cause mastitis.
2. *Streptococcus pneumoniae* is a major cause of pneumonia.
3. Certain strains of *Escherichia coli* cause severe gastritis.
4. The baby and mother are infected with *Candida albicans*.

TEST-TAKING HINT: When breastfeeding babies develop thrush, the mothers are at high risk for developing a very painful yeast infection of the breast. Because both mother and baby are infected, it is critical that they both be treated simultaneously for a minimum of 2 weeks. If they are not treated aggressively, they will continue to reinfect each other.

90. 0.1 mL.
Because the INR is between 2.1 and 3, the nurse must administer 2,500 units of heparin subcutaneously.
Standard formula:
To determine the quantity of heparin that the nurse must administer, a ratio and proportion equation should be set up:

$$\frac{\text{Known dose}}{\text{Known volume}} = \frac{\text{Desired dose}}{\text{Desired volume}}$$

$$\frac{5{,}000 \text{ units}}{0.2 \text{ mL}} = \frac{2{,}500 \text{ units}}{x \text{ mL}}$$

$$5{,}000x = 2{,}500 \times 0.2$$

$$x = \frac{2{,}500 \times 0.2}{5{,}000}$$

$$x = 0.1 \text{ mL}$$

Dimensional analysis formula:

$$\frac{\text{Known volume}}{\text{Known dosage}} \left| \frac{\text{Desired dosage}}{} \right. = \text{Desired volume}$$

$$\frac{0.2 \text{ mL}}{5{,}000 \text{ units}} \left| \frac{2{,}500 \text{ units}}{} \right. = x \text{ mL}$$

$x = 0.1$ mL

TEST-TAKING HINT: The test taker should not be confused by the titration protocol. The test taker simply must choose the dosage that meets the given criteria. Because the INR in the scenario is 2.6, the test taker can quickly see that the dosage that must be administered is the third option of 2,500 units because the client's INR of 2.6 is between 2.1 and 3.

91. 1. Although it is likely that the mother has narcotic dependency, the nurse should wait to report the family to child protective services until further evidence such as a newborn toxicology screen is obtained.
2. This statement is correct. The pediatric and obstetric healthcare providers should be advised of the noteworthy behaviors.
3. Although the nurse may discuss concerns about the client's behaviors with the primary healthcare provider and suggest a change in medication, it is not appropriate for the nurse to "prescribe" a medication by asking the provider to order a specific medication and dose. Prescribing medications is outside of a nurse's scope of practice.
4. Advising the client to take the oxycodone less frequently is not appropriate. The client may legitimately need the medication to alleviate her pain.

TEST-TAKING HINT: It is a strong likelihood that the postpartum client is dependent on a narcotic and that the neonate is exhibiting signs of withdrawal. When the nurse notifies the client's healthcare providers about the client's behaviors of concern, it would be appropriate for the nurse to recommend a toxicology screen for the baby to provide additional information. The mother will need to give her approval of this test. The nurse and provider must be transparent and point out the baby's symptoms of concern. If the evidence shows that the baby is withdrawing from an addictive substance, the mother must be told that by law, a report must be submitted to a child protective services agency. A social worker is often the professional who takes care of these details.

92. 1. Asking the young woman when her boyfriend will be visiting is inappropriate. The young woman may not have a boyfriend. It is likely that she did not choose to have the sexual experience, since she is below the age of consent.
2. **This statement is correct. Because this young woman is well below the age of consent, she must be informed that the nurse is required by law to report her pregnancy to the local child protective agency *in order to make sure she is safe*. A social worker is often the professional who takes care of talking with the client, investigating, and reporting the pregnancy and birth to authorities in the interests of child protective services.**
3. This statement is inappropriate. Because the young woman is well below the age of consent, it is inappropriate to assume she did so voluntarily and plans to do so, again.
4. This statement is inappropriate. Although the young woman is well below the age of consent, it is likely that she did not choose to have the sexual experience, and it is inappropriate to assume she did so voluntarily and plans to do so, again.

TEST-TAKING HINT: Any young woman who is found to have been sexually active should be queried regarding her experience. Girls who are below the age of consent, usually considered to be 16 years of age, may have been forced to have intercourse. Even if she states that she wanted to have intercourse, in the United States it is generally considered to be statutory rape if her partner was 16 years old or older, although this may not be the same in all states. Some may use the age of 18 or older for male partners before rape is alleged. The safety of the newborn is also at risk, as children of adolescent parents are at high risk of being abused or neglected. The young woman should be informed that the nurse or social worker is required by law to report the pregnancy and birth to a child protective services agency in order to keep her safe. The young woman should be supported and not shamed or led to believe she is in trouble with the law or is in more danger.

93. 1. **The client will likely be referred to a cardiologist.**
2. There is no need for the client to be referred to a gastroenterologist.
3. There is no need for the client to be referred to a hepatologist.
4. There is no need for the client to be referred to an immunologist.

TEST-TAKING HINT: Women who have been diagnosed with hypertensive illnesses of pregnancy are at high risk of developing cardiovascular disease. They should be monitored throughout their lives for signs of chronic hypertension, left ventricular dysfunction, right ventricular dysfunction, and other conditions (Melchiorre et al., 2014).

94. 1. Although the client does have the right to determine which type of feeding method she wishes to use for her baby, this statement does not provide the client with important information to help her choose the best feeding method.
2. **This statement is correct. Because breast milk contains many anti-infective properties, preterm babies are less likely to develop severe illnesses, most notably necrotizing enterocolitis, if breastfed.**
3. There is no evidence to show that mothers who pump milk for their babies are prepared to take their babies home sooner than those who bottle feed.
4. The charge for neonatal care is no different whether a mother feeds her baby breast milk or formula.

TEST-TAKING HINT: It is strongly advised that all women, whether they had previously planned to or not, provide breast milk for their preterm babies. However, because pumping milk for a baby in the NICU will be necessary, the decision requires commitment on the mother's part. It can be helpful for mothers to know that when given

their mother's milk, the babies are less likely to develop life-threatening infections and tend to gain weight more quickly than those who are fed formula (Herrmann & Carroll, 2014; Underwood, 2013). More recently, many NICUs use donated, pasteurized human milk for supplemental feedings in the NICU as a standard of care (Underwood, 2013). The mother must never be made to feel that she is not a good mother if she continues to refuse to breastfeed, as that can interfere with bonding.

95. 1. There is no reason to limit the baby's time at the breast to 30 minutes. It is never recommended that a mother limit the time a baby suckles at the breast.
2. This is not appropriate. Mothers who are breastfeeding babies with Down's syndrome often need additional assistance.
3. It would be appropriate for the nurse to assist the mother to latch her baby to the breast and educate her regarding how to assess for effective milk transfer.
4. Babies with Down's syndrome are not especially at high risk of becoming anemic. They, like all breastfed newborns, should receive a supplement of vitamin D, however.

TEST-TAKING HINT: In addition to the facial characteristics, children with Down's syndrome have very poor muscle tone. Because of the poor tone, babies often have difficulty maintaining a strong latch in order to suckle effectively. Because of this, the mother may need additional assistance. The baby's weight gain should be monitored carefully.

96. 1. It should never be recommended that a mother breastfeed one twin and bottle feed the other.
2. It is not appropriate for the nurse to recommend bottlefeeding versus breastfeeding. Because twins can often be breastfed simultaneously, it may actually be easier for the mother to breastfeed rather than to bottle feed.
3. Switching days that each baby bottle feeds or breastfeeds is not the best recommendation. The benefits of exclusive breastfeeding would be missed by both babies. In addition, so-called "nipple confusion" may occur, because the action of the baby's tongue is different for breast versus bottle. As a result, it is possible the babies will reject the breastfeeding method in favor of bottle feeding, since it is easier to get milk from the bottle than from the breast.
4. There are a number of breastfeeding positions that mothers can use to feed their babies simultaneously, and mothers are able to make plenty of milk for both babies.

TEST-TAKING HINT: Mothers of twins should be encouraged to breastfeed their children. Because twins are often smaller than singletons, they can benefit from the nutritional and anti-infective properties of breast milk. There are a number of breastfeeding positions such as double football hold, that make simultaneous feeding practical. A visit with a lactation consultant is often very beneficial to mothers of twins.

12 Comprehensive Examination

The previous chapters have divided maternal–newborn nursing questions by category and phase of pregnancy. This chapter will provide a different approach. It includes a combination of both low-risk and high-risk antepartum, intrapartum, and postpartum questions as well as gynecological and genetic questions in no particular order, moving back and forth from one topic to another. This is the approach the test taker will find in the Next Generation NCLEX© (NCN) examination.

QUESTIONS

1. The nurse is caring for a client at 37 weeks' gestation, who was just told that she is group B streptococcus + (positive). The client states, "How could that happen? I only have sex with my husband. Will my baby be OK?" Based on this information, which of the following should the nurse communicate to the client?

1. The client's partner must have acquired the bacteria during a sexual encounter.
2. The bacteria do not injure babies, but they could cause the client to have a bad sore throat.
3. The client is at high risk for developing pelvic inflammatory disease from the bacteria.
4. Antibiotics will be administered during labor to prevent vertical transmission of the bacteria.

2. The nurse is caring for a client in labor and delivery with the following history: G2 P1000, 39 weeks' gestation in transition phase. Fetal heart rate (FHR) 135 with early decelerations. The client states, "I'm so scared. Please make sure the baby is OK!" Which of the following responses by the nurse is appropriate?

1. "There is absolutely nothing to worry about."
2. "The fetal heart rate is within normal limits."
3. "How did your first baby die?"
4. "Did your first baby die during labor?"

3. A certified nursing assistant (CNA) is working with a registered nurse in the neonatal nursery. It would be appropriate for the nurse to delegate which of the following actions to the assistant?

1. Admission assessment on a newly delivered baby.
2. Client teaching of a neonatal sponge bath.
3. Placement of a bag on a baby for urine collection.
4. Hourly neonatal blood glucose assessments.

CASE STUDY: *The next three questions are related to the case study given below.*

The nurse is caring for a client at 40 weeks' gestation with an obstetrical history of G2 P1001. She previously had a cesarean section for breech presentation and wishes to have a trial of labor after c-section (TOLAC). The client's oxytocin induction is for postdates. She had a nonreactive nonstress test (NST) at 0800. She has an unremarkable medical history. Maternal vital signs are T 100.2° F (37.8 C°), P 90, R 20, BP 140/88. Fetus is in vertex presentation. Her cervix is 6 cm, 100% effaced, 0 station. The oxytocin was increased from 10 mU/min to 12 mU/min at 0300. It is now 0330 and the nurse is interpreting this strip. See the fetal monitor strip below.

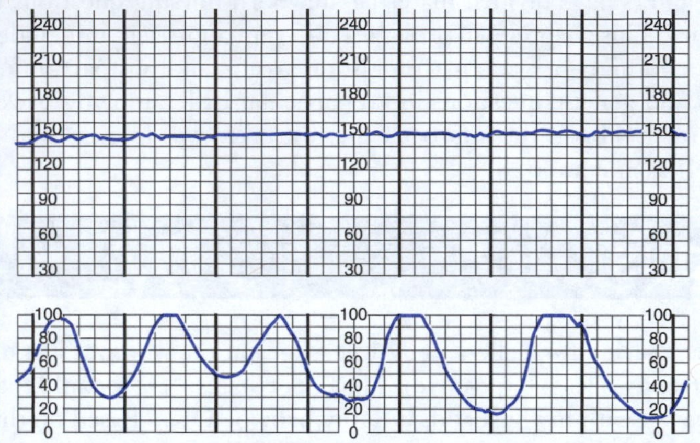

4. Select a complication for which the client and/or her fetus is at increased risk.
1. Precipitous delivery.
2. Tachysystole.
3. Hypoxemia.

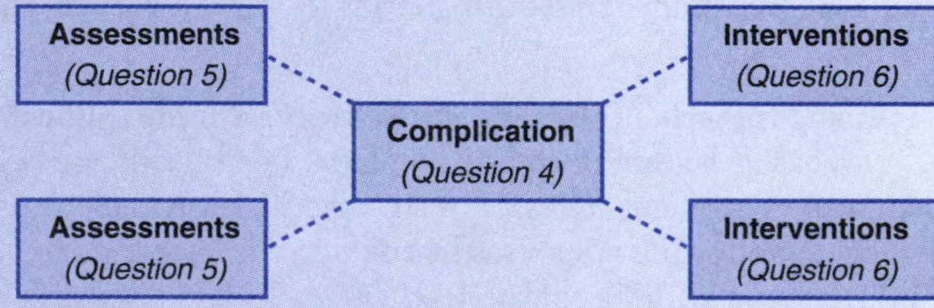

5. Which of the following assessments are most important for the nurse to manage and/or monitor to reduce the risk for the identified complication? **Select two.**
1. Contraction pattern.
2. Fetal heart rate.
3. Maternal temperature.
4. Fetal movement.

6. Specify two interventions the nurse should perform right away to reduce the risks of the identified complication.
1. Offer the client apple juice.
2. Turn off the oxytocin.
3. Administer oxygen by nonrebreather mask.
4. Change maternal position.

7. A fetus is in the left occiput anterior (LOA) position in utero. Which of the following findings would the nurse observe when doing Leopold maneuvers?
   1. Hard, round object in the fundal region.
   2. Flat object above the symphysis pubis.
   3. Soft, round object on the left side of the uterus.
   4. Small objects on the right side of the uterus.

8. A woman is being interviewed by a triage nurse at a medical doctor's office. Which of the following signs/symptoms by the client would warrant the nurse to suggest that a pregnancy test be done? **Select all that apply.**
   1. Amenorrhea.
   2. Fever.
   3. Fatigue.
   4. Nausea.
   5. Dysuria.

9. A woman is seeking counseling regarding tubal ligation. Which of the following should the nurse include in the discussion?
   1. The woman will no longer menstruate.
   2. The surgery should be done when the woman is ovulating.
   3. The surgery is easily reversible.
   4. The woman will be under anesthesia during the procedure.

10. A client has just received synthetic prostaglandins for the induction of labor. The nurse plans to monitor the client for which of the following side effects?
    1. Nausea and uterine tetany.
    2. Hypertension and vaginal bleeding.
    3. Urinary retention and severe headache.
    4. Bradycardia and hypothermia.

11. The triage nurse in an obstetric clinic received the following four messages during the lunch hour. Which of the women should the nurse telephone first?
    1. "My c-section incision from last week is leaking a whitish-yellow discharge and I have a fever. What should I do?"
    2. "I am 39 weeks pregnant with my first baby. I am having contractions about every twenty minutes."
    3. "My boyfriend and I had intercourse this morning and our condom broke. What should we do?"
    4. "I started my period yesterday. I need some medicine for these terrible menstrual cramps."

12. The primary healthcare provider caring for a pregnant client diagnosed with gonorrhea writes the following order: ceftriaxone 250 mg IM × one dose. The medication is available in 1-gram vials. The nurse adds 8 mL of normal saline to the vial. How many mL of the medication should the nurse administer? **Calculate to the nearest whole.**

    _____ mL

13. A newborn at 42 weeks' gestation is being assessed. Which of the following findings would the nurse expect to see?
    1. Folded and flat pinnae.
    2. Smooth plantar surfaces.
    3. Loose and peeling skin.
    4. Short pliable fingernails.

14. A client at 39 weeks' gestation is admitted to the labor and delivery unit for a scheduled cesarean delivery. The nurse should inform the surgeon regarding which of the following admission laboratory findings?
    1. Potassium 4.9 mEq/L.
    2. Sodium 136 mEq/L.
    3. Platelet count 75,000 cells/mm³.
    4. White blood cell count 15,000 cells/mm³.

15. A mother questions the nurse about when the newborn screening tests for inborn errors of metabolism will be performed. Which of the following is an appropriate response by the nurse?
    1. The doctor took blood from the baby's umbilical cord at birth.
    2. The pediatrician will take a blood sample at the baby's first visit.
    3. A vial of blood was drawn and sent when the baby was admitted to the nursery.
    4. Blood from the baby's heel was sent after the baby had been fed a few times.

16. On vaginal examination it is noted that the fetus is in the LSA position and −2 station. Place an "X" on the diagram in the quadrant where the fetal heart would best be assessed.

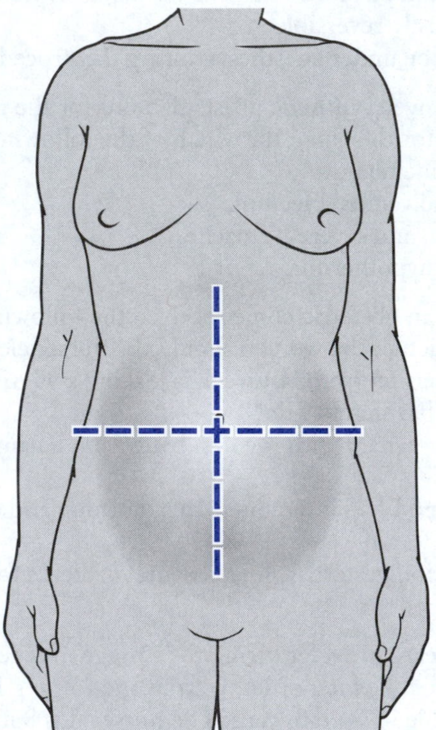

17. A young man is planning to use the condom as a contraceptive device. The nurse should teach him that which of the following actions is needed to maximize the condom's effectiveness?
    1. Use only water-soluble lubricants.
    2. Use only natural lambskin condoms.
    3. Apply the condom to a flaccid penis.
    4. Apply it tightly to the tip of the penis.

18. Which of the following electronic fetal monitor tracings shown would the nurse interpret as indicating umbilical cord compression?

1.

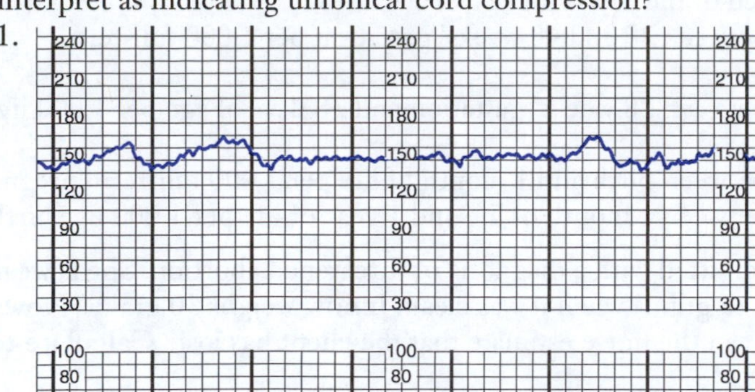

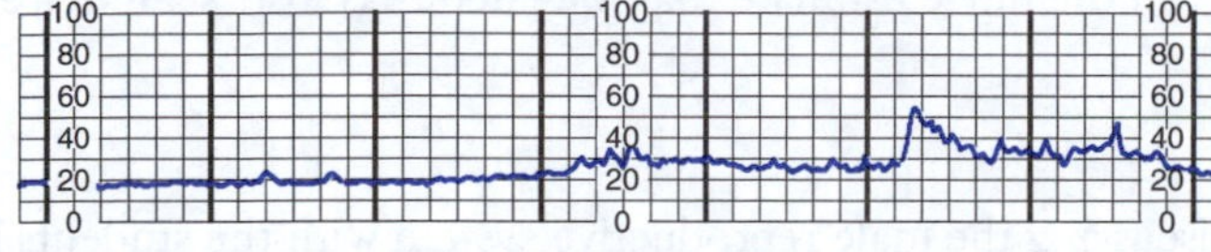

2.

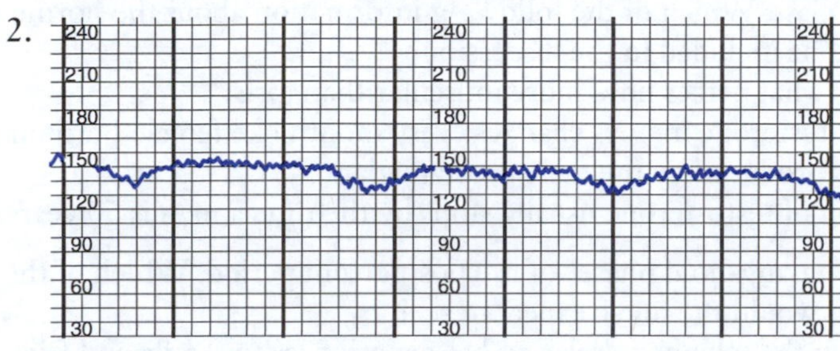

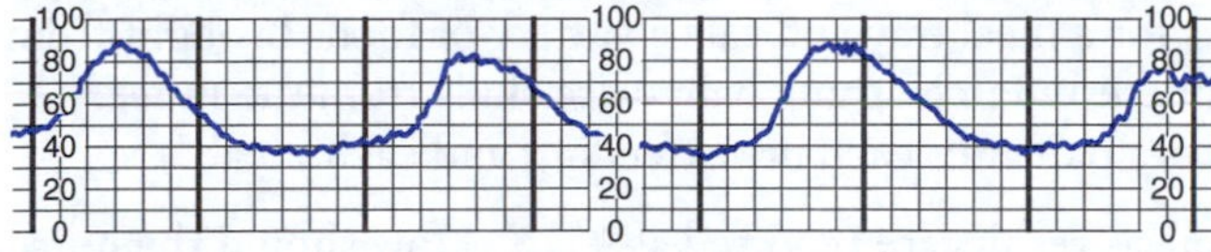

3.

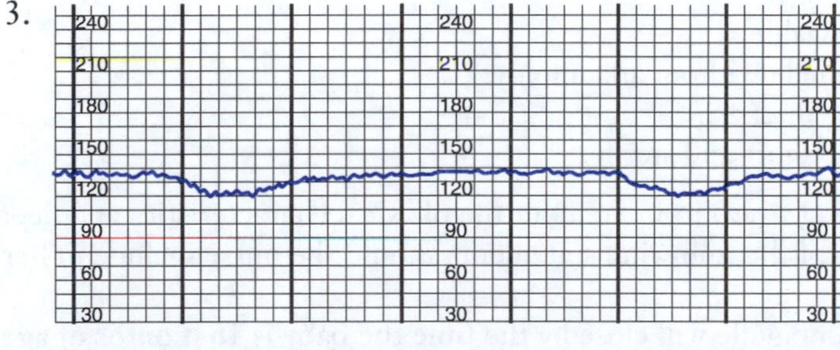

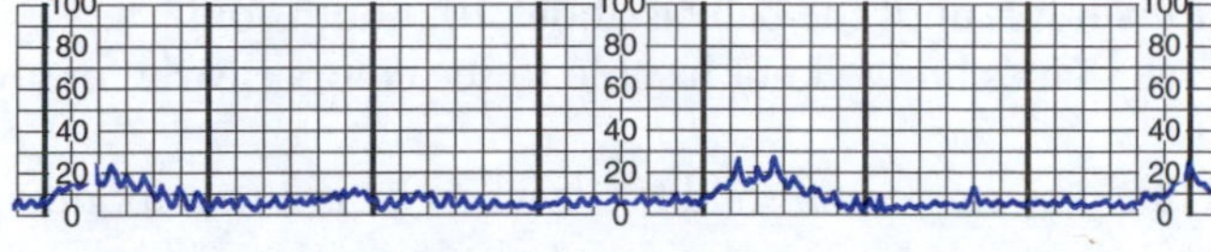

4.

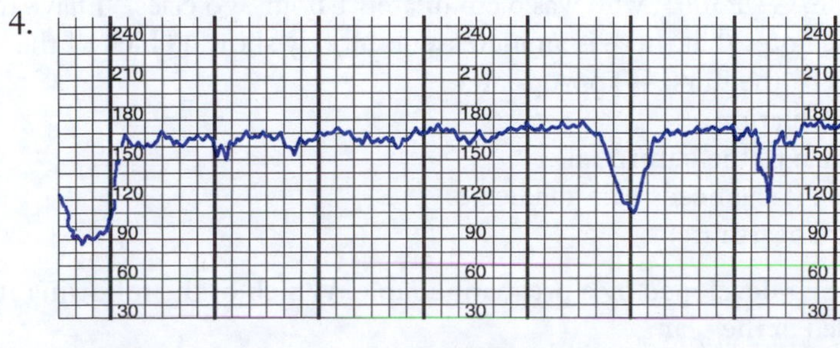

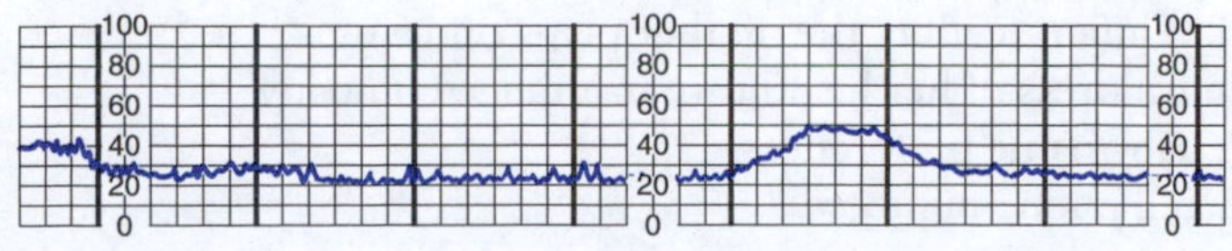

19. In 2000, the perinatal mortality rate in one county was 16. The nurse interprets that information as which of the following?
    1. 16 babies died between 28 and 40 weeks' gestation per 1,000 full-term pregnancies.
    2. 16 babies died between 28 weeks' gestation and 28 days of age per 1,000 live births.
    3. 16 babies died between birth and 1 month of life per 1,000 full-term pregnancies.
    4. 16 babies died between 1 month of life and 1 year of life per 1,000 live births.

20. A client has been admitted with a diagnosis of threatened abortion. She is wearing a pad that weighed 15 grams when it was clean. It now weighs 30 grams. How many mL of blood can the nurse estimate that the client has lost? **Calculate to the nearest whole.**

    _____ mL

21. A school nurse is discussing the male reproductive system with the students in a high school health class. Which of the following information about the hormone testosterone should be included in the discussion?
    1. "Testosterone is what makes boys more muscular than girls."
    2. "The level of testosterone in boys changes every month like female hormones do."
    3. "Testosterone is produced by the male prostate gland."
    4. "The production of testosterone usually stops by the time a man is 50 years old."

22. A woman is in the "taking-hold phase" of the postpartum period. Which of the following behaviors would the nurse expect to see?
    1. The woman is on the telephone relating her experiences to family and friends.
    2. The woman asks for a meal tray and eats a variety of foods brought from home.
    3. The woman is interested in learning baby-care skills from the nurse.
    4. The woman takes a nap after each breastfeeding and each meal.

23. A client's amniocentesis results are reported as 45, X. How should the nurse interpret these findings?
    1. The fetus is nonviable.
    2. The fetus is a female without aneuploidy.
    3. The baby will be intersex.
    4. The baby will be short and sterile.

24. The nurse is teaching a new mother about the physical characteristics and needs of her baby. Which of the following statements should the nurse include in her discussion?
    1. "The anterior fontanelle will close by the time the baby is 18 months of age."
    2. "The grasp reflex will last until the baby is about 10 months old."
    3. "Your baby can see shapes but will not be able to see colors clearly for about 6 months."
    4. "Your baby will likely be started on solid foods when he is 2 to 3 months of age."

25. A laboring woman, G4 P3003, who was 6 cm dilated 1 hour ago cries, "I have to poop!" The nurse notes that there is an increase in bloody show. Which of the following actions by the nurse is appropriate?
    1. Assess cervical dilation.
    2. Help the woman to the bathroom.
    3. Ask the woman if she needs pain medicine.
    4. Check the fetal heart rate.

26. A birth plan is being developed by a pregnant couple. Which of the following items should be included in the plan?
    1. The method of infant feeding the mother plans on using.
    2. The name and address of her healthcare insurance company.
    3. The couple's baby name preferences.
    4. The couple's cell phone numbers.

27. When providing contraceptive counseling to a woman, which of the following factors should the nurse consider? **Select all that apply.**
1. Age.
2. Obstetric history.
3. Religious beliefs.
4. Employment.
5. Body structure.

28. A baby is diagnosed with neonatal abstinence syndrome (NAS). Which of the following signs/symptoms would the nurse expect to see?
1. Hyperreflexia.
2. Anorexia.
3. Constipation.
4. Hypokalemia.

29. A woman is contracting every 3 min × 60 seconds and suddenly develops an amniotic fluid embolism (AFE), more recently referred to as anaphylactoid syndrome of pregnancy (ASP). Which of the following signs/symptoms would the nurse observe?
1. Sudden gush of fluid from the vagina.
2. Intense and unrelenting uterine pain.
3. Precipitous dilation and expulsion of the fetus.
4. Chest pain with dyspnea and cyanosis.

30. A client complaining of frequency, urgency, and burning on urination is seen by her primary healthcare practitioner. Which of the following factors in the client's history places her at risk for these complaints?
1. The client urinates immediately after every sexual encounter.
2. The client uses the diaphragm as a family planning method.
3. The client wipes from front to back after every toileting.
4. The client changes her peripads every two hours during her menses.

31. On the third postpartum day a client tells the nurse that she feels sad and that she cries easily. The nurse should explain about which of the following?
1. These feelings are normal and should diminish within a couple of weeks.
2. The physician will likely order an antidepressant for the client to take at home.
3. If the client focuses on the fact that she has a healthy baby, the feelings will cease.
4. When the client is home with her family and friends, her sad feelings will disappear.

32. A nurse is reading a research study that states, "There is a strong negative correlation between the independent and dependent variables ($r = -0.85$)." The nurse interprets the statement as which of the following?
1. The dependent variable caused a change in the independent variable.
2. The independent and dependent variables are significantly different.
3. As values of the independent variable go up, values of the dependent variable go down.
4. When the confidence interval is computed, the negative value will change to positive.

33. A nurse notes that a baby is lying in a crib in the tonic neck position. In which of the following positions is the baby lying?
1. The baby is on its back with its head turned to one side, facing his outstretched arm. The opposite arm is bent across the baby's chest.
2. When the baby faces straight ahead, the baby's head tilts toward one side.
3. Both the baby's back and head are sharply arched backward and resist being moved to midline.
4. When the baby lies prone, the baby's body arches to one side.

34. A doula is working with a laboring woman during an induction with oxytocin. The client is 6 cm dilated and is contracting every 3 min × 60 sec. Which of the following interventions should the nurse suggest the doula perform?
1. Regulate the oxytocin drip rate.
2. Check the vaginal dilation of the client.
3. Encourage the woman to use breathing techniques.
4. Monitor the client for uterine hyperstimulation.

35. A pregnant woman is complaining of ptyalism. The nurse should teach the woman to try which of the following self-care measures?
1. Use an astringent mouthwash.
2. Elevate her legs frequently.
3. Eat high-fiber foods.
4. Void when the urge is felt.

36. The nurse is counseling a woman who has been diagnosed with mild osteoporosis. Which of the following should be included in the counseling session?
1. Begin a regimen of walking each day.
2. Refrain from drinking chocolate milk.
3. Increase her daily intake of red meat.
4. Only wear shoes with rubber soles.

37. It is noted that a baby admitted to the nursery has translucent skin with visible veins. Because of this finding, the nurse should monitor this baby carefully for which of the following?
1. Polycythemia.
2. Hypothermia.
3. Hyperglycemia.
4. Polyuria.

CASE STUDY: *The next three questions refer to the case study that follows.*

A client is brought from the emergency room to the labor and delivery unit grimacing and moaning in obvious pain with her hands on her abdomen. She manages to state that she is 32 weeks pregnant and was in a motor vehicle accident while driving. This is her second pregnancy. Her abdomen is rigid and the emergency nurse reports the client is actively bleeding. The client's vital signs just before transfer were T 98.6° F (37° C), P 100, R 20, BP 110/70. The client is wearing a medic alert bracelet.

38. Select the most likely complication for which the client is at increased risk.
1. Placenta previa.
2. Placental abruption.
3. Ruptured uterus.

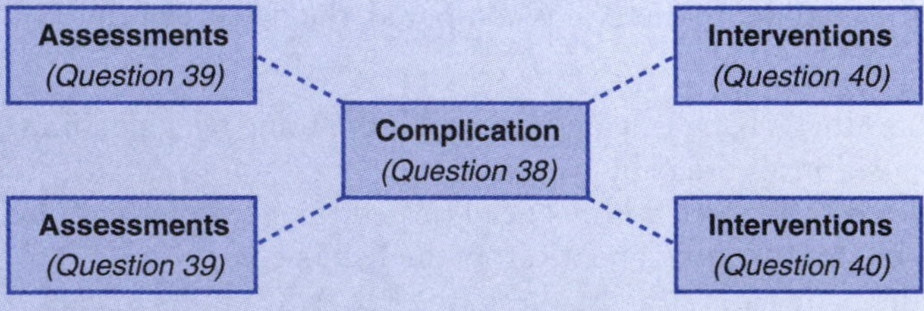

39. Which of the following assessments are most important for the nurse to monitor at this time in relation to the identified complication? **Select two.**
  1. Fetal heart rate (FHR).
  2. Pain level.
  3. Vaginal bleeding.
  4. Laboratory data.

40. The nurse is reviewing the provider's orders in preparation for an emergent caesarean section. Which orders should the nurse complete right away? **Select two.**
  1. Weigh all pads and monitor intake and output.
  2. Review the information on the medic alert bracelet with the client.
  3. Insert peripheral IV and run lactated ringer's solution bolus.
  4. Clip pubic hair and insert indwelling catheter.

41. The doctor has ordered a nonstress test (NST) for a client at 39 weeks' gestation. The nurse should interpret which of the following as a reactive test?
  1. The fetal heart rate (FHR) remains stable throughout the test period.
  2. The uterine contractions last longer than 90 seconds.
  3. The mother reports a pain level that is less than 5 on a 10-point scale.
  4. The baby moves spontaneously 3 times in 20 minutes.

42. A nurse who is creating a pedigree of a woman's family tree includes the following symbols. The symbols represent which of the following relationships?

  1. A healthy sister and brother.
  2. A couple who has mated.
  3. A grandmother and grandson.
  4. A father and daughter.

43. A woman who is in pain from a diagnosis of mastitis has abruptly weaned her baby to a bottle. Her actions place the woman at high risk for which of the following?
  1. Mammary rupture.
  2. Postpartum psychosis.
  3. Supernumerary nipples.
  4. Breast abscess.

44. The triage nurse is interviewing a 19-year old, unmarried client who states, "I felt a hard thing on the lip of my vagina this morning. It doesn't hurt." Which of the following questions is most important for the nurse to ask at this time?
  1. "Have any of your partners ever hurt you?"
  2. "Do you ever have unprotected intercourse?"
  3. "Have you ever had a baby?"
  4. "Do you think you may be pregnant?"

45. A breastfeeding mother and her baby are being discharged home after delivery. The nurse is providing anticipatory guidance about what signs the mother should expect the baby to exhibit every 24 hours by the end of the first week. Which of the following should the nurse include in his/her instructions?
  1. The baby should have at least 6 wet diapers.
  2. The baby should have at least 6 pasty stools.
  3. The baby should breastfeed at least 6 times.
  4. The baby should gain at least 6 ounces.

46. Please indicate the frequency and duration of the contraction pattern shown below.

Every ________ min × ________ sec

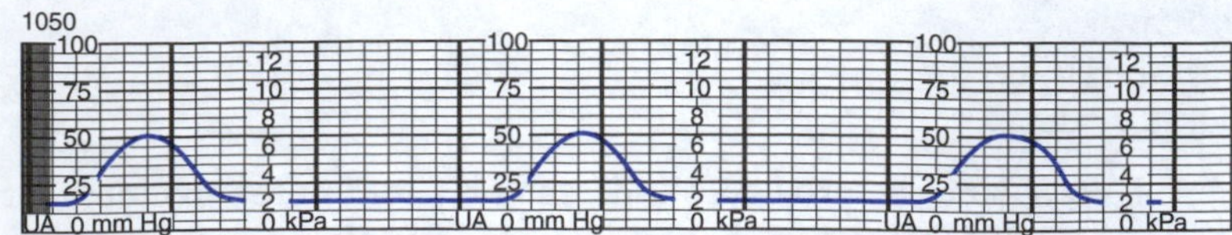

47. The nurse documents a woman's gravidity and parity as G6 P3214. Which of the following obstetric histories is consistent with this notation?
1. The woman is currently pregnant, and has 3 living children.
2. The woman is currently pregnant, and had 2 full-term pregnancies.
3. The woman is not currently pregnant, and had 4 preterm babies.
4. The woman is not currently pregnant, and had 1 abortion.

48. The nurse is teaching a woman how to do the pelvic tilt exercise. In the teaching session, which of the following should the nurse tell the woman to do?
1. Stand with the back of her heels and shoulders touching a wall.
2. Bend laterally back and forth from one side to the other.
3. Move so that her back is alternately concave and convex.
4. Lie flat on her back and move her hips from side to side.

49. A 6-month-old child has been diagnosed with a significant hearing loss. Which of the following complications could have resulted in this condition?
1. Necrotizing enterocolitis.
2. Hypoglycemia.
3. Bronchopulmonary dysplasia.
4. Kernicterus.

50. During a vaginal delivery of a macrosomic baby, the nurse midwife requests nursing assistance. Which of the following actions by the nurse would be appropriate?
1. Estimate fetal length and weight.
2. Assess intensity of contractions.
3. Provide suprapubic pressure.
4. Assist woman with breathing.

CASE STUDY: *The next three questions refer to the case study that follows.*

A client who delivered her first baby 1 week ago calls her obstetrician's office and tells the advice nurse, "I'm a breastfeeding mother and my right nipple is cracked and bleeding. Should I feed the baby on that side?"

51. Select the most likely complication for which the client is at increased risk.
1. Engorgement.
2. Mastitis.
3. Thrush.

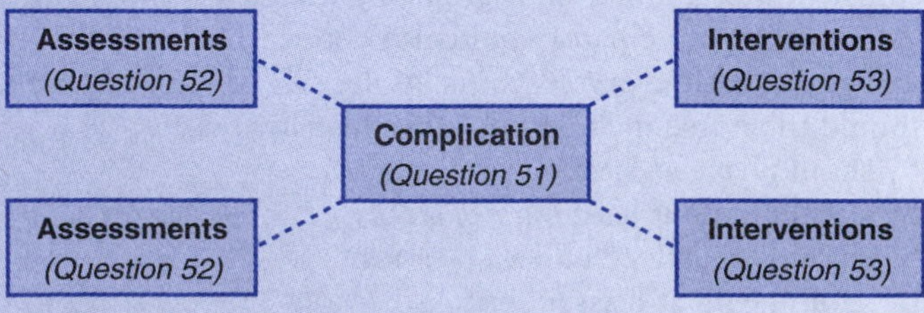

52. Which of the following comments are appropriate for the nurse to make at this time, in order to reduce the complication identified above? **Select two.**
   1. You will need to be seen by the midwife today.
   2. You should pump and dump so the baby does not swallow your blood.
   3. You should nurse the baby on both sides.
   4. You should apply lanolin cream after each feeding.

53. The nurse is reviewing the plan of care with the client. **Specify two** interventions the nurse should recommend to the client.
   1. Weigh the baby daily.
   2. Wash the nipples gently before and after each feeding.
   3. Alternate breastfeeding positions.
   4. Call the office if you develop a fever and flu-like symptoms.

54. A fetal fibronectin assessment of the cervicovaginal fluids of a client at 28 weeks gestation is positive. Based on the results, which of the following complaints should the nurse advise the client to report immediately to the healthcare provider?
   1. Headache.
   2. Visual disturbances.
   3. Uterine cramping.
   4. Oliguria.

55. A breastfeeding client asks the nurse to confirm that her newborn is positioned and latched well at the breast. Which of the following assessments would indicate that the baby is poorly latched?
   1. The baby swallows after every suckle.
   2. The baby's body is facing the mother's body.
   3. The baby's lower lip is curled under.
   4. The baby is lying at the level of the mother's breasts.

56. A fetus descending through the birth canal is going through the cardinal movements of labor. Please place the following moves in chronological order.
   1. External rotation.
   2. Flexion.
   3. Extension.
   4. Internal rotation.
   5. Expulsion.

57. The nurse is working with a pregnant woman who states that she is vegan. Which of the following actions by the nurse is appropriate?
   1. Advise the mother that she must eat some animal protein during her pregnancy.
   2. Refer the woman to a nutritionist for diet counseling.
   3. Remind the mother that cashews and coconut are excellent sources of calcium.
   4. Congratulate the woman on agreeing to eat eggs and milk.

CASE STUDY: *The next six questions refer to the case study that follows.*

A postpartum client with gestational diabetes and an obstetrical history of G5 P5004 delivered her baby vaginally 2 hours ago after a precipitous delivery. The baby weighed 9 lbs 12 ounces (4,422 grams). The client just walked to the bathroom and passed a large clot in her pad, followed by a gush of blood. She voided 100 mL in the toilet. After the client returned to bed, the nurse made the following assessment: fundus massaged to firm, 4 cm above the umbilicus and deviated to the right with moderate to heavy lochia rubra. Temp 98.6° F (37° C), P 108, R 18, BP 108/60.

58. Identify the 4 top findings that require immediate follow-up.
1. Client sensorium.
2. Urinary output.
3. Blood glucose.
4. Fundal assessment.
5. Pulse.
6. Blood pressure.

59. The nurse should first assess the client's **(select one item from the first column)**, followed by **(select one item from the second column).**

Assess first (Select one, below)	Followed by (Select one, below)
1. Residual urine	a. Residual urine
2. Total blood loss	b. Total blood loss
3. Fluid intake	c. Fluid intake
4. Medication list	d. Medication list

60. The client is at highest risk for developing **(select one item from the first column)**, as evidenced by **(select one item from the second column).**

At risk for developing . . . (Select one, below)	As evidenced by . . . (Select one, below)
1. Urinary retention	a. Blood pressure
2. Hypoglycemia	b. Fundal assessments
3. Pulmonary edema	c. Gestational diabetes
4. Postpartum hemorrhage	d. Urinary output

61. What would be the primary goal(s) of care at this time? **Select all that apply.**
1. Reduce maternal anxiety.
2. Stabilize vital signs.
3. Prevent falling.
4. Improve fundal tone.
5. Monitor intake and output.

62. For each potential nursing intervention, specify whether the intervention is indicated or contraindicated for the care of the client. Interventions are not given in the order in which they should be performed. **Each column must have a response.**

Potential Intervention	(a) Indicated	(b) Contraindicated
1. In and out catheterization		
2. Sustained fundal massage		
3. Weigh pads		
4. Insert indwelling catheter		
5. Administer uterotonic medication		
6. Administer IV bolus		

63. The nurse inserted an in-and-out catheter and obtained 500 mL urine. A solution of 1,000 lactated ringer's solution with 20 units of oxytocin was hung and a 500 mL bolus was administered. The nurse is now reassessing the client. For each assessment finding below, specify if the finding indicates that the nurse's intervention was effective, ineffective, or unrelated.

Assessment Finding	(a) Effective	(b) Ineffective	(c) Unrelated
1. Fundus boggy			
2. Fundus at umbilicus			
3. Moderate lochia			
4. Temp 98.6° F (37° C), P 100, R 18			
5. BP 120/60			
6. Unable to palpate bladder			

64. When caring for a woman whom a nurse suspects is being abused by her partner, the nurse should do which of the following?
1. Ask the client directly about how she sustained her injuries.
2. Counsel the client on how her behavior probably provoked the attack.
3. Inform the client that the police must arrest her partner.
4. Give the client a pamphlet with the names of matrimonial attorneys.

65. The nurse is caring for a baby whose blood type is A+ (positive) and direct Coombs test (DAT) is + (positive) and whose mother's blood type is O+ (positive). Which of the following risks apply for this baby? **Select all that apply.**
1. Hyperbilirubinemia.
2. Dehydration.
3. Anemia.
4. Weight loss.

66. Which of the following complications of labor and delivery may develop when a baby enters the pelvis in the left mentum posterior (LMP) position? **Select all that apply.**
1. Cephalopelvic disproportion.
2. Placental abruption.
3. Breech presentation.
4. Prolapsed cord.
5. Severe pre-eclampsia.

67. A client at 36 weeks' gestation is having an amniocentesis. For which of the following reasons is the test likely being conducted?
1. Genetic evaluation.
2. Assessment of intrauterine growth restriction.
3. Assessment of fetal lung maturation.
4. Hormonal studies.

68. A client asks the nurse to explain what luteinizing hormone (LH) does in the body. The nurse should make which of the following statements?
1. "It accelerates the growth and maturation of an egg in your ovary."
2. "It enhances the potential for the sperm to fertilize the mature egg."
3. "It promotes the movement of the egg through the fallopian tube."
4. "It stimulates the monthly release of a mature egg from your ovary."

69. A couple has decided not to have their son circumcized. Based on this decision, which of the following instructions should the nurse include in the parent teaching?
1. The couple should check their son's temperature every evening because he will be at high risk for urinary tract infections.
2. The couple should fully retract the foreskin to assess for the presence of exudate every morning.
3. The pediatrician will observe the baby void during each well-baby examination to assess for a phimosis.
4. The prepuce should be cleansed with soap and water during the baby's sponge bath.

70. A client whose most recent cervical exam was 6 cm and 90% effaced has just received fentanyl 50 micrograms IV for pain. Which of the following fetal heart changes would the nurse expect to observe on the internal fetal monitor tracing?
1. Drop in baseline heart rate.
2. Increase in number of variable decelerations.
3. Decrease in variability.
4. Rise in number of early decelerations.

71. Which of the following features are present in an embryo at 8 weeks' gestation? **Select all that apply.**
1. Four-chambered heart.
2. Fingers and toes.
3. Fully formed genitalia.
4. Facial features.

CASE STUDY: *The next six questions refer to the case study that follows.*

The nurse is caring for an 18-year-old, pregnant, African American client with an obstetrical history of G1 P0. She has no known underlying medical issues of concern.

Nurse's notes 2200: "Admitted to labor and delivery triage at 35 weeks' gestation with right upper quadrant (RUQ) pain and nausea. Vital signs are T 100.4° F (38° C), P 82, R 16, BP 160/100. O2 saturation is 94% on room air. DTRs 2+, 1 beat of clonus. The client denies a headache. Her cervical exam is 2 cm, 50% effaced, ballotable. FHR is 140 bpm with moderate variability and no decelerations. Intravenous fluid of lactated ringer's solution is running at 125 ml/hour in left hand."

2215: BP 152/110
2230: BP 170/120

The fetal monitor strip is shown below.

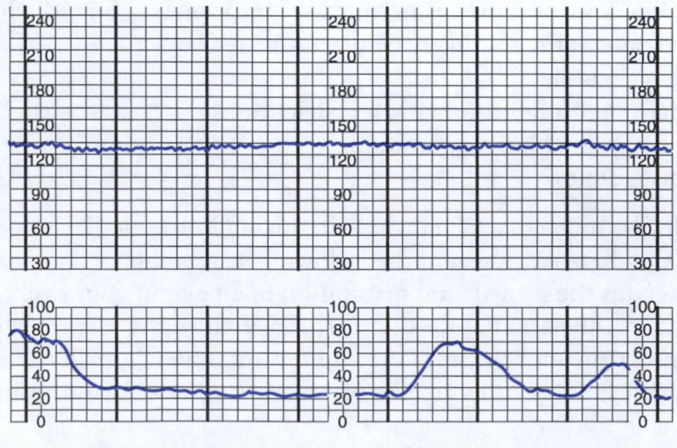

72. Highlight the findings in the nurse's notes that would require follow-up: **Select all that apply.**
1. RUQ pain and nausea.
2. Temperature.
3. Pulse.
4. Respiratory rate.
5. Blood pressure.
6. Oxygen saturation.
7. DTRs.
8. Cervical exam.

73. The client is at highest risk for **(select one answer from column 1 below)** as evidenced by **(select one answer from column 2 below).**

Column 1 Highest client risk	Column 2 As evidenced by client's . . .
1. Placental abruption	a. Vital sign assessments
2. Stroke	b. Neurological assessments
3. Prolapsed cord	c. Cervical assessment
4. Eclampsia	d. Fetal assessments

74. The nurse should first address the client's **(select one answer from column 1 below)** followed by **(select one answer from column 2 below)**

Column 1 Address this condition first	Column 2 Followed by this condition
1. Blood pressure	a. Blood pressure
2. Oxygen saturation	b. Oxygen saturation
3. DTRs	c. DTRs
4. Contractions	d. Contractions

75. The nurse is speaking with the provider about the client's plan for care. The client's laboratory values are provided below. For each potential order, indicate whether it is anticipated or contraindicated.

CLIENT'S LABORATORY VALUES

Platelet count 98,000

Aspartate aminotransferase (AST, SGOT) 45 IU/L

Alanine aminotransferase (ALT) 60 IU/L

Lactate dehydrogenase (LDH) 550 IU/L

3RD TRIMESTER REFERENCE RANGES

Platelet Count 146,000–429,000

AST 4–32 IU/L

ALT 2–25 IU/L

LDH 82–524 IU/L

Retrieved from http://perinatology.com/Reference/Reference%20Ranges/Reference%20for%20Serum.htm

Potential Order	(a) Anticipated	(b) Contraindicated
1. 24-hour urine for creatinine clearance and protein		
2. Oxytocin induction per protocol		
3. Misoprostol 25 mcg vaginally Q 4 hours per protocol		
4. Epidural when requested in labor		
5. Magnesium sulfate 4 gm IV loading dose over 30 minutes followed by 2 gm/hour maintenance dose		
6. Hydralazine 10 mg slow IV push over 2 minutes per protocol		
7. Acetaminophen 650 mg po Q 4 hours for fever or headache		

76. Select 3 orders the nurse should perform right away.
1. Begin 24-hour urine for creatinine clearance and protein.
2. Oxytocin induction per protocol.
3. Misoprostol 25 mcg vaginally q 4 hours per protocol.
4. Epidural when requested in labor.
5. Magnesium sulfate 4 gm IV loading dose over 30 minutes followed by 2 gm/hour maintenance dose.
6. Hydralazine 10 mg slow IV push over 2 minutes.
7. Acetaminophen 650 mg po q 4 hours for fever or headache.

77. **0300.** The nurse completed all of the provider's orders except the oxytocin induction and the epidural orders, which were not appropriate to complete at that time. The client required 2 doses of hydralazine 10 mg IV. Following that, the client was still hypertensive and the nurse notified the provider and obtained an order for 2 doses of labetalol 20 mg IV per protocol for BP stabilization. The client's last dose of labetalol was at 2345. Magnesium sulfate is infusing per pump at 2 gm/hour, following the initial 4 gm bolus. In the nurse's notes below, highlight the findings that indicate the client is not progressing as expected. **Select all that apply.**

Nurse's notes 0300: Irregular contractions continue, FHR 120 bpm with minimal variability, recurrent late decelerations. Cervical exam 2 cm, 50% effaced, ballotable. T 98.6° F (37° C), P 60, BP 150/90. DTRs 3+, 2 beats clonus. Oxygen saturation 95% on room air.

1. Irregular contractions continue.
2. FHR 120 bpm
3. Minimal FHR variability with recurrent late decelerations.
4. Cervical exam 2 cm, 50% effaced, ballotable.
5. T 98.6° F (37° C), P 60, BP 150/90.
6. DTRs 3+, 2 beats clonus.
7. Oxygen saturation 95% on room air.

78. A client at 39 weeks' gestation with an obstetrical history of G2 P1001, is admitted to the labor suite with rupture of membranes 15 minutes earlier and contractions q 8 minutes × 30 seconds. On vaginal exam, the cervix is 4 cm dilated and 90% effaced. The fetus is in the LSP position at −2 (minus 2) station. The fetal heart rate is 145 bpm with moderate variability and recurrent, variable decelerations. Which of the following complications of labor must the nurse assess this client for at this time?

1. Precipitous delivery.
2. Chorioamnionitis.
3. Uteroplacental insufficiency.
4. Prolapsed cord.

79. Young pregnant adolescents have increased nutritional needs as compared with pregnant adults. Which of the following foods would meet those needs?

1. Banana.
2. Cheeseburger.
3. Strawberries.
4. Rice.

80. The nurse is caring for a client and her partner who had a fetal demise. The client just gave birth to a 33-week stillborn baby. Which of the following actions by the nurse is appropriate at this time?

1. Recommend that the woman be moved to a medical unit.
2. Refrain from discussing the loss with the couple.
3. Ask the couple if they would like to hold their baby.
4. Obtain an order for a milk suppressant for the mother.

81. A woman asks the nurse to recommend the best douche for use after menstruation. Which of the following responses by the nurse is appropriate?

1. "Tap water with white vinegar is most refreshing and least allergenic."
2. "It is really best for women not to douche."
3. "Any of the over-the-counter douches is satisfactory."
4. "It is best to douche during menstruation rather than after it is over."

82. During a postpartum examination, the nurse notes that a client's left calf is warm and swollen. Which of the following actions by the nurse is appropriate at this time?

1. Notify the client's primary healthcare provider.
2. Teach the client to massage her leg.
3. Apply ice packs to the client's leg.
4. Encourage the client to ambulate.

83. A nurse sees an overweight woman looking at the babies through the nursery window. The woman asks the nurse when the babies go to their mothers for feedings and about the location of the nearest stairwell. Which of the following replies by the nurse is most appropriate at this time?

1. "The babies go to their mothers whenever they seem hungry."
2. "Please let me escort you to the mother's room you are here to visit."
3. "The babies are in the mothers' rooms for the majority of the day."
4. "Most of our visitors prefer to use the elevator to return to the lobby."

84. Without doing a vaginal examination, a nurse concludes that a primigravida who has received no medications during her labor is in transition. Which of the following signs/symptoms would lead a nurse to that conclusion?

1. The woman fell asleep during a contraction.
2. The woman yelled at her partner and vomited.
3. The woman laughed at something on the television.
4. The woman began pushing with each contraction.

85. A male baby is born with scant amounts of vernix caseosa in his axillae and groin, scant amounts of lanugo on his shoulders, testes in his scrotum, and a strong suck. The nurse would estimate that the baby is which of the following gestational ages?
1. 22 weeks.
2. 28 weeks.
3. 32 weeks.
4. 38 weeks.

86. The mother of a neonate with Down's syndrome wishes to breastfeed. Which of the following considerations should the nurse make in relation to the mother's wishes?
1. The mother should be encouraged to feed expressed breast milk via a bottle.
2. Babies with Down's syndrome consume more calories than unaffected neonates.
3. Because of the weight of the neonatal head, the side-lying position must be used.
4. The baby will likely have a weak suck due to congenitally poor muscle tone.

87. A neonate in the nursery whose mother had no prenatal care has been diagnosed with macrosomia. For which of the following signs/symptoms should the nurse carefully monitor this baby?
1. Jaundice.
2. Jitters.
3. Blepharitis.
4. Strabismus.

88. A woman has been diagnosed with chlamydia. The nurse would expect the client to complain of which of the following signs/symptoms?
1. No signs or symptoms.
2. Painful lesions on the labia.
3. Foul-smelling discharge.
4. Severe lower abdominal pain.

89. A pregnant woman and her partner have the following genotypes for an autosomal dominant disease: Aa and Aa. If asked, which of the following should the nurse say is the probability of their child having the disease?
1. 25% probability.
2. 50% probability.
3. 75% probability.
4. 100% probability.

90. The nurse is providing information to a client who plans to bottle feed her newborn infant. Which of the following should be included in the education session?
1. The baby should be burped after every 3 ounces of formula.
2. If the bottle nipple is not filled with formula throughout the feeding, the baby may take in a large amount of air.
3. The best way to heat formula for the baby is in the microwave.
4. If the mother is busy with her other children, she can prop the baby bottle up on a blanket or towel.

91. The nurse has received change of shift report on the following 4 clients. Which of the clients should the nurse assess first?
1. G1 P0000, 9 weeks' gestation, hyperemesis gravidarum, vomited twice during the last shift.
2. G2 P0101, 24 weeks' gestation, on bedrest for placenta previa, no bleeding or cramping during last shift.
3. G3 P3003, 1 day postpartum, vacuum extraction, NPO in preparation for a bilateral tubal ligation during this shift.
4. G2 P1101, 2 days postpartum, spontaneous delivery, had asthma attack during last shift.

92. Using the graph that follows, which weight for a 34-week neonate would indicate the neonate was average for gestational age?
1. 500 grams.
2. 1,700 grams.
3. 2,900 grams.
4. 4,100 grams.

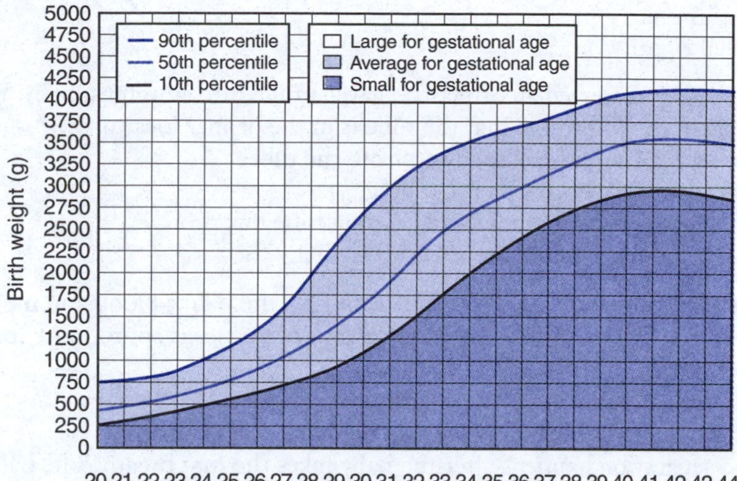

93. A provider has ordered carboprost for a client who is actively hemorrhaging during the immediate postpartum phase of care. Which of the following maternal findings would warrant questioning the order?
1. Fever.
2. History of asthma.
3. Blood pressure 90/60.
4. Hypocalcemia.

94. A breastfeeding client who delivered 6 days ago, calls the postpartum unit from home. She states, "I think I am engorged. My breasts are very hard and hot and they really hurt." Which of the following questions should the nurse ask at this time?
1. "Have you taken a warm shower this morning?"
2. "Do you have an electric breast pump?"
3. "How much did you have to drink yesterday?"
4. "When was the last time you fed the baby?"

95. A client's vital signs during labor and delivery included the following ranges: BP 100/58 to 110/66, T 98.6° F to 98.8° F (37° C–37.1° C), P 72 to 80 bpm, R 20 to 24. Two hours after a spontaneous vaginal delivery, the client's vital signs are BP 100/56; TPR 99.4° F (37.4° C), P 70 bpm, R 20; her fundus is firm and her lochia is light. Which of the following actions should the nurse perform at this time?
1. Massage the client's uterus.
2. Ask the client if she is having chills.
3. Encourage the client to drink fluids.
4. Assess the client's lung fields.

96. A G1 P1001 client whose labor was uneventful, delivered 1 minute ago. The nurse dried, suctioned, and stabilized the baby. The baby's Apgar score at this time is 3. Which of the following actions is appropriate for the nurse to do next?
1. Administer ophthalmic prophylaxis.
2. Place the baby on the abdomen of the mother.
3. Obtain assistance for full neonatal resuscitation.
4. Repeat the score to confirm its accuracy.

97. An infant of a mother with type 2 diabetes mellitus (T2DM) delivered at 40 weeks' gestation. The baby weighed 9 lbs (4,082 grams) and has just been admitted to the neonatal nursery. The neonatal intensive care nurse will monitor this baby for which of the following? **Select all that apply.**
1. Hyperreflexia.
2. Hypoglycemia.
3. Respiratory distress.
4. Opisthotonus.
5. Nuchal rigidity.

98. A nurse has just inserted an orogastric gavage tube into a preterm baby. When would the nurse determine that the tube is in the proper location?
1. When gastric aspirate is removed from the tube.
2. When the baby suckles on the tubing.
3. When respirations are unlabored during tube insertion.
4. When the tubing can be inserted no farther.

99. A client asks the nurse, "Could you explain how the baby's blood and my blood separate at delivery?" Which of the following responses is appropriate for the nurse to make?
1. "When the placenta is delivered, the circulatory systems separate."
2. "When the doctor clamps the cord, the blood stops mixing."
3. "The separation happens after the baby takes the first breath. The baby's oxygen no longer has to come from you."
4. "The blood actually never mixes. Your blood supply and the baby's blood supply are completely separate."

100. A 4-day-old breastfeeding neonate whose birth weight was 5 lbs 9 oz (2,678 grams) has lost 286 grams since the baby's cesarean birth. Which of the following actions should the nurse take?
1. Nothing, because this is an acceptable weight loss.
2. Advise the mother to stop breastfeeding and give formula.
3. Notify the primary healthcare provider of the excessive weight loss.
4. Give the baby dextrose water between breast feedings.

101. A nurse has provided a young woman with preconception counseling. Which of the statements by the woman indicates that the teaching was successful? **Select all that apply.**
1. "As soon as I think I may be pregnant, I should stop drinking alcohol."
2. "It is important for me to see my medical doctor for a complete physical."
3. "I should make sure that my daily multivitamin contains folic acid."
4. "When I go to my dentist for a checkup I should state that I may be pregnant."
5. "From now until I deliver I should refrain from eating sushi and rare meat."

102. A client who had a vaginal delivery 2 hours earlier has just been transferred to the postpartum unit from labor and delivery. Which of the following nursing care goals is of highest priority?
1. The client will breastfeed her baby every 2 hours.
2. The client will consume a nutritious diet.
3. The client will have a moderate lochial flow.
4. The client will ambulate in the hallways every shift.

103. The nurse who has just performed a vaginal examination notes that the fetus is in the left occiput posterior (LOP) position. Which of the following clinical assessments would the nurse expect to note at this time?
1. Complaints of severe back pain.
2. Rapid descent and effacement.
3. Irregular and hypotonic contractions.
4. Rectal pressure with bloody show.

104. A client who is at 8 weeks' gestation has been diagnosed with a hydatidiform mole (gestational trophoblastic disease). In addition to vaginal loss, which of the following signs/symptoms would the nurse expect to see?
1. Hyperemesis and hypertension.
2. Diarrhea and hyperthermia.
3. Polycythemia.
4. Polydipsia.

105. A woman who states that she smokes 2 packs of cigarettes each day is admitted to the labor and delivery suite in labor. The nurse should monitor this labor for which of the following?
1. Delayed placental separation.
2. Late decelerations.
3. Shoulder dystocia.
4. Precipitous fetal descent.

106. A nurse has just received report on 4 neonates in the newborn nursery. Which of the babies should the nurse assess first?
1. Neonate whose mother is HIV positive.
2. Neonate whose mother is group B streptococcus (GBS) positive.
3. Neonate whose mother's labor was 12 hours long.
4. Neonate whose mother gained 45 pounds during her pregnancy.

107. The umbilical cord is being clamped by the obstetrician. Which of the following physiological changes is taking place at this time?
1. The baby's blood bypasses the pulmonary system.
2. The baby's oxygen level begins to drop.
3. Bacteria begin to invade the baby's bowel.
4. Bilirubin rises in the baby's bloodstream.

ANSWERS AND RATIONALES

The correct answer number and rationale for why it is the correct answer are given in **boldface blue type**. Rationales for why the other possible answer options are incorrect are also given, but they are not in boldface type.

1. 1. This statement is incorrect. Approximately 1 out of every 4 women carries group B streptococcus (GBS) as normal flora. This is not a sexually transmitted infection.
2. This statement is incorrect. Group B strep can seriously injure babies. Group A beta hemolytic strep causes strep throat.
3. This statement is incorrect. The bacteria rarely cause illness in the mother.
4. This statement is accurate. Antibiotics will be administered to the mother during labor and delivery to prevent vertical transmission.

TEST-TAKING HINT: Vertical transmission refers to the transmission of disease from the mother to the baby through the vagina. Group B strep has been called the "baby killer" in the past, before antibiotics were given routinely when indicated. If a mother is colonized with the bacteria, the baby may be exposed if the membranes rupture or when the baby passes through the birth canal.

2. 1. This is an inappropriate response. Even though it is very likely that the baby will be fine, the nurse does not know for certain that the baby will be well.
2. This is the best response for the nurse to make. The nurse is providing the client with accurate, reassuring information without guaranteeing that there will definitely be a positive outcome.
3. This response is inappropriate. The client is in the transition phase of labor. She is not in a position to discuss the circumstances of her first baby's death.
4. This response is inappropriate. The client is in the transition phase of labor. She is not in a position to discuss the circumstances of her first baby's death.

TEST-TAKING HINT: Clients who have experienced fetal loss or the loss of a newborn are often very anxious during pregnancy, labor and delivery, and the early newborn period. Statistics that indicate a likelihood that there will be a good outcome often mean nothing to a person who has trusted statistics before yet experienced tragedy. The nurse must accept the client's concern and acknowledge the client's grief. It is also important for the nurse to keep the client well informed of all assessments and interventions related to the baby.

3. 1. An admission assessment should be performed by the nurse.
2. Client teaching should be performed by the nurse.
3. A urine collection bag may be put in place by the CNA.
4. The nurse should perform the hourly blood glucose assessments.

TEST-TAKING HINT: Nursing assistants do not have the education to perform sophisticated client care skills. An initial assessment, client teaching, and invasive neonatal procedures should all be performed by a skilled professional. Even though the CNA may collect blood glucose assessments on an adult, it is not appropriate for the CNA to perform them on a neonate. However the placement of a urine collection bag on a baby is a task that the CNA could be taught to perform.

4. 1. The client is not at risk of a precipitous delivery. Although this is her second baby, her first one was delivered by cesarean section. As such, her anticipated labor pattern will be one of a woman having her first baby because the birth canal has not been stretched by the previous baby.
2. The client currently has tachysystole; it is not a risk, it's a fact.
3. The fetus is at risk of hypoxemia due to tachysystole.

TEST-TAKING HINT: This question requires the test taker to recognize tachysystole and connect the associated risk of fetal hypoxemia to the contraction pattern. The client has tachysystole. As a result of inadequate uterine rest between contractions, the intervillous space from where the placenta draws oxygen does not have time to refill adequately with oxygenated maternal blood for uptake by the placenta. This results in fetal hypoxemia, or low oxygenated blood, as evidenced by minimal variability and late decelerations if the tachysystole persists.

5. **Answers 1 and 2 are correct.**
   1. **The client has tachysystole. The nurse must manage the contraction pattern and reduce the contraction frequency.**
   2. **The fetal heart rate is the only assessment the nurse can do to monitor for current or pending fetal hypoxemia that could lead to hypoxia and birth asphyxia.**
   3. The maternal temperature must be monitored, but it is unrelated to tachysystole and the risk of birth asphyxia in this case.
   4. Fetal movement is an antenatal assessment of fetal wellbeing, not an intrapartum one.

TEST-TAKING HINT: The test taker must identify contraction frequency as the place to intervene in order to reduce the risk of fetal hypoxemia.

6. **Answers 2 and 3 are correct.**
   1. Juice is not an appropriate intervention at this time. The prudent nurse would keep the client NPO in case the tachysystole could not be controlled and a cesarean section became necessary for fetal intolerance of labor.
   2. **Turn off the oxytocin to reduce contraction frequency. This is the most prudent and responsible intervention to manage tachysystole.**
   3. **Because the tachysystole interferes with adequate oxygen uptake at the placenta between contractions, supplementary oxygen is thought to increase the maternal oxygen saturation as a mitigating factor in fetal oxygenation and is the current standard of care.**
   4. A maternal change of position could be helpful in fetal oxygenation, but the test-taker must select only 2 answers. Turning off the oxytocin and administering oxygen are the most important interventions.

TEST-TAKING HINT: The FHR shows minimal variability. This could indicate that the fetus is sleeping at this time. However, it is more likely an indication of fetal hypoxemia related to tachysystole. Management of tachysystole and provision of oxygen to the fetus are the nurse's primary responsibilities. The nurse must turn off the oxytocin to reduce the contraction frequency, and administer oxygen to ensure adequate perfusion of the placenta and ultimately to the fetus. While administration of maternal oxygen is the current standard of care in this situation, the benefits of this practice have been questioned more recently, and this standard could change in the future. The prudent nurse must remain informed of changes in practice standards.

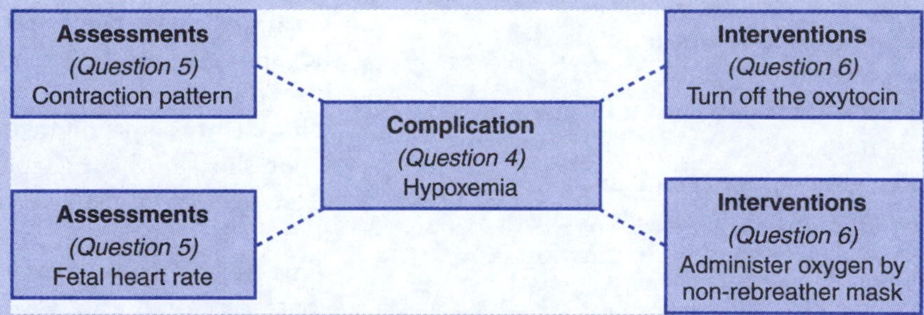

7. 1. If a hard, round object—the fetal head—was felt in the fundal region, the nurse would conclude that the fetus was in the breech position with sacral presentation.
   2. If a flat object—the fetal back—was felt above the symphysis, the nurse would conclude that the fetus was in a horizontal lie.
   3. If a soft, round object—the fetal buttocks—was felt on the left side of the uterus, the nurse would conclude that the fetus was in a horizontal lie.
   4. **A nurse could conclude that a fetus is in the LOA when feeling small objects—the fetal arms and legs—on the right side of the uterus.**

TEST-TAKING HINT: This is a difficult question. The test taker must clearly understand that in the LOA position the baby's back is on the left side of the mother's uterus as indicated by the letter "L," and the back of the baby's head, the occiput ("O") is facing the mother's anterior ("A"), or front side. This is the most common fetal presentation and is ideal. Because the baby's back is felt on the left side of the uterus, the small parts of the baby, the hands and feet, are felt on the right side.

8. **Answers 1, 3, and 4 are correct.**
   1. **Pregnancy is the most common cause of amenorrhea.**
   2. Although a client's temperature is slightly elevated during pregnancy, a nurse would not associate a fever with pregnancy.
   3. **A common complaint of women in early pregnancy is fatigue.**
   4. **A common complaint of women in early pregnancy is nausea.**
   5. Although pregnant women complain of urinary frequency early in pregnancy, they should not complain of pain with urination (dysuria).

TEST-TAKING HINT: This question is easily answered if the test taker is familiar with the presumptive signs of pregnancy—that is, the subjective complaints of pregnancy.

9. 1. This response is incorrect. Women who have bilateral tubal ligations (BTL) do still menstruate until they reach menopause.
   2. The surgery can be performed at any time, but is more easily performed the day after the birth during the postpartum hospital stay.
   3. Although BTLs have been reversed, the pregnancy success rate after reversals is variable.
   4. **This response is correct. BTL surgery is generally done under general anesthesia.**

TEST-TAKING HINT: Because scar tissue forms at the site of the BTL, it can be difficult to have a successful reversal of the procedure. Even though a sperm may be able to traverse the tube after reconstructive surgery has taken place, the fertilized egg is often too large to migrate through the tube to the uterus for implantation. Women are at high risk for ectopic pregnancies after tubal reconstructive surgery.

10. 1. **Two side effects of prostaglandin administration are nausea and uterine tetany.**
    2. Hypertension and vaginal bleeding are not associated with prostaglandin administration.
    3. Urinary retention and severe headache are not associated with prostaglandin administration.
    4. Bradycardia and hypothermia are not associated with prostaglandin administration.

TEST-TAKING HINT: The nurse must be familiar with the side effects of commonly administered medications. Prostaglandins are frequently administered to women who are to be induced but who have low Bishop scores. Prostaglandins help to ripen the cervix and soften it so it responds to uterine contractions by thinning (effacing) and dilating.

11. 1. **The nurse should call the postoperative cesarean client back first. It sounds from her description that she has a wound infection.**
    2. This client is a primigravida and if she is in labor, she is in the early phase of the first stage. Her call must be returned, but it can wait.
    3. This client should be offered emergency contraception. Although the medicine must be taken within 72 hours of intercourse, the nurse can wait to return her call.
    4. This client is complaining of menstrual pain. Although she needs pain medicine, the nurse can wait to return her call.

TEST-TAKING HINT: To answer this question, the nurse must prioritize care. The woman who is most vulnerable at this time is the woman with a wound infection. If she truly does have a wound infection, she will need to be seen by the primary healthcare provider, have a culture of the wound taken, and be put on antibiotics. For most NCLEX questions, the correct answer is the answer that responds to the most serious, life-threatening condition.

12. 2 mL.

The standard formula for this question is:

$$\frac{\text{Known dose}}{\text{Known volume}} = \frac{\text{Desired dose}}{\text{Desired volume}}$$

$$\frac{1\text{ gram}}{8\text{ mL}} = \frac{250\text{ mg}}{x\text{ mL}}$$

$$\frac{1{,}000\text{ mg}}{8\text{ mL}} = \frac{250\text{ mg}}{x\text{ mL}}$$

$$1{,}000x = 2{,}000$$
$$x = 2\text{ mL}$$

The dimensional analysis formula for this question is:

Known volume	Desired dosage	Unit conversion	Time conversion	= Desired volume
Known dosage		(if needed)	(if needed)	

8 mL	250 mg	1 g	= x mL
1 g		1,000 mg	

$$\frac{2{,}000}{1{,}000} = x\text{ mL}$$
$$x = 2\text{ mL}$$

TEST-TAKING HINT: If the nurse always uses the formula—inserting the correct values into the respective locations—calculation errors are unlikely. The known dosage and volume are given; that is, 1 gram in 8 mL. Although pre-mixed medications are prepared by the pharmacist in the hospital, a nurse in a clinic will likely need to prepare the injections and knowing the correct formula is key.

13. 1. Folded and flat pinnae are seen in preterm newborns, not postmature babies.
2. Smooth plantar surfaces are seen in preterm newborns, not postmature babies.
3. **The skin of the post-term baby is loose because the baby has depleted most of the subcutaneous fat stores and is peeling because of dehydration related to the post-term changes in the placenta.**
4. The nurse would expect to see long fingernails that may be tinged green from exposure to meconium.

TEST-TAKING HINT: Post-term babies are in utero while the placenta ages. As a result of calcifications in the placenta, the fetal supply of nourishment, hydration, and oxygen is reduced. Loose skin often connotes a loss of weight, and peeling skin is the result of poor nutrition and poor hydration.

14. 1. The client's potassium level is normal.
2. The client's sodium level is normal.
3. **The platelet count is well below normal.**
4. The white blood cell count is normal for a 38-week-gestation woman.

TEST-TAKING HINT: The normal platelet count is 150,000 to 400,000 cells/mm^3. This client's cell count is well below normal showing thrombocytopenia. Clients with low platelet counts are at high risk for bleeding spontaneously. Although thrombocytopenia could be the client's sole problem, the nurse should also assess the client for any other signs of HELLP syndrome. Although the white blood cell count is elevated for a nonpregnant woman, it is normal for a perinatal client.

15. 1. A sample of cord blood is taken but it is not used to check for inborn errors of metabolism and other diseases. Rather, the baby's blood type and Coombs test are assessed from the cord blood sample.
2. The blood must be obtained prior to the baby's discharge from the hospital.
3. This answer is incorrect. Admission blood is not used to check for inborn errors of metabolism and other diseases.
4. **This answer is correct. Because many of the inborn diseases are related to metabolism of foods, the baby must be fed a few times before the blood is drawn.**

TEST-TAKING HINT: The genetic disease phenylketonuria (PKU) is one of the many metabolic illnesses that babies are assessed for. Babies with PKU lack the enzyme needed for fully metabolizing phenylalanine, an essential amino acid. To accurately assess whether the baby lacks the enzyme or not, the baby must have consumed the proteins that are present in breast milk or formula before the blood test is performed.

16. **The test taker should place an "X" in the diagram's left upper quadrant.**

TEST-TAKING HINT: The best way to remember the placement of the fetal heart Doppler device is to remember that the heartbeat is best heard through the fetal back. This baby is in a breech position of *left sacrum anterior* (LSA). The baby's back is on the mother's left, as indicated by the letter L. The sacrum (S), or baby's bottom, is presenting and is aligned toward the front, or anterior (A), of the mother's abdomen, as indicated by the letters S and A. The sacrum presentation indicates the baby is breech. Because the baby is in the breech position and is not yet engaged at –2 station, the baby is up quite high. Because the baby's back is on the mother's left side, the fetal heart would be located in the upper left quadrant.

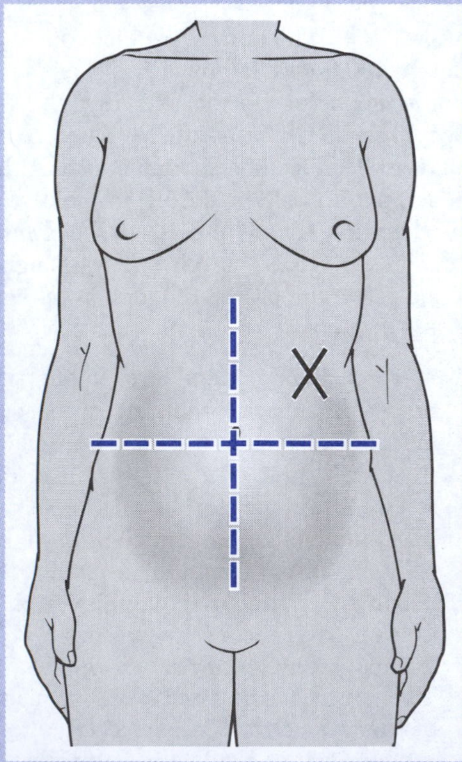

17\. 1. **This response is correct. Only water-based lubricants should be used with the condom.**
2. Natural lambskin condoms do not protect the wearer from viral sexually transmitted illnesses. Latex condoms do protect the wearer.
3. The condom should be applied to an erect penis.
4. A small reservoir should be left in the condom at the tip of the penis.

TEST-TAKING HINT: The condom is an excellent birth control and infection control device if it is used properly. The nurse must be prepared to educate clients, both male and female, in its correct use.

18\. 1. This fetal heart tracing shows a healthy fetus with good variability and accelerations.
2. This fetal heart tracing indicates that the fetus is experiencing head compression—early decelerations.
3. This fetal heart tracing indicates the presence of uteroplacental insufficiency—late decelerations.
4. **This fetal heart tracing indicates the presence of cord compression—variable decelerations.**

TEST-TAKING HINT: One way to remember why variable decelerations indicate cord compression is the fact that the cord is a free-floating object in the uterine cavity. As such, it can be compressed at various times. For example, if the baby moves a certain way, the cord can be compressed between the baby's body and the uterine wall. Some fetuses have been seen on ultrasound scans to have their hands around the cord, and they may squeeze it involuntarily. Additionally, when the mother moves to a new position, the cord can be compressed in similar ways. The decelerations seen, therefore, occur at times independent of timing of the contractions. In addition, one must consider the etiology of variable decelerations. Because of the cord compression, the blood flow within the cord is temporarily blocked. The heart protects itself from pumping against a "roadblock" by slowing down the number of heartbeats it makes until after the "roadblock" is cleared.

19. 1. This statement is incorrect. A perinatal mortality rate of 16 means that 16 babies died between 28 weeks' gestation and 28 days of age per 1,000 live births.

2. This statement is correct. A perinatal mortality rate of 16 means that 16 babies died between 28 weeks' gestation and 28 days of age per 1,000 live births.

3. This statement is incorrect. A perinatal mortality rate of 16 means that 16 babies died between 28 weeks' gestation and 28 days of age per 1,000 live births.

4. This statement is incorrect. A perinatal mortality rate of 16 means that 16 babies died between 28 weeks' gestation and 28 days of age per 1,000 live births.

TEST-TAKING HINT: The perinatal period is defined as the time period between 28 weeks' gestation and 4 weeks (or 28 days) after delivery. The best way to remember that definition is to remember that the prefix "peri" means "around" and the word "natal" refers to "birth." The perinatal period, therefore, is the time period around the birth.

20. 15 mL.

30 grams − 15 grams = 15 grams

The client has lost approximately 15 mL of blood.

TEST-TAKING HINT: The nurse must remember that 1 mL of fluid = 1 gram of fluid. This is true of blood, water, breast milk, or any other natural fluid.

21. 1. This response is true. Testosterone is responsible for the development of the male secondary sex characteristics.

2. This response is incorrect. Unlike the monthly hormonal fluctuations seen in the female, testosterone levels are relatively constant at all times.

3. This response is incorrect. Testosterone is produced by the testes.

4. Although the level of testosterone does drop slightly with age, the testes will produce the hormone throughout life.

TEST-TAKING HINT: It is important for the obstetrical nurse to be familiar with the anatomy and physiology of both the male and the female reproductive systems, since both contribute to procreation.

22. 1. Mothers who discuss their labor and delivery experiences are exhibiting a characteristic of the "taking-in" postpartum phase.

2. Mothers who eat quantities of food are exhibiting a characteristic of the "taking-in" postpartum phase.

3. When mothers are interested in learning baby-care skills from the nurse, they are exhibiting signs of the "taking-hold" postpartum phase.

4. Mothers who express intense fatigue and take naps throughout the day are exhibiting a characteristic of the "taking-in" postpartum phase.

TEST-TAKING HINT: The "taking-hold" phase is the postpartum period when mothers regain their independence and express interest in caring for their neonate. Prior to that time, during the "taking-in" phase, mothers express the need to be cared for while they internalize their labor and delivery experience.

23. 1. The amniocentesis results indicate Turner syndrome—45, X, a genetic anomaly—but the fetus is viable.

2. The fetus is a female with one of 46 chromosomes partially or completely missing. This is referred to as aneuploidy.

3. The child will be phenotypically female.

4. Babies with Turner syndrome are characterized by short stature, broad chests, and the inability to conceive.

TEST-TAKING HINT: The genetic anomaly 45, X is one of the few monosomies that are viable. There is no intellectual disability associated with Turner syndrome.

24. 1. The anterior fontanelle will close by the time the baby is about 18 months of age.

2. The grasp reflex will disappear when the baby is about 3 months of age.

3. Babies see colors at birth. And they see quite well when they are about 12 to 18 inches away from an object.

4. Babies are usually started on solids at 4 to 6 months of age.

TEST-TAKING HINT: The obstetric nurse must be familiar with normal growth and development. It is essential that nurses provide parents with anticipatory guidance regarding their child's normal growth and development milestones.

25. 1. This action is appropriate. It is very likely that this client is fully dilated. The urge to push is very similar to the urge to have a bowel movement.

2. This action is appropriate only if the nurse, after examining the woman, determines that she is not fully dilated.

3. This action is inappropriate. Not only has the client not complained of pain, but she is likely fully dilated and ready to push.
4. There is nothing in the scenario that indicates that the fetus is in danger at this time.

TEST-TAKING HINT: This client is a multipara. This is her 4th baby and her labor could go quickly. Even though her last vaginal examination indicated that she entered active labor 1 hour ago, it is very likely that this client has experienced very rapid cervical change and is now in the second stage of labor. The urge to push, a classic sign of the second stage of labor, feels very similar to the urge to have a large bowel movement. In addition, the presence of increased bloody show helps to confirm advanced cervical dilation versus a need for a bowel movement.

26. **1. The couple should include in the birth plan whether the mother plans to breastfeed or bottle feed the baby.**
2. It is unnecessary to include in the birth plan the name and address of the woman's health insurance company.
3. It is unnecessary to include in the birth plan the couple's baby name preferences.
4. It is unnecessary to include in the birth plan the couple's cell phone numbers.

TEST-TAKING HINT: A test taker who remembers the rationale for the birth plan will find the correct response to this question an easy one. The birth plan is a document that a couple creates to facilitate communication between themselves and healthcare professionals in relation to the couple's wishes for the birth. It is always important, however, to remind the couple that not all of their wishes may be possible, and that in the event of emergency the primary healthcare provider must make medical decisions that may change the plans they have made.

27. Answers 1, 2, and 3 are correct.
1. The client's age should be considered by the nurse.
2. The client's obstetric history should be considered by the nurse.
3. The client's religious beliefs should be considered by the nurse.
4. The client's employment is not usually relevant in relation to her choice of family planning method.
5. The client's body structure is not usually relevant in relation to her choice of family planning method.

TEST-TAKING HINT: Many issues will determine a client's willingness and ability to use family planning methods. For example, a client's religious beliefs may rule out any method other than a natural family planning method. If a client states that she feels she has completed her family, she may be interested in a permanent family planning method. A woman over 35 who smokes should be advised not to use a hormonally based method for health considerations.

28. **1. The nurse would expect that the baby would be hyperreflexic.**
2. Babies who are showing signs of NAS often seek urgently to suck or feed. They do not show signs of anorexia.
3. Babies who are showing signs of NAS often have diarrhea, not constipation.
4. Hypokalemia is not related to NAS.

TEST-TAKING HINT: Babies who are withdrawing from addictive substances exhibit agitated behaviors, including hyperreflexia, high-pitched crying, and disorganized behavioral states.

29. 1. These signs are evident when the amniotic sac ruptures, not when a client experiences an amniotic fluid embolism.
2. Intense, unrelenting uterine pain is seen with placental abruption and uterine rupture, not with amniotic fluid embolism.
3. Precipitous dilation and expulsion of the fetus describes a precipitous delivery.
4. Chest pain with dyspnea and cyanosis are the classic signs of amniotic fluid embolism, also referred to as "anaphylactoid syndrome of pregnancy" (ASP).

TEST-TAKING HINT: Amniotic fluid embolism (AFE) is an extremely rare, catastrophic calamity in obstetrics. It happens as a result of fluid, fetal cells, hair, and/or other debris entering the mother's pulmonary circulation. The results can be on a continuum of mild organ damage, through coagulopathy, cardiovascular collapse, or death (Kaur et al., 2016). As more is learned about the condition, it has become referred to more recently as "anaphylactoid syndrome of pregnancy" (ASP), since the body's response is one of anaphylaxis rather than mechanical pulmonary blockage due to embolism. It may occur up to 48 hours after a delivery (Kaur et al., 2016).

30. 1. Voiding after each sexual encounter decreases women's chances of developing a urinary tract infection.
2. Clients who use the diaphragm as a family planning device are at high risk for urinary tract infections.

3. To prevent the introduction of rectal flora into the urinary tract, it is important for women to wipe from front to back after toileting.
4. Because blood is an ideal medium for bacterial growth, it is recommended that women change their peripads frequently.

TEST-TAKING HINT: Women are at higher risk for urinary tract infections (UTI) than men because of the close proximity of the urethra to the vagina and rectum. The primary infective agent for bladder infections is E coli, which resides in the colon and rectum. The diaphragm is used with a spermicide. The use of spermicides changes the pH of the vagina and can kill off the protective vaginal bacteria as a result, allowing E coli to proliferate and migrate from the vagina to the urethra and ultimately to the bladder. Women should be counseled on ways to prevent UTI, and women who are prone to UTI should consider changing their family planning method from the diaphragm to another method.

31. 1. **This statement is true. The client's feelings are normal.**
2. Because the postpartum blues usually last less than 2 weeks, it is unlikely that the physician will order antidepressants for the client.
3. This statement is incorrect. It is not possible to change one's feelings by merely "thinking" positive thoughts.
4. This statement is inappropriate. The blues may continue for up to 10 days, well after the client returns home.

TEST-TAKING HINT: Postpartum blues are considered normal. About 80% of women experience them. They are related to the hormonal shifts that occur after delivery as well as fatigue and the emotional stress of having full responsibility for the care and well-being of a neonate. The finality of motherhood with no option to change one's mind also makes some women feel trapped initially until they become familiar with the new routine, become bonded with the baby, and feel more confident about their ability to handle the new role.

32. 1. Correlational statistics never indicate cause and effect relationships.
2. There is no indication of a significant relationship—designated by a *P* value—in the scenario.
3. **This statement is accurate. In a negative correlation, as the values of one variable rise, the values of the other variable drop.**
4. This statement is meaningless.

TEST-TAKING HINT: The nurse must be very careful when interpreting correlational statistics. Correlations merely communicate whether variables are related. They should never be interpreted as cause and effect relationships. Correlations may be positive, negative, or zero. In a positive correlation, both the independent and dependent variables move together. A negative correlation occurs when one variable goes up and the other goes down, much like a teeter totter on a playground. In a zero correlation, two items are not at all related. Because this question refers to a negative correlation, the nurse understands that the independent variable goes up as the dependent variable goes down.

33. 1. **This is an accurate description of the tonic neck position.**
2. This is a description of a child with torticollis.
3. This is a description of a child with opisthotonus.
4. This is a description of a baby exhibiting the trunk incurvation reflex.

TEST-TAKING HINT: Tonic neck position is a very common neonatal reflex. It is also called the fencing position and lasts until the baby is 5 to 7 months old. It has been suggested that the reflex developed to prevent babies from rolling over onto their bellies, a high-risk position that predisposes babies to sudden infant death syndrome.

34. 1. A doula is not a nurse. It is not appropriate for the nurse to delegate the regulation of the oxytocin drip rate to the doula.
2. A doula is not a nurse. It is not appropriate for the nurse to delegate the monitoring of the client's vaginal dilation to the doula.
3. **The doula is an expert in assisting laboring clients to work with their labors.**
4. A doula is not a nurse. It is not appropriate for the nurse to delegate the monitoring for hyperstimulation to the doula.

TEST-TAKING HINT: The role of the doula is as a labor support person. For the doula, assisting the client to cope with labor is the essence of the role. It is inappropriate for doulas to perform any professional nursing care such as evaluating electronic monitor tracings,

administering medications, and performing physical assessments. The nurse has the ultimate responsibility for clinical evaluations and may also help the doula to support the client in coping with labor, providing education, re-positioning, and information as needed.

35. 1. **This response is correct. Women who complain of ptyalism should be advised to use an astringent mouthwash.**
2. Elevating one's legs will not alleviate a woman's complaint of ptyalism.
3. Eating high-fiber foods will not alleviate a woman's complaint of ptyalism.
4. Voiding when the urge is felt will not alleviate a woman's complaint of ptyalism.

TEST-TAKING HINT: Some women complain of ptyalism, described as excessive salivation, during pregnancy. The condition is caused by the increase in vascularity of the mucous membranes as a result of elevated estrogen levels in the bloodstream. An astringent mouthwash can have a drying effect on the salivary glands.

36. 1. **Walking is an excellent preventive exercise for women who are at high risk for osteoporosis.**
2. Chocolate milk contains calcium and vitamin D. The intake of both substances is important in the prevention of osteoporosis.
3. Red meat is not high in calcium or vitamin D.
4. The type of shoe worn by a woman will not affect her bone density.

TEST-TAKING HINT: A woman's bone health is positively affected by her participation in exercise. Weight-bearing exercises, such as walking, jogging, running, and weight lifting, provide the most benefit for women who are at high risk for osteoporosis.

37. 1. The nurse would not expect the baby to be polycythemic.
2. **The nurse should watch for hypothermia in the baby who has transparent skin with visible veins.**
3. The nurse would expect the baby to be hypoglycemic rather than hyperglycemic.
4. The nurse would not expect the baby to have polyuria.

TEST-TAKING HINT: Translucent skin with visible veins, a sign of prematurity, indicates that the subcutaneous fat has yet to be deposited. Because subcutaneous fat is an insulating substance and the baby has very little, the baby is at high risk for hypothermia.

38. 1. A motor vehicle accident is a risk factor for placental abruption, not placenta previa.
2. **The client is at risk for a placental abruption.**
3. Although a ruptured uterus is possible after a motor vehicle accident, this client's symptoms of a rigid uterus and bleeding do not suggest that.

TEST-TAKING HINT: See the bowtie diagram on the next page. A placental abruption is always a differential diagnosis when a pregnant client has a motor vehicle accident. The placenta has been referred to by some as a large potato chip in the uterus. When the uterus is injured with force, as in a motor vehicle accident, portions of the "potato chip" can break and lift away from the uterine wall as a result. This leaves the fetus with inadequate oxygen, and puts the mother at risk of hemorrhage.

A placenta previa is a biological condition that occurs early in the pregnancy and is unrelated to a motor vehicle accident. If the client's uterus had ruptured as a result of the accident, it is not likely the client would be conscious enough to talk or that her vital signs would be in this range. She would likely have exsanguinated at the site of the accident.

39. Answers 1 and 3 are correct.
1. **By reducing the attached surface area of the placenta to its oxygen source, placental abruption can reduce the fetal oxygen supply. The nurse can only assess fetal well-being by assessing the FHR.**
2. Although the client's pain level is important to assess, it is not one of the most important assessments because it does not guide life-saving interventions.
3. **The amount of vaginal bleeding is an important assessment. The nurse should weigh all pads to calculate cumulative blood loss, which can guide further clinical treatment decisions. Most—but not all—placental abruptions are accompanied by vaginal bleeding. Because this client is bleeding, as noted in the stem, the bleeding should be monitored. If there were no bleeding, the pain level would be one of the 2 most important assessments to monitor for worsening status. This client's pain should also be assessed and monitored, but the bleeding is one of the 2 most important assessments in this case.**
4. It is not likely there are clinical labs to assess on admission. The laboratory data will be

assessed once the client is stabilized, to guide in further clinical treatment decisions.

TEST-TAKING HINT: When caring for a pregnant client who has been involved in a motor vehicle accident, the two most serious questions to answer are, "Is the fetus alive?" and "Is the mother's circulating blood quantity adequate to sustain both her and the fetus?" Finding answers to those two questions about survival are priorities. We are not given the FHR in this case study. As such, we don't know whether or not the fetus was affected by the accident. Fetal assessment should be one of the first assessments to be completed.

40. Answers 2 and 3 are correct.

1. Weighing all pads and keeping strict intake and output is important, but the pads can be weighed later, once the client is transferred to the operating room.
2. **Before the client undergoes general anesthesia, any drug allergies or serious medical conditions listed on her medic alert bracelet must be reviewed and clarified, if possible.**
3. **Insertion of an IV line is essential. A large gauge must be used in the likely need for blood transfusions.**
4. While the surgical prep and catheter insertion are important, they are tasks, not potentially life-saving interventions. Although the hair clipping is best done outside of the operating room, in an emergency it may be done in the operating room by one nurse in tandem with the catheter insertion by another nurse, just before the procedure begins.

TEST-TAKING HINT: Placental abruption is an obstetric emergency. The client may or may not have visible bleeding. This client is actively bleeding and all signs and risk factors point to a placental abruption. The client's rapid heart rate and a blood pressure that is lower than expected for a client at 32 weeks' gestation, suggests severe hypovolemia. An IV fluid bolus can perfuse the placenta and bring needed oxygen to the fetus, as well, although a blood transfusion will likely be necessary to add oxygen-carrying red blood cells to the circulation. In an emergent situation like this, a full medical history is not possible, but if the client has a life-threatening condition as suggested by her medic-alert bracelet, that must be clarified before she receives general anesthesia. The nurse must often make decisions between competing priorities in an emergent situation such as this.

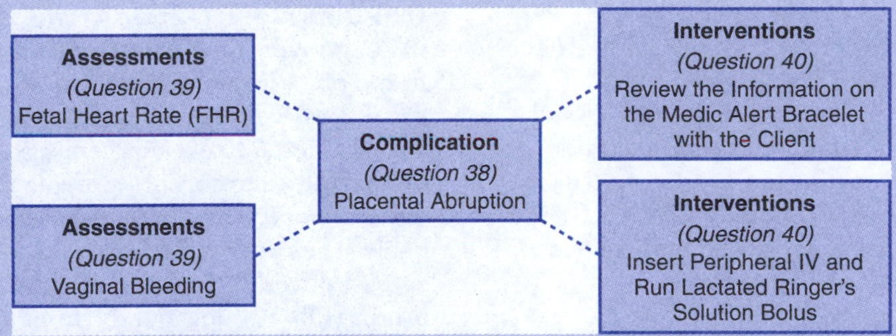

41. 1. A non-reactive nonstress test (NST) result is characterized by a stable fetal heart rate throughout the test period.
2. The length of contractions is not considered when a nonstress test is performed.
3. The mother's pain level is not considered when a nonstress test is performed.
4. A reactive nonstress test is characterized by at least 2 spontaneous fetal movements in a 20-minute time period.

TEST-TAKING HINT: A nonstress test (NST) is performed to assess the well-being and oxygenation of the fetus during pregnancy. A reactive test is a reassuring test, indicating fetal well-being. A stable FHR without accelerations is also reassuring, but the purpose of the test is to assess the FHR during periods of fetal movement. The test assesses whether or not the fetal heart rate goes up with exercise, a normal, physiologic response for all of us, in the setting of adequate oxygenation. It is important to note, however, that the NST results are not predictive of continued fetal well-being and only indicate the presence or absence of fetal hypoxemia at the time of the test (Umana & Siccardi, 2020).

42. 1. The symbol represents a couple who has mated, not a healthy sister and brother.
2. The symbol represents a couple who has mated.
3. The symbol represents a couple who has mated, not a grandmother and grandson.
4. The symbol represents a couple who has mated, not a father and daughter.

TEST-TAKING HINT: When a female (circle) and a male (square) are connected with a single line on a pedigree, a couple who has mated is represented. A circle and square connected by a double line indicates a consanguineous couple (blood relatives) who has mated.

43. 1. She is not at high risk for mammary rupture.
2. She is not at high risk for postpartum psychosis.
3. She is not at high risk for supernumerary nipples.
4. The client is at high risk for the development of a breast abscess.

TEST-TAKING HINT: When clients wean abruptly, the breasts become engorged with milk. Mastitis is a breast infection usually caused by *Staphylococcus aureus*. When the milk is not removed from the breast, an abscess, or collection of pus, can develop in the breast.

44. 1. Although it is important to ask if any of her partners have hurt her, it is not the best question to ask at this time. In addition, an injury would be painful.
2. Asking if she ever has unprotected intercourse is the best question to ask at this time.
3. Whether or not she has had a baby is not the best question to ask at this time.
4. Although asking if she thinks she may be pregnant is important, it is not the best question to ask at this time.

TEST-TAKING HINT: This is an unmarried woman who may be having intercourse with people who are intimate with others. The young woman may be feeling a lesion caused by a sexually transmitted infection, such as a syphilitic chancre or a perineal wart. This is the only question that pertains to a client's reason for coming to the clinic and must be addressed first.

45. 1. The baby should have a minimum of 6 wet diapers during each 24-hour period.
2. The baby should have 3 to 4 loose, bright yellow stools during each 24-hour period. Babies who consume formula often have pasty, brownish-colored stools.
3. The baby should breastfeed a minimum of 8 times in a 24-hour period.
4. Neonates gain, on average, about 5 oz per week, not 6 oz in a 24-hour period.

TEST-TAKING HINT: In answering this question, the test taker must pay attention to the time frame of 24 hours over a span of the first week of life. Breastfeeding mothers often worry whether their babies are receiving enough to eat. It is important, therefore, to provide the mothers with objective assessments that inform them that their babies are receiving enough fluids and nutrition: at least 6 wet diapers per day and 3 to 4 loose, bright yellow stools per 24-hour day. In addition, if the mother is still concerned about her baby's health, she can take the baby to the pediatrician's office for periodic weight evaluations. Babies generally lose 7% to 10% of their birth weight within the first week of life and then begin gaining about 4 ounces a week. However, it is not uncommon for babies to take up to 2 weeks to regain birth weight (Paul et al., 2016).

46. Every 3 min × 60 sec.

TEST-TAKING HINT: Frequency (always measured in minutes [min]) is defined as the time period from the beginning of one contraction to the beginning of the next contraction. That is, a time frame that includes the start of a contraction and

the rest period that follows. Duration (always measured in seconds [sec]) is defined as the time period from the beginning of one contraction to the end of the same contraction.

47. 1. The client is not currently pregnant and has 4 living children.
2. The client is not currently pregnant and has had 3 full-term pregnancies.
3. The client is not currently pregnant and has had 2 preterm deliveries.
4. The client is not currently pregnant and has had 1 abortion.

TEST-TAKING HINT: Gravidity (G) is defined as the total number of pregnancies a woman has had, including a current pregnancy. Parity (P) refers to deliveries. The four numbers following the P refer to the following obstetrical history, using the letters T, P, A, L. It is helpful to keep those letters in mind when assessing a client's obstetrical history. They indicate full-term pregnancies (T), preterm pregnancies (P), abortions and/or miscarriages (A), and living children (L). The client in the scenario, therefore, has been pregnant 6 times (G6). She has had 3 full-term deliveries (T3), 2 preterm deliveries (P2), 1 abortion (A1), and has 4 living children (L4). The client is not currently pregnant. The first 3 numbers of parity (Term 3 + Preterm 2, + Abortion 1) equal 6, the total number of pregnancies, which matches the gravidity (G6). If she were pregnant, her pregnancy count would be larger by 1 number (G7). Sadly, only 4 of her children are living (L4).

48. 1. A woman should be encouraged to stand erect to improve her posture but this action is not related to the pelvic tilt.
2. Bending at the waist from one side to the other can be a valuable exercise but it is not the pelvic tilt.
3. The woman successively changes her back from a concave to a convex posture when doing the pelvic tilt. This is sometimes described as arching one's back like an "angry cat" and then relaxing the back.
4. It is recommended that pregnant women not lie flat on their back.

TEST-TAKING HINT: The pelvic tilt is an excellent exercise for pregnant women. It helps to strengthen as well as to relax the muscles of the lower back. The nurse should be familiar not only with the name of exercises or other procedures but also with the way each is performed.

49. 1. Necrotizing enterocolitis does not result in hearing loss.
2. Hypoglycemia does not result in hearing loss.
3. Bronchopulmonary dysplasia does not result in hearing loss.
4. A baby who has had kernicterus can develop hearing loss.

TEST-TAKING HINT: Kernicterus occurs when bilirubin in the bloodstream reaches toxic levels beyond neonatal physiologic jaundice. Bilirubin is neurotoxic. Early signs of kernicterus are lethargy, sleepiness, and poor feeding. Severe kernicterus, when babies develop seizures and opisthotonus, can result in a number of neurological problems, including cerebral palsy, sensory deficits, and behavioral disorders.

50. 1. Estimating fetal length and weight will not assist the midwife with the delivery of the baby.
2. Assessing the intensity of the contractions will not assist the midwife with the delivery of the baby.
3. Suprapubic pressure can help to dislodge the shoulders of a macrosomic baby and facilitate the delivery.
4. Assisting the woman with breathing will not assist the midwife with the delivery of the baby.

TEST-TAKING HINT: Macrosomia can lead to shoulder dystocia during a delivery. This is a "mechanical" emergency where the vertical position of the fetal shoulders has trapped the fetus behind the horizontal pubic bone. One can visualize the letter "T," with the fetus represented by the up-and-down vertical line, and the pubic bone as a solid, crossbar that blocks the fetal descent. Suprapubic pressure just above the pubic bone helps to dislodge the shoulders and enable the baby to be delivered. The goal of suprapubic pressure is to press the upper fetal shoulder down so that the lower shoulder moves forward into an oblique, or slanted position, releasing the upper shoulder. Think of it as changing a solid, capital "T" into an italic letter "*f*." This dislodges the stuck shoulder and the baby slides out for delivery. Nurses must not apply *fundal* pressure at the top of the uterus, in this situation. Rather than facilitating delivery of the shoulders, fundal pressure can actually worsen the dystocia.

51. 1. The client is most likely at risk of engorgement.
2. Mastitis may occur if the client develops an infection, but there is no indication of an infection in the question stem, just a cracked and bleeding nipple.
3. There is no indication that the client is at risk of thrush.

TEST-TAKING HINT: It is important to focus on just what the question is asking and not to broaden it to the wider option of complications that could happen. A client can have cracked and bleeding nipples that heal without leading to mastitis. In this case, if the mother does not nurse on one side, that side can become engorged, initially. The combination of engorgement and cracked nipples may eventually lead to an abscess or mastitis if the condition does not improve.

52. Answers 3 and 4 are correct.
1. Cracked and bleeding nipples are not an emergency that requires a provider's visit.
2. There is no need to pump and dump the milk. If the baby swallows some of the mother's blood it is not a problem.
3. **The baby's strongest suck is at the beginning of the feeding. The vigor may cause unnecessary pain and trauma to the already-tender nipple. However, to reduce the risk of engorgement, the mother should nurse the baby on both sides, beginning on the unaffected side.**
4. **Lanolin cream can protect the skin and promote healing.**

TEST-TAKING HINT: Emptying the breasts and healing the skin are the two goals for this client. Other information the nurse can give the client during the conversation may include using an alternative breastfeeding position in order to change the location of the strongest suction from the baby's mouth.

53. Answers 3 and 4 are correct.
1. The baby's weight is not of concern in this scenario.
2. Washing the nipples before and after feedings is not necessary and may in fact dry out the skin, causing further cracking.
3. **Alternating breastfeeding positions can assist by providing variable positioning of the baby's mouth on the breast. This can reduce damage to the nipple.**
4. **It is always prudent to include next steps in client communication. The client's current symptoms do not suggest mastitis, but she should be advised of the risk and the symptoms that may suggest this condition, and the recommendation to call the office if the symptoms occur.**

TEST-TAKING HINT: While the initial question was focused on the client's current symptoms and concerns, the plan of care often includes the wider possibility of complications that the client should be aware of, such as mastitis. The baby's weight is not of concern, and washing the nipples frequently can disturb the natural flora and the antibiotic properties of breast milk, itself. The best answers are #3 and #4.

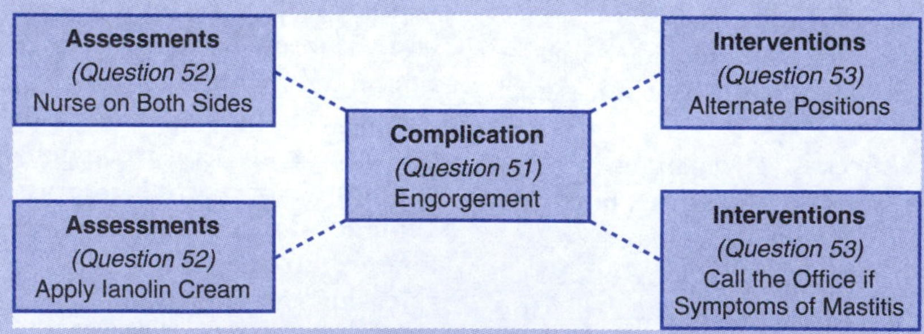

54. 1. Fetal fibronectin is an assessment of preterm labor. Headache is associated with pre-eclampsia, not preterm labor.
2. Visual disturbances are associated with pre-eclampsia, not preterm labor.
3. The nurse should advise the client to report any uterine cramping immediately.
4. Oliguria is associated with pre-eclampsia, not preterm labor.

TEST-TAKING HINT: As noted in chapter 9, question 88, fetal fibronectin is the biologic glue that attaches the fetal sac to the uterine lining. Its presence indicates the uterus might be preparing to release the fetus through contractions. As a result, a positive fetal fibronectin assessment between 22 and 37 weeks' gestation puts a client at high risk for preterm labor.

55. 1. Babies who swallow after every suck usually are latched well.
2. To latch well, babies should face their mother's body.
3. When babies' lips are curled under, they are unable to create a satisfactory suck. In addition, it is usually painful for the mother.
4. Neonates should be placed at the level of their mother's breasts to breastfeed.

TEST-TAKING HINT: Improper latching is the most common cause of breast discomfort and can cause sore nipples. To create a good latch, babies should have a large quantity of breast tissue in their mouth, lips should be wide open like a yawn, and surround both the nipple and much or all of the areola. This facilitates correct movement of the tongue. With a correct latch, the action of the mouth, tongue, and lips will massage the milk out of the milk ducts and eliminate a "chewing" action on the nipple by the baby.

56. The correct order is 2, 4, 3, 1, 5.

TEST-TAKING HINT: For the fetus to traverse the birth canal easily, the baby must first flex the head so that the chin is on the chest (flexion). This allows the fetal head to fit the oval, left-to-right shape of the pelvic inlet. With continuing descent through the pelvis, the contractions force the head to turn (internal rotation), in order to fit the lower portion of the pelvis, the pelvic outlet. Unlike the pelvic inlet's left-to-right oval, the pelvic outlet has a front-to-back oval shape. With crowning, the baby's head appears and is released from the birth canal in its face down position (extension). Once freed from the constraints of the birth canal, the head moves back into the original position in alignment with the body (external rotation). The shoulders are still in their original position. As they slide under the pubic bone, the baby is delivered (expulsion).

57. 1. Although it is not easy, it is possible to consume enough protein to sustain a pregnancy on a vegan diet.
2. This action is essential. Women's protein demands increase during pregnancy. Registered dietitians are qualified to evaluate a pregnant woman's total protein and essential amino acid intake.
3. This response is incorrect. Cashews and coconut are not excellent sources of calcium.
4. This response is incorrect. Vegans eat no animal protein.

TEST-TAKING HINT: Nurses do receive nutrition education during their nursing programs. They are not, however, experts in the field. It is very important for nurses to know the limits of their knowledge. Because protein, as well as calcium intake, is essential for a healthy pregnancy, it is important for the nurse to refer the client to the expert in the field.

58. Answers 2, 4, 5, and 6 are correct.
1. Because there is no indication that the client passed out, her sensorium is not of immediate importance.
2. The client's urinary output of 100 mL requires follow-up, especially in light of the deviated, boggy fundus. A full bladder can prevent the uterus from contracting adequately.
3. The client's blood glucose is not of concern and is not related to her bleeding or urinary output.
4. The client's fundal assessment requires follow-up assessments at least every 15 minutes, to confirm that it has moved lower and remains firm.
5. The client's rapid pulse rate and low blood pressure suggest hypovolemia.
6. Same as above. The client's rapid pulse rate and low blood pressure suggest hypovolemia.

TEST-TAKING HINT: The test taker must understand that the term "follow-up" doesn't necessarily mean the nurse must complete another assessment. To follow up on a condition may include reviewing the chart for trends, provider's orders, additional interventions, and so forth. This client has several risk factors for, and cues related to hypovolemia. The test taker should take each option and determine whether or not it requires immediate intervention and could impact the lowest step on Maslow's hierarchy of needs, that of survival.

59. Answers 1 and (d) are correct.

Assess first (Select one, below)	Followed by (Select one, below)
1. Residual urine	a. Residual urine
2. Total blood loss	b. Total blood loss
3. Fluid intake	c. Fluid intake
4. Medication list	**d. Medication list**

1. **It is unlikely the client had only 100 mL of urine in her bladder at this point; the actual volume is no doubt much larger than that. Although the client's total blood loss is of concern, the fundus cannot contract fully unless the bladder is emptied. Of these 4 options, the possible residual urine amount is the most pressing assessment that requires intervention since it can affect uterine contractility.**
2. The client's total blood loss is important, but until the bladder is emptied, the client may continue losing blood. A full bladder is likely a contributing cause of the bleeding and must be addressed promptly.
3. The client's total intake is important, but neither dehydration nor hypervolemia are of immediate concern at this time.
4. It is prudent to assess the uterotonic medication options for this client, but emptying the bladder is of primary importance initially.

d. **Once the bladder is emptied, the nurse can determine the appropriate uterotonic to administer next, followed by the intake and output assessments.**

TEST-TAKING HINT: Although postpartum hemorrhage (PPH) can be life-threatening, it is also treatable and reversible before it results in death. That is the situation in this scenario. The nurse can only do one thing at one time. The fact that the client walked to the bathroom and has not passed out is reassuring. Interventions are focused on assessing and treating the most likely contributing factor right now, a full bladder and its affect on uterine contractility. Adequate bladder emptying is the first step the nurse must take.

60. The correct answers are 4 and (b).

At risk for developing . . . (Select one, below)	As evidenced by . . . (Select one, below)
1. Urinary retention	a. Blood pressure
2. Hypoglycemia	**b. Fundal assessments**
3. Pulmonary edema	c. Gestational diabetes
4. Postpartum hemorrhage	d. Urinary output

1. She likely already has urinary retention; it is not just a risk.
2. The client is not at risk of hypoglycemia.
3. The client is not a risk of pulmonary edema.
4. **The client's most serious risk is postpartum hemorrhage. For this client, the hemorrhage is evidenced by a boggy uterus. Because the fundus requires massage to keep it firm, a boggy uterus is the most likely contributing factor, rather than a vaginal wall laceration or hematoma. All the nurse's efforts go toward achieving adequate uterine tone, beginning with bladder catheterization for residual urine.**

a. The client's blood pressure does not put her at risk of postpartum hemorrhage. Falling blood pressure is a symptom, not a risk factor for postpartum hemorrhage.
b. **The client's fundus has needed massage to remain firm. This is direct evidence that the client is at risk of postpartum hemorrhage. As such, the nurse's interventions should include treatments, such as medication, to keep the fundus firm without massage. The client has several risk factors for postpartum hemorrhage, including her multiparity, the baby's size, and the precipitous delivery.**
c. Gestational diabetes does not put the client at risk of postpartum hemorrhage.
d. Although the client's urinary output does not seem adequate and although a full

bladder can contribute to postpartum hemorrhage, that is not the primary evidence of a hemorrhage.

TEST-TAKING HINT: The test taker must read the stem of this question carefully. Both the highest risk and the evidence for that risk must be connected.

61. Answers 2 and 4 are correct.

1. There is nothing in the case study to indicate the client is anxious.
2. **The client's rising pulse and falling blood pressure correlate with severe blood loss. Her vital signs must be stabilized and supported to maintain organ perfusion.**
3. Preventing falls is a general goal for every client. The question asks for specific, primary goals for this client. There is nothing in the case study to suggest the client was unstable.
4. **Improving fundal tone is essential.**
5. *Monitoring* intake and output is an important nursing intervention, not a clinical client goal. "Equal intake and output" would be a client goal.

TEST-TAKING HINT: All of the answers should relate to measureable client conditions.

62. Answers 1(a), 2(b), 3(a), 4(b), 5(a), and 6(a) are correct.

Potential intervention	(a) Indicated	(b) Contraindicated
1. In and out catheterization	X	
2. Sustained fundal massage		X
3. Weigh pads	X	
4. Insert indwelling catheter		X
5. Administer uterotonic medication	X	
6. Administer IV bolus	X	

1(a). The bladder must be emptied to allow the uterus to fully and efficiently contract and control the bleeding in order to prevent postpartum hemorrhage.

2(b). Sustained fundal massage is contraindicated because it can cause worsening uterine atony. Brief periods of fundal massage are best.

3(a). It is important to weigh the pads and the clot to determine the amount of blood loss the client has sustained in order to guide treatment.

4(b). The client does not need an indwelling catheter at this point. It would lead to an unnecessary risk of infection.

5(a). The nurse's interventions must be focused on improving uterine contractility in order to prevent postpartum hemorrhage. Appropriate medication administration is an important part of the toolkit.

6(a). An IV bolus is appropriate to raise the client's blood pressure in light of apparent hypovolemia.

TEST-TAKING HINT: Rationales for the right answers are given in the descriptions for each answer above.

63. Answers 1(b), 2(a), 3(a), 4(c), 5(a), and 6(a) are correct.

1(b). The fundus remains boggy, indicating that beyond emptying the bladder, additional uterotonic medication is indicated. This is consistent with the client's risk factors for postpartum hemorrhage which include multiparity, large baby, and precipitous delivery.

2(a). The fundus has moved down to an expected location after the bladder was emptied, indicating that this intervention was effective.

3(a). Moderate lochia is expected at this point. It was heavy to moderate previously so the flow has been reduced from heavy, indicating an effective intervention.

4(c). The client's TPR is essentially unchanged, and these findings are unrelated to the bladder emptying and IV fluid bolus.

5(a). The client's blood pressure has improved following the IV fluid bolus, rendering it an effective intervention.

6(a). The bladder should not be palpable, so this is an expected finding that indicates the nurse's interventions were effective.

TEST-TAKING HINT: See the rationales given with each response above. The completed table is shown on the next page.

Assessment Finding	(a) Effective	(b) Ineffective	(c) Unrelated
1. Fundus boggy		X	
2. Fundus at umbilicus	X		
3. Moderate lochia	X		
4. Temp 98.6° F (37° C), P 100, R 18			X
5. BP 120/60	X		
6. Unable to palpate bladder	X		

64. 1. This action is appropriate. The client must be asked about her injuries.
2. Counseling the client on how her behavior may have provoked the attack is inappropriate. No one deserves to be abused.
3. It is inappropriate to inform the client that the police must arrest her partner. Although the nurse can recommend to the client that the police arrest her partner, they can only do so if there is sufficient evidence that the injuries were inflicted by the partner and/or the client presses charges against her partner.
4. It is inappropriate to encourage the client to get a divorce and to hand her a pamphlet with divorce attorney names.

TEST-TAKING HINT: Clients rarely discuss domestic violence issues unless they are asked directly about them. Even if the nurse does not see evidence of injury, he or she should inquire about the client's relationship during each healthcare encounter. When a healthcare professional suspects the client might be in an abusive situation, all questions about injuries or abuse must be asked when the client is alone. This question's stem does not indicate whether or not the client is alone. Unless it says she is with her partner, the test taker must not assume the partner is there, and must answer the question broadly as a general true or false question.

65. Answers 1 and 3 are correct.
1. This baby is at high risk for developing kernicterus.
2. This baby is not at risk for dehydration.
3. Anemia is a risk factor because of the pathophysiology of red blood cell destruction with ABO incompatibility.
4. This baby is not at high risk for weight loss.

TEST-TAKING HINT: The hemolytic incompatibility in this question is an ABO incompatibility due to the mother's type O blood and the baby's blood type of A. The Coombs test may be "indirect" or "direct." The *indirect* Coombs test is performed on women during pregnancy to look for antibodies floating in their blood that may attack the baby's blood if maternal and fetal blood mix. The *direct* Coombs test (DAT) is done on the baby's blood and confirms whether or not antibodies are already present and are stuck to the baby's red blood cells (RBCs). Because this baby's direct Coombs test is positive, the nurse should conclude that anti-A antibodies are present on the baby's red blood cells. If the baby's red blood cells are hemolyzed, or broken down as a result, the baby can become anemic. In addition, high levels of bilirubin (the waste product of RBC destruction), will be released into the baby's bloodstream, causing hyperbilirubinemia. If this is untreated, the baby may develop kernicterus, causing damage to the central nervous system. The positive test doesn't mean that this will definitely happen, but it is a warning to healthcare providers that it could happen. See "ABO Incompatibility" in the appendix for more information.

66. Answers 1 and 4 are correct.
1. Because a larger diameter of the fetal head is presenting to the pelvis in the LMP position, cephalopelvic disproportion is possible.
2. Placental abruption does not occur more frequently during the labor and delivery of a baby in LMP position than it does when the baby is in any other position.
3. LMP is a vertex, not a breech, position.
4. Prolapsed cord does occur more frequently when babies are in malpresentations.
5. Women are not at higher risk for pre-eclampsia when the baby is in the LMP position than they are when a baby is in any other position.

TEST-TAKING HINT: When presented with questions on fetal presentation, the second letter indicates what fetal part is presenting; look at

that first. In this question, the letter M indicates the mentum is presenting. The mentum refers to the protruding part of the baby's chin, seen in a face presentation. This baby's back is toward the mother's left side as indicated by the letter L. The letters M and P indicate that the baby's chin (M) is down posteriorly (P), toward the mother's back. If this baby were born vaginally, the entire face would present at the vaginal opening at once, with the mouth toward the bed. When a baby's mentum is presenting in the birth canal, it indicates that the baby's head failed to flex before engagement. As a result, rather than the smallest diameter of the fetal head presenting to the pelvis, a larger diameter is presenting. Cephalopelvic disproportion is a possible consequence. In addition, the fetal cord can become prolapsed more easily when the fetal face is presenting. It is generally accepted that a fetus in LMP must be delivered by cesarean section. A baby in the LMA (anterior) position, with the chin facing up, may deliver vaginally (Fomukong et al., 2019).

67. 1. A genetic amniocentesis is performed between 12 and 16 weeks' gestation.
2. Intrauterine growth restriction is detected via ultrasound.
3. A lecithin/sphingomyelin ratio and/or a shake test can be performed on amniotic fluid to determine whether the fetal lung fields are mature. These tests are performed during the third trimester.
4. Hormonal studies would not be conducted on the amniotic fluid.

TEST-TAKING HINT: To answer this question correctly, the test taker must attend carefully to the gestational age when the test is being conducted. In this question, it is being performed at 36 weeks, near the time when the fetus might be delivered. As such, it makes sense that the test is being performed to assess fetal lung maturity. Even though amniocenteses are performed to obtain fetal cells for genetic analysis, those tests are not performed during the third trimester.

68. 1. Follicle-stimulating hormone (FSH), not LH, accelerates the growth and maturation of an egg in the ovary.
2. This response is untrue. LH does not enhance the potential of the sperm to fertilize an egg.
3. This response is untrue. LH does not facilitate the egg's movement through the fallopian tube.
4. This response is correct. LH stimulates the release of a mature egg from the ovary each month.

TEST-TAKING HINT: FSH stimulates the growth and maturation of the egg, while LH stimulates the egg's release from the ovary and promotes development of a cluster of working cells called the corpus luteum. These cells are formed in the follicle that housed the egg before it popped out at ovulation. The word "lutein" comes from the Latin word, "luteus," which means "yellow." The corpus luteum is also yellow. As such, "luteinizing hormone" means the hormone that stimulates ovulation and then creates the yellow corpus luteum within the now-empty follicle. The corpus luteum stays behind in the ovary when the egg is released. If the egg is fertilized, the corpus luteum sustains the pregnancy with progesterone until the placenta takes over this function at around 12 weeks. The woman's temperature will drop slightly when she experiences the LH surge. Around 24 hours after ovulation, the woman's temperature will rise and will stay elevated for several days before returning to normal. If fertilization occurs, the temperature will remain elevated. This is the basis for the basal body temperature (BBT) charts some women are advised to keep when planning a pregnancy.

69. 1. The incidence of UTIs is slightly higher in boys who have not been circumcised, but there is no need to check the baby's daily temperature.
2. The prepuce should not be fully drawn back during the newborn period because of the potential for inducing pain and scarring.
3. The pediatrician will not have to evaluate the baby. Phimosis, or a tightened prepuce, may be present at birth or may develop subsequent to an infection. The mother, therefore, should be advised to watch that the baby's urine flows freely when he voids.
4. This response is correct. Care of the uncircumcised newborn's penis is the same as for a circumcised newborn. The baby's genitals should be cleansed with soap and water during the bath. The mother should not force the foreskin to retract, but if it does naturally loosen from the glans, she and, in later years, the boy should gently clean the exposed tissue underneath.

TEST-TAKING HINT: This question can be misleading to a test taker who assumes that by mentioning the prepuce (foreskin) the answer

implies that it must deserve special care. The best approach is to read each answer as a stand-alone true or false question. Certainly the penis, including the foreskin, or "prepuce," would be cleansed during the baby's bath, making option 4 a "true" question.

Whether or not to circumcise a male child is a decision the parents are asked to make. There is some evidence that males are less at risk of developing sexually transmitted infections if they are circumcised, and the incidence of UTI is slightly higher in boys who have not been circumcised. The American Academy of Pediatrics, however, does not recommend that all males be circumcised.

70. 1. The nurse would not expect to see a drop in the baseline fetal heart rate.
2. The nurse would not expect to see an increase in variable decelerations.
3. The nurse would expect to see a decrease in the baseline variability.
4. The nurse would not expect to see an increase in early decelerations.

TEST-TAKING HINT: Fentanyl is a narcotic analgesic. Narcotics are central nervous system (CNS) depressants. The baseline variability is an expression of the interaction between the parasympathetic and sympathetic nervous systems of the fetus. Because the narcotic enters the fetal vascular system through the placenta, the fetal CNS is depressed. As a result, the variability drops.

71. Answers 1, 2, and 4 are correct.
1. The four-chambered heart is present by 8 weeks' gestation.
2. Although webbed and short, fingers and toes are visible by 8 weeks' gestation.
3. The genitalia are not fully formed until about 12 weeks' gestation.
4. The facial features are all present by 8 weeks' gestation.

TEST-TAKING HINT: By the time the embryo reaches 8 weeks' gestation virtually all organ systems are present. Male genitalia will be differentiated by 12 weeks if testosterone is produced. If no testosterone is produced, female genitalia develop. Maturation continues in all organ systems through the remainder of the pregnancy.

72. Answers 1, 2, 5, 6, and 7 are correct.
1. The client's risk factors of age, ethnicity, and primiparity in combination with her symptoms point to possible pre-eclampsia. Right upper quadrant pain and nausea can indicate liver involvement.
2. Although the client's temperature is not related to pre-eclampsia, it suggests a differential diagnosis of flu, and follow-up is indicated to avoid fever and fetal tachycardia.
3. The client's pulse is within normal limits.
4. The client's respiratory rate is within normal limits.
5. The client's blood pressure is rising rapidly, requiring follow-up.
6. The client's oxygen saturation is on the low side and trouble-shooting is indicated.
7. The client's DTRs are consistent with the differential diagnosis of pre-eclampsia.
8. The client's cervical exam is not of primary importance at this point.

TEST-TAKING HINT: This is the step called "Recognize Cues" in the NGN test format. In this step, the nurse recognizes what is not right? What matters most? A mental checklist of normal and abnormal is a good place to start.

73. Answers 2 and (a) are correct.

Column 1 Highest client risk	Column 2 As evidenced by client's . . .
1. Placental abruption	**a. Vital sign assessments**
2. Stroke	b. Neurological assessments
3. Prolapsed cord	c. Cervical assessment
4. Eclampsia	d. Fetal assessments

1. Placental abruption is a risk associated with pre-eclampsia and hypertension. However, the client's reported RUQ pain does not suggest placental abruption.
2. The risk of stroke is a more likely complication for this client given her blood pressure readings.
3. A prolapsed cord is not a risk factor with intact membranes.
4. The client's DTRs do not suggest neurological pathology that would lead to eclamptic seizures at this point.
a. The client's blood pressures put her at risk of a stroke. This answer does not specifically indicate "blood pressure," but the test taker must understand that it is part of vital sign assessments.

b. The client's DTRs do not suggest neurological pathology that would lead to eclamptic seizures at this point, although that could change.
c. The cervical assessment is not of concern.
d. The FHR is not worrisome.

TEST-TAKING HINT: The nurse must differentiate between risk (what could happen with this diagnosis) versus symptomatology (what is happening now).

74. Answers 1 and (c) are correct.

Column 1 Address this condition first	Column 2 Followed by this condition
1. Blood pressure	a. Blood pressure
2. Oxygen saturation	b. Oxygen saturation
3. DTRs	**c. DTRs**
4. Contractions	d. Contractions

1. **The client's blood pressure carries the highest risk at this time.**
2. The oxygen saturation should be at least 95% so a reading of 94% isn't life threatening at this point.
3. The client's DTRs are within the normal range but should be closely monitored. The blood pressure is of primary importance. If it is not treated, neurological symptomatology may occur, leading to worsening DTRs and seizures.
4. The client's contractions are irregular at this time, and the fetus is coping well without decelerations.

a. The client's blood pressure will be assessed first.
b. The client's oxygen saturation does not put her life at risk.
c. **Although the client's DTRs are currently within the normal range, they could change rapidly, as the client's blood pressure rises.**
d. The client's contractions are not a threat at this time because they're irregular.

TEST-TAKING HINT: This client's most pressing risks are stroke and seizure. Both can be prevented by prompt medication—antihypertensives to prevent stroke, and magnesium sulfate to prevent eclamptic seizures.

75. The correct answers are 1(a), 2(b), 3(a), 4(b), 5(a), 6(a), and 7(a).

Potential Order	(a) Anticipated	(b) Contraindicated
1. 24-hour urine for creatinine clearance and protein	X	
2. Oxytocin induction per protocol		X
3. Misoprostol 25 mcg vaginally q 4 hours per protocol	X	
4. Epidural when requested in labor		X
5. Magnesium sulfate 4 gm IV loading dose over 30 minutes followed by 2 gm/hour maintenance dose	X	
6. Hydralazine 10 mg slow IV push over 2 minutes per protocol	X	
7. Acetaminophen 650 mg po q 4 hours for fever or headache	X	

1(a). A 24-hour urine collection for creatinine and protein is standard of care to assess kidney function and confirm a diagnosis of pre-eclampsia versus HELLP syndrome.

2(b). Due to the client's 36-week gestational age and serious symptoms, induction of labor is indicated. However, the client's cervix is not effaced adequately for oxytocin induction at this time, so the nurse should not begin the oxytocin. The cervix must be ripened first.

3(a). Misoprostol is an appropriate cervical ripening agent.

4(b). An epidural is contraindicated for this client because her platelet count is below 100,000. The nurse should remind the provider of this lab finding during the phone call.

5(a). Magnesium sulfate is appropriate to prevent eclamptic seizures.

6(a). **The client is having an acute hypertensive emergency. Hydralazine is recommended as a first-line medication for treatment.**

7(a). **Acetaminophen is appropriate to anticipate for this client, to prevent a worsening fever and accompanying fetal tachycardia, which would stress the fetus further.**

TEST-TAKING HINT: Rationales for the answers are included with each response above.

76. **The correct answers are 1, 5, and 6.**
1. **The 24-hour urine collection should start immediately.**
2. Oxytocin is contraindicated until after the cervix is ripened.
3. Cervical ripening is appropriate, but the start of the 24-hour urine collection, and administration of magnesium sulfate, and hydralazine should be given priority.
4. The client is not in labor. The nurse should question that order since the client's platelets are less than 100,000, making an epidural a contraindication. The client will be limited to inhaled analgesia such as nitrous oxide, or IV narcotics, instead of an epidural.
5. **Magnesium sulfate IV administration is appropriate to prevent eclamptic seizures.**
6. **Hydralazine or labetalol are recommended to reduce the client's blood pressure and prevent strokes.**
7. Acetaminophen is appropriate, but the 24-hour urine, magnesium sulfate, and hydralazine must take priority. The American College of Obstetricians and Gynecologists (ACOG) defines "isolated maternal fever" as a temperature of 100.4° F (38° C) to 102.2°3 F (39° C) with no additional risk factors (ACOG, 2017c).

TEST-TAKING HINT: Medications such as hydralazine and magnesium sulfate that are ordered to prevent morbidity or promote the client's survival, must be completed first. Because the 24-hour urine collection assists in the client's diagnosis and possibly further required treatments, it is also a priority.

77. **Answers 2, 3, 4, and 6 are correct, as findings that indicate the client is not progressing as expected.**
1. Irregular contractions are not unusual after misoprostol administration.
2. **The FHR shows changes toward a worsening fetal condition. The FHR is down from 140 bpm to 120 bpm, and the variability has changed from moderate variability to minimal variability.**
3. **Recurrent late decelerations are another indicator of worsening fetal condition, no doubt a response to maternal hypertension which reduces the already sub-optimal oxygen-carrying capacity of the placenta.**
4. **The cervical exam indicates no cervical change in response to the misoprostol.**
5. The vital signs indicate improvement as expected. The temp is within the normal range and the BP is lower in response to the anti hypertensive medications.
6. **The DTRs and clonus indicate the client's condition is not progressing as expected. The expectation would be that with the magnesium sulfate, the DTRs and clonus would be reduced, not increased.**
7. Oxygen saturation has improved.

TEST-TAKING HINT: Rationales for the correct answers are given in the responses above. In this type of question, the test taker is required to re-read the nurses' notes and make assessments about client progress or lack of progress and a worsening condition, the same way the nurse would assess a client in a real-world situation. Rather than recognizing the "right" answer, the test-taker is required to make an assessment about the client's condition.

If this were a "real world" case, this client would no doubt be taken to the operating room for a cesarean section, since both maternal and fetal conditions are worsening and will likely continue to worsen. Allowing for 18 to 24 hours or more to pass for her cervix to ripen, followed by several more hours of labor, would cause undue stress on both the mother and baby, leading to a more-than-likely tragic outcome.

78. 1. At –2 station, the baby is not yet engaged. Because the baby is so high, it is very unlikely that the client will experience a precipitous delivery.
2. The membranes have been ruptured a very short time. The client is not at high risk for infection at this time.
3. The fetal heart rate is showing recurrent variable decelerations. Because the baby is not post dates, and there is no evidence of other placental issues, the client is not at high risk for uteroplacental insufficiency. As such, the variable decelerations are most likely related to fetal positioning. Because the fetus is at –2 station, it is possible the umbilical cord is compressed between the fetal buttocks and the cervix, a situation referred to as an "occult prolapse" because it is unseen and/or uncertain.
4. **The membranes are ruptured, the baby is not engaged, the baby is in the sacral position, and the fetal heart rate is showing variable decelerations. The nurse should assess this client carefully for prolapsed cord.**

TEST-TAKING HINT: With a given position of LSP, the test taker knows by the second letter (S) that the sacrum is presenting; the baby is breech. The test taker must methodically consider the many factors in the scenario before determining the correct answer to this question. The key items in the order they are presented are 1) term pregnancy at 39 weeks; 2) multigravida, which could mean short labor; 3) rupture of membranes less than an hour, rules out risk of infection; 4) irregular contractions, rules out risk of precipitous delivery; 5) cervical dilation of 4 cm rules out precipitous delivery because it's early in the labor; 6) minus 2 (–2) station rules out precipitous labor, but carries a risk of prolapsed cord because nothing is blocking the cervix; 7) the baby is breech, which increases the risk of prolapsed cord and rules out precipitous labor; 8) FHR is reassuring with a normal rate and moderate variability, which rules out uteroplacental insufficiency; 9) variable decelerations indicate cord compression somewhere, including the possibility of the cord lying near the cervix and compression by the fetal buttocks with contractions. The first 3 answer options have been ruled out, but the last answer has been ruled in. By taking each possible answer and assessing it in light of the given case information, the test taker can determine the correct answer. As a reminder, in the left sacrum posterior (LSP) position, the fetal back is to the mother's left (L), the buttocks (S) are presenting at the cervix, and are toward the mother's back (P), meaning the baby is facing the front of the mother.

79. 1. A banana is an excellent fruit choice, but it does not meet the young woman's iron or calcium needs.
2. **Cheeseburgers meet both iron and calcium needs.**
3. Strawberries are an excellent fruit choice, but they do not meet the young woman's iron or calcium needs.
4. Rice is high in protein and does contain some calcium, but it is not a good iron source.

TEST-TAKING HINT: The best way to remember the special nutritional needs of young pregnant adolescents is to remember that they are still growing, themselves. As a result, they need the minerals calcium and iron, as well as protein for their own growth and development and to meet the needs of the growing fetus. Of the choices, only cheeseburgers meet all those needs.

80. 1. This action is not advisable unless the woman requests the move.
2. This action is inappropriate. The nurse must acknowledge the loss of the baby.
3. **This action is appropriate. The nurse should offer the couple the opportunity to hold their baby.**
4. This action is inappropriate. The administration of milk suppressants is not recommended because of the adverse side effects of the medications.

TEST-TAKING HINT: Holding the baby should be an option for every new parent experiencing a fetal demise, but should not be forced on them. The literature is mixed about the benefits or negative impact of seeing the baby (Farrales et al., 2020). Couples who are hesitant to see the baby may benefit from having the nurse describe the baby to them before they see it, such as skin may be purple, may be peeling, lips may be very red, etc. Some parents have reported that they appreciated the nursing staff offering repeated opportunities to see and hold the baby, even though they initially refused (Kingdon et al., 2015). Counterbalancing these findings is one in which parents reported a negative impact on their mental health after seeing and holding their stillborn baby (Redshaw et al., 2016). This demonstrates that there is no one "right" way to support families of stillborn babies, and nurses must allow the parents to lead, while

offering support and opportunity. In addition, it is very important for clients who have had a fetal loss to know that they may lactate. This can be very stressful for a grieving woman if she is unprepared. She will need information about engorgement. Some women choose to pump and donate their breastmilk to a milk bank for a few weeks, in honor of their baby. This helps them to feel like a mother as they work through their grief (Carroll, 2013).

81. 1. It is recommended that women not douche.
2. It is recommended that women not douche.
3. It is recommended that women not douche.
4. It is recommended that women not douche.

TEST-TAKING HINT: Douching not only adversely affects the vaginal environment, it also can force endometrial tissue into the tubes and onto the ovaries, resulting in endometriosis, especially when performed during the menses.

82. 1. The client's primary healthcare provider should be notified.
2. It is inappropriate to massage the client's leg.
3. It is inappropriate to apply ice packs to the leg.
4. It is inappropriate to encourage the client to walk.

TEST-TAKING HINT: Clients who exhibit any or all of the following symptoms—erythema, warmth, edema, pain—in one or both calves may have a deep vein thrombosis. The primary healthcare provider should be notified so that diagnostic tests can be ordered. If the woman were to ambulate or if she were to massage her leg, the thrombus could become dislodged.

83. 1. The nurse should refrain from giving any information to the woman regarding the babies' schedules.
2. The nurse should politely escort the woman to a postpartum room, if appropriate, or off the unit if she is not visiting a patient.
3. The nurse should refrain from giving any information to the woman regarding the babies' schedules.
4. The nurse should politely escort the woman to a postpartum room, if appropriate, or off the unit if she is not visiting a patient.

TEST-TAKING HINT: The physical characteristics and actions of the woman in the scenario are consistent with those of women who abduct neonates. By asking the woman which patient the woman wishes to visit, the nurse will be able to determine whether the woman is a legitimate visitor.

84. 1. It is very unlikely that a woman in transition would fall asleep during contractions.
2. These are characteristic actions of laboring women who are in transition.
3. It is very unlikely that a woman in transition would be watching television.
4. Pushing is characteristic of stage 2 of labor.

TEST-TAKING HINT: Transition is the most forceful phase of the first stage of labor. The contractions are strong and frequent and mothers, especially primigravidas, are usually fatigued and very uncomfortable during the phase. Vomiting is commonly seen during this phase. The pressure of vomiting on the uterus sometimes moves the baby against the cervix strongly enough to complete dilation and the woman suddenly reports an urge to push.

85. 1. At 22 weeks, testes are not yet descended, the suck is weak, and lanugo and vernix are present.
2. At 28 weeks, testes may begin to descend, the suck is weak, and lanugo and vernix are abundant.
3. At 32 weeks, testes may have descended, the suck is improving but still poor, and lanugo and vernix are abundant.
4. At 38 weeks, testes are fully descended, the suck is strong, and the amount of lanugo and vernix is minimal.

TEST-TAKING HINT: The test taker should be familiar with major fetal development milestones and consider each of these gestational ages individually. At 22 weeks' gestation the fetus is covered in lanugo, so scant amounts rule out this answer. Lanugo is also present at 28 and 32 weeks, so scant amounts rule out these answers. Preterm babies have weak sucks, and, if male, have not developed sufficiently to have their testes present in their scrotal sacs. All of these facts make answers 1, 2, and 3 incorrect, leaving 4 the correct answer.

86. 1. If a mother wishes to breastfeed, the nurse should assist her to do so.
2. Babies with Down's syndrome require the same number of calories as do other babies.
3. The mother can breastfeed the baby with Down's syndrome in any position—side-lying, cradle, cross-cradle, or football—as long as she provides the jaw support that the baby needs. Mothers of babies with Down's syndrome often find that the football hold works best.
4. Babies with Down's syndrome are hypotonic. They often have a weak suck at birth.

TEST-TAKING HINT: It would be wrong to assume that simply because a baby has a congenital defect it will be unable to breastfeed. The nurse should assess each situation individually and provide assistance when needed. If additional help is required, a lactation consultant should be recommended.

87. 1. Macrosomic babies are no more at high risk for jaundice than babies of average weight.
2. Macrosomic babies are at high risk for jitters due to hypoglycemia.
3. Macrosomic babies are no more at high risk for blepharitis, inflammation of the eyelash follicles, than babies of average weight.
4. All babies are born with a pseudostrabismus. The muscles of the eyes usually mature by 6 months when the strabismus ceases.

TEST-TAKING HINT: To answer this question correctly, the test taker must fully understand the physiology of pregnancy and the pathophysiology of a major cause of macrosomia—namely, maternal gestational diabetes. The clue is the macrosomic baby. Because the mother in this scenario had no prenatal care, it is very possible that she had undiagnosed gestational diabetes and hyperglycemia. The high glucose levels in the maternal bloodstream easily cross the placenta, resulting in high glucose levels in the fetus. The babies metabolize the glucose, resulting in a proportionate increase in body weight. When the babies deliver, their bodies continue to secrete high levels of insulin for up to 48 hours, but the high levels of maternal glucose are no longer available. Hypoglycemia and jitters (a symptom of hypoglycemia) result. Because the mother in this scenario had no prenatal care, it is very possible that she had undiagnosed gestational diabetes and hyperglycemia.

88. 1. Most women have no complaints.
2. Most women have no complaints.
3. Most women have no complaints.
4. Most women have no complaints.

TEST-TAKING HINT: Chlamydia is known as a "silent" disease because about 75% of infected women and about 50% of infected men have no symptoms. If symptoms do occur, they usually appear within a few weeks of the exposure (CDC, n.d.-b).

89. 1. There is a 75% probability that their child will have the disease.
2. There is a 75% probability that their child will have the disease.
3. There is a 75% probability that their child will have the disease.
4. There is a 75% probability that their child will have the disease.

TEST-TAKING HINT: The test taker should create and analyze a Punnett square:

Father:	A	a
Mother: A	AA	Aa
a	Aa	aa

Because only 1 dominant gene need be present for a dominant disease to be exhibited, each child has a ¾, or 75%, probability of having the disease.

90. 1. Newborn babies should be burped after consuming every 1/2 to 1 ounce of formula.
2. This statement is true. To prevent ingestion of air, the bottle nipple should be filled with formula throughout the feeding.
3. Formula should never be heated in the microwave.
4. Because of the potential for aspiration, baby bottles should never be propped.

TEST-TAKING HINT: Mothers who decide to bottle feed their babies must be educated regarding safe bottle feeding practices. Not only is propping unsafe but it also decreases the amount of quality time the mother has with her baby.

91. 1. This client did vomit twice last shift, but she is not the nurse's client of highest risk.
2. This client is at high risk for preterm labor, but she is not the nurse's client of highest risk.
3. This client does need to be given preoperative teaching and be prepared for surgery, but she is not the nurse's client of highest risk.
4. This client should be seen first. Although obstetrically she is not at high risk, her care must take priority because she had a pulmonary episode during the prior shift.

TEST-TAKING HINT: This is a complex question that requires the test taker to consider a variety of issues including antepartum clients versus postpartum clients, obstetric complications versus medical complications, and preoperative issues versus standard care issues. Although many hospitals have separate antepartum, postpartum, and intrapartum units, some smaller hospitals may have all obstetric clients on the same unit, so it is important for the nurse to consider client conditions in all phases of maternity care.

92. 1. A baby at 34 weeks, gestation that weighs 500 grams would be classified as small for gestational age.
2. A baby at 34 weeks, gestation that weighs 1,700 grams would be classified as small for gestational age.
3. A baby at 34 weeks, gestation that weighs 2,900 grams would be classified as average for gestational age.
4. A baby at 34 weeks, gestation that weighs 4,100 grams would be classified as large for gestational age.

TEST-TAKING HINT: The test taker must be prepared to interpret simple graphs. Babies who are average for gestational age weigh between the 10th and 90th percentile for a specific gestational age. Note that the 50th percentile is indicated by a light blue line within the area that designates "average for gestational age." To answer this question, identify 34 weeks' gestation on the bottom. Note the definitions of the shaded areas: large for gestational age (white) at the top; average for gestational age (light blue) in the middle; small for gestational age (dark blue) at the bottom. Take each weight and determine what shaded area it is in. Of these four options, only the 2,900-gram weight is within the light blue area that indicates "average for gestational age."

93. 1. Fever is not a contraindication for carboprost.
2. A history of asthma or other breathing problems is a contraindication for carboprost.
3. The blood pressure may rise. A blood pressure of 90/60 is not a contraindication for carboprost.
4. Hypocalcemia is not a contraindication for carboprost.

TEST-TAKING HINT: Carboprost is a powerful prostaglandin that is used for treating postpartum hemorrhage after other medications such as oxytocin and methylergonovine have been used without success. It is contraindicated for use in clients with a history of asthma, diabetes, liver, cardiac disease, and other disorders because it causes systemic vasoconstriction.

94. 1. A warm shower may help to promote the milk ejection reflex, but this is not the question the nurse should ask at this time.
2. The client may need to pump her breasts to soften them enough for the baby to latch well, but this is not the question the nurse should ask at this time.
3. Unless a client has a very low intake, the quantity of fluids that the client consumes is not related to the quantity of milk she will produce.
4. The nurse should ask the client when she fed the baby last.

TEST-TAKING HINT: Engorgement rarely develops if a mother breastfeeds frequently. Breastfeeding mothers should be encouraged to feed the baby at least 8 times in 24 hours. This equates to approximately every 2 to 3 hours. It is especially important to encourage the mothers to never skip a feeding. Until the baby is showing adequate weight gain (usually in the first two weeks), mothers are generally advised to wake the baby for a feeding if more than 4 hours have passed. If they must give the baby a bottle in place of a breastfeeding, they should pump their breasts immediately after the missed feeding. If this mother has been trying to feed the baby regularly, but the baby refuses because of engorgement, the suggestions of taking a warm shower, which can stimulate the breasts to let down, and expressing some of the milk, or pumping to soften the breasts, can be of benefit as an intervention once the possible cause of the engorgement is determined.

95. 1. The fundus is firm and the lochia is scanty. There is no need for the nurse to massage the client's fundus.
2. The client's temperature, although higher than during labor, is not elevated significantly. It is not necessary to ask her if she is having chills.
3. The only significant change in vitals is a rise in temperature to 99.4° F (37.4° C). Because the client has recently delivered, it is likely that the elevation is related to dehydration. The nurse should encourage the client to drink fluids.
4. There is nothing in the scenario that indicates that the client may have a pulmonary problem. Assessing the client's lung fields is not necessary at this time.

TEST-TAKING HINT: The only significant change in the client's vital signs from the intrapartum period to the postpartum period is the elevation in the temperature. Since the temperature is not high enough to signal an infection, it is likely related to dehydration. She should drink fluids. If the client were becoming hypovolemic from blood loss, the nurse would have noted a marked elevation in pulse rate but likely no change in blood pressure at this point. Postpartum clients are able to compensate for an extended period of time before hypotension is noted because the blood volume increases by around 50% during pregnancy.

96. 1. It is inappropriate to insert eye prophylaxis when the baby needs resuscitation.

2. This action is inappropriate. The baby needs to be resuscitated.
3. **An Apgar score of 3 after initial stabilization and resuscitative efforts is an indication for a full neonatal resuscitation. The nurse begins initial resuscitative interventions such as drying, suctioning, and stimulating the baby immediately after the birth. At 1 minute of age, if the baby has not responded to those efforts as evidenced by an Apgar score of 3, the nurse needs additional help to provide further resuscitation interventions.**
4. There is no need to repeat the score until 5 minutes after birth. The score of 3 at 1 minute is enough evidence to warrant resuscitation.

TEST-TAKING HINT: Stabilization and resuscitation, if needed, begin immediately after the birth, before the first Apgar score is completed. An Apgar score of 8 or above is common, and indicates that the baby is making a smooth transition into extrauterine life. A score of 3 indicates a baby who is severely compromised. A full resuscitation team should be called immediately.

In a real life situation, the nurse would no doubt have called for a full resuscitation team before the first minute had passed, if the baby was not responding to initial care. The intent of this question is for the test taker to demonstrate an understanding of normal Apgar scores and appropriate interventions.

97. Answers 2 and 3 are correct.
1. The baby is no more at high risk for hyperreflexia than other neonates.
2. **The nurse should monitor the baby for respiratory distress and hypoglycemia.**
3. **The nurse should monitor the baby for respiratory distress and hypoglycemia.**
4. The baby is no more at high risk for opisthotonus than other neonates.
5. The baby is no more at high risk for nuchal rigidity than other neonates.

TEST-TAKING HINT: A sometimes overlooked complication for babies of mothers with diabetes is respiratory distress. High levels of insulin reduce the production of surfactant in the baby's lungs before birth. As a consequence, even full-term infants of mothers with diabetes sometimes have respiratory difficulties in addition to the risk of hypoglycemia for reasons discussed previously.

98. 1. **The tube is placed through the mouth into the baby's stomach. When gastric juices are aspirated, the nurse knows that the tubing is in the stomach.**
2. Babies will often suck on items in their mouths. This does not mean, however, that the tubing is in place.
3. Even if the tubing is inserted correctly into the stomach, the baby may exhibit some respiratory difficulties.
4. Even though the nurse meets resistance when inserting the tube, this does not mean that it has been inserted into the stomach.

TEST-TAKING HINT: When a tube is inserted into a baby for a gavage feeding, the nurse must be certain that the tube has entered the stomach and not the lung fields.

99. 1. This response is incorrect. The maternal and fetal circulatory systems are independent throughout pregnancy.
2. This response is incorrect. The maternal and fetal circulatory systems are independent throughout pregnancy.
3. This response is incorrect. The maternal and fetal circulatory systems are independent throughout pregnancy.
4. **This response is correct. The maternal and fetal circulatory systems are independent throughout pregnancy.**

TEST-TAKING HINT: The fetal circulation and maternal circulation are independent of each other. The baby's heart pumps its blood through the umbilical arteries to the placenta and back again through the umbilical vein to the heart. Oxygen and nutrients enter into the fetal system across cell membranes in the placenta. Similarly, waste products from the fetus are eliminated through the maternal system across the same cell membranes.

100. 1. The weight loss is excessive. This response is not acceptable.
2. It is inappropriate to recommend that the woman stop breastfeeding. It may be appropriate to add supplementation, however.
3. **The nurse should notify the primary healthcare provider of the excessive weight loss.**
4. It is inappropriate for the baby to receive dextrose water between feedings.

TEST-TAKING HINT: Babies can safely lose between 5% and 10% of their birth weight in the first few days of life. Instead of calculating the exact weight loss for this baby, however, the test taker can determine what a 10% weight loss would be for the baby and compare that figure to the child's actual weight loss: $2678 \times 0.1 = 267.8$. Because the baby has lost more than 10% of the birth weight (286 is greater than 267.8), it is easy to determine that the weight loss is excessive.

101. Answers 2, 3, 4, and 5 are correct.

1. Because the majority of fetal development occurs during the embryonic period, and many women are unaware that they are pregnant until well into that period, it is too late to stop drinking alcohol when the woman "thinks" that she may be pregnant.
2. **To make sure that a woman is not suffering from a disease that could adversely affect a pregnancy, or that pregnancy would adversely affect a woman's health, it is important for a woman to have a complete medical checkup prior to becoming pregnant.**
3. **Because folic acid supplementation has been found to reduce the incidence of some birth defects, women should begin taking a daily multivitamin that includes folic acid when they are trying to become pregnant.**
4. **Because dental x-rays could injure the developing embryo, a woman should tell her dentist that she is trying to become pregnant so that the dentist can shield her abdomen during the x-ray.**
5. **Pregnant women are especially at high risk for contracting listeriosis. The offending organism, *Listeria monocytogenes*, is found in sushi and rare meat as well as in a number of other foods.**

TEST-TAKING HINT: Embryogenesis often occurs before a woman is aware that she is pregnant. Because teratogenic insults can injure the developing embryo, it is essential that women plan their pregnancies and avoid teratogens when attempting to become pregnant.

102.

1. It is not necessary to breastfeed every 2 hours. The baby should breastfeed at least eight times in 24 hours, which could be approximately every 3 hours.
2. A nutritious diet is an important nursing care goal for a postpartum client, but it is not the highest priority.
3. **The nursing care goal of "moderate lochial flow" for a postpartum client is of highest priority.**
4. Walking in the hallways every shift is an important nursing care goal for a postpartum client, but it is not the highest priority.

TEST-TAKING HINT: The nurse should consider the acronym CAB (circulation, airway, breathing) to determine which nursing care goals are of highest priority. The care goal related to lochial flow is directly related to circulation (C). If the client were to bleed heavily, her circulation would be compromised.

103.

1. **The nurse would expect the client to complain of severe back pain.**
2. Descent is often slowed when the baby is in a posterior position.
3. The nurse would not expect to see hypotonic or irregular contractions.
4. The nurse would not expect rectal pressure or an increase in bloody show.

TEST-TAKING HINT: This baby's head, or occiput, is presenting, as indicated by "O," the occiput—the back of the baby's skull. In an LOP position, the "P" indicates the baby's occiput is at the posterior side of the pelvis, at the mother's back. The occiput of the baby's head presses against the mother's coccyx during every contraction, bone on bone. This action is very painful. None of the other responses is directly linked to a posterior fetal position.

104.

1. **Hyperemesis and hypertension are often seen in clients with hydatidiform mole.**
2. Neither diarrhea nor hyperthermia is associated with hydatidiform mole.
3. Polycythemia is not associated with hydatidiform mole.
4. Polydipsia is not associated with hydatidiform mole.

TEST-TAKING HINT: Because the levels of human chorionic gonadotropin are markedly elevated with hydatidiform mole, women often experience excessive vomiting. In addition, signs of pre-eclampsia, such as hypertension, appear before 20 weeks' gestation in clients with molar pregnancies.

105.

1. Delayed placental separation is not associated with maternal cigarette smoking.
2. **The nurse should carefully monitor the labor for late decelerations.**
3. Shoulder dystocia is not associated with maternal cigarette smoking.
4. Precipitous fetal descent is not associated with maternal cigarette smoking.

TEST-TAKING HINT: Smoking affects the ability of the placenta to provide adequate oxygen to the fetus. The placentas of women who smoke are often small, infarcted, and/or calcified. During labor, therefore, there is a strong likelihood that uteroplacental insufficiency will be evident. Late decelerations are indicative of uteroplacental insufficiency.

106. 1. Babies whose mothers are HIV positive are not at high risk during the immediate neonatal period.

2. This is the correct response. Babies who are born to mothers who are GBS positive are at high risk for sepsis. The incidence of sepsis is reduced, however, when the mother receives IV antibiotics during labor.

3. Twelve hours is not an abnormal length for a client's labor.

4. Although 45 pounds is higher than the recommended weight gain for pregnancy, this baby is not the highest priority.

TEST-TAKING HINT: Each of the responses includes either a number or a disease process. To answer the question, the nurse must determine which of the answer options is a high-risk state during the immediate neonatal period. Even though babies born to women who are HIV positive may acquire the infection, the baby will not be adversely affected by the virus immediately after birth. (In fact, if mothers and babies are treated, transmission rates are almost zero.) Babies born to mothers who are GBS positive, however, may develop early-onset neonatal sepsis (EOS) within the first 3 days of life.

107. 1. This is an incorrect answer. The majority of fetal blood bypasses the pulmonary system during fetal circulation.

2. This is a correct answer. When the cord is clamped, the blood is no longer being oxygenated through the placenta. The baby's oxygen levels, therefore, begin to drop.

3. Bacteria will not colonize the bowel until the baby has been in the extrauterine environment and has eaten.

4. Bilirubin levels usually begin to rise on day 2.

TEST-TAKING HINT: If the nurse remembers the role of the umbilical cord, the answer becomes very clear. The change in the blood gases—a drop in oxygen levels with a concomitant rise in carbon dioxide levels—is one of the important triggers that stimulates babies to breathe.

Appendix

Think of the information in this appendix as "learning hacks." Because nursing assessments require a deep understanding of physiology, the topics chosen for elaboration here are those that are often difficult or complicated for many healthcare professionals to grasp, especially at the start of their careers. Sometimes, learning is enhanced by hearing the same information in familiar terms without scientific jargon, a format referred to as "plain language" (NIHa, n.d.).

In addition to plain language, some physiological concepts are presented in allegorical story form. The use of stories as a teaching pedagogy for transformative learning is an old technique (Day, 2009). It has been shown to be useful in making client education memorable and understandable (Day, 2009). The same outcome has been reported to the author by nurses and other healthcare professionals who have said they have benefited from hearing these allegories. The reader may find that a retelling of these concepts in plain language or allegory provides a wonderful "Aha!" moment in linking or understanding physiological ramifications of disease states. The selected concepts are listed alphabetically, as follows.

ABO INCOMPATIBILITY

Primary blood types are identified by the presence or absence of ABO and Rh antigens. The term "blood type" is used broadly to refer to eight blood groups: A, B, AB, or O, and the Rh factor that may be present or absent (Rh positive or Rh negative) with each one, giving 2 iterations of each letter group. ABO incompatibility is determined separately from Rh incompatibility. ABO incompatibility is specific to babies with blood types of group A, B, or AB, whose mothers are group O, regardless of Rh type.

To understand the condition, let's start with a simple definition of an antigen: a protein that causes an immune response if it is foreign to the body. The body's responses to both ABO and Rh antigens are similar in that they are based on immune responses, but the Rh response is more serious than the ABO response (Wagle, 2017). This discussion will cover ABO incompatibility only, not Rh factor. Not all babies with ABO incompatibility develop pathologic jaundice that requires extensive treatment (Thilo, n.d.). However, mother/baby dyads with maternal blood types that are 0 and/or Rh negative (Rh-) require extra screening and assessments after the birth in order to prevent problems from happening.

Blood type antigens are genetically inherited. ABO blood types are identified by the *presence or absence* of A or B antigens (or both, as in blood type AB) on the surface of the red blood cell. Note that ABO antigens are carried on the cell itself, which is different from *antibodies*, which are carried in the plasma. Antibodies (immunoglobulins) in the plasma fight against unfamiliar, or foreign RBC antigens. It's a simple form of individual discrimination, with the antigens on your RBCs telling the unfamiliar antigens on the fetal or transfusion RBCs, "If you don't look like me (with the same antigens, or blood type), my antibodies will destroy you."

The following list may help define the details.

- Red blood cell with "A" antigen means type "A" blood.
  - Plasma carries the "B" antibody—the "soldiers" to attack any "B" antigen, including that in "AB" type blood.
- Red blood cell with "B" antigen means type "B" blood.
  - Plasma carries the "A" antigen to attack any "A" antigen, including that in "AB type blood.

- Red blood cell with "AB" antigens means type "AB" blood.
  - Plasma carries no antibodies against A or B, because it recognizes them both.
  - This is why "AB" blood type is the universal *plasma* donor (as opposed to *red cell* donor. That's another complication not covered here).
- Red blood cell with "O," no antigen, means type "O" blood.
  - Plasma carries antibodies against "A," "B," and "AB," risking ABO incompatibility.

Why Does This Happen Only With Maternal Type O Blood?

Antibodies of mothers with blood types A or B are of an immune globulin type (IgM) that does not cross the placenta (Wagle, 2017). This is different from antibodies of a very small percentage of mothers (1%) with type O blood, who have a high titer of an immune globulin type (IgG) that *does* cross the placenta (Wagle, 2017).

Why Isn't ABO Incompatibility Often Seen in Fetuses?

The hemolytic disease of ABO incompatibility is primarily seen in the newborn rather than the fetus (Akanmu et al., 2015). This is because, due to immature A and B antigen development during gestation, a smaller number of A and B antigenic sites are present on fetal RBCs, reducing the severity of a fetal immune reaction (Dean, 2005). In addition, unlike the Rh antigens, which are present only on RBCs, the ABO antigens are present in a number of other tissues, which reduces the number of antibodies that attack RBCs only (Dean, 2005).

Why Are These Babies at Higher Risk of Pathologic Jaundice?

The combination of both ABO incompatibility and *normal* physiological RBC breakdown and stabilization of RBC volume after birth results in a higher number of RBCs destroyed at the same time (Dean, 2005). As a result, the affected newborn suffers from a more serious condition of anemia and jaundice.

What Stops the Immune Reaction?

Maternal antibodies are present in the newborn for several weeks to months after birth to protect the newborn until his own immune system matures. Maternal hemolytic antibodies are generally inactive in the newborn after 2 to 3 months (Thilo, n.d.), when the condition resolves itself.

No metaphor is perfect, but if you're scratching your head in confusion, see if the story below is helpful. Let's compare ABO incompatibility to four restaurants that carry various protein options (the antigens) and how they deal with food salesmen. Refer to the following table as you follow along.

The "Story" of ABO Incompatibility

This is a town where all animal protein options must be advertised by restaurants. The first restaurant we'll call "A"; it serves only antelope, and that is identified by the sign outside the door. The second one is "B" and it serves only bear. This is also advertised by a sign outside the door. Restaurant "AB" advertises that it serves both bear and antelope. Finally, there's restaurant "O." Its sign indicates it carries no animal protein at all; it's vegan.

If a salesman walks into restaurant "A" trying to sell bear (B) or vegan (O) options, measures will be taken to destroy him forever (antibodies) because this restaurant serves only antelope. (Yes, it's a cutthroat town.) Restaurant "B" will have no problem with the bear (B) salesman, but it will destroy both the antelope (A) and vegan (O) salesmen because it serves only bear. Restaurant "AB" is a little different: it invites both the antelope (A) and bear (B) salesmen in but destroys the vegan (O) salesman. What about the vegan restaurant, "O"? This restaurant will destroy both antelope (A) and bear (B) salesmen and will accept only those offering vegan (O) products.

Blood Type (Antigens on outside of RBC)	A	B	AB	O
Antigen Metaphor	Restaurant A sign says, "Ante-lope dishes only"	Restaurant B sign says "Bear dishes only"	Restaurant AB sign says, "Both antelope and bear dishes"	Restaurant O sign says, "No animal proteins"
Antibodies *in plasma*	B, O	A, O	O	A, B, AB
Metaphor	Fights bear (B) and vegan (O) salesmen	Fights antelope (A) and vegan (O) salesmen	Fights only vegan salesmen (O)	Fights ante-lope and bear salesmen A, B, AB

To summarize, a mother with type O blood has antibodies in her plasma against A, B, and the combination of AB antigens. If the mother's type O blood carries the IgG antibodies that cross the placenta, her antibodies will destroy the neonate's RBCs once he is born, as more A and B antigens develop on the neonate's RBCs as he matures. If a newborn baby develops hyperbilirubinemia as a result, phototherapy can reduce the bilirubin levels until the maternal antibodies are no longer active and the physiologic jaundice resolves. Rarely, an exchange transfusion may be necessary for the neonate.

ACID–BASE BALANCE

This is a concept that is difficult for even experienced nurses to understand fully. First, a review of the science, followed by application of that information in story form.

Acid–base balance is a balance between acids and antacids, aka *base*. Bases are chemically opposite from acids, rather like black and white.

Why Is it Called Respiratory Acidosis?

Respiratory acidosis means that there is a buildup of carbon dioxide, the acid waste product of normal aerobic metabolism, after burning glucose for energy. Because carbon dioxide is expelled through breathing, a buildup of this acid is called "respiratory acidosis." This fairly benign condition is quite common at birth and is very quickly reversed (Azhibekov & Seri, 2019; Carbonne et al., 2016).

Why Is it Called Metabolic Acidosis?

Metabolic acidosis is a more serious, "deeper" condition due to hypoxemia within the metabolism of the cell. The word "metabolism" refers to the chemical reactions inside the cells that convert fuel to energy. Metabolic acidosis means that because of inadequate oxygen delivery, a different, nonoxygen energy source other than glucose is used for cellular energy. This could be either the result of inadequate uteroplacental function related to maternal pre-eclampsia and/or diabetes, blood flow related to recurrent cord occlusion for a prolonged period of time, diabetic ketoacidosis (DKA), all of the above, or a number of other conditions. Without adequate oxygen, the cell cannot break down glucose—there's a missing ingredient. Thankfully, metabolic processes can then switch to anaerobic metabolism to keep the cells functioning. However, unlike the easily excreted waste products of carbon dioxide and water from aerobic metabolism, anaerobic metabolism reactions release lactic acid, which is not as readily expelled by the placenta, so the levels of acid rise in the fetal blood. In addition, three toxic acids, or ketones (think of this as "smoke" that comes with burning "wet firewood") are released. These are acetone, acetoacetate, and beta-hydroxybutyrate. The pH of the blood falls into the acidemic range. In response, higher amounts of bicarbonate (base) are needed to reduce the levels of acid in the blood. The immature fetal kidney must replenish the body's supply of sodium bicarbonate base. Because of kidney immaturity, production of base may not be able to keep up with demand, and a base deficit ensues.

When this condition is prolonged and the deficit is too great to restore the pH to normal levels, the pH continues to drop and cell death along with postnatal complications can occur (Carbonne et al., 2016). Even after the baby is born and breathing oxygen, metabolic acidosis can linger for several hours after birth (Carbonne et al., 2016) as the cells work to restore order.

Although the presence of metabolic acidosis by itself is not diagnostic of permanent fetal damage, severe sequelae may develop if metabolic acidosis is persistent (Azhibekov & Seri, 2019). For this reason, nurses and primary healthcare providers must be vigilant during labor and delivery to recognize symptoms that suggest acidemia or acidosis and to understand the physiology of acidemia in order to intervene appropriately.

How Can I Determine if the Baby Is at Risk?

In labor, the presence of late decelerations and deep variables can suggest fetal risk, although a tracing with the presence of FHR decelerations or minimal variability does not predict an adverse fetal outcome (Phelan, 2019). Retrospective reviews of electronic fetal monitoring strips have shown that the duration and persistence of these "abnormal" findings is most important. Newborn acidemia has been correlated with a sustained and decreasing FHR variability in association with *recurrent* FHR decelerations over the span of approximately 1 hour (Parer et al., 2006). The accepted definition of "recurrent" as defined by the National Certification Corporation is, decelerations that "occur with 50% or more of uterine contractions in any 20-minute segment (NCC, 2010, p. 4; NCC monograph, 2016). Blood from the umbilical cord is drawn after the birth and is sent for cord blood gas analysis. This gives an objective measure of the fetal acid/base balance at the time of delivery to confirm fetal acidosis.

Cord gases don't stand alone, however. They must be considered in the context of all abnormal findings, including abnormal fetal heart tracings, low Apgar scores, and the baby's requirement for intubation (Saneh et al., 2020). Taken together, these findings can assist the primary healthcare providers in identifying within the first hour of life, the newborns that are at highest risk of seizures related to asphyxia (Saneh et al., 2020).

When a quick assessment is necessary and the nurse must identify the type of acidosis at a glance, the use of single-digit values gleaned from the literature can assist in seeing the differences easily. The primary blood gas values the nurse will refer to initially are quite simple, as noted in Table 1. The nurse must remember just two *normal* values: less than 60 for normal PCO2 and less than or equal to 12 for the normal base deficit. (See first column below.)

Table 1: Single-Digit Values for Blood Gas Analysis. Given the pH is low with acidosis, then additionally, respiratory acidosis is easily recognizable by a PCO2 that is greater than 60. Metabolic acidosis is recognized by a base deficit greater than or equal to 12. If *both* of these parameters are present, it's a mixed acidosis. (AWHONN FHMPP, 2015; Andres et al., 1999; Low, et al., 1997).

	Normal Values	Respiratory Acidosis	Metabolic Acidosis	Mixed Acidosis
pH	≥7.10	<7.10	<7.10	<7.10
PCO_2 (mm Hg)	<60	>60	<60	>60
Base deficit (mEq/L)	≤12	<12	>12	>12

The presence of carbon dioxide and base deficit levels helps to determine the type, extent, and chronicity of the acidosis. Using these numbers as a baseline, the nurse can then ask, "Is the CO2 higher than 60?" If so, the newborn has respiratory acidosis. A carbon dioxide level higher than normal (CO2 greater than 60) and accompanied by a *normal base deficit*, indicates the baby has respiratory acidosis. Translated, this means that carbon dioxide is building up in his blood, but the baby still has enough bicarbonate (base) stores.

The nurse then asks, "Is the base deficit greater than 12?" When the *CO2 is normal* but the *base deficit is abnormally high*, at 12 or above, the baby has metabolic acidosis. Note the *deficit* is high; there's a *shortage* of bicarbonate to offset the acids.

When *both* the CO2 and the base deficit are higher than normal, the baby has a mixed acidosis, meaning high levels of both carbon dioxide from respiratory acidosis and lactic acid from metabolic acidosis are likely, and the baby has a shortfall of sodium bicarbonate to balance the acids. To confirm the presence of lactic acid, some providers will obtain a sample of blood from the fetal scalp before the birth, to measure the lactate levels (Carbonne et al., 2016).

Once the nurse has quickly identified respiratory, metabolic, or mixed acidosis, a closer assessment of other values can be made. Table 2 includes the full list of blood gas results. The nurse will see that both "base deficit" and "base excess" are included for clarity. Only one or the other is necessary to use, since they indicate the same number in either positive or negative terms. The choice of terms is made by the laboratory in reporting. The description of "base deficit" is straightforward in declaring "We have a deficit. We're this low on bicarbonate." In contrast, use of the term "base excess" requires a translation from what the word "excess" means (more than enough), to what the lab result actually means: "We have an excess! No, just kidding! We're in default. This is a negative number!"

The oxygen levels (PO2) are variable, so they are not necessary to assess at first glance. Same with the normal sodium bicarbonate levels of 22. The normal levels are good to know, but the base *deficit* gives more information on how well the baby's body has coped with the bicarbonate demands within the environment of the laboring uterus. The higher the base deficit, the more chronic the acidosis has been.

Table 2: Full Reference Guide for Blood Gas Analysis (AWHONN FHMPP, 2015; Andres et al., 1999; Low et al., 1997)

	Normal Values	Respiratory Acidosis	Metabolic Acidosis	Mixed Acidosis
pH	≥ 7.10	< 7.10	< 7.10	< 7.10
PCO_2 (mm Hg)	< 60	> 60	< 60	> 60
Bicarbonate (mEq/L)	≥ 22	≥ 22	< 22	< 22
Base deficit (mEq/L)	≤ 12	< 12	> 12	> 12
Base excess (mEq/L)	≥ -12	≥ -12	< -12	< -12
PO_2 (mm Hg)	> 20	Variable	Variable	Variable

The "Stories" of Acidosis

In addition to normal values, the nurse must remember the physiology that relates to each type of acidosis. No metaphor is perfect, as the author has noted in an allegorical retelling of acid–base balance related to variable decelerations and fetal acidemia (Irland, 2009a), but allegories share broad concepts that may shed light on physiology. Both aerobic and anaerobic acidosis result from an inadequate supply of oxygen, regardless of the reason, but the condition of aerobic (respiratory) acidosis is more easily reversed than that of anaerobic (metabolic) acidosis.

In an allegory of variable decelerations and fetal acidemia, the body is referred to as a village filled with busy restaurants (cellular activity).

> *In the restaurant, the garbage from food prep (carbon dioxide) is bagged and placed along the street (circulatory system) for garbage truck pickup (hemoglobin, which brings oxygen from the placenta and exchanges it for carbon dioxide). The garbage trucks travel back and forth on a road (umbilical cord) from the restaurants (cells) to the landfill (placenta). When the road*

> *to the village is blocked, as with cord compression, the garbage trucks cannot move back and forth, so garbage (carbon dioxide) builds up in the street, causing respiratory acidosis (Irland, 2009a).*

In a similar allegory, metabolic acidosis is described as worsening garbage maintenance issues within the *restaurants*—the cells.

> *With few sanitation workers (oxygen) coming in from the landfill (placenta), garbage builds up in the street, or backs up into the restaurant kitchens (metabolic acidosis). The kitchens become sour (metabolic acidosis) and the chef sprinkles baking soda (sodium bicarbonate base) around, to absorb the smell. Pantry inventory calls for 22 boxes of baking soda at all times (normal sodium bicarbonate is 22 meq/L). But, having used up more and more boxes, the chef discovers he has a deficit of more than 12 boxes as a result of garbage backup and the use of more boxes (base deficit of > 12). (Irland, 2009b).*

The nurse who anticipates the type of acidosis reflected by an accurate interpretation of the FHR understands that ". . . variable decelerations indicate a problem in the *street* (the umbilical cord) . . . late decelerations indicate a problem at the *landfill* (placenta). . . (Irland, 2009b, p. 336).

Once the baby is born, or "rescued" from the uterine environment, the so-called garbage, or anaerobic problems, are history. To use the language of the allegories, the "garbage along the streets" can be cleaned (reversing respiratory acidosis) and the "kitchens" can be restored to order (reversing metabolic acidosis) once adequate oxygen is taken in.

DIABETES

Gestational Diabetes

ONE TEASPOON OF SUGAR

Let's start with a review of physiologic blood sugar levels. In this section, the terms "sugar" and "glucose" are used interchangeably. The total amount of baseline sugar circulating in the blood is less than 1 teaspoon, or about 4-5 grams of carbohydrates (see the calculation at https://proteinpower.com/a-spoonful-of-sugar/). The calculation is based on the American Diabetes Association's definition of pre-diabetes as a fasting blood sugar reading of more than 100 mg/dL (5.5 mmol/L) in 5 liters of blood. That level rises during and after a meal. As an example, a spaghetti dinner of 2 cups of spaghetti and sauce with 2 slices of garlic bread can raise the blood sugar to around 118 grams of carbohydrate (23 teaspoons, or around half a cup of sugar), which must be reduced back down to 1 teaspoon (4 grams) within 2 to 3 hours. One can see the benefit to the pancreas of a meal with 45 grams of carbohydrates (9 teaspoons of glucose) instead, as recommended in carbohydrate counting for clients with diabetes.

Between meals and overnight, as blood sugar levels drop and the demand for glucose rises, the liver responds by breaking down stored glucose (glycogenolysis) and releasing it in order to maintain the blood sugar at the level of 1 teaspoon (100 mg/dL or 5.5 mmol/L) in 5 liters of blood.

INSULIN—NOT A "ONE AND DONE" RESPONSE

Since glucose is the primary stimulus for insulin secretion, it follows that if maintenance levels of glucose are constantly circulating, maintenance levels of insulin are also present. The pancreas maintains a continuous *background* level of insulin throughout the day and night. This is the so-called "basal insulin." This is supplemented with bursts of higher insulin *boluses* at mealtimes, the "first-phase" and "second-phase" insulin responses. First-phase insulin secretion begins within 2 minutes of eating, and continues for the first 10 minutes of a meal (Cavaghan, 2004). The insulin in the first phase is primarily preformed, stored insulin granules (Cavaghan, 2004).

The first phase of insulin secretion is followed by a prolonged second phase that consists of periodic puffs of additional insulin granules every 10 to 15 minutes for 2 to 3 hours, based on glucose levels assessed by the pancreas (Parkensen et al., 2002; Satin et al., 2015). Second phase insulin contains both stored and/or newly made insulin (Wilcox, 2005). The process continues until the glucose levels within the blood are within normal, or back to the previously described 100 g/dL (5.5 mmol/L). Because this can take 2 to 3 hours, the timeframe chosen for the diagnostic Oral Glucose Tolerance Test (OGTT) is 2 hours (some labs do a 3-hour test). The OGTT demonstrates how well the pancreas can reduce the blood sugar to normal levels within the normal timeframe after a glucose load.

Why Does Gestational Diabetes Mellitus (GDM) Happen?

The etiology of gestational diabetes is thought to be the result of limited reserves of stored insulin, which impacts the first-phase release (Saisho et al., 2010). The first phase is either delayed, or the bolus of insulin released at the start of the meal is inadequate (Saisho et al., 2010). The 2-to-3-hour postprandial timeframe for glucose level reduction is prolonged with GDM or type 2 diabetes mellitus (T2DM) since insulin plays "catch-up" due to the inadequate first-phase insulin release. The pancreas is continually behind in glucose reduction for longer than normal.

What Determines the Amount of Insulin Released?

An important point to remember is that the pancreas determines the amount of insulin to release, based on a calculation of circulating glucose levels (Röder et al., 2016; Satin, 2015). As glucose is moved from the circulation and is taken in by the cells, the blood glucose levels continue to decrease, and less insulin is needed. For the client whose cells are insulin resistant and do not respond well to the insulin in the blood vessels (where the glucose leaves the blood), and then at the cells, where glucose enters for energy, higher *blood glucose* levels persist in the circulation and the pancreas must continue to create and pump out higher levels

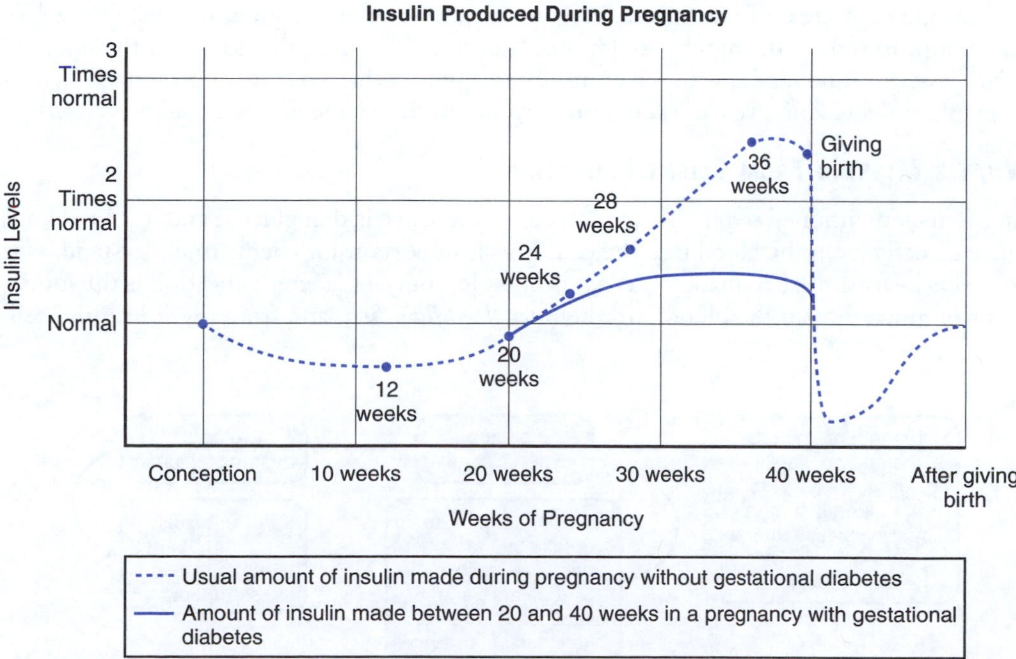

Figure 1. In the last trimester, pregnancy hormones cause increased insulin resistance. As a result, the pancreas must produce nearly 2-3 times more insulin than normal, as indicated by the dotted line in the figure above. In most pregnant women, this is no problem. Some women, however, cannot keep up with the insulin demand, as indicated in the solid line above. These women have gestational diabetes. This may be the first indication that a woman is at risk of type 2 diabetes mellitus in the future, as her pancreas eventually becomes exhausted and beta cells are destroyed as a result of hyperglycemia.

of insulin *for a longer period of time.* If the pancreas cannot meet the demand, gestational diabetes and eventually type 2 diabetes mellitus (T2DM) can result as a consequence. In this way, the normal insulin resistance of pregnancy is thought to unmask previously unknown T2DM and/or the risk of T2DM in the future, due to the inability of the pancreas to create and/or store adequate amounts of insulin for secretion.

The differences in the amounts of insulin produced by a pregnant woman without gestational diabetes and a pregnant woman with the condition are illustrated in Figure 1. One can see that the pancreas must produce nearly three times as much insulin during pregnancy in order to overcome the normal insulin resistance of pregnancy.

A first step in reducing the demands on the pancreas is nutritional education and the addition of exercise. Both of these interventions can reduce the strain on the pancreas by reducing the amount of insulin required in the first and second phases of insulin release.

INSULIN DOESN'T "UNLOCK" THE CELL DOORS—IT SIMPLY KNOCKS AT THE DOORS

Insulin receptors, which may number 15,000 to 30,000 per cell (Blackard, 1977) are temporary docking sites formed by each cell, as needed (Flier, 1983). Note they are temporary, not constant; their numbers can fluctuate. In addition, insulin is cleared from the circulation within10 to 15 minutes from release, so it must be continually replaced (Duckworth et al., 1998; Hall, 2011). When the insulin docks on the insulin receptor like a door-to-door salesman, it signals a GLUT-4 (glucose transport) receptor from the inside of the cell (a butler) to move to the cell membrane, surround the glucose molecules, and bring them inside the cell (Hod et al., 2008). The insulin is degraded, or broken down, and the insulin receptor is returned to the outside of the cell (Duckworth et al., 1998) for the next knock at the door.

As with so many things, too much of something results in resistance. With the chronic hyperglycemia of diabetes, the insulin signaling cascade that calls the glucose carrier GLUT-4 is impaired (Hod et al., 2008). The carrier resists and does not respond to the "knock on the door," resulting in a condition of "insulin resistance." Apparently, the cells' glucose stores are adequate and the pantries are full! Eventually, in response to high levels of circulating insulin, the cells create fewer insulin receptor sites (Wang et al., 2006) in what seems like an attempt to reduce the number of glucose "salesmen" (insulin) that knock at the door. As such, hyperinsulinemia leads to fewer insulin receptors, which results in prolonged hyperglycemia and a vicious cycle of even more insulin resistance (see Figure 2, below).

WHAT'S MISSING FROM CLIENT EDUCATION?

An often-unmentioned step in blood glucose maintenance is that glucose and insulin do not move directly from the blood into the cell. This is important for clients to understand, as it connects heart disease to diabetes. What is often left out of diabetes education is the movement of glucose from the blood into the *interstitial fluid first*, and from there into the cell.

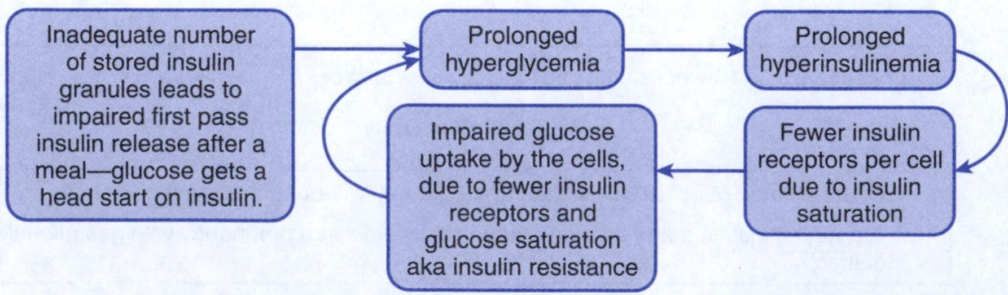

Figure 2. Cycle of Insulin Resistance. Impaired first-phase insulin release leads to prolonged hyperglycemia and prolonged hyperinsulinemia as more and more insulin is pumped into the circulation after a meal. Unfortunately, higher levels of insulin inhibit the number of insulin receptors on each cell, resulting in further prolongation of hyperglycemia. In addition, because the cell is saturated with glucose, it does not accept more. Because the process of restoring lowered blood glucose is slow, and so much demand for insulin is placed on the pancreas, it eventually becomes exhausted and begins to burn out, leading to the risk of type 2 diabetes (Catalano, et al., 1999).

Insulin receptors are present on the endothelium, the inner lining of blood vessels (Barrett & Liu, 2013; Kolka & Bergman, 2013; Masahiro et al., 2017; Richards et al., 2010; Wang et al., 2006). When released during a meal, insulin floods the blood, ready to assist the walls of the blood vessels to release insulin into the interstitial fluid (Barrett et al., 2011), and from there, to dock on the insulin receptors covering the cells so the cells can take in the glucose if they need it (Wang et al., 2006). Unused glucose in the interstitial fluid is removed through the lymph system and returns to the circulatory system through the subclavian vein. The liver converts some of it to triglycerides (hence, a higher level of cholesterol in diabetes).

The harm in hyperglycemia comes from the prolonged presence of glucose in the circulatory system. Glucose participates in chemical reactions that release free radicals, which act like an acid spill in the blood vessels. These reactions cause injury, blood clots, and stiffening of the blood vessels, leading to hypertension (Wang et al., 2006). The body can repair itself fairly well if blood glucose levels are reduced within the normal 2-to-3-hour range after a meal. But, if the levels or persistence of blood glucose are chronically high for longer periods of time, the cardiovascular system can be permanently injured by chronic hyperglycemia.

The "Story" of Gestational Diabetes Mellitus (GDM)

In this allegory, insulin molecules are described as "deliverymen."

> *The deliverymen bring produce (glucose) to the restaurants (cells) in town so the restaurants can maintain their businesses. Mysteriously, the restaurants begin refusing the produce (insulin resistance of pregnancy). In an investigation, the big city learns that a waterpark (has) . . . invaded the big city and expanded the park rapidly (pregnancy). Shuttle drivers (hormones of pregnancy) from the waterpark have bribed the restaurants in the big city to refuse more and more deliveries and have diverted the deliverymen to the shuttle drop-off center (placenta), so that most of the produce (glucose) is delivered to the waterpark (fetal circulation). Eventually, the waterpark outgrows its space and leaves town (baby's birth), and things in the big city return to normal (Irland, 2010, p. 149).*

Diabetic Ketoaocidosis

For clients with type 1 diabetes mellitus (T1DM) primarily, and for some with type 2 diabetes mellitus (T2DM) (Hamdy, 2019) a hostile environment known as diabetic ketoacidosis (DKA), occurs when insulin is either absent or inadequate in bringing glucose into the cells. This is a medical emergency for both mother and fetus.

Getting the signal that cells need glucose, the liver initially breaks down stored glycogen to release glucose. Blood sugar rises. But, without exogenous insulin for the client with T1DM, or in the face of severe insulin resistance and illness, the glucose does not enter the cell. Both maternal and fetal blood sugars rise higher and higher as the liver responds to the cells' need for glucose. Still, the cells cannot take in the glucose. With no apparently available glucose, the cells switch from *aerobic* metabolism to *anaerobic* metabolism. Instead of using glucose for fuel, they break down and burn available fatty acids in stored fat. In laymen's terms, it can be considered the body's move to "plan B" for energy when insulin is not available or is unable to release enough glucose for the cells.

Unlike the "clean" fuel of glucose, however, which breaks down into CO_2 for elimination through the lungs, and water for elimination through the kidneys, fatty acids break down into acids known as ketone bodies. Three toxic acids—acetone, acetoacetate, and beta-hydroxybutyrate—are released, creating acidemia. Normal body pH is alkaline, from 7.35 to 7.45. When the pH drops below normal levels into the acidemic range of 7.2 or less, the chemical reactions required for body organ functioning start to shut down. A dangerous spiral continues as the acidemia worsens and the blood glucose rises, untapped. This is obviously a hostile environment for both mother and fetus and is a medical emergency for them both.

DKA is always accompanied by dehydration, a result of hyperglycemia. The blood is like syrup, and pulls fluid from the extracellular fluid by osmosis in an effort to thin out the osmolarity, or concentration of the plasma. Some of the sugar overflows into the urine, taking salt and potassium with it. All of this takes a toll on cellular function. The rising levels of ketone bodies in the blood contribute to worsening acidemia, leading to vomiting, which contributes to further fluid loss and dehydration.

For the fetus, the maternal dehydration leads to decreased uteroplacental blood flow at the intervillous space. This, combined with maternal acidosis can cause impaired oxygen delivery to the fetus, with resulting fetal hypoxia and fetal acidosis. In addition, fetal hyperglycemia leads to fetal hyperinsulinemia, with an increased metabolism and demand for oxygen. Treatment consists of careful fluid replacement, insulin, electrolytes, and correction of acid–base balance.

In the case study in chapter 8 (questions 1–6), these were the steps to the client's diabetic ketoacidosis:

- Because she was not eating, she stopped administering insulin, thinking it was unnecessary. This is where she needs more education.
- Without insulin, the cells sent signals to the liver indicating they needed glucose.
- In response, the liver broke down (lysed) stored glycogen (glycogenolysis) and released it into the blood as glucose. This did not help the cells get glucose, since they didn't need glucose; they needed insulin to transfer the glucose into the cells. This situation has been referred to as "starving in a sea of plenty."
- The client's cells began breaking down fatty acids for energy, since fatty acids do not require insulin for cellular use.
- The end product of fatty acid fuel was the release of toxic ketone bodies, one of which is acetone. These circulated throughout her blood, making her even more nauseated, and she began vomiting.
- The liver continued to break down glycogen, making her blood sugar go higher and higher, leading to increased urination and dehydration.
- Her acidemic, hyperglycemic blood carried less oxygen to the placenta, and less oxygen to her major organs.
- As a result of poor placental perfusion, the fetus likely experienced hypoxia, as evidenced by minimal variability.
- Maternal treatment is focused on aggressive rehydration, followed by insulin administration, which will stop the liver's continued release of glucose once the pancreas signals the liver that normoglycemia has been restored.

Oral Glucose Tolerance Test (OGTT)

To make a diagnosis of gestational diabetes mellitus, the American College of Obstetricians and Gynecologists (ACOG) has endorsed a two-step plasma glucose measurement process for pregnant clients not previously diagnosed with diabetes. Because the one-step process endorsed by the ADA uses lower cut-off values, ACOG was concerned that an unnecessarily large group of women might be needlessly identified. This could have a negative consequence of medicalizing their pregnancies and increasing health care utilization and costs. Because ACOG's current practice of using higher thresholds to diagnose maternal hyperglycemia has been effective in reducing the rates of fetal macrosomia and shoulder dystocia ACOG chose to continue using the two-step approach instead of casting a wider net by the use of lower values (ADA, 2021a).

The two-step process begins with a *screening* exam, using a 50-gram glucose solution for clients at 24-28 weeks gestation. The client is not required to fast before the test.

The client's blood is drawn one hour after her first swallow of the solution. If her plasma glucose reading is greater than or equal to 130, 135, or 140 mg/dL (7.2, 7.5, or 7.8 mmol/L), a 100-gram *diagnostic* test is indicated within a few days. This test requires an overnight fast.

Before the client drinks the 100-gram glucose solution, a baseline, fasting blood sample is drawn. This is followed at 1, 2, and 3 hours after her first swallow of the solution.

A diagnosis of gestational diabetes mellitus (GDM) is made if at least two of the following results are met or exceeded:

- Fasting: 95 mg/dL (5.3 mmol/L)
- 1 hour: 180 mg/dL (10.0 mmol/L)
- 2 hour: 155 mg/dL (8.6 mmol/L)

FETAL CIRCULATION

Cardiac Shunting

To interpret the meaning and significance of the terms, "left-to-right shunt" or "right-to-left shunt," one must begin with the following:

1. For cardiologists, a reference to the "left side" of the heart means oxygenated blood.
2. References to the "right side" indicate oxygen-depleted blood.
   Note: One must not try to literally visualize the left and right sides of the heart in understanding *all* uses of the phrases "left-to-right shunt" or "right-to-left shunt" when used to describe cardiac conditions. The terms are used to describe both a *literal,* right-to-left, physical shunt between the fetal atria through the foramen ovale, and *figuratively* to denote whether oxygenated blood is moving into oxygen-depleted blood, or vice versa as with a patent ductus arteriosus (PDA).
3. When used to describe the condition of a neonate's patent ductus arteriosus (PDA), which is outside the heart and not on either side of the heart, the broad, figurative references of "left means oxygenated" and "right means oxygen-depleted" are used. So, as described in chapter 10, question 106, with a PDA the oxygenated blood in the aorta is shunted down through the still-open ductus arteriosus (PDA) back into the oxygen-depleted blood of the pulmonary veins, making this a "left-to-right" shunt—"oxygenated to oxygen-depleted" blood movement.
   The learner will recall that before birth, the fetal circulation is referred to as a literal "right-to-left" shunt. Oxygenated blood comes from the placenta through the umbilical vein to the vena cava and into the right atrium. From there, it is shunted to the left atrium through the foramen ovale. From the left atrium the blood is pumped down to the left ventricle, then into the aorta and out to the body. The ductus arteriosus is a shortcut that bypasses the lungs, because they are not yet oxygenating the blood.

How Do The Fetal Lungs Get Oxygenated Blood?

While *most* of the fetal blood is shunted through the foramen ovale, not all of it is. Some of it goes down, into the right ventricle and into the pulmonary arteries. There, in spite of high resistance to blood in the lungs (because they're filled with fluid at this time), a small amount of blood gets through to nourish them. However, *because* of the high resistance in the lungs, most of this oxygenated blood bypasses the lungs and finds the path of least resistance—the ductus arteriosus—into the aorta and then to the systemic circulation. After passing through the body, oxygen-depleted blood is eventually emptied into two umbilical arteries that carry it back to the placenta (the so-called "fetal lung") where it picks up oxygen and the journey starts all over again.

What Causes Closure of the Shunts?

At birth, the lungs inflate and pulmonary resistance decreases. This leads to higher pressures in the left ventricle against the foramen ovale and the flap begins to close. At the same time, the pressure against the ductus arteriosus reverses direction there. Where the highest pressure was once from the pulmonary artery (prenatally), it is now coming from the other direction within the aorta, closing the flap (the ductus arteriosus). With these changes, "normal" cardiac function begins. The right side of the heart receives oxygen-depleted blood from the vena cava and sends it to the lungs for oxygen uptake and then for distribution throughout the body.

WHY IS PDA CALLED A "LEFT-TO-RIGHT" SHUNT?

If the ductus arteriosus flap stays open after the birth, the higher pressures within the aorta push oxygenated blood through the still-patent shunt. This is when the figurative description of a "left-to-right" shunt (oxygenated-to-oxygen-depleted) is used. Within the aorta, the higher pressures push oxygenated (left) blood back down through the ductus arteriosis into the pulmonary artery's oxygen-depleted (right) blood. This previously oxygenated blood re-enters the lungs, overloading them. If uncorrected, this can cause pulmonary hypertension and eventually right-sided heart failure.

Fetal Oxygenation

As a reminder, the maternal and fetal blood circulations are separate. Oxygen from the mother and carbon dioxide waste from the fetus are exchanged through the placental membranes, in a region called the intervillous space, or *placental lake*.

Maternal blood flows through the uterine spiral arteries and is emptied into the intervillous space. Spiral arteries are just that—spirals—before pregnancy. It is these arteries that also contribute to menstrual flow when the woman is not pregnant. As a result of the pregnancy, the mother's spiral arteries become straightened and dilated, in order to provide adequate blood to the placenta for oxygen and carbon dioxide exchange, among other substances.

Note that maternal blood does not go straight from the mother's heart to the intervillous space. As maternal blood makes its way from her heart to the intervillous space, it delivers oxygen to the mother's own cells. By the time the blood reaches the intervillous space for oxygen uptake by the placental capillaries, its oxygen saturation has decreased considerably, but still has enough to adequately oxygenate the fetus if the mother is healthy (Ross et al., 2012).

Between contractions, the oxygen on the maternal side of the placental membrane rushes across to enter the fetal blood, seeking equilibrium because oxygen levels on the fetal side of the placental membrane are even lower than the mother's. Maternal health issues such as diabetes and pre-eclampsia can reduce the fetal oxygen reserve if available oxygen at the placenta is reduced due to the mother's circulatory issues.

Fetal blood draws oxygen by osmosis from the maternal blood in the intervillous space and carries it to the fetal heart through the umbilical vein. In order to recover enough oxygen from what's left in maternal blood, the fetal hemoglobin is equipped with a higher oxygen affinity (or ability to bind to oxygen) and oxygen-carrying capacity than that of the mother. The fetus depends on this supply, also called "fetal reserve" during the contraction when maternal oxygen is temporarily not available due to constriction of the spiral arteries. During strong labor contractions, as the spiral arteries are compressed by the uterus, the maternal blood supply to the intervillous space decreases at the start of the contraction, and then stops temporarily at the peak of the contraction (Ross et al., 2012). Here is where the benefit of fetal hemoglobin (Hb F) comes into play (Ross et al., 2012), as it carries a large supply of oxygen to fetal cells during the contraction. As a result, fetal cellular function continues aerobically throughout contractions.

One can see that contractions greater than 90 seconds can be stressful for the fetus, since there is temporarily no fresh oxygen available during the peak and the fetus must draw on its "fetal reserves" of oxygen throughout the contraction. For some babies, their fetal reserves cannot comfortably provide enough oxygen throughout contractions of this duration. The prudent nurse recognizes this as a factor in late decelerations and intervenes appropriately with a focus on improved fetal oxygenation, if possible, to tank up the fetal reserve.

Umbilical Cord Blood Flow

Knowing how to differentiate the umbilical arteries from the umbilical vein is important when drawing umbilical cord blood for laboratory assessments. A sample from each type of vessel is important to compare the pH differences—the arteriovenous difference—between the blood from the placenta versus the blood within the umbilical artery that comes from the baby. The blood within the umbilical *artery* is most helpful clinically, as it reflects the level and type of acids coming from the baby by measuring carbon dioxide and base deficit levels, along with other chemistry analyses.

An Artery Doesn't Always Carry Oxygenated Blood

Let's review. Within the umbilical cord, one large vein carries blood from the placenta to the fetus, and two smaller umbilical arteries carry blood from the fetus to the placenta for oxygen replenishment and carbon dioxide elimination.

We generally think of veins as carrying oxygen-depleted blood, and arteries carrying oxygenated blood. In the umbilical cord, this is just the opposite: *umbilical* arteries carry *oxygen-depleted* blood, and the *umbilical* vein carries *oxygenated* blood. Use of the word "vein" is temporarily nonsensical in an oxygen-carrying sense, but because the umbilical vein empties into the vena cava; it is part of the fetal venous system, so it's called a vein. Because umbilical arteries are part of the arterial system, carrying blood away from the heart and to the placenta, they are called arteries, even though within the umbilical cord they carry oxygen-depleted blood.

An easy way to remember how many veins and arteries are in the umbilical cord is that arteries come from the baby, so they're baby-sized. As such, two of them are required. Consider that arteries carry blood *away* from the heart. Both of the words *artery* and *away* begin with the letter "a." The umbilical *vein,* coming from the placenta, is the largest of the three blood vessels within the umbilical cord. It is also the most compressible during cord compression, since it is a vein with softer walls than the arteries. Since it carries blood from the mother's direction toward the baby, an easy way to remember its size is that the mother is larger, so this vessel is the largest, and carries nutrients from the mother to the fetus. When drawing umbilical cord blood for gases, it is recommended that one draws from one of the smaller, umbilical arteries first, followed by the larger, umbilical vein sample.

Doppler Flow Studies

Blood flow from the fetus through the placenta and back again is a closed system powered by the fetal heart; maternal and fetal blood do not mix. When there is a concern about placental blood flow resistance, especially with intrauterine growth restriction (IUGR) or preeclampsia with severe features, the provider will often order Doppler flow studies.

Doppler ultrasound measures the waveforms of each fetal cardiac cycle consisting of cardiac contraction (systole) followed by a rest for filling (diastole). Three types of waveforms may be seen. Each one helps the provider assess placental sufficiency or a move toward placental insufficiency. With an increase in placental vessel resistance due to maternal disease, the diastolic flow may be reduced initially. It later becomes absent. When the flow reverses, a decision is often made to deliver the baby to save its life. A description of these waveforms follows.

In a healthy placenta, the Doppler reveals that the waves of blood follow each other smoothly in forward succession as the fetal blood flows to the placenta and enters the vast system of low-resistance blood vessels. The waves appear on the screen as a sort of series of tall, solid evergreen trees in a row, their tips touching, one tree right next to the other. The rise of each wave indicates the speed of the blood following each beat of the fetal heart (Berkley et al., 2012).

If the blood meets resistance at the placenta (due to vasoconstriction), the Doppler waveform shows a pause between the Doppler waves (evergreen trees), as though they've all been planted a short distance apart. This is called absent end-diastolic flow (AEDF). Because the blood meets resistance at the placenta, its speed slows dramatically, making it appear there's a pause. AEDF can indicate beginning issues with placental circulation and fetoplacental vasoconstriction in response to hypoxia (Sebire, 2003). AEDF may be documented as intermittent or persistent. Understandably, a persistent pattern that occurs with each cardiac cycle is more ominous than an intermittent pattern (Baschat, 2004; Rosner et al., 2014).

As the condition worsens, the ultrasound may show reverse end-diastolic flow (REDF), seen as additional waveforms below the line of each previous wave—an upside-down bush, as it were, between and below the line of the upright trees. This indicates that the blood approaching the placental vessels has difficulty entering the placenta, resulting in "splash back" or reverse movement of the blood, like hitting a wall. This finding will often lead to a decision to deliver the fetus (see https://www.fetalhealthfoundation.org/blogs/what-are-doppler-ultrasound-tests/).

INDUCED HYPOTHERMIA

How Does it Work?

Neurological damage results from a deprivation of oxygen and glucose availability to the brain cells as a result of cord occlusion, placental dysfunction, maternal hemorrhage, or sepsis. In response to this energy failure, hypothermia works by slowing down the cellular metabolism, reducing the demand for oxygen, and slowing down the cycle of waste product generation from anaerobic metabolism, cell dysfunction followed by cell death, and further release of cellular sodium that leads to intracranial edema (Polderman, 2009; Shah et al., 2007; Zanelli et al., 2011). A drop in the core temperature to 89.6° F (32° C) slows the metabolic rate to 50% to 65% of normal (Polderman, 2009). Oxygen consumption and CO2 production also drop at the same rate (Polderman, 2009).

Treatment must be started within 6 hours of birth, with the goal of reducing the newborn's rectal temperature and maintaining that temp for at least 72 hours (Peliowski-Davidovich & Canadian Paediatric Society, Fetus and Newborn Committee, 2012). Continuous temperature monitoring with either an esophageal or rectal probe is essential (Mosalli, 2012). The neonate may be treated with head cooling only, or with whole body hypothermia with a cooling blanket (Peliowski-Davidovich & Canadian Paediatric Society, Fetus and Newborn Committee, 2012). Because hypothermia can be painful, neonates are sedated and ventilated and kept comfortable with morphine as needed (Mosalli, 2012). After 72 hours of hypothermic treatment, neonates are rewarmed over a 4-hour period of time. Throughout the treatment, vital signs and laboratory studies that include coagulation studies, CBC and differential, electrolytes, and liver function tests must be monitored vigilantly (Mosalli, 2012).

Complications related to the therapy may include a decreased heart rate and increased blood pressures initially due to an increase in peripheral vasoconstriction, increase in urine output initially, and unstable glucose levels related to factors that include insulin resistance, decreased metabolic rate and shivering (Mosalli, 2012).

Overall, experts agree that the benefits of hypothermic treatment are positive. Large outcome studies have concluded that when hypothermic treatment is initiated as soon as possible within the first 6 hours of life for neonates who meet criteria, mortality rates and severe, long-term neurodevelopmental disabilities are significantly reduced (Peliowski-Davidovich & Canadian Paediatric Society, Fetus and Newborn Committee, 2012).

JAUNDICE

Before birth, the newborn experiences polycythemia, an increase in red blood cells. This is thought to be in response to higher fetal demands for oxygen, referred to as mild hypoxia, which becomes more pronounced as the fetus grows (Jacob, 2016). Hypoxia is a trigger for increased secretion of erythropoietin, which stimulates the release of more oxygen-carrying RBCs.

At birth, the newborn no longer needs the extra red blood cells. The physiologic environment changes and the dependence on oxygenation from the placenta is replaced by increased tissue oxygenation by the lungs. Increased oxygen tension suppresses erythropoietin production, which is followed by destruction of extra RBCs and increased bilirubin production (Jacob, 2016). The accumulation of blood in a cephalohematoma can contribute to a reduction in *circulating* RBCs, and replacement through erythropoesis during the first 1 to 2 weeks of life. This can also contribute to higher jaundice levels.

The short explanation for newborn jaundice is that the immature liver cannot keep up with the elimination of bilirubin. The human body continuously forms bilirubin as the waste product of expired red blood cells (RBCs) when they die. It comes from the body's normal, physiologic maintenance and transient hemolysis of "old" red blood cells by the liver. The lifespan of an RBC is approximately 120 days in the adult, 60 to 90 days in term newborns, and 35 to 50 days in preterm newborns (Steiner & Gallagher, 2007, p. 2).

How Is Bilirubin Destroyed Before the Baby's Birth?

Before birth, as old red blood cells were hemolyzed and the bilirubin was produced, it was carried to the placenta, which transferred it to the mother's blood for further breakdown by her liver and eventual elimination in her stools. (Fun fact: It is bilirubin that gives the brown color to feces.) After the birth, the newborn's immature liver must do the entire process for the first time. With delayed cord clamping, an additional number of RBCs are transferred from the cord to the baby before the cord is cut and clamped.

How Long Does "Physiologic Jaundice" Last?

Transient physiologic jaundice is normal during the first days or up to 2 weeks after birth. Until the postbirth levels of RBCs are established, the newborn liver may be a bit overwhelmed. As a result, the bilirubin circulates throughout the baby's blood for a longer time, causing a yellow hue to the skin. The newborn's body generally completes the breakdown of this large fetal quantity of RBCs and establishes normal levels by around 2 weeks of age (Jacob, 2016).

Adequate intake is necessary for bilirubin excretion. If the newborn does not take in enough milk, reduced meconium and bilirubin levels can remain elevated due to reabsorption of bilirubin from the intestines. For this reason, adequate breastmilk intake and the passage of meconium stools are important to monitor (see https://www.cdc.gov/breastfeeding/breastfeeding-special-circumstances/maternal-or-infant-illnesses/jaundice.html).

References

Aberg, K., Norman, M., Pettersson, K., & Ekéus, C. (2016). Vacuum extraction in fetal macrosomia and risk of neonatal complications: A population-based cohort study. *Acta Obstetriciae et Gynecologica Scandinavica, 95*(10), 1089–1096. https://doi.org/10.1111/aogs.12952

Abramowski, A., Ward, R., & Hamdan, A. (2020). Neonatal hypoglycemia. StatPearls Publishing. https://www.ncbi.nlm.nih.gov/books/NBK537105

Achong, N., Duncan, E. L., McIntyre, H. D., & Callaway, L. (2014). Peripartum management of glycemia in women with type 1 diabetes. *Diabetes Care, 37*(2), 364–371. https://doi.org/10.2337/dc13-1348

Adams, E. D., Stark, M. A., & Low, L. K. (2016). A nurse's guide to supporting physiologic birth. *Nursing for Women's Health, 20*(1), 76–86. https://doi.org/10.1016/j.nwh.2015.12.009

Agency for Healthcare Research and Quality. (n.d.). *Tool: Safe magnesium sulfate administration*. https://www.ahrq.gov/hai/tools/perinatal-care/modules/strategies.html

Agerson, A. N., & Scavone, B. M. (2012). Prophylactic epidural blood patch after unintentional dural puncture for the prevention of postdural puncture headache in parturients, *Anesthesia & Analgesia, 115*(1), 133–136. https://doi.org/10.1213/ANE.0b013e31825642c7

Aguree, S., & Gernand, A. D. (2019). Plasma volume expansion across healthy pregnancy: A systematic review and meta-analysis of longitudinal studies. *BMC Pregnancy and Childbirth, 19*, Article 508. https://doi.org/10.1186/s12884-019-2619-6

Akanmu, A. S., Oyedeji, O. A., Adeyemo, T. A., & Ogbenna, A. A. (2015). Estimating the risk of ABO hemolytic disease of the newborn in Lagos. *Journal of Blood Transfusion*, Article 560738. https://doi.org/10.1155/2015/560738

Akinmoladun, J. A., & Olukemi Bello, O. (2018). Prevalence of prenatal ultrasound diagnosed single umbilical artery in a cohort with associated congenital malformations. *Tropical Journal of Obstetrics & Gynaecology, 35*(3), 304–309. https://doi.org/10.4103/TJOG.TJOG_22_18

Allen, R. E. (2004). Diaphragm fitting. *American Family Physician, 69*(1), 97–100. https://www.aafp.org/afp/2004/0101/p97.html

American Academy of Pediatrics. (n.d.) *Newborn screening: Critical congenital heart defects*. https://www.aap.org/en-us/advocacy-and-policy/aap-health-initiatives/PEHDIC/Pages/Newborn-Screening-for-CCHD.aspx

American Academy of Pediatrics. (2011, reaffirmed 2015). Postnatal glucose homeostasis in late-preterm and term infants. *Pediatrics, 127*(3), 575–579. https://doi.org/10.1542/peds.2010-3851

American Academy of Pediatrics. (2012). Breastfeeding and the use of human milk. *Pediatrics, 129*(3), e827–e841. https://doi.org/10.1542/peds.2011-3552

American Academy of Pediatrics. (2013, reaffirmed 2018). The transfer of drugs and therapeutics into human breast milk: An update on selected topics. *Pediatrics, 132*(3), e796–e809. https://doi.org/10.1542/peds.2013-1985

American Academy of Pediatrics. (2014). Policy statement: Contraception for adolescents. *Pediatrics, 134*(4), e1244–e1256. https://doi.org/10.1542/peds.2014-2299

American Academy of Pediatrics. (2016). HealthyChildren.org. https://www.healthychildren.org/english/health-issues/vaccine-preventable-diseases/pages/default.aspx

American Academy of Pediatrics, Subcommittee on Hyperbilirubinemia. (2004). Management of hyperbilirubinemia in the newborn infant 35 or more weeks of gestation. *Pediatrics*, *114*(1), 297–316. https://doi.org/10.1542/peds.114.1.297

American College of Nurse-Midwives. (2015). Intermittent auscultation for intrapartum fetal heart rate surveillance. *Journal of Midwifery & Women's Health*, *60*(5), 626–632. https://doi.org/10.1111/jmwh.12372

American College of Nurse-Midwives. (2017). A model practice template for hydrotherapy in labor. *Journal of Midwifery & Women's Health*, *62*(1), 120–126. https://doi.org/10.1111/jmwh.12587

American College of Obstetricians and Gynecologists. (2009). Practice Bulletin No. 107: Induction of Labor. https://www.acog.org/clinical/clinical-guidance/practice-bulletin/articles/2009/08/induction-of-labor

American College of Obstetricians and Gynecologists. (2013a). Committee Opinion No. 548: Weight gain during pregnancy. *Obstetrics & Gynecology*, *121*(1), 210–212. https://doi.org/10.1097/01.AOG.0000425668.87506.4c

American College of Obstetricians and Gynecologists. (2013b). Hypertension in pregnancy: Report of the American College of Obstetricians and Gynecologists' Task Force on Hypertension in Pregnancy. *Obstetrics & Gynecology*, *122*(5), 1122–1131. https://doi.org/10.1097/01.AOG.0000437382.03963.88

American College of Obstetrics and Gynecology. (2015, reaffirmed 2018). Committee Opinion No. 633. Alcohol abuse and other substance use disorders: Ethical issues in obstetric and gynecologic practice. *Obstetrics & Gynecology*, *125*(6), 1529–1537. https://doi.org/ 10.1097/01.AOG.0000466371.86393.9b

American College of Obstetricians and Gynecologists. (2016a). Practice Bulletin No. 165: Prevention and management of obstetric lacerations at vaginal delivery. *Obstetrics & Gynecology*, *128*(1), e1–e15. https://doi.org/10.1097/AOG.0000000000001523

American College of Obstetricians and Gynecologists. (2016b). Practice Bulletin No. 171: Management of preterm labor. *Obstetrics & Gynecology*, *128*(4): e155–e164. https://doi.org/10.1097/AOG.0000000000001711

American College of Obstetricians and Gynecologists. (2017a). ACOG Committee Opinion No. 689 summary: Delivery of a newborn with meconium-stained amniotic fluid. *Obstetrics & Gynecology*, *129*(3), 593–594. https://doi.org/10.1097/AOG.0000000000001946

American College of Obstetricians and Gynecologists. (2017b). ACOG Committee Opinion No. 712: Intrapartum managment of intraamniotic infection. https://www.acog.org/clinical/clinical-guidance/committee-opinion/articles/2017/08/intrapartum-management-of-intraamniotic-infection

American College of Obstetricians and Gynecologists. (2017c). ACOG Committee Opinion No. 713: Antenatal corticosteroid therapy for fetal maturation. *Obstetrics & Gynecology*, *130*(2), e101–109. https://doi.org/10.1097/AOG.0000000000002237

American College of Obstetricians and Gynecologists. (2017d). ACOG Practice Bulletin No. 183: Postpartum hemorrhage. https://clinicalinnovations.com/wp-content/uploads/2017/10/ACOG_Practice_Bulletin_No_183_Postpartum-Hemorrhage-2017.pdf

American College of Obstetricians and Gynecologists. (2019a, reaffirmed 2021). Committee Opinion No. 766: Approaches to limit intervention during labor and birth. https://www.acog.org/clinical/clinical-guidance/committee-opinion/articles/2019/02/approaches-to-limit-intervention-during-labor-and-birth

American College of Obstetricians and Gynecologists. (2019b, reaffirmed 2020). ACOG Committee Opinion No. 781: Infertility workup for the women's health specialist. https://www.acog.org/clinical/clinical-guidance/committee-opinion/articles/2019/06/infertility-workup-for-the-womens-health-specialist

American College of Obstetricians and Gynecologists. (2020a). ACOG Committee Opinion No. 797: Prevention of group B streptococcal early-onset disease in newborns. *Obstetrics & Gynecology*, *135*(2), e51–e72. https://doi.org/10.1097/AOG.0000000000003668

American College of Obstetricians and Gynecologists. (2020b). ACOG Practice Bulletin No. 217: Prelabor rupture of membranes. http://unmfm.pbworks.com/w/file/fetch/140666496/Prelabor%20Rupture%20of%20Membranes_ACOG%20Practice%20Bulletin%2C%20Number%20217.pdf

American College of Obstetricians and Gynecologists. (2020c). ACOG Practice Bulletin No. 222: Gestational hypertension and preeclampsia. *Obstetrics & Gynecology, 135*(6), e237–e260. https://doi.org/10.1097/AOG.0000000000003891

American Diabetes Association. (2021a). Classification and diagnosis of diabetes: *Standards of Medical Care in Diabetes—2021. Diabetes Care, 44*(Suppl. 1), S15–S33. https://care.diabetesjournals.org/content/diacare/44/Supplement_1/S15.full.pdf

American Diabetes Association. (2021b). Management of diabetes in pregnancy: *Standards of Medical Care in Diabetes—2021. Diabetes Care, 44*(Suppl. 1), S200–S210. https://care.diabetesjournals.org/content/diacare/44/Supplement_1/S200.full.pdf

American Heart Association. (2015). 2015 AHA guidelines update for CPR and ECC (pp. S501–S518). https://www.cercp.org/images/stories/recursos/Guias%202015/Guidelines-RCP-AHA-2015-Full.pdf

Amir, L. H., & The Academy of Breastfeeding Medicine Protocol Committee. (2014). ABM Clinical Protocol #4: Mastitis. *Breastfeeding Medicine, 9*(5), 239–243. https://doi.org/10.1089/bfm.2014.9984

Andres, R. L., Saade, G., Gilstrap, L. C., Wilkins, I., Witlin, A., Zlatnik, F., & Hankins, G. V. (1999). Association between umbilical blood gas parameters and neonatal morbidity and death in neonates with pathologic fetal acidemia. *American Journal of Obstetrics and Gynecology, 181*(4), 867–871. https://doi.org/10.1016/s0002-9378(99)70316-9

Anthony, J., & Schoeman, L. K. (2013). Fluid management in pre-eclampsia. *Obstetric Medicine, 6*(3), 100–104. https://doi.org/10.1177/1753495X13486896

Archer, T., & Champagne, H. (2013). Fluid management in preeclampsia toolkit. *California Maternal Quality Care Collaborative*. https://www.cmqcc.org/resource/fluid-management-preeclampsia-toolkit-pdf

Arslanoglu, S., Boquien, C.-Y., King, C., Lamireau, D., Tonetto, P., Barnett, D., Bertino, E., Gaya, A., Gebauer, C., Grovslien, A., Moro, G. E., Weaver, G., Wesolowska, A. M., & Picaud, J.-C. (2019). Fortification of human milk for preterm infants: Update and recommendations of the European Milk Bank Association (EMBA) Working Group on Human Milk Fortification. *Frontiers in Pediatrics*, 7, Article 76. https://doi.org/10.3389/fped.2019.00076

Ashwal, E., Salman, L., Tzur, Y., Aviram, A., Bashi, T. B.-M., Yogev, Y., & Hiersch, L. (2018). Intrapartum fever and the risk for perinatal complications: The effect of fever duration and positive cultures. *The Journal of Maternal-Fetal & Neonatal Medicine, 31*(11), 1418–1425. https://doi.org/10.1080/14767058.2017.1317740

Association of Women's Health, Obstetric, and Neonatal Nurses. (2015). *Fetal heartrate monitoring principles and practices (FHMPP)* (5th ed.). Author.

Association of Women's Health, Obstetric, and Neonatal Nurses. (2021). Guidelines for active management of the third stage of labor using oxytocin: AWHONN Practice Brief Number 12. *Journal of Obstetric, Gynecologic, and Neonatal Nurses, 50*, 499–502. https://doi.org/10.1016/j.jogn.2021.04.006

Azad, M. B., Movce, B. L., Guillemette, L., Pascoe, C. D., Wicklow, B., McGavock, J. M., Halayko, A. J., & Dolinsky, V. W. (2017). Diabetes in pregnancy and lung health in offspring: Developmental origins of respiratory disease. *Paediatric Respiratory Reviews, 21*, 19–26. https://www.azadlab.ca/uploads/8/9/1/2/89121762/azad_2017_-_maternal_diabetes___lung_health_in_offspring__review___paediatric_resp_reviews.pdf

Azhibekov, T., & Seri, I. (2019). Acid-base homeostasis in the fetus and newborn. In W. Oh & M. Baum (Eds.), *Nephrology and fluid/electrolyte physiology* (3rd ed., pp. 85–95). https://www.sciencedirect.com/science/article/pii/B9780323533676000066

Aziz, K., Lee, H. C., Escobedo, M. B., Hoover, A. V., Kamath-Rayne, B. D., Kapadia, V. S., Magid, D. J., Niermeyer, S., Schmölzer, G. M., Szyld, E., Weiner, G. M., Wyckoff, M. H., Yamada, N. K., & Zaichkin, J. (2020). Part 5: Neonatal resuscitation: 2020 American

Heart Association guidelines for cardiopulmonary resuscitation and emergency cardiovascular care. *Circulation*, *142*(Suppl. 2), S524–S550. https://doi.org/10.1161/CIR.0000000000000902

Baby-Friendly USA. (2021). *The baby-friendly hospital initiative: Guidelines and evaluation criteria* (6th ed.). Author. https://www.babyfriendlyusa.org/wp-content/uploads/2021/07/Baby-Friendly-GEC-Final.pdf

Baker, B. (2015). Evidence-based practice to improve outcomes for late preterm infants. *Journal of Obstetric, Gyncologic, and Neonatal Nurses*, *44*, 127–134. https://doi.org/10.1111/1552-6909.12533

Balest, A. L. (2021). Respiratory support in neonates and infants. In *Merck manual*. https://www.merckmanuals.com/professional/pediatrics/perinatal-problems/respiratory-support- in-neonates-and-infants

Ballard, J. L., Khoury, L. C., Wedig, K., Wang, L., Eilers-Walsman, B. L., & Lipp, L. (1991). New Ballard Score, expanded to include extremely premature infants. *Journal of Pediatrics*, *19*(3), 417–423. With permission.

Barnhart, M. L., & Rosenbaum, K. (2019). Anaphylactoid syndrome of pregnancy. *Nursing for Women's Health*, *23*(1), 38–48. https://doi.org/10.1016/j.nwh.2018.11.006

Barrett, E. J., & Liu, Z. (2013). The endothelial cell: An "early responder" in the development of insulin resistance. *Reviews in Endocrine & Metabolic Disorders*, *14*(1), 21–27. https://doi.org/10.1007/s11154-012-9232-6

Barrett, E. J., Wang, H., Upchurch, C. T., & Liu, Z. (2011). Insulin regulates its own delivery to skeletal muscle by feed-forward actions on the vasculature. *American Journal of Physiology. Endocrinology and Metabolism*, *301*(2), E252–E263. https://doi.org/10.1152/ajpendo.00186.2011

Basaldella, L., Marton, E., Bekelis, K., & Longatti, P. (2011). Spontaneous resolution of atraumatic intrauterine ping-pong fractures in newborns delivered by cesarean section. *Journal of Child Neurology*, *26*(11), 1449–1451. https://doi.org/10.1177/0883073811410058

Baschat A. A. (2004). Doppler application in the delivery timing of the preterm growth-restricted fetus: Another step in the right direction. *Ultrasound in Obstetrics & Gynecology*, *23*(2), 111–118. https://doi.org/10.1002/uog.989

Beall, M. H., van den Wijngaard, J. P., van Gemert, M. J., & Ross, M. G. (2007). Regulation of amniotic fluid volume. *Placenta*, *28*(8–9), 824–832. https://doi.org/10.1016/j.placenta.2006.12.004

Beattie, S. (2007). Bedside emergency: Wound dehiscence. *RN*, *70*(6), 34–37.

Benitz, W. E., Wynn, J. L., & Polin, R. A. (2015). Reappraisal of guidelines for management of neonates with suspected early-onset sepsis. *The Journal of Pediatrics*, *166*(4), 1070–1074. https://doi.org/10.1016/j.jpeds.2014.12.023

Berg, O., Lee, R. H., & Chagolla, B. (2013). Magnesium sulfate. *Improving Health Care Response to Preeclampsia: A California Quality Improvement Toolkit*. California Maternal Quality Care Collaborative. https://www.cmqcc.org/resource/2826/download

Berkley, E., Chauhan, S. P., & Abuhamad, A. (2012). Doppler assessment of the fetus with intrauterine growth restriction. *American Journal of Obstetrics & Gynecology*, *206*(4), 300–308. https://doi.org/10.1016/j.ajog.2012.01.022

Bishop, E. H. (1964). Pelvic scoring for elective induction. *Obstetrics & Gynecology*, *24*, 266. https://journals.lww.com/greenjournal/Citation/1964/08000/Pelvic_Scoring_for_Elective_Induction.18.aspx

Blackard, W. G. (1977). Insulin receptors. *Medical College of Virginia Quarterly*, *13*(1), 12–16. https://scholarscompass.vcu.edu/mcvq/vol13/iss1/5/

Boettiger, M., Tyer-Viola, L., & Hagan, J. (2017). Nurses' early recognition of neonatal sepsis. *Journal of Obstetric, Gynecologic, and Neonatal Nurses*, *46*, 834–845. doi:10.1016/j.jogn.2017.08.007

Boorsma, E. M., ter Maaten, J. M., Damman, K., Dinh, W., Gustafsson, F., Goldsmith, S., Burkhoff, D., Zannad, F., Udelson, J. E., & Voors, A. A. (2020). Congestion in heart failure: A contemporary look at physiology, diagnosis and treatment. *National Reviews Cardiology*, *17*, 641–655. https://doi.org/10.1038/s41569-020-0379-7

Borghesi, A., Stronati, M., & Fellay, J. (2017). Neonatal group B streptococcal disease in otherwise healthy infants: Failure of specific neonatal immune responses. *Frontiers in Immunology*, *8*, Article 215. https://doi.org/10.3389/fimmu.2017.00215

Brace, R. A., Cheung, C. Y., & Anderson, D. F. (2018). Regulation of amniotic fluid volume: Insights derived from amniotic fluid volume function curves. *American Journal of Physiology: Regulatory, Integrative and Comparative Physiology*, *315*(4), R777–R789. https://doi.org/10.1152/ajpregu.00175.2018

Brinkman, J. E., & Sharma, S. (2020). Physiology, metabolic alkalosis. StatPearls Publishing. https://www.ncbi.nlm.nih.gov/books/NBK482291

Brown University Psychopathology Update. (2013). Guidance issued on the use of SSRIs in pregnancy, *124*(3), 1–8.

Burt, C. C., & Durbridge, J. (2009). Management of cardiac disease in pregnancy. *Continuing Education in Anaesthesia, Critical Care & Pain*, *9*(2), 44–47. https://doi.org/10.1093/bjaceaccp/mkp005

Cagir, B. (2018). Postoperative ileus treatment & management. *Medscape*. https://emedicine.medscape.com/article/2242141-treatment#d6

Cahill, A. G., Roehl, K. A., Odibo, A. O., & Macones, G. A. (2012). Association and prediction of neonatal acidemia. *American Journal of Obstetrics & Gynecology*, *207*(3), 206.e1–206.e8. https://doi.org/10.1016/j.ajog.2012.06.046

California Maternal Quality Care Collaborative. (2015). *OB Hemorrhage Toolkit V 2.0. OB Hemorrhage Toolkit V 2.0*. https://www.cmqcc.org/resources-tool-kits/toolkits/ob-hemorrhage-toolkit

Carbonne, B., Pons, E., & Maisonneuve, E. (2016). Foetal scalp blood sampling during labour for pH and lactate measurements. *Best Practice & Research in Clinical Obstetrics and Gynaecology*, *30*, 62–67. http://doi.org/10.1016/j.bpobgyn.2015.05.006

Carroll, K. (2013). Donating breast milk helps bereaved mothers deal with loss. *The Milk Bank*. https://www.themilkbank.org/blog-2/donating-breastmilk-helps-bereaved-mothers-heal

Casey, C. F., Slawson, D. C., & Neal, L. R. (2010). Vitamin D supplementation in infants, children, and adolescents. *American Family Physician*, *81*(6), 745–748. https://www.aafp.org/afp/2010/0315/p745.html

Catalano, P. M., Huston, L., Amini, S. B., & Kalhan, S. C. (1999). Longitudinal changes in glucose metabolism during pregnancy in obese women with normal glucose tolerance and gestational diabetes mellitus. *American Journal of Obstetrics & Gynecology*, *180*(4), 903–916. https://doi.org/10.1016/s0002-9378(99)70662-9

Cavaghan, M. K. (2004). The beta cell and first-phase insulin secretion. *Medscape*, *6*(2). http://cme.medscape.com/viewarticle/483307

Centers for Disease Control and Prevention. (n.d.-a). *Breast surgery*. https://www.cdc.gov/breastfeeding/breastfeeding-special-circumstances/maternal-or-infant-illnesses/breast-surgery.html

Centers for Disease Control and Prevention. (n.d.-b). *Chlamydia—CDC fact sheet*. https://www.cdc.gov/std/chlamydia/stdfact-chlamydia.htm

Centers for Disease Control and Prevention. (n.d.-c). *Genital herpes*. https://www.cdc.gov/std/Herpes/default.htm

Centers for Disease Control and Prevention. (n.d.-d). *Human papillomavirus (HPV)*. https://www.cdc.gov/hpv/

Centers for Disease Control and Prevention. (n.d.-e). Listeria *(listeriosis): People at risk—pregnant women and newborns*. https://www.cdc.gov/listeria/risk-groups/pregnant-women.html#:~:text=Pregnant%20women%20with%20a%20Listeria,and%20even%20death

Centers for Disease Control and Prevention. (n.d.-f). *Pregnancy and whooping cough: Get the whooping cough vaccine during each pregnancy.* https://www.cdc.gov/pertussis/pregnant/mom/get-vaccinated.html

Centers for Disease Control and Prevention. (n.d.-g). *Rubella (German measles, three-day measles): Pregnancy and rubella*. https://www.cdc.gov/rubella/pregnancy.html#:~:text=Congenital%20Rubella%20Syndrome%20(CRS)&text=Pregnant%20women%20who%20contract%20rubella,in%20the%20developing%20baby's%20body)

Chapman, S. C. (2016). The decompensated neonate in the first week of life. *Clinical Pediatric Emergency Medicine, 17*(2), 134–139. https://doi.org/10.1016/j.cpem.2016.04.003

Chauhan, G., & Tadi, P. (2020). *Postpartum changes*. StatPearls Publishing. https://www.ncbi.nlm.nih.gov/books/NBK555904

Chawanpaiboon, S., Vogel, J. P., Moller, A.-B., Lumbiganon, P., Petzold, M., Hogan, D., Landoulsi, S., Jampathong, N., Kongwattanakul, K., Laopaiboon, M., Lewis, C., Rattanakanokchai, S., Teng, D. N., Thinkhamrop, J., Watananirun, K., Zhang, J., Zhou, W., & Gülmezoglu, A. M. (2019). Global, regional, and national estimates of levels of preterm birth in 2014: A systematic review and modelling analysis. *Lancet Global Health*, 7, e37–e46. http://doi.org/10.1016/S2214-109X(18)30451-0

Choe, J., Shanks, A. L., & De Jesus, O. (2020). *Early decelerations*. StatPearls Publishing. https://www.ncbi.nlm.nih.gov/books/NBK557393

Chollat, C., Sentilhes, L., & Marret, S. (2018). Fetal neuroprotection by magnesium sulfate: From translational research to clinical application. *Frontiers in Neurology*, *9*, Article 247. https://doi.org/10.3389/fneur.2018.00247

Colditz, M. J., Lai, M. M., Cartwright, D. W., & Colditz, P. B. (2014). Subgaleal haemorrhage in the newborn: A call for early diagnosis and aggressive management. *Journal of Paediatrics and Child Health, 51*, 140–146. https://doi.org/10.1111/jpc.12698

Cornell University. (2000). Pressure conversion. *Critical Care Pediatrics.* http://www-users.med.cornell.edu/~spon/picu/calc/pressure.htm

Coustan, D. R., Lowe, L. P., Metzger, B. E., & Dyer, A. R. (2010). The Hyperglycemia and Adverse Pregnancy Outcome (HAPO) study: Paving the way for new diagnostic criteria for gestational diabetes mellitus. *American Journal of Obstetrics & Gynecology*, *202*(6), 654.e1–654.e6. https://doi.org/10.1016/j.ajog.2010.04.006

da Costa, T. X., Azeredo, F. J., Ururahy, M., da Silva Filho, M. A., Martins, R. R., & Oliveira, A. G. (2020). Population pharmacokinetics of magnesium sulfate in preeclampsia and associated factors. *Drugs in R&D*, *20*(3), 257–266. https://doi.org/10.1007/s40268-020-00315-2

Davis, A. L., Carcillo, J. A., Aneja, R. K., Deymann, A. J., Lin, J. C., Nguyen, T. C., Okhuysen-Cawley, R. S., Relvas, M. S., Rozenfeld, R. A., Skippen, P. W., Stojadinovic, B. J., Williams, E. A., Yeh, T. S., Balamuth, F., Brierley, J., de Caen, A. R., Cheifetz, I. M., Choong, K., Conway, E. Jr., … Zuckerberg, A. L. (2017). American College of Critical Care Medicine clinical practice parameters for hemodynamic support of pediatric and neonatal septic shock. *Critical Care Medicine*, *45*(6), 1061–1093. https://doi.org/10.1097/CCM.0000000000002425

Davis, S. (2011). Do diaphragms cause urinary tract infections? *Medscape.* https://www.webmd.com/urinary-incontinence-oab/features/do-diaphragms-cause-urinary-tract-infections

Day, V. (2009). Promoting health literacy through storytelling. *The Online Journal of Issues in Nursing*, *14*(3). https://ojin.nursingworld.org/MainMenuCategories/ANAMarketplace/ANAPeriodicals/OJIN/TableofContents/Vol142009/No3Sept09/Health-Literacy-Through-Storytelling.html

Dean L. (2005). *Blood groups and red cell antigens.* National Center for Biotechnology Information. https://www.ncbi.nlm.nih.gov/books/NBK2266

Dekker, R. (2012). *What is the evidence for perineal massage during pregnancy to prevent tearing?* https://www.lamaze.org/Connecting-the-Dots/what-is-the-evidence-for-perineal-massage-during-pregnancy-to-prevent-tearing

Desseauve, D., Fradet, L., Gherman, R. B., Cherni, Y., Gachon, B., & Pierre, F. (2020). Does the McRoberts' manoeuvre need to start with thigh abduction? An innovative biomechanical study. *BMC Pregnancy and Childbirth, 20*, Article 264. https://doi.org/10.1186/s12884-020-02952-6.

De Silva, D. A., Synnes, A. R., von Dadelszen, P., Lee, T., Bone, J. N., MAG-CP, CPN and CNN collaborative groups, & Magee, L. A. (2018). MAGnesium sulphate for fetal neuroprotection to prevent cerebral palsy (MAG-CP)—implementation of a national guideline in Canada. *Implementation Science, 13*, Article 8. https://doi.org/10.1186/s13012-017-0702-9

Dickison, P., Haerling, K., & Lasater, K. (2019). Integrating the National Council of State Boards of Nursing Clinical Judgment Model into nursing educational frameworks. *Journal of Nursing Education, 58*(2), 72–78. https://doi.org/10.3928/01484834-20190122-03

Dosanjh, A. (2018). Neonatal cyanosis: A clinical diagnosis. *EC Paediatrics*, 7(12), 1164–1168. https://www.ecronicon.com/ecpe/pdf/ECPE-07-00378.pdf

Dubil, E., & Magann, E. F. (2013). Amniotic fluid as a vital sign for fetal wellbeing. *Australasian Journal of Ultrasound in Medicine, 16*(2), 62–70. https://doi.org/10.1002/j.2205-0140.2013.tb00167.x

Duckworth, W. C., Bennett, R. B., & Hamel, F. G. (1998). Insulin degradation: Progress and potential. *Endocrine Reviews, 19*(5), 608–624. https://doi.org/10.1210/edrv.19.5.0349

Duerbeck, N. B., Chaffin, D. G., & Seeds, J. W. (1992). A practical approach to umbilical artery pH and blood gas determinations. *Obstetrics & Gynecology, 79*(6), 959–962.

Durbin, D. R., Hoffman, B. D., & Council on Injury, Violence, and Poison Prevention. (2018). Child passenger safety. *Pediatrics, 142*(5), e20182460. https://doi.org/10.1542/peds.2018-2460

Eichenwald, E. C. (2020). Overview of cyanosis in the newborn. *UpToDate*. https://www.uptodate.com/contents/overview-of-cyanosis-in-the-newborn

Enkhmaa, D., Wall, D., Mehta, P. K., Stuart, J. J., Rich-Edwards, J. W., Merz, C. N., & Shufelt, C. (2016). Preeclampsia and vascular function: A window to future cardiovascular disease risk. *Journal of Women's Health, 25*(3), 284–291. https://doi.org/10.1089/jwh.2015.5414

Escobedo, M. B., Aziz, K., Kapadia, V. S., Lee, H. C., Niermeyer, S., Schmolzer, G. M., Szyld, E., Weiner, G. M., Wyckoff, M. H., Yamada, N. K., & Zaichkin, J. G. (2019). 2019 American Heart Association focused update on neonatal resuscitation: An update to the American Heart Association guidelines for cardiopulmonary resuscitation and emergency cardiovascular care. *Circulation, 140*, e922–e930. https://doi.org/10.1161/CIR.0000000000000729

Fakih, H. M. (2014). Spontaneous neonatal subgaleal hematomas after caesarian section. *Journal of Case Reports, 4*(2), 359–362. http://doi.org/10.17659/01.2014.0091

Farrales, L. L., Cacciatore, J., Jonas-Simpson, C., Dharamsi, S., Ascher, J., & Klein, M. C. (2020). What bereaved parents want health care providers to know when their babies are stillborn: A community-based participatory study. *BMC Psychology, 8*, Article 18. https://doi.org/10.1186/s40359-020-0385-x

Farrar, D. (2016). Hyperglycemia in pregnancy: Prevalence, impact, and management challenges. *International Journal of Women's Health, 8*, 519–527. https://doi.org/10.2147/IJWH.S102117

Feig, D. S., Zinman, B., Wang, X., & Hux, J. (2008). Risk of development of diabetes mellitus after diagnosis of gestational diabetes. *Canadian Medical Association Journal, 179*, 229–234. https://doi.org/10.1503/cmaj.080012

Feldman, A. Z., & Brown, F. M. (2016). Management of type 1 diabetes in pregnancy. *Current Diabetes Reports, 16*, Article 76. https://doi.org/10.1007/s11892-016-0765-z

Flier, J. S. (1983). Insulin receptors and insulin resistance. *Annual Review of Medicine, 34*, 145–160. https://www.annualreviews.org/doi/pdf/10.1146/annurev.me.34.020183.001045

Fomukong, N. H., Edwin, N., Edgar, M., Nkfusai, N. C., Ijang, Y. P., Bede, F., Shirinde, J., & Cumber, S. N. (2019). Management of face presentation, face and lip edema in a primary healthcare facility case report, Mbengwi, Cameroon. *The Pan African Medical Journal*, *33*, 292. https://doi.org/10.11604/pamj.2019.33.292.18927

Forray, A., & Foster, D. (2015). Substance use in the perinatal period. *Current Psychiatry Reports*, *17*(11), Article 19. https://doi.org/10.1007/s11920-015-0626-5

Gallacher, D. J., Hart, K., & Kotecha, S. (2016). Common respiratory conditions of the newborn. *Breathe*, *12*(1), 30–42. https://doi.org/10.1183/20734735.000716

García-Patterson, A., Gich, I., Amini, S. B., Catalano, P. M., de Leiva, A., & Corcoy, R. (2010). Insulin requirements throughout pregnancy in women with type 1 diabetes mellitus: Three changes of direction. *Diabetologia*, *53*, 446–451. https://doi.org/10.1007/s00125-009-1633-z

Geis, G. M., & Clark, D. A. (2017). Meconium aspiration syndrome workup. *Medscape*. https://emedicine.medscape.com/article/974110-workup

Gill, P., Tamirisa, A. P., & Van Hook, J. W. (2020). *Acute eclampsia*. StatPearls Publishing. https://www.ncbi.nlm.nih.gov/books/NBK459193

Gillies, D., Wells, D., & Bhandari, A. P. (2012). Positioning for acute respiratory distress in hospitalised infants and children. *Cochrane Database of Systematic Reviews*. https://www.cochranelibrary.com/cdsr/doi/10.1002/14651858.CD003645.pub3/full

Hale, T. W., & Rowe, H. E. (2014). *Medications and mother's milk* (16th ed.). Hale.

Hall, J. E. (2011). *Guyton and Hall textbook of medical physiology* (13th ed., pp. 983–994). W.B. Saunders.

Hamdan, A. H. (2017). Pediatric hydrops fetalis. *Medscape*. https://emedicine.medscape.com/article/974571-overview#a7

Hamdy, O. (2019). Diabetic ketoacidosis (DKA). *Medscape*. https://emedicine.medscape.com/article/118361-overview

Hammer, E. S., & Cipolla, M. J. (2015). Cerebrovascular dysfunction in preeclamptic pregnancies. *Current Hypertension Reports*, *17*, Article 64. https://doi.org/10.1007/s11906-015-0575-8

Hamza, A., Herr, D., Solomayer, E. F., & Meyberg-Solomayer, G. (2013). Polyhydramnios: Causes, diagnosis and therapy. *Geburtshilfe und Frauenheilkunde*, *73*(12), 1241–1246. https://doi.org/10.1055/s-0033-1360163

Hansen, T. W. R. (2017). Neonatal jaundice. *Medscape*. https://emedicine.medscape.com/article/974786-overview

Heitzmann, D., & Warth, R. (2007). No potassium, no acid: K+ channels and gastric acid secretion. *Physiology*, *22*, 335–341. https://doi.org/10.1152/physiol.00016.2007

Henderson, W. (2017). 5 facts about cystic fibrosis and fertility. *Cystic Fibrosis News Today*. https://cysticfibrosisnewstoday.com/2017/11/08/5-facts-about-cystic-fibrosis-and-fertility

Herrmann, K., & Carroll, K. (2014). An exclusively human milk diet reduces necrotizing enterocolitis. *Breastfeeding Medicine*, *9*(4), 184–190. https://doi.org/10.1089/bfm.2013.0121

Hill, M. G., & Cohen, W. R. (2016). Shoulder dystocia: Prediction and management. *Women's health*, *12*(2), 251–261. https://doi.org/10.2217/whe.15.103

Hillman, N. H., Kallapur, S. G., & Jobe, A. H. (2012). Physiology of transition from intrauterine to extrauterine life. *Clinics in Perinatology*, *39*(4), 769–783. https://doi.org/10.1016/j.clp.2012.09.009

Hod, M., Jovanovic, L., Di Renzo, G. C., de Leiva, A., & Langer, O. (Eds.). (2008). *Textbook of diabetes and pregnancy* (2nd ed.). Informa Healthcare USA.

Holtzmann, M., Wretler, S., Cnattingius, S., & Nordström, L. (2015). Cardiotocography patterns and risk of intrapartum fetal acidemia. *Journal of Perinatal Medicine*, *43*, 473–479. https://doi.org/10.1515/jpm-2014-0105

Hua, M., Odibo, A. O., Macones, G., Roehl, K. A., Crane, J. P., & Cahill, A. G. (2010). Single umbilical artery and its associated findings. *Obstetrics & Gynecology 115*, 930–934. https://doi.org/10.1097/AOG.0b013e3181da50ed

Huang, H.-C., Yang, H.-I., Chang, Y.-H., Chang, R.-J., Chen, M.-H., Chen, C.-Y., Chou, H.-C., Hsieh, W.-S., & Tsao, P.-N. (2012). Model to predict hyperbilirubinemia in healthy term and near-term newborns with exclusive breast feeding. *Pediatrics and Neonatology*, *53*(6), 354–358. https://doi.org/10.1016/j.pedneo.2012.08.012

Huybrechts, K. F., Bateman, B. T., Palmsten, K., Desai, R. J., Patorno, E., Gopalakrishnan, C., Levin, R., Mogun, H., & Hernandez-Diaz, S. (2015). Antidepressant use late in pregnancy and risk of persistent pulmonary hypertension of the newborn. *Journal of the American Medical Association*, *313*(21), 2142–2151. https://doi.org/10.1001/jama.2015.5605

Irland, N. (2009a). The story of variable decelerations and acid-base balance. *Nursing for Women's Health*, *13*(2), 159–161. https://doi.org/10.1111/j.1751-486X.2009.01408.x

Irland, N. (2009b). Late decelerations and acid-base balance. *Nursing for Women's Health*, *13*(4), 335–340. https://doi.org/10.1111/j.1751-486X.2009.01444.x

Irland, N. (2010). The story of gestational diabetes. *Nursing for Women's Health*, *14*(2), 147–155. https://doi.org/10.1111/j.1751-486X.2010.01529.x

Irland, N. (2018). Case report of spontaneous skull fracture in a newborn with cesarean birth for persistent occiput posterior position. *Nursing for Women's Health*, *22*(3), 250–254. https://doi.org/10.1016/j.nwh.2018.03.003

Jacob, E. A. (2016). Hematological differences in newborn and aging: A review study. *Hematology & Transfusion International Journal*, *3*(3), 178–190. https://medcraveonline.com/HTIJ/HTIJ-03-00067.pdf

Jha, K., Nassar, G. N., & Makker, K. (2020). *Transient tachypnea of the newborn*. StatPearls Publishing. https://www.ncbi.nlm.nih.gov/books/NBK537354

Jeavons, W. (2005). Sterile speculum exams & fFN collection. *Nursing for Women's Health*, *9*(3), 237–240. https://doi.org/10.1177/1091592305279119

Kaur, K., Bhardwaj, M., Kumar, P., Singhal, S., Singh, T., & Hooda, S. (2016). Amniotic fluid embolism. *Journal of Anaesthesiology Clinical Pharmacology*, *32*(2), 153–159. https://doi.org/10.4103/0970-9185.173356

Kim, K.-H., & Steinberg, G. (2019). Preeclampsia. *Medscape*. https://emedicine.medscape.com/article/1476919-overview#a1

Kingdon, C., O'Donnell, E., Givens, J., & Turner, M. (2015). The role of healthcare professionals in encouraging parents to see and hold their stillborn baby: A meta-synthesis of qualitative studies. *PLoS One*. https://doi.org/10.1371/journal.pone.0130059

Kocherlakota, P. (2014). Neonatal abstinence syndrome. *Pediatrics*, *134*(2), e547–e561. https://doi.org/10.1542/peds.2013-3524

Kolka, C. M., & Bergman, R. N. (2013). The endothelium in diabetes: Its role in insulin access and diabetic complications. *Reviews in Endocrine & Metabolic Disorders*, *14*(1), 13–19. https://doi.org/10.1007/s11154-012-9233-5

Kumar, V., Shearer, J. C., Kumar, A., & Darmstadt, G. L. (2009). Neonatal hypothermia in low resource settings: A review. *Journal of Perinatology*, *29*, 401–412. https://www.nature.com/articles/jp2008233.pdf

Lakshmanan, J., & Ross, M. (2008). Mechanism(s) of *in utero* meconium passage. *Journal of Perinatology*, *28*, S8–S13. https://doi.org/10.1038/jp.2008.144

Likis, F. E., Andrews, J. A., Collins, M. R., Lewis, R. M., Seroogy, J. J., Starr, S. A., Walden, R. R., & McPheeters, M. L. (2012). Nitrous oxide for the management of labor pain. *Comparative Effectiveness Review No. 67* [AHRQ Publication No. 12-EHC071-EF] (pp. ES-1–E18). Agency for Healthcare Research and Quality. https://effectivehealthcare.ahrq.gov/sites/default/files/related_files/labor-nitrous-oxide_executive.pdf

Lim, K.-H., & Steinberg, G. (2018). Preeclampsia. *Medscape*. https://emedicine.medscape.com/article/1476919-overview

Low, L. A., Lindsay, B. G., & Derrick, E. J. (1997). Threshold of metabolic acidosis associated with newborn complications. *American Journal of Obstetrics & Gynecology*, *177*(6), 1391–1394. https://doi.org/10.1016/s0002-9378(97)70080-2

Maakaron, J. E. (2020). Sickle cell anemia clinical presentation. *Medscape*. https://emedicine.medscape.com/article/205926-clinical

Macones, G. A, Caughey, A. B., Wood, S. L., Wrench, I. J., Huang, J., Norman, M., Pettersson, K., Fawcett, W. J., Shalabi, M. M., Metcalfe, A., Gramlich, L., Nelson, G., & Wilson, R. D. (2019). Guidelines for postoperative care in cesarean delivery: Enhanced Recovery After Surgery (ERAS) Society recommendations (part 3). *American Journal of Obstetrics & Gynecology*, *221*(247), 247.E1–247.E9. http://doi.org/10.1016/j.ajog.2019.04.012

March of Dimes. (n.d.). *Neonatal abstinence syndrome (NAS)*. https://www.marchofdimes.org/complications/neonatal-abstinence-syndrome-(nas).aspx

Marron, R. L., Lanphear, B. P., Kouides, R., Dudman, L., Manchester, R. A., & Christy, C. (1998). Efficacy of informational letters on hepatitis B immunization rates in university students. *Journal of American College Health*, *47*(3), 123–127. https://doi.org/10.1080/07448489809595632

Martin, J. A., & Osterman, M. J. K. (2018). *Describing the increase in preterm births in the United States, 2014–2016* [NCHS Data Brief No. 312]. https://www.cdc.gov/nchs/data/databriefs/db312.pdf

Masahiro, K., Sakaguchi, M., Lockhart, S. M., Cai, W., Li, M. E., Homan, E. P., Rask-Madsen, C., & Kahn, C. R. (2017). Endothelial insulin receptors differentially control insulin signaling kinetics in peripheral tissues and brain of mice. *Proceedings of the National Academy of Sciences*, *114*(40), E8478–E8487. https://doi.org/10.1073/pnas.1710625114

McGuire, S. F. (2017). Understanding the implications of birth weight. *Nursing for Women's Health*, *21*(1), 45–49. https://doi.org/10.1016/j.nwh.2016.12.005

Mechcatie, E. (2013). FDA warns about magnesium sulfate effects on newborns. *OB/Gyn News*. https://www.mdedge.com/obgyn/article/58987/womens-health/fda-warns-about-magnesium-sulfate-effects-newborns

Melchiorre, K., Sharma, R., & Thilaganathan, B. (2014). Cardiovascular implications in preeclampsia. *Circulation*, *130*, 703–714. http://circ.ahajournals.org/content/130/8/703.full.pdf+html

Miftahof, R. N., & Nam, H. G. (2011). *Biomechanics of the gravid human uterus* (pp. 129–154). Springer.

Mohan, M., Baagar, K. A. M., & Lindow, S. (2017). Management of diabetic ketoacidosis in pregnancy. *The Obstetrician & Gynaecologist*, *19*, 55–62. https://doi.org/10.1111/tog.12344

Morfaw, F., Fundoh, M., Bartoszko, J., Mbuagbaw, L., & Thabane, L. (2018). Using tocolysis in pregnant women with symptomatic placenta praevia does not significantly improve prenatal, perinatal, neonatal and maternal outcomes: A systematic review and meta-analysis. *Systematic Reviews*, 7, Article 249. https://doi.org/10.1186/s13643-018-0923-2

Morton, S., & Brodsky, D. (2016). Fetal physiology and the transition to extrauterine life. *Clinics in Perinatology*, *43*(3), 395–407. https://doi.org/10.1016/j.clp.2016.04.001

Mosalli, R. (2012). Whole body cooling for infants with hypoxic-ischemic encephalopathy. *Journal of Clinical Neonatalogy*, *1*(2), 101–106. https://doi.org/10.4103/2249-4847.96777

Muppidi, V., Meegada, S., Challa, T., Siddamreddy, S., & Samal, S. (2020). Euglycemic diabetic ketoacidosis in a young pregnant woman precipitated by urinary tract infection. *Cureus*, *12*(3), e7331. https://doi.org/10.7759/cureus.7331

Murray, M., & Huelsmann, G. (2009). *Labor and delivery nursing: A guide to evidence-based practice* (1st ed., pp. 38, 39). Springer Publishing Company.

National Certification Corporation. (2010). NICHD definitions and classifications: Application to electronic fetal monitoring interpretation. *NCC Monograph*, *3*(1), 1–20. https://www.nccwebsite.org/resources/docs/final_ncc_monograph_web-4-29-10.pdf

National Collaborating Centre for Women's and Children's Health. (2007). *Intrapartum care: Care of healthy women and their babies during childbirth*. RCOG Press. https://www.ncbi.nlm.nih.gov/books/NBK49388

National Council of State Boards of Nursing. (2019a). Approved NGN item types. *Next Generation NCLEX News*. https://www.ncsbn.org/NGN_Fall19_ENG_final.pdf

National Council of State Boards of Nursing. (2019b). *NCLEX-RN® examination: Test plan for the National Council Licensure Examination for Registered Nurses*. Chicago. https://www.ncsbn.org/2019_

National Council of State Boards of Nursing. (2020). The NGN case study. *NCLEX News*. https://www.ncsbn.org/NGN_Spring20_Eng_02.pdf

National Council of State Boards of Nursing. (2021). Next Generation NCLEX®: Standalone items. *NCLEX News*. https://www.ncsbn.org/NGN_Spring21_Eng.pdf

National Institutes of Health. (n.d.-a). *Drugs and lactation database (LactMed)*. National Library of Medicine. https://www.ncbi.nlm.nih.gov/books/NBK501922

National Institutes of Health. (n.d.-b). *Plain language at NIH*. https://www.nih.gov/institutes-nih/nih-office-director/office-communications-public-liaison/clear-communication/plain-language

Nicholson, L. (2007). Caput succedaneum and cephalohematoma: The Cs that leave bumps on the head. *Neonatal Network*, *26*(5), 277–281. http://www.academyofneonatalnursing.org/NNT/Nervous_Caput.pdf

Nick, J. M. (2006). Deep tendon reflexes, magnesium, and calcium: Assessments and implications, *Journal of Obstetric, Gynecologic, & Neonatal Nursing*, *33*(2), 221–230. https://doi.org/10.1177/0884217504263145

Nkadi, P. O., Merritt, A., & Pillers, D.-A. M. (2009). An overview of pulmonary surfactant in the neonate: Genetics, metabolism, and the role of surfactant in health and disease. *Molecular Genetics and Metabolism*, *97*(2), 95–101. https://doi.org/10.1016/j.ymgme.2009.01.015

Noctor, E., & Dunne, F. (2015). Type 2 diabetes after gestational diabetes: The influence of changing diagnostic criteria. *World Journal of Diabetes*, *6*(2), 234–244. https://doi.org/10.4239/wjd.v6.i2.234

Parer, J. T., King, T., Flanders, S., Fox, M., & Kilpatrick, S. J. (2006). Fetal acidemia and electronic fetal heart rate patterns: Is there evidence of an association? *Journal of Maternal-Fetal and Neonatal Medicine*, *19*(5), 289–294. https://doi.org/10.1080/14767050500526172

Patel, E. A. (2020). Macrosomia. *Medscape*. https://emedicine.medscape.com/article/262679-overview

Paul, I. M., Schaefer, E. W., Miller, J. R., Kuzniewicz, M. W., Li, S. X., Walsh, E. M., & Flaherman, V. J. (2016). Weight change nomograms for the first month after birth. *Pediatrics*, *138*(6), e20162625. https://doi.org/10.1542/peds.2016-2625

Peliowski-Davidovich, A., & Canadian Paediatric Society, Fetus and Newborn Committee. (2012). Hypothermia for newborns with hypoxic ischemic encephalopathy. *Paediatrics & Child Health*, *17*(1), 41–46. https://doi.org/10.1093/pch/17.1.41

Pettit, J., & Wykoff, M. M. (2007). *Peripherally inserted central catheters* (2nd ed.). National Association of Neonatal Nurses. https://www.neomedinc.com/wp-content/uploads/2019/06/NANN-PICC-Guidelines-for-Practice.pdf

Phelan, J. P. (2019). Fetal considerations in the critically ill gravida. In J. P. Phelan, L. D. Pacheco, M. R. Foley, G. R. Saade, G. A. Dildy, & M. A. Belfort (Eds.), *Critical care obstetrics* (6th ed., pp. 123–150). John Wiley & Sons.

Pillarisetty, L. S., & Bragg, B. N. (2020). *Late decelerations*. StatPearls Publishing. https://www.ncbi.nlm.nih.gov/books/NBK539820

Polderman, K. H. (2009). Mechanisms of action, physiological effects, and complications of hypothermia. *Critical Care Medicine*, *37*(7 Suppl.), S186–S202. https://doi.org/10.1097/CCM.0b013e3181aa5241

Polin, R. A., Watterberg, K., Benitz, W., & Eichenwald, E. (2014). The conundrum of early-onset sepsis. *Pediatrics*, *133*(6), 1122–1123. https://doi.org/10.1542/peds.2014-0360

Politi, S., D'Emidio, L., Cignini, P., Giorlandino, M., & Giorlandino, C. (2010). Shoulder dystocia: An evidence-based approach. *Journal of Prenatal Medicine*, *4*(3), 35–42. https://www.ncbi.nlm.nih.gov/pmc/articles/PMC3279180

Pongou, R. (2013). Why is infant mortality higher in boys than in girls? A new hypothesis based on preconception environment and evidence from a large sample of twins. *Demography*, *50*(2), 421–444. https://doi.org/10.1007/s13524-012-0161-5

Pørksen, N., Hollingdal, M., Juhl, C., Butler, P., Veldhuis, J. D., & Schmitz, O. (2002). Pulsatile insulin secretion: Detection, regulation, and role in diabetes. *Diabetes*, *51* (Suppl. 1), S245–S254. https://doi.org/10.2337/diabetes.51.2007.S245

Potter, C. F., & Kicklighter, S. D. (2016). Infant of diabetic mother. *Medscape*. https://emedicine.medscape.com/article/974230-overview#a1

Powe, C. E., Levine, R. J., & Karumanchi, S. A. (2011). Preeclampsia, a disease of the maternal endothelium: The role of antiangiogenic factors and implications for later cardiovascular disease. *Circulation*, *123*(24), 2856–2869. https://doi.org/10.1161/CIRCULATIONAHA.109.853127

Preboth, M. (2000). ACOG guidelines on antepartum fetal surveillance. *American Family Physician*, *62*(5), 1184–1188. https://www.aafp.org/afp/2000/0901/p1184.html

Preti, M., & Chandraharan, E. (2018). Importance of fetal heart rate cycling during the interpretation of the cardiotocograph (CTG). *International Journal of Gynecology and Reproductive Sciences*, *1*(1), 10–12. https://ologyjournals.com/ijgrs/ijgrs_00003.pdf

Puopolo, K. M., Lynfield, R., & Cummings, J. J. (2019). Management of infants at risk for group B streptococcal disease. *Pediatrics*, *144*(2), e20191881. https://doi.org/10.1542/peds.2019-1881

Raines, D. A. (2020). *Cephalohematoma*. StatPearls Publishing. https://www.ncbi.nlm.nih.gov/books/NBK470192

Redshaw, M., Hennegan, J. M., & Henderson, J. (2016). Impact of holding the baby following stillbirth on maternal mental health and well-being: Findings from a national survey. *British Medical Journal*, *6*(8). https://doi.org/10.1136/bmjopen-2015-010996

Richards, O. C., Raines, S. M., & Attie, A. D. (2010). The role of blood vessels, endothelial cells, and vascular pericytes in insulin secretion and peripheral insulin action. *Endocrine Reviews*, *31*(3), 343–363. https://doi.org/10.1210/er.2009-0035

Röder, P. V., Wu, B., Liu, Y., & Han, W. (2016). Pancreatic regulation of glucose homeostasis. *Experimental & Molecular Medicine*, *48*(3), e219. https://doi.org/10.1038/emm.2016.6

Rodríguez-Almagro, J., Hernández-Martínez, A., Rodríguez-Almagro, D., Quirós-García, J. M., Martínez-Galiano, J. M., & Gómez-Salgado, J. (2019). Women's perceptions of living a traumatic childbirth experience and factors related to a birth experience. *International Journal of Environmental Research and Public Health*, *16*(9), 1654. https://doi.org/10.3390/ijerph16091654

Rosner, J., Rochelson, B., Rosen, L., Roman, A., Vohra, N., & Tam Tam, H. (2014). Intermittent absent end diastolic velocity of the umbilical artery: Antenatal and neonatal characteristics and indications for delivery. *The Journal of Maternal-Fetal & Neonatal Medicine*, 27(1), 94–97. https://doi.org/10.3109/14767058.2013.806475

Ross, M. G. (2019). What should be considered prior to delivery in patients with eclampsia? *Medscape*. https://www.medscape.com/answers/253960-78056/what-should-be-considered-prior-to-delivery-inpatients-with-eclampsia

Ross, M. G., Ervin, M. G., & Novak, D. (2012). Placental and fetal physiology. In S. G. Gabbe, J. R. Niebyl, J. L. Simpson, M. B. Landon, H. I. Galan, E. R. M. Jauniaux, & D. A. Driscoll (Eds.), *Obstetrics: Normal and problem pregnancies* (6th ed., pp. 23–41). Elsevier Saunders.

Saisho, Y., Miyakoshi, K., Tanaka, M., Shimada, A., Ikenoue, S., Kadohira, I., Yoshimura, Y., & Itoh, H. (2010). Beta cell dysfunction and its clinical significance in gestational diabetes. *Endocrine Journal*, *57*(11), 973–980. https://doi.org/10.1507/endocrj.k10e-231

Salvesen, K. Å., Hem, E., & Sundgot-Borgen, J. (2012). Fetal wellbeing may be compromised during strenuous exercise among pregnant elite athletes. *British Journal of Sports Medicine*, *46*, 279–283. http://doi.org/10.1136/bjsm.2010.080259

Saneh, H., Mendez, M. D., & Srinivasan, V. N. (2020). *Cord blood gas*. StatPearls Publishing. https://www.ncbi.nlm.nih.gov/books/NBK545290

Satin, L. S., Butler, P. C., Ha, J., & Sherman, A. S. (2015). Pulsatile insulin secretion, impaired glucose tolerance and type 2 diabetes. *Molecular Aspects of Medicine*, *42*, 61–77. https://doi.org/10.1016/j.mam.2015.01.003

Satou, G. M., & Halnon, N. J. (2019). Pediatric congestive heart failure. *Medscape*. https://emedicine.medscape.com/article/2069746-overview

Sayad, E. (2020). *Meconium aspiration*. StatPearls Publishing. https://www.statpearls.com/ArticleLibrary/viewarticle/24819

Schillie, S., Vellozzi, C., Reingold, A., Harris, A., Haber, P., Ward, J. W., & Nelson, N. P. (2018). Prevention of hepatitis B virus infection in the United States: Recommendations of the Advisory Committee on Immunization Practices. *Morbidity and Mortality Weekly Report*, *67*(No. RR-1), 1–31. http://doi.org/10.15585/mmwr.rr6701a1

Scott, J. R. (2014). Intrapartum management of trial of labour after caesarean delivery: Evidence and experience. *BJOG*, *121*, 157–162. https://doi.org/10.1111/1471-0528.12449

Sebire, N. J. (2003). Umbilical artery Doppler revisited: Pathophysiology of changes in intrauterine growth restriction revealed. *Ultrasound in Obstetrics & Gynecology*, *21*, 419–422. https://doi.org/10.1002/uog.133

Shah, P. S., Ohlsson, A., & Perlman, M. (2007). Hypothermia to treat neonatal hypoxic ischemic encephalopathy. *Archives of Pediatric & Adolescent Medicine*, *161*(10), 951–958. https://doi.org/10.1001/archpedi.161.10.951

Shiel, W. C., Jr. (n.d.). Hematocrit ranges and chart: Test, high, low, and normal. *MedicineNet*. https://www.medicinenet.com/hematocrit/article.htm

Sibai, B. M. (2004). Diagnosis, controversies, and management of the syndrome of hemolysis, elevated liver enzymes, and low platelet count. *Obstetrics & Gynecology*, *103*, 981–991. https://doi.org/10.1097/01.AOG.0000126245.35811.2a

Sibai, B. M., & Viteri, O. A. (2014). Diabetic ketoacidosis in pregnancy. *Obstetrics & Gynecology*, *123*(1), 167–178. https://doi.org/10.1097/AOG.0000000000000060

Simpson, K. R. (2016). *Fetal assessment and safe labor management*. National Certification Corporation. https://www.nccwebsite.org/content/documents/courses/2016_NCC_Monograph_CE_Version.pdf

Smith, J. R. (2018). Postpartum hemorrhage. *Medscape*. https://emedicine.medscape.com/article/275038-overview#a4

Spong, C. Y., Berghella, V., Wenstrom, K. D., Mercer, B. M., & Saade, G. R. (2012). Preventing the first cesarean delivery: Summary of a joint *Eunice Kennedy Shriver* National Institute of Child Health and Human Development, Society for Maternal-Fetal Medicine, and American College of Obstetricians and Gynecologists workshop. *Obstetrics & Gynecology*, *120*(5), 1181–1193. https://www.ncbi.nlm.nih.gov/pmc/articles/PMC3548444

Stanescu, A., & Stoicescu, S. M. (2014). Neonatal hypoglycemia screening in newborns from diabetic mothers—Arguments and controversies. *Journal of Medicine and Life*, 7(Spec. Iss. 3), 51–52. https://www.ncbi.nlm.nih.gov/pmc/articles/PMC4391423

Stanford School of Medicine. (n.d.). *Bhutani nomogram*. https://med.stanford.edu/newborns/professional-education/jaundice-and-phototherapy/bhutani-nomogram.html

Steiner, L. A., & Gallagher, P. G. (2007). Erythrocyte disorders in the perinatal period. *Seminars in Perinatology*, *31*(4), 254–261. https://doi.org/10.1053/j.semperi.2007.05.003

Stevens, B., Yamada, J., Ohlsson, A., Haliburton, S., & Shorkey, A. (2016). Sucrose for analgesia in newborn infants undergoing painful procedures. *Cochrane Database of Systematic Reviews*, (7), Article CD001069. https://doi.org/10.1002/14651858.CD001069.pub5

Steward, K., & Raja, K. (2019). *Physiology, ovulation, basal body temperature*. StatPearls Publishing. https://www.ncbi.nlm.nih.gov/books/NBK546686

Tang, J., Bergman, J., & Lam, J. M. (2010). Harlequin colour change: Unilateral erythema in a newborn. *Canadian Medical Association Journal*, *182*(17), E801. https://doi.org/10.1503/cmaj.092038

Thigpen, J., & Melton, S. T. (2014). Neonatal abstinence syndrome: A challenge for medical providers, mothers, and society. *Journal of Pediatric Pharmacology and Therapeutics*, *19*(3), 144–146. https://doi.org/10.5863/1551-6776-19.3.144

Thilo, E. (n.d.). *Hemolytic disease of the newborn (alloimmunization)*. https://www.cancertherapyadvisor.com/home/decision-support-in-medicine/pediatrics/hemolytic-disease-of-the-newborn-alloimmunization

Tully, H. M., & Dobyns, W. B. (2014). Infantile hydrocephalus: A review of epidemiology, classification and causes. *European Journal of Medical Genetics*, *57*(8), 359–368. https://doi.org/10.1016/j.ejmg.2014.06.002

Turner, J. M., Mitchell, M. D., & Kumar, S. S. (2020). The physiology of intrapartum fetal compromise at term. *American Journal of Obstetrics and Gynecology*, *222*(1), 17–26. https://doi.org/10.1016/j.ajog.2019.07.032

Umana, O. D., & Siccardi, M. A. (2020). *Prenatal non-stress test*. StatPearls Publishing. https://www.ncbi.nlm.nih.gov/books/NBK537123

Underwood, M. A. (2013). Human milk for the premature infant. *Pediatric Clinics of North America*, *60*(1), 189–207. http://www.ncbi.nlm.nih.gov/pmc/articles/PMC3508468

U.S. Department of Health and Human Services. (n.d.). *Health information privacy*. http://hhs.gov/ocr/privacy/hipaa/understanding/index.html

U.S. Department of Health and Human Services. (2020). *Guidelines for the use of antiretroviral agents in pediatric HIV infection* (pp. G-1–G-22). https://aidsinfo.nih.gov/guidelines/html/2/pediatric-arv/510/antiretroviral-management-of-newborns-with-perinatal-hiv-exposure-or-hiv-infection

van Dellen, S. A., Wisse, B., Mobach, M. P., & Dijkstra, A. (2019). The effect of a breastfeeding support programme on breastfeeding duration and exclusivity: A quasi-experiment. *BMC Public Health*, *19*, Article 993. https://doi.org/10.1186/s12889-019-7331-y

Verani, J. R., McGee, L., & Schrag, S. J. (2010). Prevention of pernatal group B streptococcal disease: Revised guidelines from CDC, 2010. *Morbidity and Mortality Weekly Report*, *59*(RR-10), 1–32. https://www.cdc.gov/mmwr/pdf/rr/rr5910.pdf

Vintzileos, A. M., & Smulian, J. C. (2016). Decelerations, tachycardia, and decreased variability: Have we overlooked the significance of longitudinal fetal heart rate changes for detecting intrapartum fetal hypoxia? *American Journal of Obstetrics & Gynecology*, *215*(3), 261–264. https://doi.org/10.1016/j.ajog.2016.05.046

Wagle, S., & Deshpande, P. G. (2017). Hemolytic disease of the newborn. *Medscape*. https://emedicine.medscape.com/article/974349-overview#a5

Wang, H., Liu, Z., Li, G., & Barrett, E. J. (2006). The vascular endothelial cell mediates insulin transport into skeletal muscle. *American Journal of Physiology, Endocrinology and Metabolism*, *291*, E323–E332. https://doi.org/10.1152/ajpendo.00047.2006

Wilcox, G. (2005). Insulin and insulin resistance. *The Clinical Biochemist Reviews*, *26*(2), 19–39. https://www.ncbi.nlm.nih.gov/pmc/articles/PMC1204764/pdf/cbr26_2pg019.pdf

Williams, K. P., & Galerneau, F. (2003). Intrapartum fetal heart rate patterns in the prediction of neonatal acidemia. *American Journal of Obstetrics & Gynecology*, *188*(3), 820–823. https://doi.org/10.1067/mob.2003.183

Williams, P. J., & Pipkin, F. B. (2011). The genetics of pre-eclampsia and other hypertensive disorders of pregnancy. *Best Practice and Research: Clinical Obstetrics & Gynaecology*, *25*(4), 405–417. https://doi.org/10.1016/j.bpobgyn.2011.02.007

Wong, A. W., & Rosh, A. J. (2019). Postpartum infections. *Medscape*. https://emedicine.medscape.com/article/796892-overview

World Health Organization. (1997). Care in normal birth: A practical guide. *Birth*, *24*(2), 121–123. https://doi.org/10.1111/j.1523-536X.1997.00121.pp.x

World Health Organization. (2018). Intrapartum care for a positive childbirth experience. https://apps.who.int/iris/bitstream/handle/10665/272447/WHO-RHR-18.12-eng.pdf?ua=1

Wormer, K. C., Jamil, R. T., & Bryant, S. B. (2019). *Acute postpartum hemorrhage*. StatPearls Publishing. https://www.ncbi.nlm.nih.gov/books/NBK499988

Wyckoff, M. H., Aziz, K., Escobedo, M. B., Kapadia, V. S., Kattwinkel, J., Perlman, J. M., Simon, W., Weiner, G. M., & Zaichkin, J. G. (2015). Part 13: Neonatal resuscitation: 2015 American Heart Association guidelines update for cardiopulmonary resuscitation and emergency cardiovascular care. *Circulation*, *132*(18 Suppl. 2), S543–S560. https://doi.org/10.1161/CIR.0000000000000267

Wynn, J. L., & Wong, H. R. (2010). Pathophysiology and treatment of septic shock in neonates. *Clinics in Perinatology*, *37*(2), 439–479. https://doi.org/10.1016/j.clp.2010.04.002

Yellayi, A. S. S., Aruna, S., & Devi, D. H. (2017). Role of amnioinfusion in prevention of meconium aspiration syndrome. *International Journal of Scientific Study*, *5*(5), 272–277. http://www.ijss-sn.com/uploads/2/0/1/5/20153321/ijss_aug_oa58_-_2017.pdf

Zanelli, S., Buck, M., & Fairchild, K. (2011). Physiologic and pharmacologic considerations for hypothermia therapy in neonates. *Journal of Perinatology*, *31*(6), 377–386. https://doi.org/10.1038/jp.2010.146

Zhang, J., Landy, H. J., Ware Branch, D., Burkman, R., Haberman, S., Gregory, K. D., Hatjis, C. G., Ramirez, M. M., Bailit, J. L., Gonzalez-Quintero, V. H., Hibbard, J. U., Hoffman, M. K., Kominiarek, M., Learman, L. A., Van Veldhuisen, P., Troendle, J., & Reddy, U. M. (2010). Contemporary patterns of spontaneous labor with normal neonatal outcomes. *Obstetrics & Gynecology*, *116*(6), 1281–1287. https://doi.org/10.1097/AOG.0b013e3181fdef6e

Index

References followed by the letter "f" are for figures.

D

E

F

G

H

M

N

O

P

U

V

W

X

Y

Z